MW01052655

MKSAP® for Students 4

Medical Knowledge Self-Assessment Program®

Developed by
American College of Physicians
Clerkship Directors in Internal Medicine

Publisher's Information

American College of Physicians
190 N. Independence Mall West
Philadelphia, PA 19106-1572
215-351-2600

ISBN: 978-1-934465-03-5

Printed in the United States of America

Acknowledgments

Douglas S. Paauw, MD, FACP
Medicine Clerkship Director
Professor of Medicine
Rathmann Family Foundation Endowed Chair for
    Patient-centered Clinical Education
Department of Medicine
University of Washington School of Medicine
Seattle, Washington

Carlos Palacio, MD, MPH, FACP
Assistant Professor of Medicine
Medicine Clerkship Director
University of Florida College of Medicine-Jacksonville
Jacksonville, Florida

Deborah Peltier, MD
Associate Professor of Medicine
Clerkship Director, Geriatrics and Ambulatory Medicine
Dartmouth Medical School
Hanover, New Hampshire

Nora L. Porter, MD
Co-Director, Internal Medicine Clerkship
Department of Internal Medicine and Pediatrics
St Louis University School of Medicine
St. Louis, Missouri

Jamal Qureshi, MD
Assistant Clinical Professor of Medicine
Medicine Clerkship Director
University of Wisconsin Medical School-Milwaukee Campus
Milwaukee, Wisconsin

Roshini Pinto-Powell, MD
Assistant Professor of Medicine
Inpatient Medicine Clerkship Co-director
Dartmouth Medical School
Lebanon, New Hampshire

Debra L. Stottlemyer, MD, MBA
Assistant Professor of Medicine
Associate Medicine Clerkship Director
Associate Director, Graduate Medical Education
    Core Curriculum
Loma Linda University School of Medicine
Loma Linda, California

John A. Varras, MD
Clerkship Director
Assistant Professor of Medicine
Department of Internal Medicine
University of Nevada School of Medicine
Las Vegas, Nevada

T. Robert Vu, MD
Assistant Professor of Clinical Medicine
Director, Internal Medicine Clerkships
Indiana University School of Medicine
Indianapolis, Indiana

H. Douglas Walden, MD, MPH, FACP
Professor of Medicine
Internal Medicine Clerkship Director
Department of Internal Medicine
Saint Louis University School of Medicine
St. Louis, Missouri

Leigh Watson-Ramirez, MD, FACP
Associate Professor of Medicine
Director M3 and M4 Internal Medicine Student Programs
Greenville Hospital System Campus of University of
    South Carolina School of Medicine
Greenville, South Carolina

Sean A. Whelton, MD
Assistant Professor of Medicine
Clerkship Director, Internal Medicine
Division of Rheumatology, Allergy, and Immunology
Georgetown University Hospital
Washington, DC

Kevin D. Whittle, MD
Associate Professor, Internal Medicine
3rd Year Medicine Clerkship Director
Sanford School of Medicine
University of South Dakota
Souix Falls, South Dakota

MKSAP for Student 4 Contributors

Arlina Ahluwalia, MD
Clinical Assistant Professor of Medicine
Stanford University School of Medicine
Clerkship Site Director
Palo Alto VAHCS
Palo Alto, California

Eyad Al-Hihi, MD, FACP
Associate Professor of Medicine
Clerkship Director, Ambulatory Medicine
Section Chief, Division of General Internal Medicine
Medical Director, Internal Medicine Clinics
Truman Medical Center-Hospital Hill
University of Missouri-Kansas City School of Medicine
Kansas City, Missouri

Erik K. Alexander, MD, FACP
Director, Medical Student Education
Brigham & Women's Hospital
Assistant Professor of Medicine
Harvard Medical School
Boston, Massachusetts

Irene Alexandraki, MD, FACP
Assistant Professor of Medicine
University of Florida College of Medicine
Jacksonville, Florida

Mark Allee, MD, FACP
Assistant Professor of Medicine
Department of Internal Medicine
University of Oklahoma College of Medicine
Oklahoma City, Oklahoma

Hugo A. Alvarez, MD, FACP
Associate Professor of Medicine
Sub-Internship Director
Clerkship Site Director Department of Medicine
Rosalind Franklin University of Medicine and Science
Mount Sinai Hospital
Chicago, Illinois

Alpesh N. Amin, MD, MBA, FACP
Medicine Clerkship Director
Associate Program Director, IM Residency
University of California, Irvine
Irvine, California

Mary Jane Barchman, MD, FACP, FASN
Associate Professor of Medicine
Section of Nephrology and Hypertension
Director, Introduction to Medicine Course
Clerkship Director, Internal Medicine
Brody School of Medicine at East Carolina University
Greenville, North Carolina

Seth Mark Berney, MD, FACP
Professor of Medicine
Chief, Section of Rheumatology
Director, Center of Excellence for Arthritis and
    Rheumatology
Louisiana State University Health Sciences Center
School of Medicine in Shreveport
Shreveport, Louisiana

Cynthia A. Burns, MD
Assistant Professor, Clerkship Director
Inpatient Internal Medicine
Wake Forest University School of Medicine
Dept of Internal Medicine
Section of Endocrinology and Metabolism
Winston-Salem, North Carolina

Amanda Cooper, MD
Assistant Professor of Medicine
University of Pittsburgh Medical Center
University of Pittsburgh School of Medicine
Pittsburgh, Pennsylvania

Thomas M. DeFer, MD, FACP
Clerkship Director
Division of Medical Education
Department of Internal Medicine
Washington University School of Medicine
St Louis, Missouri

Reed E. Drews, MD, FACP
Program Director
Hematology-Oncology Fellowship
Co-Director, Core Medicine 1 Clerkship
Beth Israel Deaconess Medical Center
Harvard Medical School
Boston, Massachusetts

Steven J. Durning, MD, FACP, Maj., USAF, MC
Associate Professor of Medicine
Co-Director, Intro to Clinical Reasoning Course
Uniformed Services University of the Health Sciences
Bethesda, Maryland

Richard S. Eisenstaedt, MD, FACP
Chair, Department of Medicine
Abington Memorial Hospital
Professor of Medicine
Temple University School of Medicine
Philadelphia, Pennsylvania

D Michael Elnicki, MD, FACP
Director, Ambulatory Medicine Clerkship
Director, Section of General Internal Medicine
University of Pittsburgh School of Medicine
UPMC Shadyside
Pittsburgh, Pennsylvania

Mark J. Fagan, MD, FACP
Clerkship Director
Department of Medicine
Alpert Medical School of Brown University
Providence, Rhode Island

Sara B. Fazio, MD
Assistant Professor, Harvard Medical School
Director, Core I Medicine Clerkship
Division of General Internal Medicine
Beth Israel Deaconess Medical Center
Boston, Massachusetts

J. Michael Finley, DO, FACP, FACOI
Associate Professor and Chair of Medicine
Department of Medicine
Western University
College of Osteopathic Medicine
Pomona, California

Jane P. Gagliardi, MD
Assistant Clinical Professor
Department of Internal Medicine
Department of Psychiatry and Behavioral Sciences
Duke University School of Medicine
Durham, North Carolina

Peter Gliatto, MD
Assistant Professor of Medicine
Director, Medical Clerkships
Mount Sinai School of Medicine
New York, New York

Eric H. Green, MD, MSc
Course Director, Patients, Doctors, and Communities
Assistant Professor of Medicine
Montefiore Medical Center
Albert Einstein College of Medicine
Bronx, New York

Mark C. Haigney, MD
Director of Cardiology
Professor of Medicine
Director of Cardiology
Uniformed Services University of the Health Sciences
Bethesda, Maryland

Charin L. Hanlon, MD, FACP
Assistant Professor of Internal Medicine
Clerkship Director, Internal Medicine
West Virginia University-Charleston Division
Charleston, West Virginia

Warren Hershman, MD
Director of Student Education
Department of Medicine
Boston University School of Medicine
Boston, Massachusetts

Mark D. Holden, MD, FACP
Eagle's Trace Medical Director
Erickson Retirement Communities
Houston, Texas

Ivonne Z. Jiménez-Velázquez, MD, FACP
Professor and Vice-Chair for Education
Geriatrics Program Director
Clerkship Director
Internal Medicine Department
University of Puerto Rico, School of Medicine
San Juan, Puerto Rico

Lawrence I. Kaplan, MD, FACP
Professor of Medicine
Section Chief-General Internal Medicine
Internal Medicine Clerkship Director
Temple University School of Medicine
Philadelphia, Pennsylvania

Asra R. Khan, MD
Assistant Professor Clinical Medicine
Associate Program Director, Internal Medicine
Residency
Medicine Clerkship Director
University of Illinois at Chicago College of Medicine
Chicago, Illinois

Sarang Kim, MD
Assistant Professor of Medicine
Division of General Internal Medicine
University of Medicine and Dentistry of New Jersey
Robert Wood Johnson Medical School
New Brunswick, New Jersey

Christopher A. Klipstein, MD
Internal Medicine Clerkship Director
Associate Professor
Department of Medicine
University of North Carolina School of Medicine
Chapel Hill, North Carolina

Cynthia H. Ledford, MD
Clerkship Director of Internal Medicine
Ohio State University College of Medicine
Columbus, Ohio

Bruce Leff, MD, FACP
Associate Professor of Medicine
Medicine Clerkship Director
Johns Hopkins University School of Medicine
Baltimore, Maryland

Fred A. Lopez, MD, FACP
Associate Professor and Vice Chair
Department of Medicine
Louisiana State University Health Sciences Center
Assistant Dean for Student Affairs
LSU School of Medicine
New Orleans, Louisiana

Anna C. Maio, MD, FACP
Division Chief and Associate Professor
Division of General Internal Medicine
Department of Internal Medicine
Creighton University School of Medicine
Omaha, Nebraska

Kevin M. McKown, MD, FACP
Associate Professor of Medicine
Co-Chief, Section of Rheumatology
Program Director, Rheumatology Fellowship
Co-Clerkship Director
Department of Medicine
University of Wisconsin School of Medicine and
    Public Health
Madison, Wisconsin

Janet N. Myers, MD, FACP, FCCP
Associate Professor of Medicine
Deputy Clerkship Director, Department of Medicine
Uniformed Services University of the Health Sciences
Bethesda, Maryland

Robert W. Neilson, Jr., MD
Assistant Professor
Clerkship Director
Texas Tech University Health Sciences Center
Department of Internal Medicine
Division of General Internal Medicine
Lubbock, Texas

Katherine Nickerson, MD
Vice Chair
Department of Medicine
Associate Professor of Clinical Medicine
Clerkship Director
Columbia University, College of Physicians and Surgeons
New York, New York

L. James Nixon, MD
Clerkship Director
Division of General Internal Medicine
University of Minnesota Medical School
University of Minnesota Medical Center, Fairview
Minneapolis, Minnesota

Carlos Palacio, MD, MPH, FACP
Clerkship Director
Assistant Professor of Medicine
University of Florida College of Medicine-Jacksonville
Jacksonville, Florida

Hanah Polotsky, MD
Assistant Professor of Medicine
Clerkship Director
Montefiore Medical Center
Albert Einstein College of Medicine
Bronx, New York

Nora L. Porter, MD
Co-Director, Internal Medicine Clerkship
Saint Louis University School of Medicine
St Louis, Missouri

Priya Radhakrishnan, MD
Clinical Assistant Professor
University of Arizona College of Medicine
Clerkship Director, Associate Program Director,
    Internal Medicine
St. Joseph Hospital & Medical Center
Phoenix, Arizona

Joseph Rencic, MD, FACP
Assistant Professor of Medicine
Clerkship Site Director, Associate Program Director
Department of Internal Medicine
Tufts-New England Medical Center
 Boston, Massachusetts

Kathleen F. Ryan, MD, FACP
Associate Professor of Medicine
Clerkship Director
Division of General Internal Medicine
Department of Internal Medicine Drexel University
    College of Medicine
Philadelphia, Pennsylvania

James L. Sebastian, MD, FACP
Director of Student Teaching Programs
Department of Medicine
Medical College of Wisconsin
Clement J. Zablocki Veterans Affairs Medical Center
Milwaukee, Wisconsin

Patricia Short, MD, MAJ, MC, USA
Associate Professor
Associate Clerkship Director
Department of Medicine
Uniformed Services University of the Health Sciences
Bethesda, MD
Madigan Army Medical Center
Ft. Lewis, Washington

Diane C. Sliwka, MD
Assistant Clinical Professor of Medicine
Division of Hospital Medicine
University of California San Francisco School of Medicine
San Francisco, California

Harold M. Szerlip, MD, FACP, FCCP
Professor and Vice-Chairman
Department of Medicine
Medical College of Georgia
Augusta, Georgia

Gary Tabas, MD, FACP
Associate Professor of Medicine
University of Pittsburgh School of Medicine
Pittsburgh, Pennsylvania

Tomoko Tanabe, MD, FACP
Assistant Professor of Medicine
Associate Clerkship Director
University of California, San Diego
San Diego, California

David C. Tompkins, MD
Associate Chair
Department of Medicine
SUNY, Stony Brook Health Sciences Center
Stony Brook, New York

Dario M. Torre, MD, MPH, FACP
Clerkship Director
Department of Medicine
Medical College of Wisconsin
Milwaukee, Wisconsin

H. Douglas Walden, MD, MPH, FACP
Co-Director, Internal Medicine Clerkship
Saint Louis University School of Medicine
St Louis, Missouri

Joseph T. Wayne, MD, MPH, FACP
Associate Professor of Medicine
Associate Professor of Pediatrics
Clerkship Director, Internal Medicine
Albany Medical College
Albany, New York

John Jason White, MD
Assistant Professor of Medicine
Department of Medicine
Section Nephrology
Medical College of Georgia
Augusta, Georgia

Kevin D. Whittle, MD
Associate Professor, Internal Medicine
3rd Year Medicine Clerkship Director
Sanford School of Medicine
University of South Dakota
Sioux Falls, South Dakota

The American College of Physicians gratefully acknowledges the special contributions to *MKSAP for Students 4* of Michael Ripca (design and layout), and Scott Hurd and Ricki Jo Kaufman (production systems), Lisa Rockey (editorial production support), Rosemarie Houton (editorial production support), Helen Kitzmiller (editorial production support), and Charlotte Fierman (manuscript editing). The CD-ROM product was developed by Steven Spadt, John McKnight and Christopher Forrest of the College's Electronic Product Development group. The College also wishes to acknowledge that many other persons, too numerous to mention, have contributed to the production of this product. Without their dedicated efforts, the publication would not have been possible.

Foreword

Dear Student:

As the national organization for internal medicine specialists and subspecialists, the American College of Physicians is committed to providing the highest quality educational materials and resources throughout the continuum of training and practice in internal medicine. Early in that continuum are the clinical clerkships in internal medicine for students during their third and fourth years of medical school. Recognizing the critical importance of these clerkships for all students — whether or not they plan to enter the specialty of internal medicine — the College has been collaborating with the Clerkship Directors in Internal Medicine (CDIM) to develop and produce two publications specifically targeted to medical students on their internal medicine clerkships.

This publication, *MKSAP for Students,* now in its 4th edition, employs an interactive, case-based model of topic-based questions (with accompanying answers and critiques) to teach students about the major clinical problems in internal medicine. The companion publication, *Internal Medicine Essentials for Clerkship Students,* nicely complements *MKSAP for Students,* providing a concise text that can be read from cover to cover during an internal medicine clerkship. Both *MKSAP for Students* and *Internal Medicine Essentials* are modeled after the much larger *Medical Knowledge Self-Assessment Program (MKSAP),* which has served for the past 40 years (and through 14 editions) as the gold standard for residents preparing for the certifying examination in internal medicine and for practicing physicians who wish to refresh, update, and assess their knowledge.

I wish to acknowledge the critical role of two individuals in developing this educational resource — Dr. Patrick Alguire (Editor-in-Chief of *MKSAP for Students* since its inception) and the late Dr. Herbert S. Waxman (my predecessor at the American College of Physicians). Without the vision and outstanding work of Drs. Alguire and Waxman, and without the support of the Clerkship Directors in Internal Medicine and the superb input of many of its members, *MKSAP for Students* would not be what it is today — an invaluable learning tool for students embarking on the challenging journey to link scientific principles and clinical knowledge in the care of their patients.

Internal medicine is an exciting and intellectually stimulating specialty. We hope that *MKSAP for Students* will reinforce that feeling for you, enriching your clinical experiences and serving as a useful companion as you learn the fundamental concepts of the specialty and apply them in clinical settings. Remember, the knowledge we gain is not just abstract learning — it provides the foundation for the care of our patients, who deserve only the best!

Best of luck to you in your studies and in your future career.

Steven E. Weinberger, MD, FACP
Senior Vice President for Medical Education and Publishing
American College of Physicians

Preface

Welcome to the newest print and electronic edition of *MKSAP for Students*. The fourth edition of this popular series contains over 450 **completely new** multiple-choice questions, updated references, more color photographs and ECG tracings than ever before, and a new organization. *MKSAP for Students* is intended primarily for third-year students participating in their required internal medicine clerkship. Other audiences include fourth-year students on an advanced medicine clerkship; second-year students involved in problem-based learning; and physician assistant students.

MKSAP for Students 4 is now written to support its companion textbook, *Internal Medicine Essentials for Clerkship Students 2*. Authors who contributed to the *Essentials* textbook also wrote questions for *MKSAP for Students*. Additional questions were written by internal medicine clerkship directors. Like *Essentials*, *MKSAP for Students 4* is now organized into 11 chapters that correspond to the traditional subspecialty disciplines of internal medicine and general internal medicine. This allows a one-to-one correspondence between the textbook and the self-assessment questions. The beginning of each subspecialty chapter also lists the "Training Problems" from *The Core Medicine Clerkship Curriculum Guide* that are assessed by the chapter's multiple-choice questions. *The Clerkship Curriculum Guide* is a nationally recognized curriculum for the required third-year internal medicine clerkship created and published by the Clerkship Directors in Internal Medicine and the Society for General Internal Medicine. It defines the competencies, knowledge, attitudes, and skills that medical students are expected to master by the end of their clerkship.

As in previous issues, the questions are formatted as clinical vignettes that resemble the types of questions you will encounter at the end of the clerkship subject examination and the internal medicine component of the USMLE licensing examination. Each question has a detailed answer critique that identifies the correct answer, an explanation of why that answer is correct and the other options are incorrect, and a short bibliography. New to this edition are succinct "Key Points" that summarize the important "take home messages" for each question. We anticipate that reviewing the "Key Points" will be an efficient way to prepare for upcoming examinations. We recommend that students read the clinical vignette, select an answer, and then read the associated answer critique. Each question has been specifically reviewed by at least three clerkship directors to ensure that it meets the learning needs of students participating in the medicine clerkship.

The inclusion of the CD version of *MKSAP for Students 4* gives you the option of working with printed material or an enhanced electronic version. The electronic version has search capabilities and tracks your answers to questions, as well as your score, automatically.

The fourth edition of *MKSAP for Students* would have been impossible without the valuable and entirely voluntary contributions of many people, some of whom are named in the Acknowledgments section. Others, not specifically named, were representatives of a wide spectrum of constituencies and organizations, such as the Clerkship Directors in Internal Medicine and various committees within the American College of Physicians, including the Education Committee and the Council of Student Members.

As in the past, we hope to receive more excellent feedback from students to improve future editions. Thank you for making *MKSAP for Students* such a success!

Patrick C. Alguire, MD, FACP
Editor-in-Chief

Contents

Chapter 1
Cardiovascular Medicine

Cardiovascular Medicine contains self-assessment items that correspond to the following chapters in the *Internal Medicine Essentials for Clerkship Students 2* textbook:

Approach to Chest Pain
Chronic Stable Angina
Acute Coronary Syndrome
Supraventricular Arrhythmias
Ventricular Arrhythmias
Heart Failure
Valvular Heart Disease

Cardiovascular Medicine contains self assessment items that correspond to the following Training Problems in the *Core Medicine Clerkship Guide*:

Chest Pain
Acute Myocardial Infarction
Heart Failure

Chapter 1

Cardiovascular Medicine

Questions

Item 1

A 68-year-old man is evaluated in the office for pain in his right great toe. Two days ago, he had coronary angiography from the right femoral artery that showed three widely patent bypass grafts and a total occlusion of the second diagonal artery. Percutaneous revascularization was attempted but was unsuccessful. The patient has a history of type 2 diabetes mellitus, hypertension, and exertional chest pain.

On examination, his toe is painful to touch but not warm (*See Figure 1 in Color Plates*). Laboratory studies show a normal hematocrit and leukocyte count; serum creatinine is 2.2 mg/dL (pre-procedure serum creatinine was 1.6 mg/dL). Urinalysis shows eosinophils. Electrocardiogram is unchanged from a previous tracing.

Which of the following is the most likely diagnosis?

(A) Cholesterol emboli
(B) Gout
(C) Femoral artery dissection
(D) Radiocontrast nephropathy

Item 2

A 73-year-old woman is evaluated in the office during a routine examination. She has no complaints and feels well. Her medications are levothyroxine for hypothyroidism and hydrochlorothiazide for hypertension. An electrocardiogram performed 2 years ago was normal.

On physical examination, heart rate is 42/min and regular. The remainder of the examination is normal. Her thyroid-stimulating hormone level is normal. An electrocardiogram obtained as part of the current evaluation is shown.

Which of the following diagnoses is confirmed by the electrocardiogram?

(A) First-degree atrioventricular heart block
(B) Mobitz type I second-degree atrioventricular block
(C) Mobitz type II second-degree atrioventricular block
(D) Third-degree atrioventricular block (complete heart block)

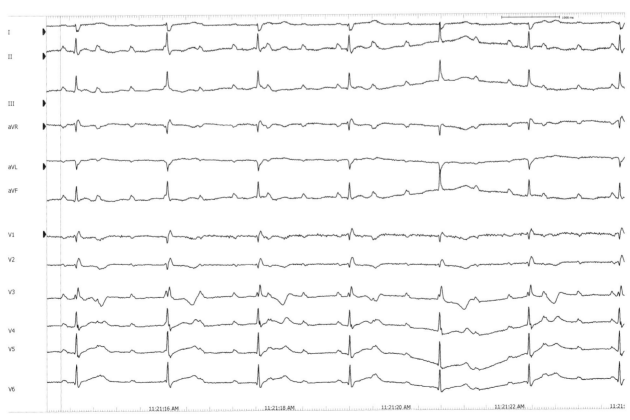

Item 2

3

Item 3

A 73-year-old woman is evaluated in the emergency department for chest pain with radiation to the back and jaw, diaphoresis, and lightheadedness of 4 hours' duration. Her medical history includes a 20-year history of hypertension and type 2 diabetes mellitus. Medications are metformin, atenolol, and aspirin.

On physical examination, blood pressure is 130/84 mm Hg and heart rate is 87/min and regular. The jugular vein is distended to 5 cm while the patient is upright. She has a faint left carotid bruit, bibasilar crackles to one quarter up from the pulmonary bases, normal S_1 and S_2, and an S_4 and an S_3 with a grade 2/6 holosystolic murmur heard best at the apex to the axilla. The electrocardiogram is shown. An electrocardiogram from 6 months ago was normal. The initial serum troponin measurement is elevated.

Which of the following is the most likely electrocardiographic diagnosis?

(A) Left bundle branch block
(B) Idioventricular tachycardia
(C) Right bundle branch block
(D) Third-degree atrioventricular block (complete heart block)

Item 4

A 72-year-old man is evaluated in the office for bilateral leg pain and cramping after walking briskly up an incline. The pain is in the distal thigh and calf and is worse on the right side. He has no pain when walking downhill. The patient has a 100-pack-year smoking history, type 2 diabetes mellitus, hypertension, and heart failure. His medications are captopril, furosemide, atenolol, atorvastatin, metformin, and aspirin.

On physical examination, the blood pressure is 146/68 mm Hg and heart rate 82/min and regular. The lungs are clear. Cardiac examination reveals an S_4. There is a right femoral artery bruit with absent pulses and mild dependent rubor. Ankle-brachial index is 0.8.

Which of the following is the most likely cause of this patient's symptoms?

(A) Arterial ischemia
(B) Osteoarthritis
(C) Peripheral neuropathy
(D) Right popliteal venous thrombosis
(E) Spinal stenosis

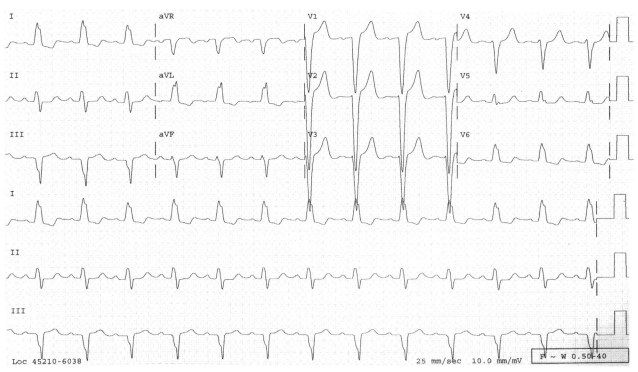

Item 3

Item 5

A 29-year-old man with a history of injection drug use is evaluated in the emergency department for fever. Five years ago, he was diagnosed with mitral valve endocarditis and underwent valve replacement with a bileaflet tilting disk prosthesis. He had been clinically stable until 3 to 4 weeks ago. He has had night sweats and has lost 3.6 kg (8 lb) over the past month. The patient has not used recreational drugs since his valve replacement and has been compliant with his warfarin regimen.

Physical examination shows a temperature of 38.1 °C (100.6 °F), heart rate of 40/min, and blood pressure of 106/62 mm Hg. Jugular venous pressure is estimated at 12 cm H_2O. Bibasilar crackles are heard. There is a mechanical S_1 and normal S_2 with no S_3 or S_4. A grade 2/6 holosystolic murmur is heard throughout the precordium. There is trace pedal edema.

The electrocardiogram is shown.

Which of the following is the most likely electrocardiographic diagnosis?

(A) First-degree atrioventricular block
(B) Mobitz type I second-degree atrioventricular block
(C) Mobitz type II second-degree atrioventricular block
(D) Third-degree atrioventricular block (complete heart block)

Item 6

A 26-year-old woman is evaluated for sharp left precordial chest pain preceded by 2 to 3 days of sore throat, diffuse myalgias, and malaise. The chest pain is nonradiating and is aggravated by deep breaths. She does not have cough, dyspnea, fever, dizziness, or palpitations. She has always been healthy and does not use illicit drugs. A member of her immediate family was recently diagnosed with infectious mononucleosis.

On physical examination, her temperature is 36.7 °C (98 °F), heart rate is 95/min, respiration rate is 24/min, and blood pressure is 110/60 mm Hg. No lymphadenopathy is present, and the jugular veins are not distended. Lungs are clear. Cardiac examination is notable for an intermittent systolic "squeaky" sound along the left sternal border.

An electrocardiogram shows diffuse 1 to 3 mm of ST elevation with an upwardly concave configuration. An echocardiogram shows no pericardial effusion.

Which of the following is the most appropriate initial treatment for this patient?

(A) Clopidogrel
(B) Heparin
(C) Indomethacin
(D) Prednisone

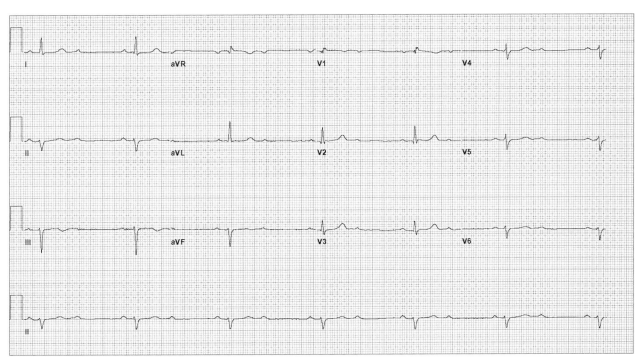

Item 5

Item 7

A 62-year-old man with chronic obstructive pulmonary disease is evaluated in the emergency department for fatigue, dyspnea, anorexia, and nausea. He has a history of mild left ventricular systolic dysfunction and has been treated with an angiotensin-converting enzyme inhibitor and digoxin for approximately 6 months.

Physical examination demonstrates a heart rate of 110/min with some irregularity. Blood pressure is 110/60 mm Hg. The jugular venous pressure is not elevated. There is mild wheezing during expiration. The cardiac examination demonstrates distant heart sounds with some irregularity but no murmurs.

Laboratory studies:

Hemoglobin	11.1 g/dL
Sodium	138 meq/L
Potassium	3.4 meq/L
Creatinine	1.6 mg/dL

The electrocardiogram is shown.

Which of the following is the most likely diagnosis?

(A) Atrial fibrillation
(B) Atrial flutter
(C) Atrial tachycardia with block
(D) Multifocal atrial tachycardia

Item 8

A 69-year-old man has been treated medically for chronic stable angina for 7 years. Over the past 6 months, he has been noticing some mild neck discomfort brought on by playing tennis. He has a 15-year history of type 2 diabetes mellitus. His medications are metoprolol, aspirin, atorvastatin, and insulin.

Results of the physical examination are unremarkable. An electrocardiogram shows a pattern of left ventricular hypertrophy. Cardiac catheterization is performed and shows 90% stenosis in the proximal left anterior descending coronary artery, 85% stenosis in the middle right coronary artery, and 70% stenosis in the proximal left circumflex coronary artery. The left ventricular ejection fraction at rest is 40%.

Which of the following treatments would offer this patient the greatest improvement in longevity?

(A) Begin clopidogrel
(B) Begin dipyridamole
(C) Coronary artery bypass graft surgery
(D) Implantable cardioverter-defibrillator

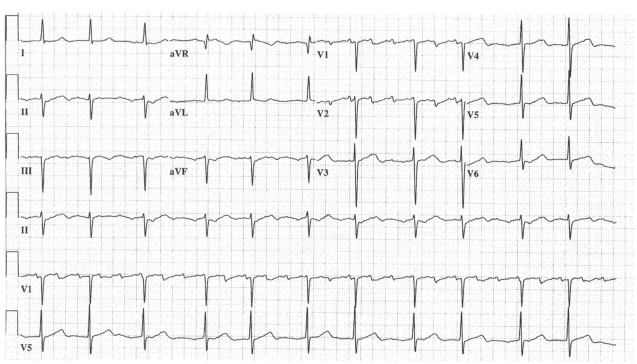

Item 7

Item 9

A 50-year-old man is evaluated in the emergency department because of a 6-hour history of "tearing" posterior chest pain, diaphoresis, and shortness of breath. He has never had this pain before and has no history of trauma. He has a 15-year history of hypertension treated with hydrochlorothiazide and enalapril and a 2-year history of heartburn treated with omeprazole.

On physical examination, the patient appears agitated. Temperature is 37.5 °C (99.5 °F), blood pressure is 113/48 mm Hg, heart rate is 115/min, respiration rate is 22/min, and oxygen saturation is 97% with the patient receiving oxygen, 2 L/min by nasal cannula. Lung examination reveals crackles at both bases. On cardiac examination, the S_1 is faint, the P_2 is accentuated, and a summation gallop (combined S_3 and S_4) is present. A grade 3/6 diastolic murmur is heard at the left upper sternal border; there are no rubs.

A chest radiograph shows only an enlarged heart. The electrocardiogram is shown.

Which of the following is the most likely diagnosis?

(A) Acute pericarditis
(B) Aortic dissection
(C) Gastroesophageal reflux disease
(D) Myocardial infarction
(E) Pulmonary embolism

Item 10

An elderly man collapses in an airport. A physician who witnesses the collapse checks his pulse and respirations and finds neither.

Which of the following is the most important determinant for short-term survival in this patient?

(A) Time to cardiopulmonary resuscitation
(B) Time to defibrillation
(C) Time to intubation
(D) Time to transport to the hospital

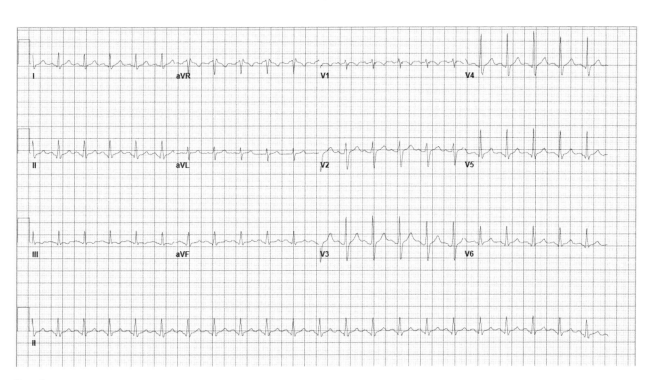

Item 9

Item 11

A 49-year-old man is evaluated in the emergency department for severe left precordial chest pain. The pain is sharp in quality and worsens with coughing or deep breathing. The chest pain has waxed and waned for the last 3 days and was preceded by a 3-day history of nonproductive cough, chills, myalgias, and fatigue. The patient has a history of cocaine use and a 60-pack-year smoking history. He has a 10-year history of hypertension and type 2 diabetes mellitus. His medications are lisinopril, low-dose aspirin, and glyburide.

On physical examination, temperature is 37.2 °C (99 °F), heart rate is 103/min, respiration rate is 22/min, and blood pressure is 153/92 mm Hg. The jugular veins are not distended. The lungs are clear. Heart sounds are distant with no evidence of murmur. A two-component rub is auscultated along the left lower sternal border. The remainder of the examination is normal. His electrocardiogram is shown.

Which of the following is the most likely diagnosis?

(A) Acute myocardial infarction
(B) Acute pericarditis
(C) Aortic dissection
(D) Costochondritis
(E) Pleuritis

Item 12

A 53-year-old man with long-standing ischemic cardiomyopathy is admitted to the intensive care unit with hypotension following a 24-hour episode of viral gastroenteritis. He is given intravenous fluids. The following day he develops chest pain, shortness of breath, and mental status changes.

On physical examination, temperature is 38.2 °C (100.8 °F), heart rate is 100/min, blood pressure is 75/45 mm Hg, respiration rate is 12/min, and he is mildly lethargic. Jugular venous pressure is difficult to assess. The lungs are clear. Cardiac examination reveals regular rhythm, a normal S_1 and S_2, and the presence of an S_3. There is peripheral edema bilaterally to the thighs, and the extremities are cool. A pulmonary artery catheter is placed and provides the following data.

Central venous pressure	12 mm Hg (normal, 0-5 mm Hg)
Pulmonary artery pressure	40/15 mm Hg (normal, 20-25/5-10 mm Hg)
Pulmonary capillary wedge pressure	18 mm Hg (normal, 6-12 mm Hg)
Cardiac output	3.5 L/min (normal, 4-8 L/min)

Which of the following is the most likely diagnosis?

(A) Cardiogenic shock
(B) Hypovolemic shock
(C) Septic shock
(D) Toxic shock

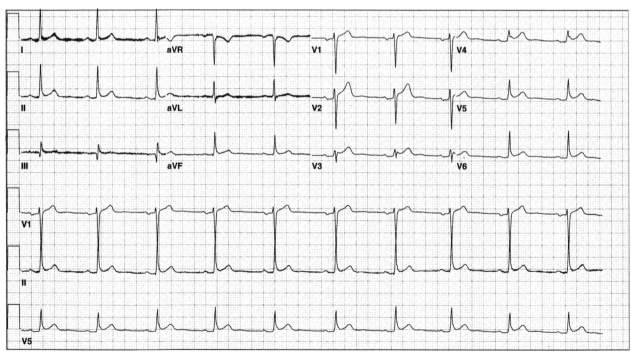

Item 11

Item 13

A 55-year-old man is evaluated in the office because of a 6-month history of substernal chest pain and dyspnea that typically occur on exertion. The pain resolves with rest, but he is not sure whether it goes away immediately or after 10 or 15 minutes. The pain may occasionally come after eating and is sometimes relieved with antacids. The symptoms have not been getting any worse. He has a 20-pack-year history of cigarette smoking and has an older brother and a father with coronary artery disease. He has no other medical problems and takes no medications.

On physical examination, blood pressure is 140/80 mm Hg, heart rate is 80/min and regular, and oxygen saturation is 98% with the patient breathing room air. There is no jugular venous distention. Heart sounds are normal without murmurs or extra sounds. The lungs are clear. Peripheral pulses are equal, and there are no bruits over the carotid and femoral arteries. There is no peripheral edema.

Resting electrocardiogram is shown.

Which of the following is the most appropriate next diagnostic test in the evaluation of this patient?

(A) Dobutamine echocardiography
(B) Exercise electrocardiography with perfusion imaging
(C) Exercise electrocardiography without perfusion imaging
(D) Pharmacologic stress myocardial perfusion imaging

Item 14

A 32-year-old woman is brought to the hospital with chest pain after a party. She has had similar pain previously, primarily in the morning and rarely with exertion. The pain usually subsides spontaneously and occasionally is associated with diaphoresis but rarely with dyspnea. She almost lost consciousness at work during the most recent episode. The patient has occasionally inhaled cocaine. She is otherwise healthy and takes no medications. She has no family history of coronary artery disease.

On physical examination, blood pressure is 128/70 mm Hg and heart rate is 72/min. There is no jugular venous distention or carotid bruits. The lungs are clear, and cardiac examination shows a normal S_1 and S_2 and a faint mid-systolic click but no murmur. Electrocardiogram taken during the chest pain shows a 1-mV inferior ST elevation; a subsequent electrocardiogram taken after resolution of the pain is normal. Serum troponin concentration is elevated. Therapy with heparin, aspirin, metoprolol, and nitroglycerin is begun.

The next morning, coronary angiography shows a normal angiographic appearance of the arteries and normal left ventricular wall motion.

Which of the following is the most likely diagnosis?

(A) Coronary artery atherosclerosis
(B) Coronary artery dissection
(C) Coronary artery vasculitis
(D) Coronary artery vasospasm

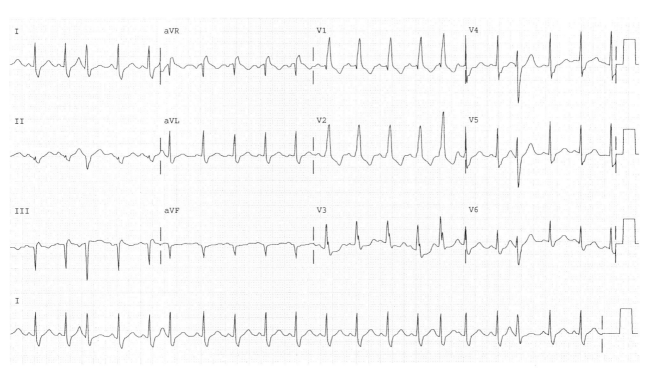

Item 13

Item 15

A 69-year-old man is evaluated in the emergency department for the acute onset of substernal chest pain radiating to the left arm. The patient is a former smoker with a history of hypertension.

On physical examination, he is diaphoretic. Blood pressure is 210/95 mm Hg in the right arm and 164/56 mm Hg in the left arm, heart rate is 90/min and regular, and respiration rate is 20/min. There is dullness half way up the right posterior thorax and a grade 2/6 diastolic murmur is present at the right upper sternal border. Electrocardiogram is shown.

Which of the following is the most likely diagnosis?

(A) Aortic dissection involving the right coronary artery
(B) Acute anteroseptal wall myocardial infarction
(C) Acute lateral wall myocardial infarction
(D) Coarctation of the aorta

Item 16

A 64-year-old woman is evaluated in the emergency department 6 hours after the onset of severe crushing chest pain associated with diaphoresis, nausea, and vomiting. Her medical history is significant only for hyperlipidemia; her medications are atorvastatin and aspirin. On physical examination, blood pressure is 140/88 mm Hg, and heart rate is 88/min. The lungs are clear, and no cardiac murmurs are heard. Examination of the abdomen and extremities is normal. Electrocardiogram shows a 3-mV ST elevation in leads II, III, and aVF, with occasional premature ventricular contractions. The hospital does not have cardiac catheterization facilities, and the patient is therefore given fibrinolytic therapy. Her chest pain resolves; she has two episodes of 6- to 10-beat ventricular tachycardia and stable hemodynamic parameters. Electrocardiogram now shows <0.5-mV ST elevation.

In addition to heparin and aspirin, which of the following approaches is the most appropriate next step in the management of this patient?

(A) Amiodarone
(B) β-Blocker
(C) Coronary angiography
(D) Lidocaine

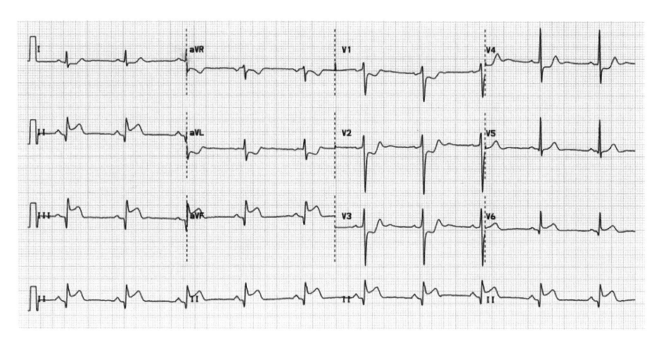

Item 15

Item 17

A 49-year-old man is evaluated in the emergency department for severe, intermittent chest pain beginning 2 days ago. His medical history includes hypercholesterolemia and hypertension and his medications are a statin and a β-blocker.

On physical examination, the blood pressure is 115/80 mm Hg and heart rate is 100/min. He has no jugular venous distention or carotid bruits. Lungs are clear, and heart sounds are faint but normal without murmurs or gallops. Electrocardiogram is shown. The serum troponin concentration is 4.8 ng/mL (normal <0.5 ng/mL).

Which of the following is the most likely diagnosis?

(A) Acute pericarditis
(B) ST elevation myocardial infarction (STEMI)
(C) Non-ST elevation myocardial infarction (NSTEMI)
(D) Variant angina

Item 18

A 49-year-old man is evaluated in the emergency department for chest discomfort accompanied by nausea and dyspnea that began 2 hours ago. On physical examination, blood pressure is 109/78 mm Hg and heart rate is 88/min. There is no jugular venous distention and no carotid bruits. The lungs are clear. Cardiac examination shows a normal S_1 and S_2 and no gallops, rubs, or murmurs. The troponin level is 6 ng/mL (normal <0.5 ng/mL). Electrocardiogram shows a 1-mV ST elevation in leads II, III, and aVF.

He is treated with enoxaparin, aspirin, metoprolol, and glycoprotein receptor blockers and is taken to the cardiac catheterization laboratory. A stent is placed in a subtotally occluded right coronary artery. A follow-up echocardiogram shows normal wall motion, normal valve function, and a normal ejection fraction. By day 4, he has no complications and is prepared to be discharged.

In addition to aspirin, clopidogrel, and metoprolol, which of the following medications should be given at discharge?

(A) Atorvastatin
(B) Gemfibrozil
(C) Niacin
(D) Warfarin

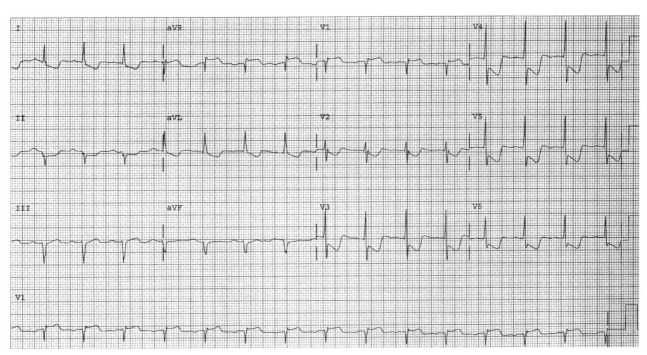

Item 17

Item 19

A 60-year-old man is evaluated in the emergency department for chest discomfort that has been present on and off for 6 hours. The patient is treated with aspirin, an intravenous β-blocker, and intravenous nitroglycerin. The initial electrocardiogram is shown. Initial troponin and creatine kinase–MB levels are elevated.

On physical examination, the heart rate is 60/min and blood pressure is 78/60 mm Hg. The jugular venous pressure is elevated to the angle of the jaw. The lungs are clear. On cardiac examination, the apical impulse is normal, and a parasternal lift is present. Normal S_1 and S_2 are heard. An S_3 and a brief systolic murmur that does not change with respiration are heard along the left sternal border.

Which of the following is the most likely cause for this patient's findings?

(A) Acute cardiac tamponade
(B) Aortic dissection
(C) Left ventricular free-wall rupture
(D) Right ventricular myocardial infarction

Item 20

A 78-year-old man is evaluated in the emergency department for a 1-week history of palpitations and weakness. He has had multiple similar episodes in the past year but has never sought treatment. His other medical problems include hypertension and type 2 diabetes mellitus, and his medications are lisinopril, hydrochlorothiazide, and metformin. He has no history of heart disease and had a normal electrocardiographic exercise stress test 1 year ago.

On physical examination, he is alert and in no acute distress. Blood pressure is 135/80 mm Hg, heart rate is 143/min and irregular, respiration rate is 14/min, and oxygen saturation is 98% with the patient breathing room air. On cardiac examination, there are no murmurs. Lungs are clear.

Electrocardiogram shows atrial fibrillation with a rapid ventricular rate without evidence of ischemic changes. Cardiac enzyme values are normal. His heart rate decreases to 74/min with administration of labetalol.

Which of the following is the most appropriate long-term treatment for this patient?

(A) Atrioventricular nodal ablation and pacemaker implantation
(B) Metoprolol and aspirin
(C) Metoprolol and warfarin
(D) Procainamide

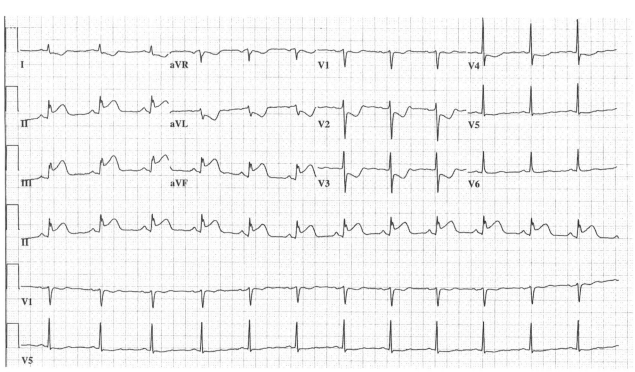

Item 19

Item 21

A 66-year-old woman is evaluated in the emergency department for severe substernal chest discomfort lasting 45 minutes. She has a 10-year history of type 2 diabetes mellitus and hypertension for which she takes metformin, aspirin, and enalapril. Physical examination shows a blood pressure of 120/60 mm Hg, heart rate of 86/min, and respiration rate of 18/min. Her lungs are clear, there is no jugular venous distention, and heart sounds are normal. There is no peripheral edema. Her electrocardiogram is shown.

Which of the following is the most likely cause of chest pain in this patient?

(A) Costochondritis
(B) Gastroesophageal reflux disease
(C) Myocardial infarction
(D) Pericarditis
(E) Pulmonary embolism

Item 22

A 56-year-old man is evaluated in the office during a routine physical examination. He has no cardiovascular complaints. His medical history is unremarkable.

On physical examination, heart rate is approximately 90/min and irregularly irregular, and blood pressure is 130/78 mm Hg. Except for the abnormal cardiac rhythm, the remainder of the examination is unremarkable.

The electrocardiogram demonstrates atrial fibrillation with a heart rate of 92/min. The chest radiograph is unremarkable. Laboratory test results, including assessment of thyroid function, are normal. The patient is not aware of the abnormal rhythm or its duration.

In addition to heart rate control, which of the following would be most appropriate for this patient?

(A) Aspirin
(B) Clopidogrel
(C) Direct-current cardioversion
(D) Warfarin

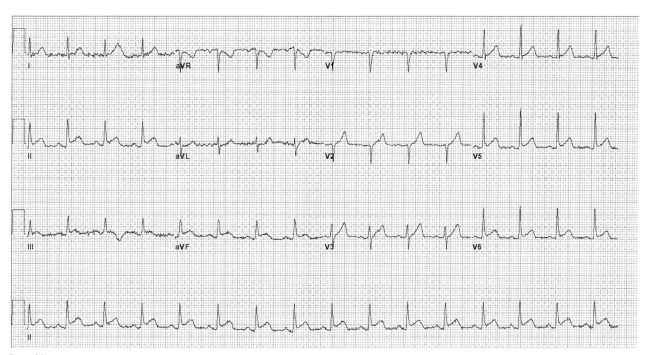

Item 21

Item 23

A 68-year-old man is evaluated in the emergency department for chest pain that has lasted 90 minutes. He was eating dinner when he had the sudden onset of sharp precordial pain radiating toward both shoulders and his back. The pain is described as 9/10 in severity. Medical history is significant for hypertension and hyperlipidemia.

Physical examination shows a heart rate of 90/min, respiration rate of 19/min, blood pressure of 110/60 mm Hg, and oxygen saturation of 94% with the patient breathing room air. Bibasilar crackles are heard. Heart sounds are distant. There is a normal S_1 and S_2 and no S_4 or S_3. An electrocardiogram is shown.

Which of the following is the most likely diagnosis?

(A) Acute anterior wall myocardial infarction
(B) Acute inferior wall myocardial infarction
(C) Acute lateral wall myocardial infarction
(D) Acute pericarditis
(E) Acute posterior wall myocardial infarction

Item 24

A 33-year-old man is evaluated in the office for palpitations. He reports intermittent symptoms that do not correlate with any particular activity. He is only mildly disturbed by the palpitations but wants to have his heart evaluated. His medical history is unremarkable, and he takes no medications. His physical examination and electrocardiogram also are unremarkable. A 24-hour electrocardiogram shows a normal sinus rhythm with 3004 total premature ventricular contractions in 24 hours. An echocardiogram shows a structurally normal heart. Thyroid function studies and electrolyte levels are normal.

Which of the following is the most appropriate treatment for this patient?

(A) Atenolol
(B) Flecainide
(C) Radiocatheter ablation
(D) Reassurance

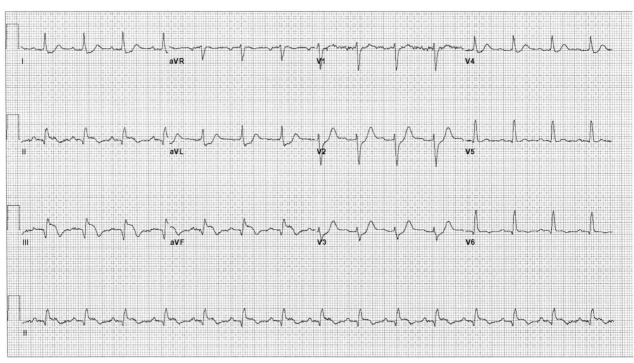

Item 23

Item 25

A 42-year-old man is evaluated at a rural emergency department for severe left shoulder and chest pain that radiates to the jaw and is associated with diaphoresis and mild dyspnea. The patient has no prior medical history and takes no medications.

In the emergency department, intravenous heparin and an aspirin are administered. On physical examination, blood pressure is 90/79 mm Hg and heart rate is 54/min. There is no jugular vein distention and no carotid bruits. The lungs are clear. Cardiac examination reveals a normal S_1 and S_2 and no murmurs. Electrocardiogram is shown.

The receiving hospital does not have a cardiac catheterization laboratory, and the closest hospital with one is 62 miles away. It usually takes at least 2 hours to arrange transfer.

Before transfer, which of the following therapeutic agents should be given?

(A) Clopidogrel
(B) Esmolol
(C) Fibrinolytic therapy
(D) Glycoprotein receptor blocker
(E) Nitroglycerin

Item 26

A 38-year-old man is hospitalized with palpitations and dyspnea. He has no significant medical history and does not take any medications. He has a 20-pack-year smoking history and drinks alcohol daily. He does not use illicit drugs.

On physical examination, temperature is 36.9 °C (98.5 °F), blood pressure is 120/80 mm Hg, and heart rate is 115/min. Jugular venous pressure is normal. The lungs are clear. Cardiac examination shows an irregularly irregular rhythm. There is trace edema at both ankles.

Laboratory studies:

Hemoglobin	14 g/dL
Mean corpuscular volume	101 fL
Aspartate aminotransferase	55 U/L
Alanine aminotransferase	45 U/L
Thyroid-stimulating hormone	4.5 µU/mL

Electrocardiogram shows normal voltage, normal axis, and atrial fibrillation. Echocardiogram shows dilated ventricles with normal wall thickness and severely decreased systolic function (left ventricular ejection fraction, 15%). The patient is started on lisinopril, carvedilol, and warfarin. Later in the hospital course, he spontaneously converts to normal sinus rhythm, he feels well, and has a blood pressure of 105/75 mm Hg and a heart rate of 63/min. Electrocardiogram confirms normal sinus rhythm.

Which of the following is the most likely type of cardiomyopathy in this patient?

(A) Alcoholic
(B) Amyloid
(C) Hypertrophic
(D) Ischemic

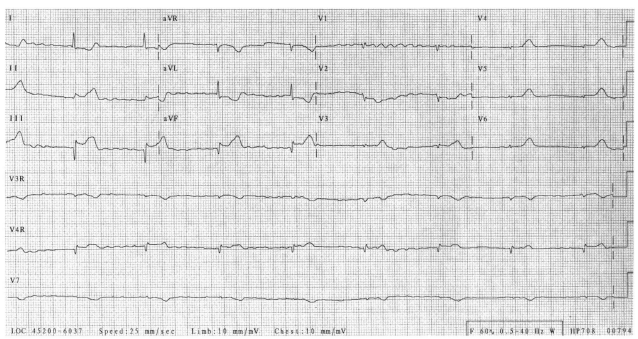

Item 25

LOC 45200-6037   Speed:25 mm/sec   Limb:10 mm/mV   Chest:10 mm/mV   F 60% 0.5-40 Hz W   HP708   00794

Item 27

A 43-year-old man is evaluated in the emergency department for palpitations. He has no prior personal or family history of cardiovascular disease, diabetes mellitus, or hypertension. On physical examination, the lungs are clear. Cardiovascular examination is unremarkable with the exception of a rapid heart rate.

The chest radiograph is normal. The electrocardiogram is shown. The patient converts to sinus rhythm spontaneously while in the emergency department, and the subsequent electrocardiogram is normal.

Which of the following is the most likely rhythm disorder responsible for this patient's symptoms?

(A) Atrial fibrillation
(B) Atrial flutter
(C) Atrioventricular nodal re-entrant tachycardia
(D) Atrioventricular re-entrant tachycardia

Item 28

A 68-year-old woman is hospitalized with palpitations and shortness of breath. She has a history of hypertension and chronic atrial fibrillation, and her medications are furosemide, candesartan, and warfarin. On physical examination, the heart rate is 120/min with an irregularly irregular rhythm, and blood pressure is 130/80 mm Hg with no evidence of pulsus paradoxus. She has an elevated jugular venous pressure with normal x and y descent, crackles in both lungs, and marked lower extremity edema. Echocardiography shows left ventricular hypertrophy, an ejection fraction of 70%, and no significant valvular disease.

After intravenous diuretics are begun, the patient's symptoms improve, and the crackles and peripheral edema resolve. Her heart rate is now 99/min, and her blood pressure is 120/75 mm Hg.

Which of the following is the most likely primary mechanism of her heart failure?

(A) Constrictive pericarditis
(B) Diastolic dysfunction
(C) Systolic dysfunction
(D) Valvular disease

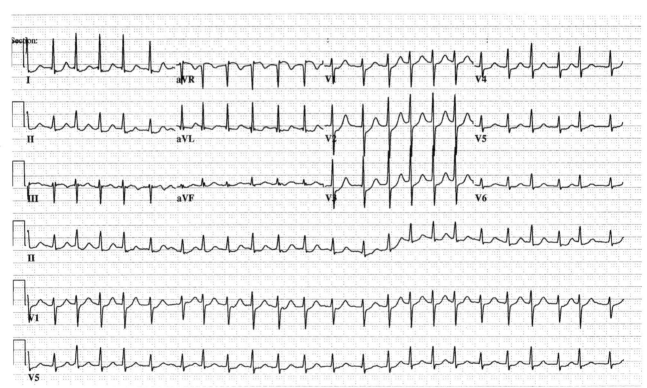

Item 27

Item 29

A 73-year-old man is evaluated in the office for shortness of breath and decreased exercise tolerance for the past 3 days. He has no other medical problems, and his only medication is low-dose aspirin daily.

On physical examination, heart rate is 148/min and blood pressure is 118/68 mm Hg. The lungs are clear. Cardiac examination demonstrates tachycardia with no murmur. The electrocardiogram is shown.

Which of the following is most likely causing this patient's symptoms?

(A) Atrial fibrillation
(B) Atrial flutter
(C) Multifocal atrial tachycardia
(D) Sinus tachycardia

Item 30

A 26-year-old woman is hospitalized because of a 7-day history of increasing shortness of breath. Two weeks ago, she had flu-like symptoms of fever, muscle aches, and chest pain, which have since resolved. She does not take any medications.

On physical examination, temperature is 37 °C (98.6 °F), blood pressure is 120/79 mm Hg, and heart rate is 100/min and regular. The lungs are clear. Cardiac examination shows a normal S_1 and S_2. Echocardiogram shows normal-sized ventricles, decreased systolic function (left ventricular ejection fraction, 40%) that is global and most severe in the anterior wall, and no significant valvular abnormalities. Coronary angiography discloses no evidence of coronary artery disease.

Which of the following is the most appropriate next step in treating this patient?

(A) Azithromycin
(B) Enoxaparin
(C) Ibuprofen
(D) Lisinopril
(E) Prednisone

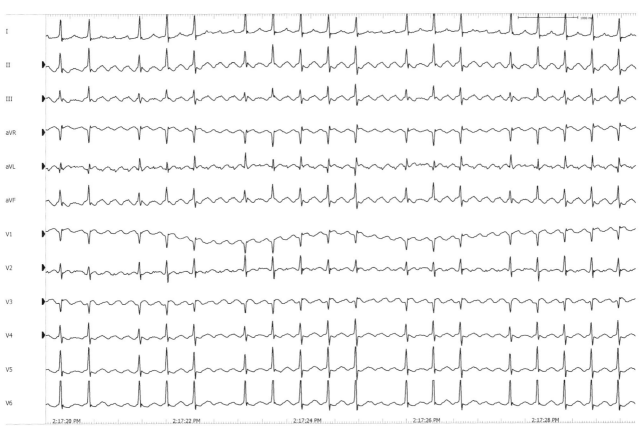

Item 29

Item 31

A 68-year-old man is evaluated in the emergency department for shortness of breath and palpitations. He reports a 3-day history of progressive shortness of breath, with productive cough and wheezing. In addition, his heart "has been racing" since last night. He has a 50-pack-year smoking history and bronchospastic lung disease, for which he uses inhaled bronchodilators.

On physical examination, temperature is 37.8 °C (100 °F), and heart rate is 122/min. The patient is in moderate respiratory distress. Examination of the chest shows decreased airflow with expiratory wheezing. The cardiac examination demonstrates distant heart sounds. Electrolytes are normal. The electrocardiogram is shown.

Which of the following is the most likely electrocardiographic diagnosis?

(A) Accelerated idioventricular tachycardia
(B) Atrioventricular nodal re-entrant tachycardia
(C) Atrioventricular re-entrant tachycardia
(D) Multifocal atrial tachycardia

Item 32

A 58-year-old man is evaluated in the office for a 3-month history of shortness of breath with exertion. He has a 10-year history of hypertension and type 2 diabetes mellitus but no history of coronary artery disease. His medications are extended-release metoprolol, aspirin, metformin, and atorvastatin.

On physical examination, blood pressure is 165/92 mm Hg and heart rate is 88/min. Jugular venous pressure is 10 cm H_2O. Bibasilar crackles are present, cardiac rhythm is regular, and an S_3 is present. Electrocardiogram shows normal sinus rhythm and left ventricular hypertrophy. Laboratory test results include potassium of 4.2 meq/L and creatinine of 1.0 mg/dL. An echocardiogram is ordered, and furosemide is prescribed.

The patient returns the following week with resolution of his symptoms. His blood pressure at this visit is 130/78 mm Hg, his heart rate is 65/min, jugular venous pressure is 4 cm H_2O, lungs are clear, and the S_3 is absent. The echocardiogram shows left ventricular hypertrophy, reduced systolic function, and inferior wall hypokinesis.

Which of the following is the most appropriate medication change at this time?

(A) Change metoprolol to carvedilol
(B) Start digoxin
(C) Start lisinopril
(D) Start spironolactone

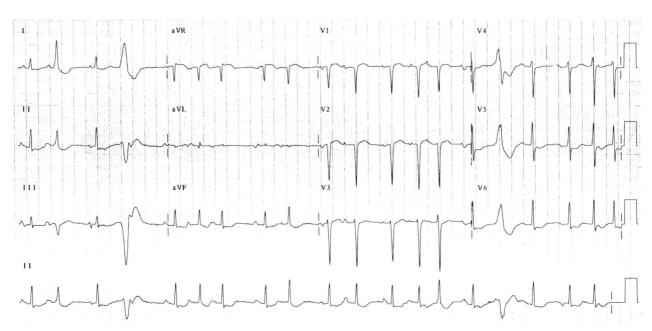

Item 31

Item 33

A 28-year-old man is evaluated in the office for a 5-year history of palpitations. These episodes used to occur once or twice a year, but over the past 6 months he has been experiencing them on a monthly basis. He reports that his heart starts "racing" suddenly for no reason, and the episode usually terminates abruptly after he takes a few deep breaths. Episodes typically last 10 to 15 minutes, although one episode last month lasted 30 minutes. He is otherwise healthy, has no other symptoms, and takes no medications. Physical examination is normal.

A baseline electrocardiogram is shown.

Which of the following is the most likely cause of his arrhythmia?

(A) Atrial flutter
(B) Atrial tachycardia with block
(C) Atrioventricular re-entrant tachycardia (Wolff-Parkinson-White syndrome)
(D) Atrioventricular nodal re-entrant tachycardia

Item 34

A 50-year-old man is evaluated during a routine follow-up office visit for heart failure, which was diagnosed 1 year ago. A stress test at the time of diagnosis was negative for ischemia. At his most recent evaluation 4 months ago, an echocardiogram showed left ventricular enlargement and hypertrophy, a left ventricular ejection fraction of 40%, and no significant valvular disease. An electrocardiogram was unchanged, showing left ventricular hypertrophy but no evidence of previous myocardial infarction. The patient is currently asymptomatic, and his medications are hydrochlorothiazide and lisinopril.

On physical examination, heart rate is 85/min and blood pressure is 135/85 mm Hg. There is no jugular venous distention or peripheral edema. The lungs are clear. There is a soft S_4 but no murmur.

Which of the following medications should be added to the patient's regimen?

(A) Carvedilol
(B) Digoxin
(C) Diltiazem
(D) Losartan
(E) Spironolactone

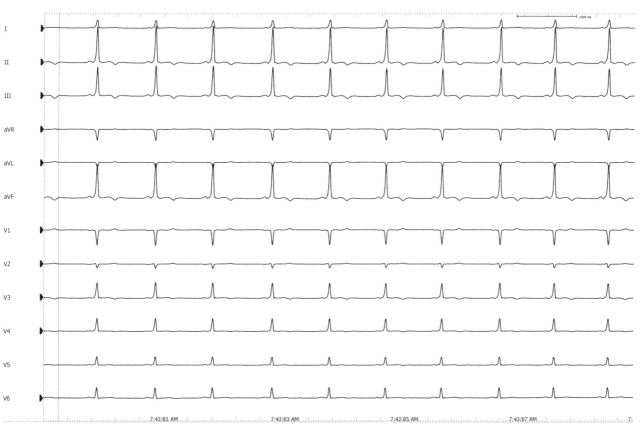

Item 33

Item 35

A 22-year-old man is evaluated in the emergency department for a rapid heart rate and lightheadedness. He reports episodes of a "racing heart" a few times each year since his early teens. He describes today's episode as different: it started as one of his regular episodes but then became erratic. In addition, the lightheadedness has never happened before. He is otherwise healthy and takes no medications.

On physical examination, the patient is diaphoretic. Blood pressure is 72 mm Hg palpable. His lungs are clear, and cardiac examination demonstrates a rapid irregular rhythm with no murmurs. The electrocardiogram is shown.

Which of the following is the most appropriate therapy for this patient?

(A) Direct-current cardioversion
(B) Intravenous procainamide
(C) Intravenous verapamil
(D) Overdrive atrial pacing

Item 36

A 43-year-old woman with idiopathic cardiomyopathy (most recent left ventricular ejection fraction, 30%) is evaluated in the office. She has fatigue and shortness of breath with minimal activity. Her medications are lisinopril, 2.5 mg daily; sustained-release metoprolol, 12.5 mg daily; digoxin, 0.125 mg daily; and furosemide, 80 mg daily.

On physical examination, blood pressure is 110/75 mm Hg and heart rate is 94/min. There is jugular venous distention to 2 cm above the clavicle at a 45-degree incline. Cardiac rhythm is regular, with normal S_1 and S_2 and no gallops. There is no peripheral edema.

Laboratory studies:

Blood urea nitrogen	43 mg/dL
Potassium	5.1 meq/L
Creatinine	2.7 mg/dL
Digoxin	0.9 µg/L

Which of the following would be the most appropriate medication change?

(A) Increase digoxin
(B) Increase furosemide
(C) Increase metoprolol
(D) Start spironolactone

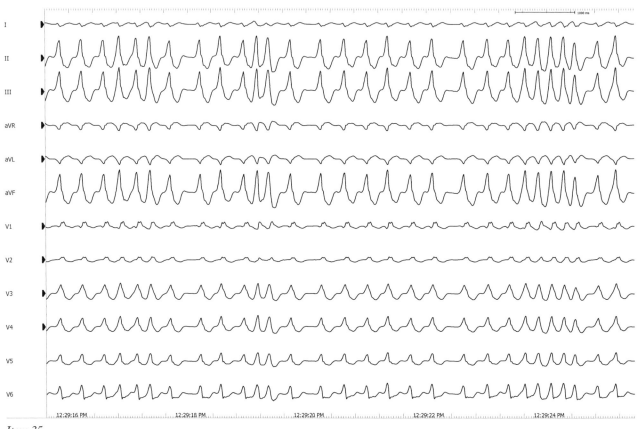

Item 35

Item 37

A 63-year-old man is evaluated in the emergency department after calling 911 for chest pain and diaphoresis. He had an anterior wall myocardial infarction 5 years ago, after which he underwent coronary artery bypass grafting. He has a history of New York Heart Association class II congestive heart failure, hypertension, and hypercholesterolemia. His current medications are furosemide, potassium chloride, enalapril, digoxin, atorvastatin, metoprolol, and aspirin.

On physical examination he is diaphoretic. Heart rate is 192/min, and blood pressure is 85/43 mm Hg. He has jugular venous distention, and the cardiac examination reveals tachycardia with no murmurs. Bibasilar crackles are heard.

The electrocardiogram is shown.

Which of the following is the most likely electrocardiographic diagnosis?

(A) Atrial fibrillation
(B) Left bundle branch block
(C) Right bundle branch block
(D) Ventricular tachycardia

Item 38

A 29-year-old woman is evaluated in the emergency department at 30 weeks gestation for increasing dyspnea on exertion. On physical examination, blood pressure is 110/70 mm Hg and heart rate is 98/min and regular. Bilateral crackles are heard. Cardiac examination shows a normal S_1, a fixed split S_2, a grade 2/6 early systolic murmur at the base, a grade 2/6 holosystolic murmur at the apex radiating to the axilla, and an S_3 gallop. There is trace peripheral edema. Echocardiography shows global left ventricular hypokinesis, with an ejection fraction of 30% and moderate mitral regurgitation. Peripartum cardiomyopathy and heart failure are diagnosed.

Which of the following medications is contraindicated at this time?

(A) Atenolol
(B) Furosemide
(C) Isosorbide dinitrate
(D) Lisinopril

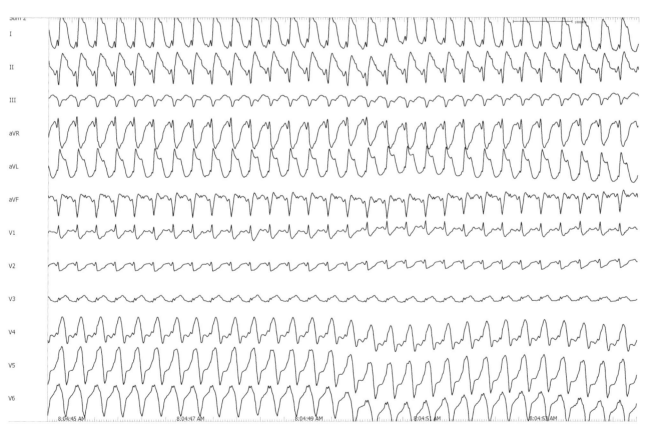

Item 37

Item 39

A 70-year-old man is evaluated in the emergency department for palpitations and substernal chest pain that began 30 minutes ago. He has a history of coronary artery disease and hypertension. His medications are hydrochlorothiazide, pravastatin, metoprolol, sublingual nitroglycerin, and aspirin.

Physical examination reveals a diaphoretic man who is anxious and short of breath. Blood pressure is 100/60 mm Hg, heart rate is 160/min, and respiration rate is 22/min. He has large jugular venous *a* waves, varying intensity of S_1, and an S_3. There are crackles at the lung bases. Bilateral lower extremity edema is present.

His electrocardiogram is shown.

Which of the following intravenous drugs should be administered at this time?

(A) Dopamine
(B) Lidocaine
(C) Tissue plasminogen activator
(D) Verapamil

Item 40

A 65-year-old woman with heart failure due to nonischemic cardiomyopathy (left ventricular ejection fraction is 25%) is evaluated in the office for a 1-week history of increasing dyspnea on exertion. Her symptoms have progressed to the point that she is no longer able to perform even minimal activities of daily living. She has not had any chest pain or pressure, and her weight has not fluctuated more than a few pounds over the past month. She takes furosemide, lisinopril, and carvedilol and is compliant with a salt-restricted diet.

On physical examination, blood pressure is 105/60 mm Hg, heart rate is 75/min and regular, and respiration rate is 18/min. Findings include jugular venous distention, scattered bibasilar crackles, an S_3 gallop, and trace bilateral pretibial edema.

Addition of which of the following medications will most likely improve this patient's symptoms and prolong her survival?

(A) Amlodipine
(B) Digitalis
(C) Metolazone
(D) Milrinone
(E) Spironolactone

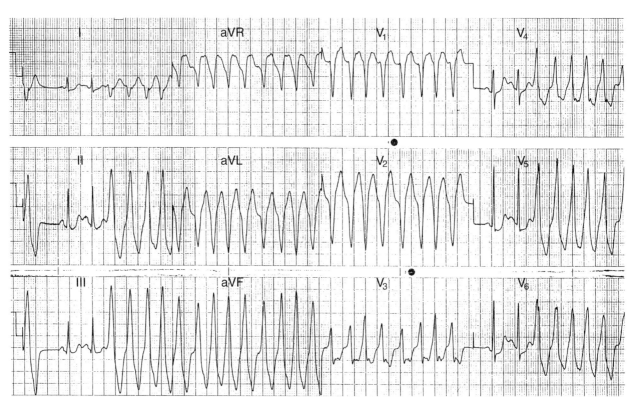

Item 39

Item 41

A 45-year-old woman with a 20-year-history of type 2 diabetes mellitus is evaluated for a 1-month history of progressive shortness of breath. Two months ago, she had a flu-like illness with nausea, vomiting, and sweating.

On physical examination, the patient is obese (BMI 32.9). Heart rate is 75/min, and blood pressure is 185/93 mm Hg. Jugular venous pressure is elevated. Bibasilar crackles are present. Cardiac examination shows regular rhythm, normal S_1 and S_2, and the presence of an S_3. There is peripheral edema. An electrocardiogram is shown. An echocardiogram is notable for left ventricular hypertrophy and severely decreased systolic function (left ventricular ejection fraction, 20%).

Which of the following is the most appropriate next diagnostic test?

(A) Cardiac catheterization
(B) Exercise stress test
(C) Endomyocardial biopsy
(D) Measurement of B-type natriuretic peptide

Item 42

A 34-year-old man is seen in the office for a routine evaluation. He is asymptomatic and has no personal or family history of cardiovascular disease. He jogs 2 to 3 miles three times per week.

On physical examination, temperature is normal, heart rate is 70/min, and blood pressure is 140/58 mm Hg. There is no jugular venous distention. Lungs are clear. Cardiovascular examination reveals a point of maximal impulse that is displaced 1 cm from the midclavicular line and is diffuse. There is an early decrescendo diastolic murmur heard at the left parasternal third intercostal space that does not radiate or change with respiration. There are brisk, prominent distal pulses throughout the extremities, with a "pistol shot" sound heard when auscultating over the peripheral arteries. A transthoracic echocardiogram is scheduled

Which of the following is the most likely diagnosis?

(A) Aortic dissection
(B) Aortic valve regurgitation
(C) Aortic valve stenosis
(D) Pulmonary valve regurgitation
(E) Pulmonary valve stenosis

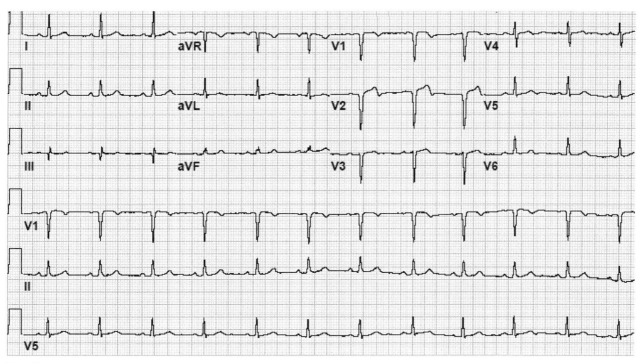

Item 41

Item 43

A 79-year-old woman is seen in the office for an annual examination. She walks regularly to and from the bus stop several times per week. It now takes her 25 minutes to get to the bus stop, whereas it only took her 10 minutes a year ago. She describes dyspnea midway in her walk, causing her to stop and catch her breath. She does not have angina, presyncope, syncope, or pedal edema.

On physical examination, heart rate is 80/min, and blood pressure is 165/86 mm Hg. Carotid artery upstrokes are delayed. The lungs are clear. There is a sustained apical impulse. S_1 is normal, and there is a single S_2 and an S_4. A grade 3/6 late-peaking systolic murmur is heard best at the right second intercostal space with radiation into the right carotid artery. Transthoracic echocardiogram is scheduled.

Which of the following is the most likely diagnosis?

(A) Aortic valve stenosis
(B) Hypertrophic cardiomyopathy
(C) Mitral valve regurgitation
(D) Tricuspid valve regurgitation
(E) Ventricular septal defect

Item 44

A 78-year-old woman is evaluated in the office for a 1-year history of progressively decreasing exercise tolerance. She has been in good health other than hypertension and osteoarthritis.

On physical examination, heart rate is 84/min and regular, respiration rate is 12/min, and blood pressure is 170/90 mm Hg. Carotid upstrokes are brisk, and jugular venous pressure is 8 cm H_2O. The lungs are clear. S_1 is soft, and there is a physiologically split S_2. A grade 2/6 mid-systolic murmur is present at the base with radiation to the apex but not to the carotid arteries, and there is a grade 1/6 early diastolic decrescendo murmur at the left sternal border. There is no peripheral edema.

Which of this patient's physical examination findings is the most helpful for excluding severe aortic stenosis?

(A) Blood pressure
(B) Carotid upstroke
(C) Murmur intensity
(D) Radiation of the murmur
(E) Second heart sound (S_2)

Item 45

A 68-year-old man is evaluated in the office during a routine physical examination. A heart murmur was diagnosed at age 28 years, and echocardiography 20 years ago revealed a bicuspid aortic valve with minimal obstruction to aortic outflow. He works full time, is very active, and has no physical limitations. He does not have chest pain, dyspnea on exertion, or syncope and takes no medications.

On physical examination, heart rate is 68/min and blood pressure is 128/78 mm Hg. The carotid pulses are full and not delayed. A long, late-peaking grade 3/6 systolic crescendo–decrescendo murmur is present at the second right intercostal space with radiation to the carotid arteries; no diastolic murmur is heard. S_1 is normal, and S_2 is diminished and paradoxically split. An S_4 gallop is heard at the cardiac apex. The lungs are clear. There is no lower extremity edema.

Electrocardiography shows a heart rate of 70/min, normal sinus rhythm, left atrial enlargement, and prominent R waves in leads V_5 and V_6.

Which of the following findings suggests the presence of advanced aortic stenosis in this patient?

(A) Absent aortic ejection click
(B) Left atrial enlargement
(C) Long, late-peaking systolic murmur
(D) Radiation of the systolic murmur to the carotid arteries
(E) S_4 gallop

Item 46

A 32-year-old man is evaluated in the office during an annual physical examination. He is asymptomatic, and there is no personal or family history of cardiovascular disease. On physical examination, vital signs are normal. S_1 and S_2 are normal, and an S_4 is present. There is a grade 2/6 crescendo-decrescendo systolic murmur heard best at the lower left sternal border. The murmur does not radiate to the carotid arteries. The Valsalva maneuver increases the intensity of the murmur, and moving from a standing to a squatting position, performing a passive leg lift while recumbent, and performing isometric handgrip exercises decrease the intensity. Rapid upstrokes of the peripheral pulses are present.

Which of the following is the most likely diagnosis?

(A) Aortic valve stenosis
(B) Atrial septal defect
(C) Hypertrophic cardiomyopathy
(D) Mitral valve prolapse
(E) Ventricular septal defect

Item 47

A 57-year-old woman with a 6-month history of progressive dyspnea on exertion is evaluated in the office. Physical examination reveals an elevated jugular venous pressure, bibasilar crackles, a grade 2/6 holosystolic murmur at the apex that radiates to the axilla and does not vary with respiration, a loud pulmonic component of S_2, an enlarged point of maximal impulse, and moderate edema up to both shins. An electrocardiogram shows left atrial and ventricular enlargement. Chest radiograph shows mild cardiomegaly and pulmonary congestion.

Which of the following is the most likely diagnosis?

(A) Aortic valve regurgitation
(B) Aortic valve stenosis
(C) Mitral valve regurgitation
(D) Mitral valve stenosis
(E) Tricuspid valve regurgitation

Item 48

A 23-year-old woman who is 23 weeks pregnant is evaluated in the office because of a 2-month history of increasing shortness of breath. On physical examination, blood pressure is 100/60 mm Hg, heart rate is 88/min and regular, and respiration rate is 26/min. Jugular venous pressure is 18 cm H_2O, carotid upstrokes are brisk, and bibasilar crackles are present. On cardiac examination, the apical impulse is faint in the mid left 6th intercostal space, and there is a forceful sternal heave. The S_1 is loud, and there is fixed splitting of S_2, a soft apical systolic murmur, and an opening snap followed by a grade 2/6 mid-diastolic murmur.

Which of the following is the most likely diagnosis?

(A) Aortic valve stenosis
(B) Mitral valve stenosis
(C) Normal findings of pregnancy
(D) Patent ductus arteriosus
(E) Peripartum cardiomyopathy

Item 49

A 19-year-old woman is evaluated in the office for palpitations described as isolated "extra beats" that do not occur with any regularity. She has no history of syncope or presyncope, no cardiovascular risk factors, and no family history of cardiovascular disease. She does not have signs or symptoms of congestive heart failure and takes no medications.

On physical examination, vital signs are normal. Her lungs are clear. There is no S_4 or S_3. A grade 2/6 late systolic murmur is present that is heard best at the cardiac apex and radiates toward the left axilla. A midsystolic click is heard. Following a Valsalva maneuver and a squat-to-stand maneuver, the midsystolic click moves closer to the S_1, but the intensity of the murmur does not change. The remainder of her examination is unremarkable.

Which of the following is the most likely diagnosis accounting for the heart murmur?

(A) Benign (innocent) flow murmur
(B) Hypertrophic cardiomyopathy
(C) Mitral valve regurgitation
(D) Mitral valve prolapse

Chapter 1

Cardiovascular Medicine
Answers and Critiques

Item 1   Answer: A

Any patient who develops a new peripheral ischemia after an invasive procedure involving arterial access should be suspected of having cholesterol emboli. In a prospective study of 1786 consecutive patients ≥40 years of age who underwent left-heart catheterization, cholesterol embolism syndrome was found in 25 patients (1.4%) including 12 (48%) with cutaneous signs and 16 (64%) with renal insufficiency. Eosinophil counts were significantly higher in patients with this syndrome. Urinary eosinophilia is also common. The in-hospital mortality rate was 16.0% (compared with 0.5% of unaffected patients). The incidence of cholesterol embolism syndrome increased in patients with atherosclerotic disease, hypertension, a history of smoking, and elevation of baseline C-reactive protein values. This patient's presentation is typical for cholesterol emboli likely related to catheter manipulation and dislodgement of an atherosclerotic plaque during cardiac catheterization. Treatment is supportive.

This patient has no history of gout; in addition, his extremity was not warm to touch, and there was evidence of ischemic necrosis of tissue. Femoral artery dissection would not be associated with renal dysfunction or urinary eosinophils. Radiocontrast nephropathy, common in elderly patients with diabetes mellitus, would not be associated with ischemic necrosis of the toe.

KEY POINT

• Peripheral ischemia after an arterial catheterization suggests cholesterol embolism syndrome.

Bibliography

1. **Fukumoto Y, Tsutsui H, Tsuchihashi M, Masumoto A, Takeshita A.** The incidence and risk factors of cholesterol embolization syndrome, a complication of cardiac catheterization: a prospective study. J Am Coll Cardiol. 2003;42:211-6. [PMID: 12875753]

Item 2   Answer: D

Third-degree atrioventricular block, or complete heart block, refers to a lack of atrioventricular conduction (characterized by lack of conduction of all atrial impulses to the ventricles), as seen in this patient's electrocardiogram. Many patients with complete heart block are symptomatic and are treated with a pacemaker. There is some evidence that pacemaker implantation may improve survival for patients with asymptomatic complete heart block; therefore, all patients with complete heart block should be treated with pacemaker implantation.

First-degree heart block is recognized electrocardiographically as a prolongation of the PR interval; all P waves are conducted and this condition requires no specific treatment. Second-degree heart block is characterized by intermittent nonconduction of P waves and subsequent "dropped" ventricular beats. Second-degree heart block is divided into types, Mobitz I and Mobitz II. Mobitz type I second-degree heart block is characterized by progressive prolongation of the PR interval until a dropped beat occurs. This type of heart block is characteristically transient and usually requires no specific treatment. Mobitz type II second-degree heart block is characterized by a regularly dropped beat (e.g., a nonconducted P wave every second or third beat) without progressive prolongation of the PR interval and is usually associated with evidence of additional disease in the conduction system, such as bundle branch block or bifascicular or trifascicular block. Mobitz type II heart block suddenly and unpredictably progresses to complete heart block and is usually treated with a pacemaker.

KEY POINT

• A pacemaker is indicated in patients with acquired third-degree atrioventricular block.

Bibliography

1. **Gregoratos G, Abrams J, Epstein AE, Freedman RA, Hayes DL, Hlatky MA, et al.** ACC/AHA/NASPE 2002 guideline update for implantation of cardiac pacemakers and antiarrhythmia devices: summary article: a report of the American College of Cardiology/American Heart Association Task Force on Practice Guidelines (ACC/AHA/NASPE Committee to Update the 1998 Pacemaker Guidelines). Circulation. 2002;106:2145-61. [PMID: 12379588]

Item 3   Answer: A

The examination shows heart failure and a murmur of mitral regurgitation, and the electrocardiogram shows a new left bundle branch block. Electrocardiographically, left bundle branch block is associated with absent Q waves in leads I, aVL, and V_6; a large, wide and positive R wave in leads I, aVL, and V_6 ("tombstone" R waves); and prolongation of the QRS complex to >0.12 sec. Repolarization abnormalities are present consisting of ST segment and T wave vectors directed opposite to the QRS complex. The presentation of acute coronary syndrome with new left bundle branch block should be considered equivalent to ST-elevation myocardial infarction and true posterior wall myocardial infarction, with management including early invasive diagnostic studies and coronary intervention. The most benefit is provided by reperfusion within 12 hours of the onset of symptoms.

In right bundle branch block, lead I will show a small Q wave and tall R wave; lead V_6 will show a small positive R wave followed by a small negative S wave followed by a large positive deflection ("rabbit ears"). There is ST depression and T-wave inversion in right precordial leads. The QRS complex is >0.12 sec. There are no clinical features to suggest idioventricular tachycardia or slow ventricular tachycardia, which is demonstrated electrocardiographically as a wide QRS complex (without conducting P waves) and a heart rate between 60 and 100/min. Third-degree atrioventricular block, or complete heart block, refers to a lack of atrioventricular conduction characterized by lack of conduction of all atrial impulses to the ventricles.

KEY POINTS

• Left bundle branch block is associated with absent Q waves in leads I, aVL, and V_6; a large, wide and positive R wave in leads I, aVL, and V6 ("tombstone" R waves); and prolongation of the QRS complex to >0.12 sec.

• The constellation of chest pain, elevated biomarkers, and new-onset left bundle branch block is considered equivalent to ST-elevation myocardial infarction.

Bibliography
1. Sgarbossa EB, Birnbaum Y, Parrillo JE. Electrocardiographic diagnosis of acute myocardial infarction: Current concepts for the clinician. Am Heart J. 2001;141:507-17. [PMID: 11275913]

Item 4   Answer: A

The patient's history of exercise-induced leg pain, its relief with rest or walking downhill, vascular bruit and absent pulses on physical examination, dependent rubor, and several major risk factors for atherosclerotic artery disease all point to arterial ischemia as the cause of his symptoms. Determination of the ankle-brachial index (ABI) is a common initial test in the evaluation for peripheral vascular disease. With a Doppler probe, the ABI is measured as the ratio of the highest right/left dorsalis pedis/posterior tibial artery systolic pressure divided by the highest right/left brachial artery systolic pressure. A normal ABI is 1.0 to 1.3. Most patients with peripheral vascular disease have an ABI <0.9, and those with severe disease (rest ischemia) have an ABI of <0.4. An ABI >1.3 suggests a calcified, noncompressible vessel, most commonly seen in patients with long-standing diabetes mellitus and hypertension.

Peripheral neuropathy would be unlikely to present as pain with exercise. Spinal stenosis commonly presents as pain with standing and after walking a variable distance, most prominently with spinal extension, and is usually relieved by flexing forward, sitting, or lying down. Like spinal stenosis, osteoarthritis may cause pain on walking but is usually independent of grade; neither condition can account for the patient's other findings including bruit, diminished pulses, dependent rubor, and abnormal ABI. Popliteal venous thrombosis may present with localized pain and erythema, but the pain would not be exertional and cannot account for bilateral pain or the physical examination findings.

KEY POINTS

• Most patients with peripheral vascular disease have an ankle-brachial index (ABI) <0.9, and those with severe disease (rest ischemia) have an ABI <0.4.

• An ABI >1.3 indicates vascular calcification.

Bibliography
1. Khan NA, Rahim SA, Anand SS, Simel DL, Panju A. Does the clinical examination predict lower extremity peripheral arterial disease? JAMA. 2006;295:536-46. [PMID: 16449619]

Item 5   Answer: C

This patient has evidence for Mobitz type II second-degree atrioventricular block. Second-degree heart block is characterized by intermittent nonconduction of P waves and subsequent "dropped" ventricular beats. Second-degree heart block is divided into types, Mobitz I and Mobitz II. Mobitz type I second-degree heart block is characterized by progressive prolongation of the PR interval until a dropped beat occurs. This type of heart block is characteristically transient and usually requires no specific treatment. Mobitz type II second-degree heart block is characterized by a regularly dropped beat (e.g., a nonconducted P wave every second or third beat) without progressive prolongation of the PR interval and is often associated with evidence of additional disease in the conduction system such as bundle branch block or bifascicular or trifascicular block. Mobitz type II second-degree heart block suddenly and unpredictably progresses to complete heart block and is usually treated with a pacemaker.

First-degree heart block is recognized, electrocardiographically, as a prolongation of the PR interval; all P waves are conducted and this condition requires no specific treatment. Third-degree atrioventricular block, or complete heart block, refers to a lack of atrioventricular conduction (characterized by lack of conduction of all atrial impulses to the ventricles).

This patient has a mechanical mitral valve. He has a recent history of fevers, night sweats, and weight loss, raising suspicion for bacterial endocarditis. The presence of valvular dysfunction (murmur and heart failure) and his electrocardiographic findings heighten concern that an underlying endocarditis of the prosthetic valve with associated paravalvular abscess is present.

Infection of a prosthetic valve is one of the more common complications of mechanical valves, occurring in up to 3% to 6% of patients. In more severe infections, a paravalvular abscess can develop and affect surrounding structures, such as the His-Purkinje pathway. Paravalvular extension of infection is a significant concern in patients with prosthetic valves. In this patient, empiric broad-spectrum antibiotics should be instituted after obtaining blood cultures from multiple sites. A temporary pacemaker can be placed to provide electrical stability with a normal-range heart rate and to pace his heart if the cardiac rhythm degenerates into complete atrioventricular block. Antibiotics can subsequently be tailored to specific coverage of the causative organism, once this is isolated.

- Bacterial prosthetic valve endocarditis should be suspected in any patient with a prosthetic heart valve and an unexplained fever.

- Second-degree atrioventricular block is characterized by intermittent nonconduction of P waves and subsequent "dropped" ventricular beats.

Bibliography

1. **Da Costa D, Brady WJ, Edhouse J.** Bradycardias and atrioventricular conduction block. BMJ. 2002;324:535-8. [PMID: 11872557]

Item 6   Answer: C

This patient's sharp, pleuritic chest pain preceded by 2 to 3 days of prodromal symptoms is characteristic of acute viral pericarditis. The pericardial friction rub is suggestive of acute pericarditis, and the presence of ST segments that are upwardly concave on electrocardiography further supports this diagnosis. The lack of a pericardial effusion on echocardiography does not exclude pericarditis, given that 40% of patients with pericarditis may not have this finding.

The recommended initial treatment for acute viral pericarditis is a high-dose nonsteroidal anti-inflammatory drug such as indomethacin or ibuprofen. Indomethacin is rapidly tapered after 5 to 7 days because of the potential for toxicity with long-term use. Aspirin may also be used, although the high doses required may cause gastrointestinal problems.

If severe chest pain remains after 2 to 3 days of nonsteroidal anti-inflammatory drug treatment in patients with acute pericarditis, a 7- to 10-day tapering course of corticosteroids should be considered. However, corticosteroids such as prednisone have associated toxicity and are not recommended as first-line agents in the treatment of uncomplicated acute pericarditis. Low-dose colchicine may be used as an alternative to corticosteroids.

An acute myocardial infarction should always be considered in the setting of chest pain with ST elevation on electrocardiography. However, this patient's young age, viral prodrome, quality of the pain, and friction rub point to a diagnosis of acute pericarditis, and anticoagulation in a patient with known acute pericarditis is contraindicated because of the potential for hemopericardium.

Clopidogrel has no benefit as an anti-inflammatory agent for the treatment of acute pericarditis and is not indicated.

- The initial treatment for acute viral pericarditis is a high-dose nonsteroidal anti-inflammatory drug.

Bibliography

1. **Lange RA, Hillis LD.** Clinical practice. Acute pericarditis. N Engl J Med. 2004;351:2195-202. Erratum in: N Engl J Med. 2005;352:1163. [PMID: 15548780]

Item 7   Answer: C

This patient has atrial tachycardia with variable block, which is a classic electrocardiographic finding for digitalis toxicity. Atrial tachycardias usually appear as a "long RP" tachycardia, with a PR interval equal to or slightly longer than normal. The P-wave morphology may be upright, biphasic, or inverted in the inferior leads, depending on the site of origin. In this patient, atrioventricular block is manifested by conduction of every other P wave (2:1 atrioventricular block). Digoxin should be discontinued immediately, and the diagnosis should be confirmed by measurement of a serum digoxin level. Additionally, the serum potassium level should be restored to >4.0 meq/L, and calcium and magnesium levels and acid-base status should be checked and corrected if abnormal. Bradyarrhythmias may be treated with atropine or ventricular pacing. Digoxin-specific antibody fragments (digitalis-binding agents) should be administered for life-threatening digitalis toxicity; that is, toxicity associated with life-threatening arrhythmias (ventricular tachycardia or fibrillation), refractory hyperkalemia, absolute digoxin level >10 µg/L regardless of the clinical status, ingestion of a lethal digoxin dose, or an arrhythmia with associated hypotension. Risk factors for digitalis toxicity include hypokalemia, hypomagnesemia, hypercalcemia, renal insufficiency, hypothyroidism, advanced pulmonary disease, and pharmacologic interactions with other drugs, notably verapamil, quinidine, and amiodarone.

Atrial fibrillation is characterized by an irregularly irregular rhythm with atrial fibrillatory waves seen at a rate of 300–600/min, causing the baseline to be irregular. Atrial flutter is characterized by jagged "sawtooth" flutter waves between QRS complexes. Multifocal atrial tachycardia characteristically occurs in the setting of severe illness and is manifested by three or more P-wave configurations and PR intervals on the electrocardiogram with associated tachycardia.

- Atrial tachycardia with variable block is a classic electrocardiographic finding for digitalis toxicity.

- Digitoxin-specific antibody fragments (digitalis-binding agents) should be administered for life-threatening digitalis toxicity.

Bibliography

1. **Hauptman PJ, Kelly RA.** Digitalis. Circulation. 1999;99:1265-70. [PMID: 10069797]

Item 8   Answer: C

This fit, elderly man with no contraindications to coronary revascularization has the clinical features (three-vessel coronary artery disease [CAD] and left ventricular dysfunction) that warrant an invasive treatment approach rather than simply adjusting his medications. Patients who have CAD with large zones of ischemia benefit the most from interventional approaches added to their existing medical treatment. Patients with obstructive left main CAD and/or three-vessel CAD with a reduced left ventricular ejection fraction (≤40%) or a moderate to large amount of myocardial ischemia have improved survival rates with coronary artery bypass grafting (CABG) in combination with medical therapy as compared with medical therapy alone. Patients with multivessel CAD and diabetes mellitus have better outcomes with CABG compared with percutaneous angioplasty. Thus, CABG is preferable to a percutaneous intervention in these patients.

The implantable cardioverter-defibrillator has emerged as an important prophylactic treatment option for reducing sudden cardiac death in selected patients with CAD. An ejection fraction ≤30% helps to identify patients likely to benefit from this procedure. In this patient, the ejection fraction was reduced but remained above 30%. In addition, in patients with an ejection fraction ≤30% who are being considered for an implantable cardioverter-defibrillator, CABG remains the primary treatment when multivessel CAD is present. Thus, placement of an implantable cardioverter-defibrillator is not the best choice for this patient.

KEY POINTS
- Coronary artery bypass grafting improves survival in patients with obstructive left main and/or three-vessel coronary artery disease and reduced ejection fraction.
- Coronary artery bypass grafting improves survival in comparison to percutaneous intervention in patients with diabetes mellitus and multivessel coronary artery disease.

Bibliography
1. **Stone KE, Chiquette E, Chilton RJ.** Diabetic endovascular disease: role of coronary artery revascularization. Am J Cardiol. 2007;99:105B-112B. [PMID: 17307063]

Item 9   Answer: B

This patient most likely has aortic dissection at the level of the ascending aorta. Aortic dissection is life-threatening and often presents with abrupt-onset, tearing chest pain and acute hemodynamic compromise. Propagation of the dissection can occur both distally and proximally to the intimal tear and is responsible for many of the clinical manifestations, including ischemia (coronary, cerebral, or spinal), aortic regurgitation, and cardiac tamponade. The patient's increased P$_2$ suggests pulmonary hypertension due to acute left heart failure precipitated by acute volume overload. The chest radiograph may show widening of the mediastinum, a helpful diagnostic clue, and there may be considerable variation (>20 mm Hg) in the right and left arm blood pressures. This patient needs an emergent imaging study: contrast-enhanced CT of the chest, transesophageal echocardiography, and thoracic magnetic resonance angiography have similar accuracy, and the choice often depends on availability.

The absence of fever, pleuritic chest pain (typically relieved by the patient sitting up and leaning forward), and a pericardial friction rub makes acute pericarditis unlikely. Furthermore, the electrocardiogram does not show the characteristic findings of acute pericarditis: diffuse ST-segment elevations that

are concave upward and in no particular anatomic distribution and PR-segment depression, especially in leads II and III. Chest pain due to gastroesophageal reflux disease (GERD) can mimic cardiac pain. However, chest pain due to GERD, often described as burning or stabbing, typically occurs after meals and is worse when lying down. Finally, GERD cannot explain the patient's abnormal vital signs or cardiac findings.

Acute myocardial infarction is not an unreasonable diagnosis, but the electrocardiogram fails to show the characteristic findings of ST-segment elevations >1 mm in two or more contiguous leads or a new left bundle branch block. Also, acute myocardial infarction cannot explain the increased P$_2$ or the findings of acute aortic regurgitation. Patients with pulmonary embolism often develop acute dyspnea-associated chest pain, but the chest pain is typically pleuritic, not tearing. The electrocardiogram in patients with pulmonary embolism often shows a nonspecific sinus tachycardia, as in this patient, but pulmonary embolism cannot explain the physical examination findings.

KEY POINTS
- Aortic dissection can propagate both distally and proximally to the intimal tear and is often associated with signs of acute ischemia (coronary, cerebral, or spinal), aortic regurgitation, and cardiac tamponade.
- Widening of the mediastinum on chest radiography and variation (>20 mm Hg) in the right and left arm blood pressures are helpful diagnostic clues for acute aortic dissection.

Bibliography
1. **Ince H, Nienaber CA.** Diagnosis and management of patients with aortic dissection. Heart. 2007;93:266-70. [PMID: 17228080]

Item 10   Answer: B

Because most adults who suffer cardiac arrest initially demonstrate ventricular arrhythmias, time to defibrillation is the most important determinant of survival. Defibrillation within the first 4 minutes of ventricular fibrillation results in high survival rates, and the availability of automated external defibrillators in many public settings such as airports has made early defibrillation possible. Each minute that defibrillation is delayed reduces the chance of eventual hospital discharge by 8% to 10%.

Bystander cardiopulmonary resuscitation has been shown to improve survival, but prompt defibrillation is more important. Time to transport to the hospital does not correlate with survival—it is restoration of normal blood flow that is critical. Intubation helps provide adequate oxygenation but also is not as important as restoration of a normal cardiac rhythm.

KEY POINT
- Time to defibrillation is the most important determinant of survival in cardiac arrest.

Bibliography
1. **Ali B, Zafari AM.** Narrative review: cardiopulmonary resuscitation and emergency cardiovascular care: review of the current guidelines. Ann Intern Med. 2007;147:171-9. [PMID: 17679705]

Item 11   Answer: B

Acute viral pericarditis is the most likely diagnosis in this patient with a several-day prodrome of constitutional symptoms, pleuritic chest pain, and a pericardial friction rub. Acute severe chest pain has a broad differential diagnosis, which should include potentially life-threatening entities that require urgent treatment. Given this patient's history of diabetes mellitus, tobacco and cocaine use, and hypertension, the differential diagnosis includes an acute coronary syndrome (unstable angina or myocardial infarction). Additional entities include pneumonia, aortic dissection, pleuritis, costochondritis, and pulmonary embolism. However, aortic dissection, costochondritis, or pulmonary embolism would not explain the patient's constitutional symptoms or electrocardiographic findings. Pneumonia or pleuritis could explain the constitutional symptoms, but not the pericardial friction rub or electrocardiographic findings. The 12-lead electrocardiogram confirms the diagnosis of acute pericarditis with the presence of PR-segment depression and ST segments that are upwardly concave. PR-segment depression is virtually pathognomonic for acute pericarditis, although it can occur in a few other possible but rare entities (e.g., atrial myocardial ischemia). ST segments that are upwardly concave are useful findings to help distinguish acute pericarditis from an acute myocardial infarction, in which a downwardly concave pattern is seen. Finally, pericarditis is associated with diffuse ST-segment elevations as compared with localized elevations in myocardial infarction.

KEY POINT

- PR-segment depression is virtually pathognomonic for acute pericarditis.

Bibliography

1. **Little WC, Freeman GL.** Pericardial disease. Circulation. 2006;113:1622-32. Erratum in: Circulation. 2007;115:e406. [PMID: 16567581]

Item 12   Answer: A

This patient has cardiogenic shock, manifested by hypotension and evidence of hypoperfusion (decreased mental status, cool extremities). The pulmonary artery catheter data show volume overload—central venous and pulmonary capillary wedge pressures are elevated. The volume overload and low cardiac output are most consistent with cardiogenic shock.

Septic shock and toxic shock are types of distributive shock, result from a severe decrease in systemic vascular resistance, and are often associated with an increased cardiac output and low pulmonary capillary wedge pressure. Although the patient was febrile, the hemodynamic data do not support either septic shock or toxic shock. Hypovolemic shock is associated with reduced pulmonary capillary wedge pressure, cardiac output, central venous pressure, and pulmonary artery pressure. Even though the patient had a bout of viral gastroenteritis that could result in hypovolemia, the hemodynamic data are most compatible with cardiogenic shock.

KEY POINT

- The pulmonary capillary wedge pressure is elevated and the cardiac output is low in patients with primary cardiogenic shock.

Bibliography

1. **Summerhill EM, Baram M.** Principles of pulmonary artery catheterization in the critically ill. Lung. 2005;183:209-19. [PMID: 16078042]

Item 13   Answer: C

The most appropriate diagnostic test for this patient is exercise electrocardiography (ECG) without imaging. This patient is at intermediate risk for coronary artery disease. His pain has certain features consistent with angina and he has risk factors for coronary artery disease. The chronic and stable nature of his symptoms, in addition to the absence of acute changes on the resting ECG, allows for ECG stress testing instead of coronary angiography. Exercise ECG is most appropriate because the patient can exercise and his resting ECG is normal except for complete right bundle branch block (prolonged QRS complex; M-shaped QRS [rsR'] complex in lead V_1; and wide S waves in leads V_6 and I), which does not interfere with the interpretation of an exercise stress test.

Exercise ECG with myocardial imaging and exercise echocardiography are reserved for patients with an intermediate probability of coronary artery disease who can exercise and have either pre-excitation (Wolff-Parkinson-White) syndrome or more than 1 mm of ST-segment depression on resting ECG. These baseline ECG changes make it difficult to interpret possible ischemic ST-segment changes on exercise ECG. Exercise ECG with myocardial imaging and exercise echocardiography also are frequently used in patients with a history of previous revascularization procedures (percutaneous transluminal coronary angiography or coronary artery bypass grafting), in those who take digoxin, and in those who have left ventricular hypertrophy. Digoxin often causes ST-segment depression and reduces the specificity of exercise treadmill testing. Left ventricular hypertrophy with a repolarization abnormality on resting ECG also reduces the specificity of exercise treadmill testing.

Pharmacologic stress myocardial perfusion imaging and dobutamine echocardiography are performed in patients with an intermediate pretest probability of coronary artery disease and an electronically paced ventricular rhythm or left bundle branch block; exercise stress testing is associated with an increase in false-positive test results in patients with left bundle branch block. These tests are also appropriate in patients who cannot exercise.

KEY POINT

- Exercise electrocardiography is best suited for patients with an intermediate probability of coronary artery disease who can exercise, including patients with less than 1 mm ST-segment depression or complete right bundle branch block on resting electrocardiogram.

Bibliography

1. **Snow V, Barry P, Fihn SD, Gibbons RJ, Owens DK, Williams SV, Weiss KB, Mottur-Pilson C; ACP; ACC Chronic Stable Angina Panel.** Evaluation of primary care patients with chronic stable angina: guidelines from the American College of Physicians. Ann Intern Med. 2004;141:57-64. [PMID: 15238371]

Item 14   Answer: D

This patient has a presumptive diagnosis of myocardial infarction due to vasospasm of the coronary artery. Factors favoring this diagnosis are the normal angiographic appearance of the coronary arteries, use of cocaine, chest pain after a party (implying use of cocaine), and the episodic ST elevation with spontaneous resolution in the absence of fibrinolysis.

Coronary artery atherosclerotic disease is not likely, based upon the normal coronary artery catheterization. In addition to coronary artery vasospasm, other causes of myocardial ischemia or infarction in the absence of atherosclerotic coronary artery disease include coronary artery dissection, vasculitis (scleroderma and other connective tissue diseases), thromboembolism in the settings of endocarditis or paradoxical embolism, valvular disease, and hypertrophic cardiomyopathy. Spontaneous coronary artery dissection has been reported in pregnant women with or without hypertension but coronary artery dissection is unlikely in a nonpregnant woman Vasculitis seems unlikely in the absence of any additional signs or symptoms to support a diagnosis of collagen vascular disease. Endocarditis is unlikely in the absence of fever and a heart murmur, and hypertrophic cardiomyopathy is unlikely in the absence of a murmur and the normal electrocardiogram (following resolution of the chest pain).

The best treatment for coronary artery vasospasm is nitrates in the short term and calcium channel blockers over the long term. Angiotensin-converting enzyme inhibitors reduce mortality in patients with ST elevation myocardial infarction and in patients with a left ventricular ejection fraction <40% following an acute myocardial infarction. This patient meets neither of these criteria and is unlikely to benefit from this therapy. This patient should be strongly urged not to use cocaine.

KEY POINT

- Coronary artery vasospasm is treated with nitrates in the short term and calcium channel blockers in the long term.

Bibliography

1. **Mirza MA.** Angina like pain and normal coronary arteries. Uncovering cardiac syndromes that mimic CAD. Postgrad Med. 2005;117:41-6, 54. [PMID: 15948368]

Item 15   Answer: A

This patient has risk factors for both coronary artery disease and aortic dissection. The markedly disparate blood pressure between the arms and the diastolic murmur of aortic regurgitation strongly suggest acute ascending aortic dissection involving the aortic valve. Dullness of the right lung field with resting dyspnea suggests hemothorax. The most common coronary artery to be involved with ascending aortic dissection is the right coronary artery with resulting inferior wall myocardial infarction. This patient's electrocardiogram shows ST elevation in the inferior leads (II, III, aVF) and is compatible with an inferior ST elevation myocardial infarction. Treatment with β-blockers to decrease shear stress should be started.

Anteroseptal wall myocardial infarction is indicated by ST elevation in leads V_1–V_4; changes in leads V_4–V_6 indicate apical or lateral infarction. These infarction patterns are not supported by the patient's electrocardiogram, and they are not associated with aortic dissection. Coarctation of the aorta is associated with hypertension and can produce differences in the blood pressures between the upper and lower extremities, but not between the right and left arms. Coarctation is not associated with aortic insufficiency, aortic dissection, or hemothorax.

KEY POINT

- Ascending aortic dissection may lead to aortic regurgitation and obstruction of the right coronary artery.

Bibliography

1. **Ince H, Nienaber CA.** Diagnosis and management of patients with aortic dissection. Heart. 2007;93:266-70. [PMID: 17228080]

Item 16   Answer: B

This patient has features of successful reperfusion after an acute inferior ST-elevation myocardial infarction and may be treated medically until risk stratification is performed or recurrent ischemia or complications occur. The usual management consists of heparin, aspirin, β-blockers, angiotensin-converting enzyme inhibitors, and statins. Clinical trials show that β-blocker therapy reduces infarct size and the frequency of recurrent myocardial ischemia and improves short- and long-term survival.

Evidence of successful fibrinolysis involves resolution of both chest pain and ST elevation. The rapidity with which these resolve is directly related to early patency of the affected artery. Reperfusion arrhythmias, typically manifested as a transient accelerated idioventricular arrhythmia, usually do not require additional antiarrhythmic therapy with lidocaine or amiodarone.

Immediate coronary angiography is not indicated unless recurrent ischemia, persistent ST elevation, or hemodynamic instability, including heart failure, occurs.

KEY POINT

- β-Blocker therapy reduces infarct size and the frequency of recurrent myocardial ischemia and improves short- and long-term survival.

Bibliography

1. **Kopecky SL.** Effect of beta blockers, particularly carvedilol, on reducing the risk of events after acute myocardial infarction. Am J Cardiol. 2006;98:1115-9. Epub 2006 Aug 31. [PMID: 17027583]

Item 17   Answer: C

This patient has an acute coronary syndrome of non-ST elevation myocardial infarction (NSTEMI). A non-ST elevation acute coronary syndrome is recognized by ST depressions and/or T wave inversions without Q waves. These ST-T wave abnormalities may be present in many leads but must appear in at least two leads, as in this patient, and more commonly are localized to the leads associated with the region of ischemic myocardium. The electrocardiographic changes of unstable angina are indistinguishable from NSTEMI, and these two acute coronary syndromes are treated similarly. Unstable angina is usually not associated with elevated cardiac biomarkers (creatine kinase and troponin), but small elevations have been reported, and the electrocardiographic changes resolve with resolution of the ischemia.

ST elevation myocardial infarction (STEMI), variant angina, and acute pericarditis are all associated with ST elevation and are not compatible with this patient's electrocardiographic findings. The earliest change associated with STEMI is the development of a hyperacute or tall, peaked T wave. Thereafter, the ST segment elevates in the leads recording electrical activity of the ischemic myocardium. An initial Q wave (typically 0.04 sec in duration) develops over a period of several hours to days and there is a loss of R wave amplitude. Over time (weeks), the ST segment normalizes, the R wave amplitude is further reduced, the Q wave deepens, and the T wave inverts. Some patients with STEMI never develop a Q wave.

Reversible transmural ischemia, due to coronary vasospasm, may cause transient ST elevations known as Prinzmetal's variant angina. The ST elevations usually resolve completely within minutes and are not typically associated with elevated cardiac biomarkers.

The initial electrocardiographic stage of acute pericarditis is characterized by diffuse ST elevation with reciprocal ST depression in leads aVR and V_1. There is also depression of the PR segment in leads aVL, aVF, V5, and V_6.

KEY POINTS

- A non-ST elevation acute coronary syndrome is recognized by ST depressions and/or T wave inversions without Q waves.

- ST elevation myocardial infarction, variant angina, and acute pericarditis are important cardiac diagnoses associated with ST-segment elevation.

Bibliography

1. **Martinez-Rumayor A, Januzzi JL Jr.** Non-ST segment elevation acute coronary syndromes: A comprehensive review. South Med J. 2006;99:1103-10. [PMID: 17100031]

Item 18   Answer: A

This patient has survived a small inferior wall myocardial infarction and was successfully treated with a stent. At discharge, he should receive aspirin, metoprolol, clopidogrel for at least 180 days, and a statin regardless of his serum cholesterol level. In patients with coronary artery disease, especially those presenting with symptoms and those undergoing revascularization by either stenting or bypass graft surgery, statin therapy reduces late cardiovascular events despite having minimal or no effect on the angiographic appearance of the coronary arteries.

The PROVE IT-TIMI 22 study compared a moderate-dose statin (pravastatin, 40 mg/d) with a high-dose statin (atorvastatin, 80 mg/d) in patients hospitalized for acute coronary syndrome. The median LDL cholesterol levels achieved were 95 mg/dL by the pravastatin group and 62 mg/dL for the atorvastatin group. Those receiving atorvastatin had a 16% reduction in the composite endpoint of death from any cause, myocardial infarction, unstable angina requiring rehospitalization, coronary artery revascularization, and stroke during 2 years of follow-up. These results showed evidence of benefit from early aggressive LDL cholesterol lowering with high-dose atorvastatin.

Warfarin is not indicated after ST-elevation myocardial infarction treated by stenting unless there is another indication such as atrial fibrillation, deep venous thrombosis, or intracardiac thrombus.

Niacin for hypertriglyceridemia may be needed, but at this time the triglyceride values are not reported and may be falsely elevated early in the course of ST-elevation myocardial infarction. The first line of treatment would be statins even for normal LDL cholesterol levels in patients with documented coronary artery disease. The combination of statins with a fibrate (e.g., gemfibrozil) is attractive for patients who have both high cholesterol and triglyceride levels or for those who continue to have elevated triglyceride levels after reaching their LDL cholesterol target on statin therapy. However, in this patient, the best initial choice is a statin.

KEY POINT

- In patients with an acute coronary syndrome, statin therapy is indicated regardless of the serum cholesterol level.

Bibliography

1. **Ray KK, Cannon CP, Ganz P.** Beyond lipid lowering: What have we learned about the benefits of statins from the acute coronary syndromes trials? Am J Cardiol. 2006;98:18P-25P. Epub 2006 Sep 29. [PMID: 17126675]

Item 19   Answer: D

The patient has classic features of a right ventricular myocardial infarction. The characteristic features of right ventricular myocardial infarction on physical examination include progressive hypotension, jugular venous pressure elevation, and clear lung fields. In addition, a right ventricular lift is common, and tricuspid valve regurgitation may be audible on physical examination. These findings are caused by right ventricular dysfunction, right-sided cardiac enlargement, and tricuspid annular dilatation. The electrocardiogram demonstrates inferior (leads II, III, aVF) ST elevation indicative of acute ischemia in the territory of the right coronary artery (right ventricle and inferior and posterior portions of the left ventricle). The diagnosis of right ventricular myocardial infarction can be confirmed by echocardiography demonstrating right ventricular enlargement with reduced systolic function.

Aortic dissection is unlikely in this patient. The presence of elevated ST-segments on the electrocardiogram and elevated cardiac enzyme concentrations make myocardial infarction more likely. Additionally, elevated jugular venous pressure is atypical in the setting of aortic dissection, but may occur with associated cardiac tamponade. Acute cardiac tamponade and left ventricular free-wall rupture are also unlikely in this patient; both are rare late manifestations of myocardial injury, occurring on days 2 to 7 following an acute myocardial infarction. Both entities can cause sudden hypotension, and pericardial pain (pleuritic and positional) may be present.

KEY POINT

• Right ventricular infarction should be suspected in patients with inferior electrocardiographic ischemic changes who present with hypotension, clear lung fields, and elevated jugular venous pressure.

Bibliography

1. **Pfisterer M.** Right ventricular involvement in myocardial infarction and cardiogenic shock. Lancet. 2003;362:392-4. [PMID: 12907014]

Item 20   Answer: C

This patient is best treated with rate control and anticoagulation. Atrial fibrillation is the most common clinically significant arrhythmia and accounts for the most hospitalizations for cardiac arrhythmias. It occurs in less than 1% of patients ages 60 to 65 years but in 8% to 10% of patients older than 80 years. The estimated risk for stroke in affected patients is 5% per year without anticoagulation. In patients with nonvalvular atrial fibrillation, warfarin with a target INR of 2.0 to 3.0 has been shown to decrease stroke risk by an average of 62%, compared with a 19% decrease with aspirin therapy. To determine whether the risk of stroke is high enough to warrant chronic anticoagulation, risk stratification scores have been developed. One such stratification scheme is known as CHADS$_2$ score: *C*ongestive heart failure, *H*ypertension, *A*ge >75 years, *D*iabetes, *S*troke or transient ischemic attack (TIA). Patients are given 2 points for a history of stroke or TIA (the strongest risk factor) and 1 point for all other risk factors. This patient has a CHADS$_2$ score of 3. The risk of stroke is lowest in patients with a CHADS$_2$ score of 0 (1.2%). The risk is 18% for a CHADS$_2$ score of 6 (maximum score). Patients with a CHADS$_2$ score of ≥3 and patients with a history of stroke are at high risk and should be considered for chronic anticoagulation with warfarin. Patients with a CHADS$_2$ score of 1 or 2 should be assessed on an individual basis for aspirin versus warfarin therapy.

In patients who tolerate atrial fibrillation with few symptoms, restoration of normal sinus rhythm is not indicated. Strategies of rate versus rhythm control have been found to be similar with respect to symptoms, mortality, and stroke risk. More hospitalizations and adverse drug reactions occur in patients receiving rhythm control compared with rate control. This elderly patient would be at significant risk of drug side effects from anti-arrhythmic agents and would likely have breakthrough episodes of atrial fibrillation. Therefore, in addition to chronic anticoagulation with warfarin, this patient should receive medication to control the ventricular rate, such as a β-blocker.

Atrioventricular nodal ablation for atrial fibrillation with pacemaker placement should be reserved for those patients who do not tolerate pharmacologic therapy. New ablation strategies are being investigated and are increasingly recommended in clinical practice guidelines. These include catheter-directed ablation of the pulmonary vein ostia within the left atrium. The success rate of this procedure is as high as 88% at 6 months without requiring pacemaker placement.

KEY POINTS

• Strategies of rate versus rhythm control for atrial fibrillation are similar with respect to symptoms, mortality, and stroke risk.

• Most patients with atrial fibrillation are treated with a combination of rate control and long-term anticoagulation.

Bibliography

1. **Snow V, Weiss KB, LeFevre M, McNamara R, Bass E, Green LA, Michl K, Owens DK, Susman J, Allen DI, Mottur-Pilson C; AAFP Panel on Atrial Fibrillation; ACP Panel on Atrial Fibrillation.** Management of newly detected atrial fibrillation: a clinical practice guideline from the American Academy of Family Physicians and the American College of Physicians. Ann Intern Med. 2003;139:1009-17. [PMID: 14678921]

2. **Gage BF, Waterman AD, Shannon W, Boechler M, Rich MW, Radford MJ.** Validation of clinical classification schemes for predicting stroke: results from the National Registry of Atrial Fibrillation. JAMA. 2001;285:2864-70. [PMID: 11401607]

Item 21   Answer: C

The symptoms and electrocardiogram in this woman are consistent with an acute myocardial infarction, with the electrocardiogram showing ST elevation predominantly in the inferior leads (II, III, aVF). The patient's age and 10-year history of diabetes and hypertension put her at high risk for myocardial infarction.

Pericarditis can cause severe chest pain, but on electrocardiography, ST elevation is generalized in more than the inferior leads and PR depression is present. In addition, pericardial chest pain is continuous and radiates to the left shoulder and is relieved by sitting up and a two- or three-component friction rub is generally present. The possibility of pulmonary embolism must always be kept in mind, but its electrocardiographic changes are nonspecific and not localized to the inferior leads, and the pattern of chest pain usually is pleuritic. Costochondritis, a localized inflammation of the joints linking the sternum to the ribs, is a frequent cause of musculoskeletal chest pain that is associated with localized chest wall tenderness but no electrocardiographic changes. Gastroesophageal reflux disease is a common diagnosis in adults and frequently causes chest pain. The pain is intermittent, usually related to meals, and is not associated with electrocardiographic changes.

KEY POINT

• Chest pain associated with localized electrocardiographic ST changes suggests acute coronary syndrome.

Bibliography

1. Savonitto S, Ardissino D, Granger CB, Morando G, Prando MD, Mafrici A, et al. Prognostic value of the admission electrocardiogram in acute coronary syndromes. JAMA. 1999;281:707-13. [PMID: 10052440]

Item 22   Answer: A

This patient with asymptomatic atrial fibrillation has no risk factors for stroke; therefore, aspirin would be sufficient thromboembolic risk protection. The CHADS$_2$ score is used to assess stroke risk in patients with atrial fibrillation. The CHADS$_2$ score assigns 1 point each for the presence of congestive heart failure, hypertension, age 75 years or older, and diabetes mellitus and 2 points for a history of stroke or transient ischemic attack. This patient's CHADS$_2$ score is 0; therefore, risk of stroke is low and anticoagulation other than aspirin is not necessary.

Cardioversion is recommended primarily for patients with symptoms related to atrial fibrillation or patients with hemodynamic deterioration due to the loss of sinus rhythm. There are no data to suggest that conversion to sinus rhythm improves survival; cardioversion is therefore not indicated in this patient. If the patient's symptoms progressed to a point at which cardioversion would be indicated, anticoagulation with warfarin would be required first because of the potential of having an atrial clot that could embolize upon the restora-

tion of sinus rhythm. Clopidogrel has not been demonstrated to be effective thromboprophylaxis for patients with atrial fibrillation. The combination of clopidogrel and aspirin has been shown to worsen outcomes in patients with atrial fibrillation by increasing the risk of bleeding.

KEY POINT

• Aspirin is sufficient thromboembolic risk protection in patients with asymptomatic atrial fibrillation and no risk factors for stroke.

Bibliography

1. Go AS, Fang MC, Singer DE. Antithrombotic therapy for stroke prevention in atrial fibrillation. Prog Cardiovasc Dis. 2005;48:108-24. [PMID: 16253651]

Item 23   Answer: B

This patient's clinical presentation is consistent with an acute inferior wall myocardial infarction; i.e., sudden onset of anterior chest pain radiating to the shoulders and ST elevation in the inferior leads (II, III, aVF). Posterior wall myocardial infarction may be associated with ST depression in leads V_1 and V_2. Posterior wall infarction is often associated with an inferior wall infarction, but this is not the case for this patient. Anterior (anteroseptal) wall myocardial infarction is associated with ST elevation in the anterior chest leads (V_1–V_3) and lateral wall and apical infarction with ST elevation in the lateral chest leads (V_4–V_6). Acute pericarditis is associated with PR-segment depression and widespread ST segments that are upwardly concave. PR-segment depression is virtually pathognomonic for acute pericarditis, but is seen in several other possible but rare entities (e.g., atrial myocardial ischemia). ST segments that are upwardly concave are useful findings to help distinguish acute pericarditis from an acute myocardial infarction, in which a downwardly concave pattern is seen.

KEY POINTS

• Acute myocardial infarction can be localized according to ST elevation in specific electrocardiographic leads: inferior infarction in leads II, III, and aVF; anteroseptal infarction in leads V_1–V_3; lateral and apical infarctions in leads V_4–V_6.

• Acute posterior wall myocardial infarction is often associated with inferior wall infarction and may be associated with ST depression in leads V_1–V_2.

Bibliography

1. Chun AA, McGee SR. Bedside diagnosis of coronary artery disease: a systematic review. Am J Med. 2004;11:334-43. [PMID: 15336583]

Item 24   Answer: D

In healthy adults, premature ventricular contractions at rest are common and are not a cause for concern. Even very frequent premature ventricular contractions on a 24-hour electrocardiogram are not of concern in the absence of underlying structural heart disease. This otherwise healthy patient needs reassurance. Suppression of premature ventricular contractions is indicated only in patients with severe and disabling symptoms, which may include palpitations, fatigue, and light-headedness. In these patients, β-blockers are the safest initial choice. Antiarrhythmic agents such as flecainide are associated with more side effects and thus are a second-line option for patients who continue to have debilitating symptoms despite β-blocker therapy. Catheter ablation of premature ventricular contractions is feasible; however, because of the technical demands of the procedure and its variable success rate, it is reserved for the most refractory cases.

KEY POINT

• In healthy adults, premature ventricular contractions are common and are not a cause for concern.

Bibliography

1. **Ng GA**. Treating patients with ventricular ectopic beats. Heart. 2006;92:1707-12. [PMID: 17041126]

Item 25   Answer: C

The electrocardiogram shows Q waves and ST elevation in leads II, III, and aVF diagnosing an inferior ST-elevation myocardial infarction (STEMI). Patients presenting less than 12 hours after the onset of symptoms of STEMI are best treated with a percutaneous coronary intervention. However, if the receiving hospital does not have a catheterization laboratory with interventional capabilities and transfer would take more than 2 hours, the patient should undergo prompt fibrinolysis. Fibrinolytic therapy should be given within 30 minutes of arrival in the emergency department. Percutaneous coronary intervention reperfusion is achieved for 90% to 95% of vessels compared with 60% to 75% of vessels with fibrinolytic therapy. The goal of all reperfusion strategies for patients with STEMI is to achieve a patent vessel within 90 minutes from the onset of symptoms.

The patient with STEMI arriving more than 12 hours after symptom onset who is asymptomatic is not a candidate for fibrinolytic therapy. Studies have also shown that the risk of fibrinolysis outweighs the benefit in patients with ST-segment depression.

In some patient groups, percutaneous coronary intervention is preferred over fibrinolysis even when transfer to a facility with a cardiac catheterization laboratory will take more than 2 hours: 1) patients in whom fibrinolysis is contraindicated (e.g., those with recent surgery, stroke, bleeding diathesis, uncontrolled hypertension, or peptic ulcer disease); 2) STEMI patients presenting more than 12 hours after symptoms who still have residual ST-segment elevation or a complicated presentation (e.g., heart failure, high-grade ventricular arrhythmias, shock); 3) STEMI occurring in patients who have had coronary artery bypass graft surgery (owing to the high likelihood of saphenous vein graft thrombosis); and 4) patients with cardiogenic shock (pulmonary edema and systolic blood pressure <100 mm Hg), especially those <75 years old.

Although both glycoprotein receptor blockers and clopidogrel are given to patients with acute myocardial infarction undergoing percutaneous coronary intervention, these drugs should not precede or delay the administration of fibrinolytic therapy. β-Blockers are beneficial in acute STEMI. However, β-blockers do not replace prompt reperfusion therapy and are relatively contraindicated in this patient with a low heart rate and blood pressure at presentation. Nitroglycerin provides symptom relief but does not affect clinical outcome and is relatively contraindicated in patients who have marginal blood pressure (<100 mm Hg systolic in the setting of acute STEMI).

KEY POINT

• STEMI patients who cannot be reperfused by a direct coronary intervention within 90 to 120 minutes should receive fibrinolytic therapy if there are no contraindications.

Bibliography

1. **Pinto DS, Southard M, Ciaglo L, Gibson CM**. Door-to-balloon delays with percutaneous coronary intervention in ST-elevation myocardial infarction. Am Heart J. 2006;151:S24-9. [PMID: 16777506]

Item 26   Answer: A

This patient likely has alcoholic cardiomyopathy, which generally occurs after many years of heavy alcohol consumption, although it may also occur after a short period of heavy consumption. Typically, both ventricles are dilated and globally hypokinetic. The patient reports that he drinks alcohol daily, and his laboratory test results suggest chronic alcohol use (macrocytosis) and possibly an acute episode of heavy alcohol use (mild elevation of aminotransferases, new-onset atrial fibrillation). In addition to medical therapy for heart failure, therapy for alcoholic cardiomyopathy must include total abstinence from alcohol. Abstinence may reverse the cardiomyopathy in patients with less advanced disease.

Cardiac amyloidosis results in increased left ventricular wall thickness due to deposition of amyloid, and, as a result, typically presents with restrictive cardiomyopathy, which is characterized by diastolic rather than systolic dysfunction. On echocardiography, ventricular chambers are typically small with thick walls, and the atria are dilated. Because increased left ventricular wall thickness is caused by infiltration of the myocardium rather than hypertrophy, the electrocardiographic voltage is generally low.

Hypertrophic cardiomyopathy is characterized by inappropriate, marked, and asymmetric hypertrophy of the left ventricle. The hypertrophy usually involves the interventricular septum, although there is a wide range of severity and location of hypertrophy, hemodynamic consequences, and symptoms. The left ventricular cavity is small, unlike the cavity in this patient.

Ischemic cardiomyopathy is often, but not invariably, associated with symptomatic coronary artery disease. The electrocardiogram may show evidence of previous infarction and the echocardiogram typically shows focal, not global, hypokinesis.

• Alcoholic cardiomyopathy is a dilated cardiomyopathy.

Bibliography
1. **Piano MR.** Alcoholic cardiomyopathy: incidence, clinical characteristics, and pathophysiology. Chest. 2002;121:1638-50. [PMID: 12006456]

Item 27   Answer: A

The electrocardiogram is characteristic for atrial fibrillation, showing a rapid, irregularly irregular rhythm with no discernible P waves and atrial fibrillatory waves at a rate between 350 and 600 beats/min. The fibrillatory waves vary in amplitude, morphology, and intervals, creating a rough, irregular baseline between the QRS complexes. There is no evidence of structural heart disease in this patient on the basis of the history and physical examination. The follow-up normal electrocardiogram also suggests that cardiac structure and function are likely normal. These findings are most consistent with a diagnosis of lone atrial fibrillation. In this setting, aspirin and additional outpatient evaluation should be recommended. This should include a transthoracic echocardiogram to exclude occult valve or other structural heart disease and also to assess the size of the left atrial appendage. Thyroid studies and a careful family history should also be obtained to exclude familial atrial fibrillation.

Atrial flutter is recognized by its saw-tooth pattern of flutter waves most noticeable in the inferior leads II, III and aVF; flutter waves are distinctly different from the small, chaotic fibrillation waves characteristic of atrial fibrillation. In the typical form of atrioventricular (AV) nodal re-entrant tachycardia, the atria and ventricles are simultaneously activated, and either no P wave is visible, or a small pseudo r' deflection in lead V_1 and a pseudo S-wave deflection inferiorly are seen. AV nodal re-entrant tachycardia is easily distinguished from atrial fibrillation by the regularity of the rhythm and smooth baseline denoting the absence of chaotic atrial fibrillation waves. AV re-entrant tachycardia (bypass-tract-mediated tachycardia) is associated with an accessory AV pathway. Bypass-tract-mediated tachycardias are re-entrant tachycardias in which the anterograde conduction (atria-to-ventricle) is typically via the AV node, and retrograde conduction is via the bypass tract. Because bypass-tract conduction is typically faster than conduction via the AV node, atrial activation occurs rapidly after the QRS complex (within the ST segment), resulting in a "short RP" tachycardia. Only accessory pathways with anterograde conduction will show a pre-excitation (Wolff-Parkinson-White) pattern consisting of a short PR interval and a delta wave initiating the R wave deflection on the sinus rhythm electrocardiogram. Like AV nodal re-entrant tachycardia, the rhythm in AV re-entrant tachycardia is regular and the baseline is smooth, making the distinction from atrial fibrillation straightforward.

• Atrial fibrillation is characterized electrocardiographically by an irregularly irregular rhythm with no discernible P waves and atrial fibrillation waves creating an irregular baseline.

Bibliography
1. **Dewar RI, Lip GY; Guidelines Development Group for the NICE clinical guideline for the management of atrial fibrillation.** Identification, diagnosis and assessment of atrial fibrillation. Heart. 2007;93:25-8. Epub 2006 Sep 4. [PMID: 16952973]

Item 28   Answer: B

This patient has a history and echocardiographic findings consistent with diastolic dysfunction. She has hypertension, which predisposes to the development of left ventricular hypertrophy and associated impaired ventricular relaxation.

Although she presented with evidence of heart failure, the echocardiogram demonstrated normal systolic function and no significant valvular abnormalities that could account for the heart failure. Therefore, systolic dysfunction and valvular disease are unlikely. Constrictive pericarditis is also unlikely in the absence of pulsus paradoxus, normal x and y descent, and no echocardiographic evidence of constrictive pericarditis, such as pericardial thickening or abrupt posterior motion of the ventricular septum in early diastole with inspiration.

The primary treatment goals in patients with diastolic heart failure are to treat the underlying cause (if possible), manage any potentially exacerbating factors, and optimize diastolic filling by slowing the heart rate with β-blockers. To date, there have been no medications shown to reduce morbidity and mortality in patients with diastolic dysfunction.

• The diagnosis of diastolic heart failure is generally made when signs and symptoms of systolic heart failure are present but the echocardiogram shows a normal left ventricular ejection fraction and an absence of significant valvular abnormalities.

Bibliography
1. **Chinnaiyan KM, Alexander D, Maddens M, McCullough PA.** Curriculum in cardiology: integrated diagnosis and management of diastolic heart failure. Am Heart J. 2007;153:189-200. [PMID: 17239676]

Item 29   Answer: B

This patient has an electrocardiogram consistent with atrial flutter. Atrial flutter waves are evident in the inferior leads, and appear as a "saw-tooth" pattern. In this electrocardiogram, atrioventricular conduction occurs once every two flutter waves (2:1 atrioventricular conduction) and is very typical for atrial flutter.

Atrial fibrillation is characteristically associated with an irregularly irregular rhythm, no discernible P waves, and atrial fibrillatory waves at a rate between 350 and 600/min. The fibrillatory waves vary in amplitude, morphology, and intervals, creating a rough, irregular baseline between the QRS complexes. Multifocal atrial tachycardia is defined by the electro-cardiographic presence of discrete P waves with at least three different morphologic patterns with varying P-P, P-R and R-R intervals. P wave morphology is generally best seen in leads II, III and V$_1$. In adults, multifocal atrial tachycardia is often associated with other serious illnesses, often hypoxic chronic obstructive pulmonary disease. Sinus tachycardia is a sinus rhythm with a ventricular rate >100/min. The P waves have a normal morphology but can become difficult to see with heart rates >140/min since they begin to merge with the preceding T wave. Slowing the heart rate with carotid sinus massage can often reveal the hidden P waves and establish the diagnosis.

KEY POINT

• Atrial flutter is characterized by saw-tooth pattern flutter waves most noticeable in the inferior electrocardiographic leads.

Bibliography
1. Fitzpatrick AP, Earley M, Petkar S, Diab I, Fox D, Williams P. Practical management of common atrial arrhythmias 2: common atrial flutter. Br J Hosp Med (Lond). 2007;68:201-4. [PMID: 17465101]

Item 30   Answer: D

This patient's presentation, including a viral prodrome, chest pain, symptoms and findings of heart failure in the absence of significant coronary artery disease, is consistent with acute myocarditis, which can range in presentation from asymptomatic to acute cardiogenic shock. Wall motion abnormalities on echocardiography can be regional or global during acute myocarditis. There is no specific treatment for acute myocarditis other than supportive care and the usual treatment for heart failure, including an angiotensin-converting enzyme inhibitor such as lisinopril, in the absence of contraindications.

The patient's normal blood pressure is not consistent with a serious infection, such as sepsis, and in the absence of other, more concrete evidence for infection, antibiotics are not indicated. The results of the coronary angiography rule out acute coronary syndrome, and therefore enoxaparin is not indicated. Although myocarditis is characterized by inflammation, there is no proven role for ibuprofen or corticosteroids for treatment.

KEY POINT

• Therapy for acute myocarditis generally consists of standard care for heart failure tailored to the severity of the myocarditis.

Bibliography
1. Magnani JW, Dec GW. Myocarditis: current trends in diagnosis and treatment. Circulation. 2006;113:876-90. [PMID: 16476862]

Item 31   Answer: D

Multifocal atrial tachycardia is most commonly seen in acutely ill patients, most often in the setting of pulmonary disease. Multifocal atrial tachycardia is defined by the electrocardiographic presence of discrete P waves with at least three different morphologic patterns with varying P-P, P-R, and R-R intervals. P wave morphology is generally best seen in leads II, III, and V$_1$. Therapy is directed at the underlying disease process because otherwise the arrhythmia will be refractory to therapy or will recur. In this patient, treatment should be directed at the pulmonary disease and correction of any electrolyte imbalances, especially magnesium. Therefore, the treatment of choice in this patient is oxygen, inhaled bronchodilators, and possibly oral antibiotics. Second-line therapy in patients with refractory tachycardia is a calcium-channel blocker such as diltiazem or verapamil. Electrolytes should be corrected, and magnesium should be administered even if serum magnesium levels are normal.

There are no clinical features to suggest idioventricular tachycardia (slow ventricular tachycardia), which is demonstrated electrocardiographically as a wide QRS complex (without preceding conducting P waves) and a heart rate between 60 and 100/min. Atrioventricular (AV) re-entrant tachycardia is a bypass-tract-mediated re-entrant tachycardia, in which the anterograde conduction (atria-to-ventricle) is typically via the AV node, and retrograde conduction is via the bypass tract. Because bypass-tract conduction is typically faster than conduction via the AV node, atrial activation occurs rapidly after the QRS complex, resulting in a "short RP" tachycardia, and the P wave is usually located within the ST segment. In AV nodal re-entrant tachycardia, the atria and ventricles are activated simultaneously from the AV node; the QRS complex is narrow, and there are no P waves.

KEY POINT

• Multifocal atrial tachycardia is characterized on electrocardiograms by three or more P wave morphologic patterns and variable PR intervals.

Bibliography
1. McCord J, Borzak S. Multifocal atrial tachycardia. Chest. 1998;113:203-9. [PMID: 9440591]

Item 32   Answer: C

Angiotensin-converting enzyme inhibitors are indicated for all patients with systolic heart failure, regardless of the level of the ejection fraction or functional status unless there are contraindications (including hyperkalemia, acute renal failure, or a history of angioedema).

Sustained-release metoprolol and carvedilol are both approved for heart failure treatment in the United States. Currently, there is no definitive evidence indicating whether one is better than the other for the treatment of heart failure. Digoxin improves symptoms and reduces hospitalizations for patients with heart failure but is not indicated for patients with asymptomatic heart failure in the absence of other indications (such as rate control for atrial fibrillation). Spironolactone is indicated for patients with heart failure who have severe symptoms (New York Heart Association class III or IV).

KEY POINT

- Angiotensin-converting enzyme inhibitors are indicated for all patients with systolic heart failure, regardless of ejection fraction or functional status, barring contraindications.

Bibliography
1. Dagenais GR, Pogue J, Fox K, Simoons ML, Yusuf S. Angiotensin-converting-enzyme inhibitors in stable vascular disease without left ventricular systolic dysfunction or heart failure: a combined analysis of three trials. Lancet. 2006;368:581-8. [PMID: 16905022]

Item 33   Answer: C

The combination of manifest pre-excitation (short PR segment and delta wave [slurred initial upstroke of the QRS complex]) in this patient's baseline electrocardiogram plus tachycardia establishes the diagnosis of the Wolff-Parkinson-White syndrome, which can cause an atrioventricular (AV) re-entrant tachycardia. AV re-entrant tachycardia is a bypass-tract-mediated re-entrant tachycardia, in which the anterograde conduction (atria-to-ventricle) is typically via the AV node, and retrograde conduction is via the bypass tract. Because bypass-tract conduction is typically faster than conduction via the AV node, during episodes of atrial tachycardia, atrial activation occurs rapidly after the QRS complex, resulting in a "short RP" tachycardia and the P wave is usually located within the ST segment. Because the ventricle is activated normally during tachycardia, the QRS complex is narrow. Patients with Wolff-Parkinson-White syndrome should be offered radiofrequency catheter ablation as first-line therapy. This recommendation is based on the high success rate of catheter ablation and the presence of a small but persistent risk of sudden cardiac death if the arrhythmia is untreated.

Sinus tachycardia, AV nodal re-entrant tachycardia, atrial tachycardia, and atrial flutter can cause paroxysmal episodes of palpitations, but none of these conditions is associated with a short PR segment and delta wave.

KEY POINT

- Atrioventricular re-entrant tachycardia (Wolff-Parkinson-White syndrome) is characterized electrocardiographically by a short PR segment, delta wave, and tachycardia.

Bibliography
1. Esberger D, Jones S, Morris F. ABC of clinical electrocardiography. Junctional tachycardias. BMJ. 2002;324:662-5. [PMID: 11895828]

Item 34   Answer: A

Treatment with an angiotensin-converting enzyme (ACE) inhibitor and a β-blocker is indicated for all patients with any degree of systolic heart failure, including this asymptomatic patient with a low ejection fraction, because treatment with

both agents has been shown to reduce morbidity and mortality.

Losartan, an angiotensin-receptor blocker (ARB), is an acceptable alternative in a patient who cannot tolerate an ACE inhibitor, but there is no benefit to adding an ARB to an ACE inhibitor. Calcium-channel blockers are indicated in patients with heart failure who have hypertension or angina that is not adequately controlled with an ACE inhibitor or β-blocker. First-generation calcium-channel blockers, such as nifedipine, diltiazem, and verapamil, cause a reactive increase in sympathetic activity in response to peripheral vasodilatation and negative inotropic effects, whereas second-generation calcium-channel blockers, such as amlodipine, are more vasoselective, less cardiodepressant, and do not appear to have a deleterious effect on outcome in patients with heart failure. Spironolactone and digoxin are not indicated for patients with asymptomatic systolic heart failure. Spironolactone reduces mortality in patients with severe symptomatic heart failure (New York Heart Association class III or IV) and a left ventricular ejection fraction ≤35%. Digoxin alleviates symptoms and reduces hospitalizations related to heart failure, but has not been shown to reduce mortality.

KEY POINTS

- An angiotensin-converting enzyme inhibitor and a β-blocker are indicated in all patients with systolic heart failure, including asymptomatic patients with low ejection fractions.

- Spironolactone and digoxin are not indicated in patients with asymptomatic systolic heart failure.

Bibliography
1. O'Connor CM. The new heart failure guidelines: strategies for implementation. Am Heart J. 2007;153:2-5. [PMID: 17394896]

Item 35   Answer: A

This patient is unstable, as demonstrated by his symptoms and low blood pressure. In unstable patients, electrical cardioversion should always be considered the treatment of choice regardless of the tachycardia mechanism. This electrocardiogram is consistent with atrial fibrillation in a patient with an accessory atrioventricular pathway. In patients with atrial fibrillation and an accessory pathway (bypass tract), the rapid atrial impulses travel to the ventricle through both the normal conduction system and the accessory pathway. Because of the chaotic electrical activity in the atria, the degree of conduction via both pathways is quite variable. Therefore, the electrocardiogram shows variable degrees of pre-excitation (manifested by variable QRS complex widths) and great irregularity.

Verapamil and other atrioventricular nodal blocking drugs should not be given to patients with pre-excitation tachycardias, especially pre-excitation atrial fibrillation, because blocking the atrioventricular nodal conduction may enhance conduction down the accessory pathway, leading to faster heart rates and, possibly, hemodynamic collapse. For such patients, drugs capable of directly slowing conduction on the pathway, such as procainamide and ibutilide, are the best options, provided the patient is stable and does not require immediate cardioversion. Overdrive atrial pacing is not possible; this patient is in atrial fibrillation, therefore, pacing would not result in capture of the electrical impulse.

KEY POINT

- Tachycardic patients who are unstable should undergo immediate direct-current cardioversion.

Bibliography

1. Blomstrom-Lundqvist C, Scheinman MM, Aliot EM, Alpert JS, Calkins H, Camm AJ, et al. ACC/AHA/ESC guidelines for the management of patients with supraventricular arrhythmias—executive summary: a report of the American College of Cardiology/American Heart Association Task Force on Practice Guidelines and the European Society of Cardiology Committee for Practice Guidelines (Writing Committee to Develop Guidelines for the Management of Patients With Supraventricular Arrhythmias). Circulation. 2003;108:1871-909. [PMID: 14557344]

Item 36   Answer: C

In general, β-blockers for the treatment of systolic heart failure should be up-titrated toward the doses used in clinical trials, with the aim of achieving the morbidity and mortality benefits demonstrated by such increases. However, this dose increase may be limited by the patient's blood pressure, heart rate, or symptoms. There is evidence that heart rate response to the dose of β-blocker may be more indicative of an adequate level of treatment than the absolute dose itself. This patient is on the lowest dose of sustained-release metoprolol, and her blood pressure and heart rate are well within ranges that would tolerate a higher dose at this time. In contrast, there is no definitive dose-dependent benefit when using angiotensin-converting enzyme inhibitors, and the patient's elevated serum potassium and creatinine concentrations limit the ability to increase the dose.

Although spironolactone is indicated for patients with severe heart failure, it is important to be aware of the other criteria for using spironolactone: left ventricular ejection fraction ≤35%, serum creatinine ≤2.5 mg/dL, and serum potassium ≤5 meq/L. This patient's creatinine and potassium levels are too high to start spironolactone. Her digoxin level is therapeutic, and thus there is no need to increase the digoxin dose; in fact, higher therapeutic levels of digoxin have been associated with greater mortality. The physical examination and laboratory test results suggest a stable state of euvolemia, and there is no need to change the furosemide dose at this time.

KEY POINT

- In patients with systolic heart failure, β-blocker therapy should be titrated to heart rate.

Bibliography

1. O'Connor CM. The new heart failure guidelines: strategies for implementation. Am Heart J. 2007;153:2-5. [PMID: 17394896]

Item 37   Answer: D

This patient has ventricular tachycardia. Ventricular tachycardia is defined as three or more consecutive beats originating below the atrioventricular node (wide-complex beats not associated with a conducted P wave), with a heart rate >100–120/min. Patients with sustained ventricular tachycardia in the setting of significant structural heart disease have a high risk of future recurrence, with a mortality rate as high as 25% per year. An implantable cardioverter-defibrillator reduces sudden cardiac death in patients with ventricular fibrillation or sustained ventricular tachycardia associated with hemodynamic compromise and is superior to amiodarone therapy. It is therefore recommended in this population unless there is a contraindication.

The electrocardiogram for a patient with atrial fibrillation shows a rapid, irregularly irregular rhythm with no discernible P waves and atrial fibrillatory waves at a rate between 350 and 600/min. The fibrillatory waves vary in amplitude, morphology, and intervals, creating a rough, irregular baseline between the QRS complexes. Unless there is co-existing bundle branch block, the QRS complex is narrow. Electrocardiographically, left bundle branch block is associated with absent Q waves in leads I, aVL, and V_6; a large, wide, and positive R wave in leads I, aVL, and V_6 ("tombstone" R waves); and prolongation of the QRS complex to >0.12 sec. Repolarization abnormalities are present consisting of ST segment and T wave vectors directed opposite to the QRS complex. In right bundle branch block, lead I will show a small Q wave and tall R wave; lead V6 will show a small positive R wave and a small negative S wave followed by a large positive deflection (the "rabbit ear"). There is ST depression and T wave inversion in right precordial leads and upright T waves in left precordial and limb leads. The QRS complex is >0.12 sec.

KEY POINTS

- Patients with sustained ventricular tachycardia in the setting of significant structural heart disease are at high risk of future recurrence with a high mortality rate.

- An implantable cardioverter-defibrillator improves survival in patients with sustained ventricular tachycardia and concomitant structural heart disease.

Bibliography

1. Kokolis S, Clark LT, Kokolis R, Kassotis J. Ventricular arrhythmias and sudden cardiac death. Prog Cardiovasc Dis. 2006;48:426-44. Erratum in: Prog Cardiovasc Dis. 2006;49:58. [PMID: 16714162]

Item 38   Answer: D

The principles of management of heart failure in the pregnant patient parallel therapy in the nonpregnant patient, with the modification that some medications should be avoided during pregnancy. This patient with a low left ventricular ejection fraction should be started on afterload reduction therapy. Because angiotensin-converting enzyme inhibitors may cause fetal renal agenesis and should be avoided during pregnancy, hydralazine is the most appropriate choice for this patient. Furosemide can be used to control volume overload, but attention must be paid to avoiding hypovolemia and its deleterious effect on the fetus. Nitrates often are added to hydralazine to improve the effectiveness of vasodilator therapy. On a long-term basis, the addition of a β-blocker may be helpful; however, β-blockers should be avoided in patients with decompensated heart failure and considered only after afterload reduction has been established and volume status has been optimized.

KEY POINTS

• The use of angiotensin-converting enzyme inhibitors should be avoided during pregnancy.

• Hydralazine and nitrates are the vasodilators of choice to treat heart failure during pregnancy.

Bibliography
1. **Sliwa K, Fett J, Elkayam U.** Peripartum cardiomyopathy. Lancet. 2006;368:687-93. [PMID: 16920474]

Item 39   Answer: B

This patient has symptomatic monomorphic ventricular tachycardia and needs emergent treatment. Sustained monomorphic ventricular tachycardia in hemodynamically stable patients is treated initially with intravenous lidocaine, procainamide, or amiodarone. If the patient is hemodynamically unstable, direct-current cardioversion is used.

Ventricular tachyarrhythmias have wide-complex QRS morphology (QRS complex >0.12 sec) and a ventricular rate greater than 100/min. Ventricular tachyarrhythmias are classified as either sustained or nonsustained and either monomorphic or polymorphic. Sustained ventricular tachycardia persists for more than 30 seconds or requires termination because of hemodynamic collapse; nonsustained ventricular tachycardia is characterized by three or more beats lasting up to 30 seconds. Ventricular tachycardia is monomorphic if the QRS complexes in the same leads do not vary in contour or polymorphic if the QRS complexes in the same leads vary in contour. Physical examination findings of cannon a waves and variable intensity S1 are suggestive of atrioventricular dissociation and support the diagnosis of ventricular tachycardia in this patient.

Thrombolytic agents such as recombinant tissue plasminogen activator (rtTPA) are not used unless a diagnosis of acute myocardial infarction is established. Although myocardial infarction is highly probable in this patient, the initial electrocardiogram is not diagnostic. If myocardial infarction is ultimately diagnosed in this patient, given the presence of ventricular tachycardia and heart failure, a primary coronary intervention (e.g., coronary angioplasty and stenting) is preferred to thrombolytic therapy. Intravenous dopamine does not terminate ventricular tachycardia and could trigger ventricular fibrillation. Verapamil does not terminate ventricular

tachycardia occurring in the setting of coronary artery disease and could trigger hemodynamic collapse. If this patient had supraventricular tachycardia with aberrant conduction, adenosine or verapamil is an acceptable treatment.

KEY POINT

• Hemodynamically stable but symptomatic monomorphic ventricular tachycardia is treated emergently with intravenous lidocaine, procainamide, or amiodarone.

Bibliography
1. **ECC Committee, Subcommittees and Task Forces of the American Heart Association.** 2005 American Heart Association Guidelines for Cardiopulmonary Resuscitation and Emergency Cardiovascular Care. Circulation. 2005;112:IV1-203. Epub 2005 Nov 28. [PMID: 16314375]

Item 40   Answer: E

The use of low-dose anti-aldosterone agents such as spironolactone should be carefully considered in selected patients with recently decompensated New York Heart Association class III–IV heart failure. When added to standard therapy of angiotensin-converting enzyme (ACE) inhibitors and β-blockers, spironolactone substantially reduces the risk of morbidity and death in patients with severe heart failure due to systolic dysfunction. ACE inhibition may not completely reduce or inhibit aldosterone production. Aldosterone causes salt and water retention and myocardial fibrosis; the addition of spironolactone may blunt these effects. The original spironolactone heart failure clinical trial included patients with serum creatinine levels <2.6 mg/dL and potassium levels <5.0 meq/L. Because the risk of hyperkalemia may be higher in patients who do not meet these criteria, spironolactone should be used with caution in these patients.

Calcium channel blockers such as amlodipine can lead to worsening heart failure and an increased risk of cardiovascular events in patients with a reduced left ventricular ejection fraction. Digitalis (e.g., digoxin) may improve symptoms and reduce the need for hospitalization in patients with current or prior symptoms of heart failure due to systolic dysfunction, but the drug's narrow risk/benefit ratio and the lack of survival benefit limit its usefulness. The addition of metolazone to a loop diuretic may help overcome diuretic resistance in patients with refractory edema, but diuretic therapy has not been shown to improve survival in patients with heart failure. Long-term studies with other oral positive inotropic agents, such as milrinone, have shown little efficacy and were terminated early because of an increased risk of death in patients with heart failure.

KEY POINT

• When added to standard therapy of angiotensin-converting enzyme inhibitors and β-blockers, spironolactone substantially reduces the risk of morbidity and death in patients with severe heart failure due to systolic dysfunction.

Bibliography

1. **Hunt SA; American College of Cardiology; American Heart Association Task Force on Practice Guidelines (Writing Committee to Update the 2001 Guidelines for the Evaluation and Management of Heart Failure)**. ACC/AHA 2005 guideline update for the diagnosis and management of chronic heart failure in the adult: a report of the American College of Cardiology/American Heart Association Task Force on Practice Guidelines (Writing Committee to Update the 2001 Guidelines for the Evaluation and Management of Heart Failure). J Am Coll Cardiol. 2005;46:e1-82. Erratum in: J Am Coll Cardiol. 2006;47:1503-1505. [PMID: 16168273]

Item 41　　Answer: A

The patient's electrocardiogram shows a previous anteroseptal myocardial infarction (Q waves in leads V_1–V_3). She may have had a myocardial infarction 2 months ago, resulting in systolic dysfunction. Her risk factors for coronary artery disease include diabetes mellitus, obesity, and hypertension. The American College of Cardiology/American Heart Association class I (evidence or general agreement that therapy is useful and effective) indications for cardiac catheterization include patients who have angina and who may be candidates for revascularization.

Measuring B-type natriuretic peptide would likely confirm mild volume overload but would not add to the diagnosis; the physical examination already suggests volume overload, and the echocardiogram already confirms severe systolic dysfunction. The priority in diagnosis should be to rule out coronary artery disease as a treatable cause of heart failure. The pretest probability of coronary artery disease is very high in this patient, and a cardiac stress test, which is most useful diagnostically for risk stratification in patients with an intermediate pretest probability of disease, would not be helpful. Few patients with new-onset heart failure require endomyocardial biopsy as part of their diagnostic evaluation. Endomyocardial biopsy is useful in patients with unexplained cardiomyopathy, in whom a definitive diagnosis, such as amyloidosis or sarcoidosis, would affect treatment and prognosis.

KEY POINT

- In patients with new-onset heart failure, ischemia should be ruled out if risk factors are present.

Bibliography

1. **Onwuanyi A, Taylor M.** Acute decompensated heart failure: pathophysiology and treatment. Am J Cardiol. 2007;99:25D-30D. Epub 2007 Jan 25. [PMID: 17378992]

Item 42　　Answer: B

This young, asymptomatic patient has a bicuspid aortic valve and significant aortic regurgitation. Transthoracic echocardiography is the diagnostic test of choice. The physical examination findings that support aortic regurgitation include the displaced and diffuse apical impulse (left ventricular dilatation), the diastolic murmur at the left sternal border, and the peripheral artery findings that include brisk pulses with rapid collapse and a "pistol shot" sound that can be auscultated over large peripheral arteries.

Aortic valve stenosis is associated with a systolic, not diastolic, murmur, and the apex beat is hyperkinetic and prolonged, not displaced and diffuse. Aortic valve stenosis is also associated with a small, delayed carotid pulse that is distinctly different from the rapidly rising and collapsing pulse of aortic regurgitation. Aortic dissection can produce acute aortic insufficiency, but patients typically have severe chest pain that radiates through to the back, an absent S_1 due to premature closure of the mitral valve, and a soft S_2. Pulmonary valve stenosis, like aortic valve stenosis, causes a systolic murmur, and murmurs of both pulmonary valve stenosis and pulmonary valve regurgitation increase with inspiration, a finding that is absent in this patient. Finally, pulmonary valve abnormalities are not associated with peripheral artery findings.

KEY POINT

- Chronic aortic valve regurgitation is associated with a basal, left-sided diastolic murmur that does not change with respiration.

Bibliography

1. **Maurer G.** Aortic regurgitation. Heart. 2006;92:994-1000. [PMID: 16775114]

Item 43　　Answer: A

This patient has severe aortic stenosis based upon her symptoms and quality of the murmur. Severe aortic stenosis is associated with carotid artery pulsations that are low volume and late (in relation to the apical impulse), a late peaking murmur (indicating an increased pressure gradient across the aortic valve), and a sustained apical impulse and absent splitting of S_2 (both indicating a prolonged ejection time). The most common cause of aortic stenosis is progressive calcific valve disease of a normal trileaflet valve. The primary indication for aortic valve replacement in patients with aortic stenosis is onset of cardiac symptoms. This patient has symptomatic disease with exertional dyspnea and decreased exercise tolerance. Referral for aortic valve replacement should be the next step in her management.

Physical examination findings in patients with hypertrophic cardiomyopathy and left ventricular outflow obstruction show a variable and dynamic systolic murmur that is increased by a Valsalva maneuver and standing and is diminished by hand gripping, leg elevation, and squatting. Carotid upstrokes are brisk. Mitral regurgitation is associated with a holosystolic murmur that radiates to the cardiac apex and is associated with a displaced, not sustained, apical impulse. Tricuspid regurgitation causes a systolic murmur heard best along the left sternal border; the murmur increases with inspiration and does not radiate to the carotid arteries. Ventricular septal defect would be an unusual cause of a systolic murmur in an elderly person in the absence of a recent myocardial infarction. Ventricular septal defects can be associated with a precordial thrill, and if pulmonary hypertension develops, fixed splitting of the S_2 occurs. The murmur of a ventricular septal defect does not radiate to the carotid arteries.

- The physical findings of severe aortic stenosis include small and late carotid pulsations, late peaking systolic murmur, absence of splitting of the S_2, and a sustained apical impulse.

Bibliography

1. **Otto CM.** Valvular aortic stenosis: disease severity and timing of intervention. J Am Coll Cardiol. 2006;47:2141-51. [PMID: 16750677]

Item 44   Answer: E

Physical examination is helpful for defining the presence of heart valve disease but is less useful for evaluation of disease severity. In this elderly woman with symptoms that may be due to aortic stenosis, the presence of a systolic murmur on examination is of concern. The most helpful physical examination finding in this patient is a physiologically split S_2, which has a specificity of 76% for excluding severe aortic stenosis. With severe stenosis, the stiff aortic valve leaflets do not "snap" shut, thus the aortic component of the S_2 is absent. In addition, a physiologically split S_2 rules out the delay in left ventricular ejection that is associated with severe aortic valve stenosis.

About one third of adults with severe aortic stenosis have systemic hypertension, so this finding does not exclude the diagnosis. In fact, concurrent hypertension and aortic stenosis "double loads" the left ventricle, resulting in increased wall stress and earlier symptom onset. In patients with hypertension, the increased stiffness of the peripheral vessels may mask the expected delay and decrease in carotid upstroke that is classically associated with severe aortic stenosis. The loudness of the murmur in aortic stenosis is only helpful when a grade 4/6 murmur (murmur and a palpable thrill) is present because this finding is specific for severe valve obstruction. Most patients with severe aortic stenosis have a grade 3/6 murmur and some have a grade 2/6 murmur. In the elderly, the murmur of aortic stenosis may radiate to the apex instead of to the carotid arteries. Severe aortic stenosis is very unlikely with a grade 1 or absent systolic murmur, but severe stenosis may be present with a grade 2 murmur.

In clinical practice, most physicians would obtain an echocardiogram in this patient because aortic valve disease almost certainly is present, even if not yet severe. Echocardiography provides prognostic information in this setting. In patients with mild aortic stenosis (aortic jet velocity <3 m/s, valve area >1.5 cm^2), progression to symptoms occurs in only 8% of patients per year. In contrast, in patients with asymptomatic severe stenosis (aortic jet velocity >4 m/s, valve area <1.0 cm^2), about 40% develop symptoms that prompt valve surgery within 1 year. Outcomes are intermediate with moderate aortic steno-

sis (jet velocity 3–4 m/s, valve area 1–1.5 cm^2), with an annual rate of symptom onset of about 17%.

- Physical examination is helpful in identifying the presence, but not the severity, of heart valve disease.

- The most sensitive physical examination finding excluding the diagnosis of severe aortic stenosis is a physiologically split S_2.

Bibliography

1. **Etchells E, Glenns V, Shadowitz S, Bell C, Siu S.** A bedside clinical prediction rule for detecting moderate or severe aortic stenosis. J Gen Intern Med. 1998;13:699-704. [PMID: 9798818]

2. **Etchells E, Bell C, Robb K.** Does this patient have an abnormal systolic murmur? JAMA. 1997;277:564-71. [PMID: 9032164]

Item 45   Answer: C

This patient's long, late-peaking systolic murmur suggests severe aortic stenosis. In adults, aortic stenosis is most commonly caused by rheumatic heart disease, a bicuspid aortic valve, and degenerative disease of a tricuspid aortic valve. Significant obstruction to aortic outflow typically develops gradually over many years. Signs of severe stenosis may include angina, dyspnea, or syncope, as well as a lengthening murmur with a peak later in systole, paradoxical splitting of S_2, and the presence of pulsus parvus et tardus (a small and slow-rising peripheral pulse). Evaluation for possible surgical valve replacement may be warranted if any of these findings are present.

Electrocardiographic evidence of left atrial enlargement and an S_4 gallop suggestive of left ventricular hypertrophy are often present years before surgical intervention for aortic stenosis is needed and do not correlate well with the severity of the obstruction. A characteristic systolic murmur at the base of the heart with radiation to the carotid arteries often is present regardless of disease severity. The primary importance of an aortic ejection click is its etiological association. In patients with aortic stenosis the presence of an ejection click implies that the stenosis is at the valvular level and there is some mobility to the valve. Elderly patients with calcific aortic stenosis and immobile valves do not have ejection clicks. The absence of an ejection click is not well correlated with severity of stenosis.

- A long, late-peaking systolic murmur is associated with advanced aortic stenosis.

Bibliography

1. **Carabello BA.** Clinical practice. Aortic stenosis. N Engl J Med. 2002;346:677-82. [PMID: 11870246]

Item 46   Answer: C

In this patient, the physical examination is most consistent with hypertrophic cardiomyopathy. Rapid upstrokes of the peripheral pulses help differentiate hypertrophic cardiomyopathy from aortic stenosis, which is characterized by low volume and delayed peripheral pulses (pulsus parvus et tardus). The murmur of hypertrophic cardiomyopathy is caused by obstruction of the left ventricular outflow tract from a thickened interventricular septum. In contrast to aortic stenosis, the murmur of hypertrophic cardiomyopathy rarely radiates to the level of the carotid arteries. The stand-to-squat maneuver and passive leg lift transiently increase venous return (preload) and therefore increase left ventricular chamber size and volume. If preload is transiently increased, the end-systolic dimension of the left ventricle increases, and there is less relative obstruction/turbulence in the left ventricular outflow tract with a resulting decrease in murmur intensity. If venous return is transiently decreased, as with the Valsalva maneuver or the squat-to-stand maneuver, left ventricular chamber size decreases and the septum and mitral leaflet are brought closer together. As a consequence, turbulent flow in the outflow tract is increased, increasing the intensity of the murmur. A murmur that increases with the Valsalva maneuver is a strong indicator that hypertrophic cardiomyopathy is present, with a positive likelihood ratio of 14.0. An absence of change in a murmur with the squat-to-stand, passive leg lift, and handgrip exercise maneuvers provides strong evidence against a diagnosis of hypertrophic cardiomyopathy, with a negative likelihood ratio of 0.1.

In contrast to the murmur of hypertrophic cardiomyopathy, the murmur associated with mitral valve prolapse and regurgitation is a holosystolic to late systolic murmur. This murmur is usually associated with a midsystolic click and is located at the apex. A Valsalva maneuver causes the click and murmur to occur earlier in systole. Having the patient squat from the standing position, perform leg raising, and do maximal isometric exercises moves the click-murmur complex toward S_2. The murmur associated with a ventricular septal defect is a harsh systolic murmur located parasternally that radiates to the right sternal edge. Maneuvers that increase afterload, such as isometric handgrip exercise, increase the regurgitant left-sided murmurs of mitral regurgitation and ventricular septal defect.

An atrial septal defect is associated with a wide, fixed split S_2 and a soft systolic murmur that may or may not be audible. If present, the murmur is heard best over the pulmonic area.

The murmur of aortic stenosis is a mid-peaking systolic murmur that often radiates superiorly, toward the carotid arteries. There are no accentuating maneuvers for the murmur of an atrial septal defect or aortic stenosis.

KEY POINT

• The murmur of hypertrophic cardiomyopathy increases after a Valsalva maneuver and decreases with standing to squatting.

Bibliography
1. Lembo NJ, Dell'Italia LJ, Crawford MH, O'Rourke RA. Bedside diagnosis of systolic murmurs. N Engl J Med. 1988;318:1572-8. [PMID: 2897627]

Item 47   Answer: C

This patient has findings consistent with chronic mitral regurgitation with associated hemodynamic and structural sequelae, ultimately leading to the development of symptomatic heart failure. The location of the murmur is characteristic of mitral valve regurgitation (holosystolic, loudest at the apex, and radiating to the axilla). The prominent pulmonic component of the S_2 suggests pulmonary hypertension secondary to chronic mitral valve regurgitation. She has evidence of left-sided heart failure, including left atrial and ventricular enlargement on the electrocardiogram, crackles on lung examination, and pulmonary congestion on the chest radiograph. The signs of right-sided heart failure (peripheral edema, jugular venous distention) are the upstream effects of elevated left-sided filling pressures.

Chronic aortic valve stenosis can also cause left-sided heart failure, but the murmur of aortic stenosis is diamond-shaped, loudest at the right sternal border, and radiates to the carotid arteries. Mitral valve stenosis is characterized by an opening snap after the S_2 followed by a low-frequency decrescendo murmur (diastolic "rumble"). Significant mitral valve stenosis results in elevated left atrial pressure, secondary pulmonary hypertension, and, ultimately, right-sided heart failure. Because the left ventricle is protected from pressure or volume overload, mitral stenosis does not lead to left ventricular hypertrophy. The murmur of aortic valve regurgitation is an early blowing diastolic murmur heard loudest at the left sternal border. Chronic aortic regurgitation may lead to left ventricular enlargement and left-sided heart failure. The murmur of tricuspid valve regurgitation is systolic, loudest at the lower left sternal border, and becomes louder with inspiration. Significant tricuspid valve regurgitation will lead to right-sided heart failure but should not cause signs and symptoms of left-sided heart failure.

KEY POINT

• Physical examination findings of mitral valve regurgitation include a holosystolic murmur at the apex that radiates to the axilla without respiratory variation.

Bibliography
1. Otto CM. Clinical practice. Evaluation and management of chronic mitral regurgitation. N Engl J Med. 2001;345:740-6. [PMID: 11547744]

Item 48   Answer: B

This patient has symptoms of mitral valve stenosis. Her physical examination shows a loud S_1 due to the forceful closing of the stenotic mitral valve. The S_2 has a fixed split due to accompanying pulmonary hypertension and a prolonged right ventricular ejection time. The classic findings of mitral stenosis, an opening snap and a low-pitched diastolic rumble, are often difficult to hear, particularly in a pregnant patient. The opening snap follows the S_2 and has an audible quality similar to a normal S_2. The opening snap may be mistaken for a split S_2 unless it is recognized that the sound is loudest at the apex, instead of the base. Both the opening snap and the diastolic rumble are heard best with the bell of the stethoscope at the apex and are enhanced when the patient is in a left lateral decubitus position. Often accompanying mitral regurgitation is easier to hear. The diagnosis can be confirmed by echocardiography.

Mitral valve stenosis is more common in women than men, and the age at symptom onset varies worldwide. Patients are often asymptomatic until there is a superimposed hemodynamic stress, such as pregnancy.

Aortic valve stenosis is characterized by a loud systolic murmur at the cardiac base. Peripartum cardiomyopathy typically presents later in pregnancy; although physical examination findings of heart failure might be similar, peripartum cardiomyopathy is not associated with an opening snap or diastolic murmur. A patent ductus arteriosus results in a continuous cardiac murmur. In pregnancy, a basal systolic ejection murmur is normal, but signs of heart failure are definitely abnormal.

KEY POINTS
- Classic findings of mitral stenosis include a loud S_1 and an opening snap followed by a rumbling diastolic murmur.
- Previously undiagnosed mitral stenosis often first becomes symptomatic during pregnancy.

Bibliography
1. Carabello BA. Modern management of mitral stenosis. Circulation. 2005;112:432-7. [PMID: 16027271]

Item 49   Answer: D

The auscultatory feature of mitral valve prolapse is a "click-murmur" complex—a midsystolic click, thought to be from the sudden tensing of the mitral subvalvular apparatus as the leaflets prolapse into the left atrium, is followed by a late systolic murmur. The Valsalva maneuver and standing from a squatting position decrease end-diastolic volume and move the click-murmur complex closer to the S_1.

Mitral valve prolapse occurs in approximately 2% of the general population and is the most common cause of mitral regurgitation. In the absence of significant mitral regurgitation, primary mitral valve prolapse is usually asymptomatic but can present with palpitations or atypical chest discomfort. Palpitations are common and are usually associated with benign premature atrial or ventricular contractions. Sustained arrhythmias are exceedingly rare.

Hypertrophic cardiomyopathy is associated with a harsh crescendo-decrescendo systolic murmur that begins slightly after S_1 and is heard best at the apex and lower left sternal border. The Valsalva maneuver and standing from a squatting position increase the intensity of the murmur. The murmur of hypertrophic cardiomyopathy is the only murmur that increases in intensity with the Valsalva maneuver. Benign (innocent) flow murmurs are typically midsystolic grade

1–2/6 murmurs associated with normal heart sounds and no other findings. The presence of a click, an S_4, abnormal splitting of S_2, or increased intensity or duration of the murmur with the Valsalva maneuver or standing are not compatible with a benign (innocent) flow murmur. The murmur of mitral valve regurgitation begins shortly after S_1 and ends just prior to S_2 (holosystolic murmur). It is not associated with clicks, and the intensity is not increased with standing from a squatting position or with the Valsalva maneuver.

KEY POINTS
- The auscultatory feature of mitral valve prolapse is a midsystolic click followed by a late systolic murmur.
- In mitral valve prolapse, the Valsalva maneuver and standing from a squatting position move the click-murmur complex closer to S_1.

Bibliography
1. Hayek E, Gring CN, Griffin BP. Mitral valve prolapse. Lancet. 2005; 365:507-18. [PMID: 15705461]

Chapter 2
Endocrinology and Metabolism

Endocrinology and Metabolism contains self-assessment items that correspond to the following chapters in the *Internal Medicine Essentials for Clerkship Students 2* textbook:

Diabetes Mellitus and Diabetic Ketoacidosis
Dyslipidemia
Thyroid Disease
Adrenal Disease
Osteoporosis

Endocrinology and Metabolism contains self assessment items that correspond to the following Training Problems in the *Core Medicine Clerkship Guide*:

Diabetes Mellitus
Dyslipidemia

Chapter 2

Endocrinology and Metabolism

Questions

Item 1

A 26-year-old woman is evaluated in the office for amenorrhea. Her last menstrual period was 3 months ago, and three home pregnancy tests have been negative. She has no other symptoms and takes no medications. Menarche occurred at age 12 years, and her menstrual cycle had been regular until 3 months ago. Upon further questioning, she recounts weekly headaches and occasional galactorrhea on breast palpation.

Physical examination, including neurologic examination and deep tendon reflexes, is normal. A pregnancy test is negative, and the prolactin level is 1665 ng/mL.

Which of the following is the most likely cause of this patient's hyperprolactinemia?

(A) Chronic renal failure
(B) Pregnancy
(C) Primary hypothyroidism
(D) Prolactin-producing pituitary tumor

Item 2

A 68-year-old woman is scheduled to undergo arteriography of the lower extremities for progressive claudication. She has type 2 diabetes mellitus (hemoglobin A_{1c} 6.4%) that is well controlled with pioglitazone and metformin. On the day of the procedure, she is to receive nothing by mouth all morning except for medications until after the procedure.

Which of the following decisions regarding her medications is most appropriate on the day of the procedure?

(A) Continue both medications
(B) Withhold both medications
(C) Withhold metformin
(D) Withhold pioglitazone

Item 3

A 32-year-old woman who has had type 1 diabetes mellitus for 20 years is evaluated during a routine office follow-up visit. She is using 32 units of premixed insulin twice daily (75/25 neutral protamine lispro/lispro mix) at her morning and evening meals. Most premeal capillary glucose readings range between 100 and 200 mg/dL. Fasting glucose readings average approximately 170 mg/dL. She does, however, have hypoglycemic reactions about once or twice a week, usually between 1:00 and 3:00 AM. The most recent hemoglobin A_{1c} was 7.4%. Examination reveals normal weight and blood pressure and no evidence of diabetic complications.

Which of the following would be most appropriate to improve her glucose control?

(A) Change to insulin glargine at bedtime with three premeal injections of insulin lispro during the day
(B) Change to three premeal injections of insulin lispro during the day
(C) Increase the dose of both the morning and the evening premixed insulin
(D) Reduce caloric consumption

Item 4

A 55-year-old woman asks to be tested for diabetes mellitus because she had a fasting glucose value of 130 mg/dL at a recent local health fair. She has no symptoms of polydipsia or polyuria. She has mild osteoarthritis but no other significant illnesses. Her mother and sister both developed type 2 diabetes mellitus in their 50s. She takes only occasional aspirin or acetaminophen for joint pains.

On physical examination, the blood pressure is 120/75 mm Hg, heart rate is 72/min, and BMI is 25.2. The remainder of her physical examination is normal.

Which of the following should be done next to establish a diagnosis of diabetes mellitus?

(A) Measure the hemoglobin A_{1c}
(B) Measure a fasting plasma insulin level
(C) Measure a 2-hour postprandial plasma glucose level
(D) Repeat the fasting plasma glucose measurement

Item 5

A healthy 54-year-old woman with a strong family history of type 2 diabetes mellitus requests an oral glucose tolerance test to evaluate her risk of developing diabetes. The results of a 2-hour glucose tolerance test after a 75-g oral glucose load are as follows:

Fasting glucose   104 mg/dL
2-hour glucose   168 mg/dL

Which of the following characterizes the patient's glycemic status?

(A) Impaired fasting glucose
(B) Impaired glucose tolerance
(C) Impaired fasting glucose and impaired glucose tolerance
(D) Normal glucose tolerance
(E) Type 2 diabetes mellitus

Item 6

A 45-year-old man requests advice about prevention of diabetes mellitus. He has hypertension, for which he takes a β-blocker. His father developed type 2 diabetes mellitus at age 49 years, had hypertension and hyperlipidemia, and subsequently died of a myocardial infarction.

On physical examination, the blood pressure is 150/95 mm Hg, heart rate is 80/min, and BMI is 31.8. The remainder of the physical examination is normal.

Laboratory studies:

Fasting glucose	94 mg/dL
2-Hour postprandial glucose	136 mg/dL
Total cholesterol	185 mg/dL
Triglycerides	203 mg/dL
HDL cholesterol	44 mg/dL
LDL cholesterol	100 mg/dL

Which of the following would be most appropriate in preventing the development of type 2 diabetes mellitus in this patient?

(A) Acarbose
(B) Diet, exercise, and weight loss
(C) Low-dose insulin
(D) Metformin
(E) Rosiglitazone

Item 7

A 48-year-old man with type 2 diabetes mellitus is evaluated during a routine follow-up office visit. He has had diabetes for 8 years and has no known complications. His diabetes medications are maximum dosages of metformin and pioglitazone, insulin glargine, 30 units every morning, and insulin aspart, 20 units with each meal.

On physical examination, the blood pressure is 155/95 mm Hg, heart rate is 64/min, and BMI is 34.7. The remainder of the physical examination is normal.

Glucose profile:

Fasting	Mean 213 mg/dL Range 165–233 mg/dL
Pre-lunch	Mean 220 mg/dL Range 178–251 mg/dL
Pre-dinner	Mean 211 mg/d Range 155–228 mg/dL
Bedtime	Mean 153 mg/dL Range 149–244 mg/dL
2-Hour postprandial (done twice)	202 mg/dL and 211 mg/dL

Which of the following insulin adjustments is most likely to improve this patient's blood glucose profile?

(A) Add morning NPH insulin
(B) Decrease mealtime aspart
(C) Decrease morning glargine
(D) Increase mealtime aspart
(E) Increase morning glargine

Item 8

A 54-year-old man was recently diagnosed as having type 2 diabetes mellitus. He has been treated for hyperlipidemia and hypertension for the past 2 years. He does not have cardiovascular disease. His current medications are metformin, pioglitazone, lisinopril, atorvastatin, and aspirin.

On physical examination, the blood pressure is 120/75 mm Hg, heart rate is 84/min, and BMI is 29.6. The remainder of the physical examination is normal.

Laboratory studies:

Fasting glucose	159 mg/dL
Hemoglobin A_{1c}	7.4%
Creatinine	1.1 mg/dL
Total cholesterol	142 mg/dL
Triglycerides	145 mg/dL
HDL cholesterol	48 mg/dL
LDL cholesterol	65 mg/dL
Urine albumin/creatinine ratio	13 mg/g

In addition to emphasizing diet, exercise, and weight loss, which of the following medication changes would be most appropriate at this time?

(A) Add a fibrate
(B) Add niacin
(C) Increase atorvastatin dose
(D) Increase antihyperglycemic therapy
(E) Increase lisinopril dose

Item 9

A 62-year-old man is evaluated in the office for persistent hyperglycemia. He has had type 2 diabetes mellitus for 6 years and also has hypertension, hyperlipidemia, coronary artery disease, and New York Heart Association class III congestive heart failure. His only diabetes medication is glyburide, 10 mg twice a day (maximum dose).

On physical examination, the blood pressure is 125/80 mm Hg, heart rate is 84/min, and BMI is 33.1. He has mild bibasilar crackles and 2+ pitting edema but no evidence of infection.

His fasting glucose is 298 mg/dL, hemoglobin A_{1c} is 10.2%, and creatinine is 2.0 mg/dL.

In addition to diet, exercise, and weight loss, which of the following is the most appropriate therapeutic intervention to control his blood glucose level at this time?

(A) Insulin
(B) Metformin
(C) Metformin plus pioglitazone
(D) Pioglitazone
(E) Repaglinide

Item 10

A 29-year-old woman who has had type 1 diabetes mellitus for 15 years is evaluated during a regular follow-up office visit. Her current insulin regimen consists of insulin glargine, 28 units at bedtime, and insulin lispro, 4 units three times a day with meals. She has occasional nightmares that awaken her from sleep; her blood glucose levels on two of these occasions were 53 mg/dL and 48 mg/dL.

On physical examination, the blood pressure is 115/70 mm Hg, heart rate is 80/min, and BMI is 22 (she weighs 60 kg [132 lb]). She has no evidence of retinopathy or peripheral neuropathy. Her hemoglobin A_{1c} is 7.1%.

Glucose profiles:

Fasting	Mean 210 mg/dL
	Range 51–243 mg/dL
Pre-lunch	Mean 141 mg/dL
	Range 65–203 mg/dL
Pre-dinner	Mean 125 mg/dL
	Range 68–165 mg/dL
Bedtime	Mean 130 mg/dL
	Range 71–158 mg/dL

Which of the following insulin adjustments should be made first?

(A) Increase glargine at bedtime
(B) Decrease glargine at bedtime
(C) Increase lispro at all three meals
(D) Decrease lispro at all three meals
(E) Decrease lispro at dinner

Item 11

A 57-year-old woman with type 2 diabetes mellitus is evaluated during a routine follow-up office visit. She has had diabetes for 3 years and has no known complications. Her current medications for diabetes are metformin, 1000 mg twice a day; pioglitazone, 45 mg/d; and insulin glargine, 30 units every morning.

On physical examination, the blood pressure is 140/80 mm Hg, heart rate is 80/min, and BMI is 30.5. The hemoglobin A_{1c} is 9.8%. The remainder of the physical examination is normal.

Glucose profiles:

Fasting	Mean 105 mg/dL
	Range 82–123 mg/dL
Pre-lunch	Mean 136 mg/dL
	Range 128–163 mg/dL
Pre-dinner	Mean 138 mg/dL
	Range 122–171 mg/dL
Bedtime	Mean 143 mg/dL
	Range 129–188 mg/dL
2-Hour postprandial (done 3 times)	232–295 mg/dL

Which of the following medication adjustments is most likely to improve this patient's blood glucose profile?

(A) Add acarbose
(B) Add NPH insulin at bedtime
(C) Add NPH insulin in the morning
(D) Add short-acting insulin (lispro or aspart) with meals
(E) Increase glargine dose

Item 12

A 59-year-old woman with a 12-year history of type 2 diabetes mellitus is evaluated during a routine office visit. She takes glimepiride, 4 mg/d (50% of the maximum dose), and reports fasting and premeal capillary blood glucose readings predominantly between 160 and 240 mg/dL. She has no history of cardiovascular disease. Her other medications are ramipril and rosuvastatin, and she is compliant with diet and exercise recommendations.

The physical examination is notable for a blood pressure of 132/84 mm Hg, background retinopathy, and mild loss of vibratory sensation in the feet. Laboratory testing shows a hemoglobin A_{1c} of 9.2% and serum creatinine of 1.1 mg/dL.

Which of the following interventions would improve this patient's glucose control?

(A) Continue glimepiride, add metformin
(B) Increase glimepiride dose
(C) Stop glimepiride, begin metformin
(D) Stop glimepiride, begin a thiazolidinedione

Item 13

A 48-year-old man with a history of alcoholism is evaluated after discharge from the hospital where he was admitted with acute pancreatitis. The patient was found to have a pancreatic pseudocyst on abdominal CT scan. During the hospitalization, his fasting glucose level ranged from 150 to 200 mg/dL. The patient had normal glucose concentrations before this episode and has no personal or family history of diabetes mellitus.

On physical examination, the patient is lean, and blood pressure is normal. The abdomen is soft, and the liver is enlarged.

Laboratory studies:

Fasting glucose	172 mg/dL
Triglycerides	Normal
Aspartate aminotransferase	84 U/L
Alanine aminotransferase	69 U/L
Amylase	Normal
Lipase	Normal

Which of the following types of diabetes is this patient most likely to have?

(A) Latent autoimmune diabetes of adulthood
(B) Secondary diabetes
(C) Type 1 diabetes mellitus
(D) Type 2 diabetes mellitus

Item 14

A 62-year-old woman is evaluated in the office during follow-up for type 2 diabetes mellitus. The diagnosis of diabetes was confirmed 8 months ago, when she had a fasting plasma glucose level of 141 mg/dL during routine screening. Attempts at nonpharmacologic control are started with a diet and exercise program. The patient has lost 5 kg (11 lb) and walks briskly 3 days a week for 45 minutes. She monitors her blood glucose with occasional finger-stick testing at home, and reports fasting values of 135 to 145 mg/dL. The patient's medical history is notable for hypertension, hypercholesterolemia, renal insufficiency (creatinine, 1.9 mg/dL), and heart failure. She takes furosemide, lisinopril, metoprolol, simvastatin, and aspirin daily. She does not smoke.

On physical examination, the blood pressure is 130/70 mm Hg, heart rate is 60/min, and BMI is 32. Jugular venous pressure is not elevated. Lungs are clear. Cardiac examination is normal without murmur or extra sounds. There is 1+ pitting edema of the ankles.

Fasting plasma glucose level today is 142 mg/dL and hemoglobin A_{1c} is 7.3%.

Which of the following is the most appropriate treatment option for this patient at this time?

(A) Glyburide
(B) Insulin
(C) Metformin
(D) Pioglitazone
(E) No additional intervention

Item 15

An 18-year-old man is evaluated in the emergency department for anorexia and diffuse, nonradiating abdominal pain of 24 hours' duration. He also has had six episodes of bilious vomiting beginning yesterday, but no fever or chills. His bowel habits are typically regular but he has not had a bowel movement today. He has an 8-year history of type 1 diabetes mellitus, and his medications include insulin glargine and lispro and lisinopril. He skipped his insulin yesterday when he started feeling sick. He drinks alcohol frequently, but has not had alcohol in the past week.

On physical examination, the temperature is 35.8 °C (96.5 °F), blood pressure is 110/50 mm Hg, dropping to 90/50 mm Hg upon standing, heart rate is 110/min, and respiration rate is 32/min. Cardiopulmonary examination is normal except for tachycardia. Abdominal examination reveals diminished but present bowel sounds and diffuse tenderness to deep palpation without masses, guarding, or rigidity. Rectal examination shows brown stool that is negative for occult blood.

Laboratory studies:

Hemoglobin	17 g/dL
Leukocyte count	16,000/µL
Sodium	120 meq/L
Potassium	5.6 meq/L
Chloride	96 meq/L
Bicarbonate	12 meq/L
Blood urea nitrogen	32 mg/dL
Creatinine	1.2 mg/dL
Glucose	586 mg/dL

Serum amylase, lipase, and aminotransferase concentrations are normal. Urine specific gravity is 1.032; ketones are 3+.

Which of the following is the most likely cause of the abdominal pain?

(A) Acute pancreatitis
(B) Alcoholic hepatitis
(C) Alcoholic ketoacidosis
(D) Diabetic ketoacidosis

Item 16

A 23-year-old man who has had type 1 diabetes mellitus for 19 years is evaluated during a follow-up office visit. His disease has been well controlled (latest hemoglobin A_{1c} was 6.9%) on evening insulin glargine and premeal insulin lispro.

On physical examination, his blood pressure is 120/70 mm Hg. The remainder of the examination is unremarkable, with no evidence of retinopathy or edema. The urine albumin/creatinine ratio is elevated at 133 mg/g. On repeated testing, the ratio is 146 mg/g.

Which of the following is the most appropriate next step in the management of this patient?

(A) Begin an angiotensin-converting enzyme (ACE) inhibitor
(B) Begin a calcium channel blocker
(C) Increase the evening insulin glargine dose
(D) Provide continued observation

Item 17

A 78-year-old woman with a 10-year history of type 2 diabetes mellitus is hospitalized with obtundation. She developed a fever and dyspnea 3 days before admission. Her antihyperglycemic regimen consists of glipizide and pioglitazone. Her hemoglobin A_{1c} is in the range of 7.5% to 8.5% and glucose levels range from 200 to 350 mg/dL.

On physical examination, the blood pressure is 80/50 mm Hg, and the heart rate is 122/min.

Laboratory studies:

Glucose	1245 mg/dL
Sodium	143 meq/L
Bicarbonate	25 meq/L
Urinalysis	No ketones

Which of the following is the most appropriate initial therapy for this patient?

(A) Intravenous insulin infusion
(B) Intravenous normal saline infusion
(C) Intravenous normal saline infusion followed by insulin infusion
(D) Intravenous dopamine

Item 18

A 62-year-old woman is evaluated during a routine follow-up office visit. She has a 12-year history of type 2 diabetes mellitus treated with metformin and a 40-pack-year history of cigarette smoking; she is a current smoker.

On physical examination, blood pressure is 172/92 mm Hg. The patient is obese (BMI 39). The lungs are clear. No gallops or murmurs are heard on cardiac examination. The abdomen is nontender, and peripheral pulses are normal.

The results of a lipid profile are as follows:

Total cholesterol	257 mg/dL
HDL cholesterol	43 mg/dL
LDL cholesterol	178 mg/dL
Triglycerides	182 mg/dL

Which of this patient's findings is a coronary artery disease equivalent?

(A) Cigarette smoking
(B) Diabetes mellitus
(C) Elevated LDL cholesterol
(D) Hypertension
(E) Obesity

Item 19

A 45-year-old woman undergoes evaluation in the office after learning that her random total cholesterol level, which was measured at a health screening fair 1 month ago, was 260 mg/dL. The review of systems indicates increasingly heavy menstruation and constipation. Her family history is negative for coronary artery disease. The patient is obese but is otherwise healthy and does not smoke.

On physical examination, blood pressure is 120/80 mm Hg. BMI is 31. The remainder of the examination is normal.

Laboratory studies:

Total cholesterol	256 mg/dL
Triglycerides	205 mg/dL
HDL cholesterol	40 mg/dL
LDL cholesterol	175 mg/dL

Which of the following is the most appropriate next step in the management of this patient?

(A) Fibric acid derivative
(B) Fish oil supplement
(C) Statin
(D) Thyroid-stimulating hormone measurement

Item 20

A 55-year-old woman is evaluated during a routine office visit. Her medical history includes osteopenia. She does not smoke, have any other medical problems, or take any medications. Her mother had a myocardial infarction at age 70 years.

On physical examination, the blood pressure is 132/80 mm Hg. The remainder of the examination is unremarkable.

Laboratory studies:

Total cholesterol (fasting)	220 mg/dL
Triglycerides (fasting)	140 mg/dL
HDL cholesterol (fasting)	42 mg/dL
LDL cholesterol (fasting)	150 mg/dL

Which the following is the most appropriate next step in the management of this patient?

(A) Diet rich in plant stanols or sterols
(B) Niacin therapy
(C) Repeated cholesterol measurement in 5 years
(D) Statin therapy

Item 21

A 54-year-old woman is found on routine screening to have a thyroid-stimulating hormone (TSH) level of <0.01 μU/mL. She feels well in general and has good exercise tolerance but on careful questioning states that she does have decreased ability to concentrate. Medical history is otherwise unremarkable.

On physical examination, the blood pressure is 130/70 mm Hg, heart rate is 76/min, and BMI is 22.5. The thyroid gland is slightly enlarged, firm, and irregular in consistency.

Laboratory studies:

TSH (repeated)	<0.01 μU/mL
Free T_4	1.9 ng/dL
Total T_3	165 ng/dL
Thyroid iodine (^{131}I) uptake	38% at 24 hours

Electrocardiogram is normal. Thyroid scan shows patchy uptake with focal areas of increased uptake.

Which of the following is the most likely diagnosis?

(A) Nonthyroidal illness
(B) Subclinical hyperthyroidism
(C) Surreptitious thyroid ingestion
(D) Thyroiditis

Item 22

A 75-year-old woman is admitted to the medical intensive care unit with progressive obtundation. The patient's medical records state that she is taking levothyroxine, but she has not been seen in follow-up for more than 3 years.

Physical examination reveals a nonarousable elderly woman, with core temperature of 35 °C (95 °F), blood pressure of 100/74 mm Hg, and heart rate of 48/min. The patient weighs 82 kg (180 lb). She has a 4-cm transverse scar above the suprasternal notch, cold "doughy" skin, and a delayed deep tendon reflex relaxation phase. There is no nuchal rigidity and no localizing neurologic findings.

Serum sodium is 127 meq/L. Urinalysis shows >100 leukocytes/hpf and gram-negative rods. Results of urine and blood cultures are pending.

Which of the following is the most likely diagnosis?

(A) Hypoglycemia
(B) Intracerebral hemorrhage
(C) Meningitis
(D) Myxedema coma

Item 23

A 28-year-old woman is evaluated in the office for fatigue, weight gain, and occasional constipation. The patient has a history of craniopharyngioma treated with resection and subsequent radiation therapy. She now has hypopituitarism and diabetes insipidus. Her medications are hydrocortisone, levothyroxine, oral contraceptives, and desmopressin. She does not have dizziness, nausea, vomiting, polyuria, or polydipsia. She has regular menstrual cycles. The physical examination is unremarkable.

Laboratory studies:

Electrolyte panel	Normal
Thyroid-stimulating hormone	0.1 µU/mL
Free T$_4$	0.5 ng/dL

Which of the following changes should be made to this patient's therapy?

(A) Decrease hydrocortisone dose
(B) Discontinue oral contraceptives
(C) Increase desmopressin dose
(D) Increase levothyroxine dose

Item 24

A 29-year-old woman is evaluated in the office after having missed her menses; she thinks that she is pregnant. The patient has a history of thyroid cancer that was detected 1 year ago and treated with near-total thyroidectomy and radioactive iodine ablation. She is otherwise healthy and feels well. She is now taking levothyroxine, 125 µg/d, and her serum thyroid-stimulating hormone concentration 4 months ago was 1.5 µU/mL. An office pregnancy test confirms that the patient is pregnant.

Which of the following adjustments to the patient's thyroid replacement medication will most likely be necessary?

(A) Change to a combination of levothyroxine and triiodothyronine
(B) Change to triiodothyronine
(C) Decrease the levothyroxine dosage by 30%
(D) Increase the levothyroxine dosage by 30%
(E) No change is needed

Item 25

A 24-year-old woman is evaluated in the office for palpitations and sweating that began 4 weeks after she delivered her first child 8 weeks ago. She has had occasional loose stools. Otherwise, she has generally felt well. She nursed her baby for 6 weeks but decided to stop breastfeeding 2 weeks ago. Her family history is unremarkable. She is taking multivitamins but no other supplements or medications.

On physical examination, the blood pressure is 110/60 mm Hg, heart rate is 92/min, and BMI is 23.7. The thyroid gland is of normal size, slightly firm in consistency, and nontender.

Laboratory studies:

Thyroid-stimulating hormone	<0.01 µU/mL
Free T$_4$	3.4 ng/dL
Total T$_3$	315 ng/dL
Thyroid iodine (^{131}I) uptake	<1% at 24 hours

A thyroid scan shows no visible radioiodine uptake.

Which of the following is the most likely diagnosis?

(A) Graves' thyrotoxicosis
(B) Hyperfunctioning adenomatous thyroid nodule
(C) Thyroiditis
(D) Toxic multinodular goiter

Item 26

A 35-year-old man is evaluated in the office for palpitations and difficulty sleeping. He has no eye symptoms or neck pain. He is a nonsmoker, and family history is significant only for a mother with hypothyroidism.

On physical examination, the blood pressure is 135/75 mm Hg, and heart rate is 95/min. Thyroid examination reveals a diffuse goiter without tenderness, nodules, or bruit.

Laboratory studies:

Thyroid-stimulating hormone	<0.01 µU/mL
Free T$_4$	2.7 ng/dL
Antithyroid peroxidase antibodies	180 U/mL (normal <2 U/mL)
Thyroid iodine (^{131}I) uptake	0.6% at 24 hours

Thyroid ultrasonography shows a diffusely heterogeneous thyroid parenchyma, but no nodules.

Which of the following is the most appropriate therapy for this patient's thyrotoxicosis?

(A) Atenolol
(B) Methimazole
(C) Prednisone
(D) Radioiodine ablation therapy
(E) Thyroidectomy

Item 27

A 45-year-old woman is evaluated in the office for malaise, fatigue, and a 4-kg (8.8-lb) weight loss. She has no nausea, vomiting, or diarrhea. She has autoimmune thyroiditis and takes levothyroxine, 0.1 mg daily. Six months ago, her free T_4 level was 1.3 ng/dL and thyroid-stimulating hormone level was 1.9 µU/mL.

On physical examination, the blood pressure is 98/60 mm Hg, and the heart rate is 98/min with orthostatic changes. Thyroid examination shows a firm, slightly enlarged thyroid without nodules. Cardiovascular and pulmonary examinations are normal. Skin examination shows increased pigmentation. Deep tendon reflexes are normal.

Laboratory studies:

Sodium	130 meq/L
Potassium	5.9 meq/L
Calcium	10.4 mg/dL
Thyroid-stimulating hormone	8.3 µU/mL
Free T_4	1.4 ng/dL

Which of the following is the most likely cause of this patient's symptoms?

(A) Adrenal insufficiency (Addison's disease)
(B) Antacid abuse
(C) Dysautonomia
(D) Hypothyroidism
(E) Pernicious anemia

Item 28

A 52-year-old man is evaluated in the hospital for persistent hypotension 24 hours after undergoing minor ankle surgery to repair a fracture. Before the fracture, the patient's only symptoms were chronic headache, general malaise, and fatigue over the past few months. He also has had dizziness with standing and a 3-year history of erectile dysfunction. He had not been taking any prescription medications before his hospitalization and is currently taking only acetaminophen with codeine for postoperative pain control.

Postoperative laboratory studies:

Hematocrit	35%
Leukocyte count	15,000/µL
Sodium	130 meq/L
Potassium	5.1 meq/L
Aspartate aminotransferase	25 U/L
Alanine aminotransferase	23 U/L

Chest radiograph and electrocardiogram are normal. Results of blood cultures drawn 24 hours ago show no growth.

On physical examination, he is afebrile; the blood pressure is 88/56 mm Hg, and heart rate is 110/min. He does not have hyperpigmentation, but there is decreased body hair. A cosyntropin (ACTH) stimulation test shows a cortisol level of 10 µg/dL 30 minutes after administration of 250 µg of ACTH (normal, >23 µg/dL).

Which of the following should be done immediately?

(A) Corticosteroid replacement
(B) CT scan of the abdomen
(C) Empiric antibiotic therapy
(D) MRI of the head

Item 29

A 36-year-old man is evaluated in the office for erectile dysfunction. He has noted a declining libido with difficulty attaining and maintaining an erection during intercourse.

He has gained approximately 10 kg (22 lb) over the past 18 months and was diagnosed with impaired glucose tolerance last month.

On physical examination, blood pressure is 148/93 mm Hg. Wide violaceous striae are present on the abdomen. The remainder of the examination, including examination of the genitals, is normal.

A 24-hour urine collection shows a urine free cortisol concentration three times the upper limit of normal. Serum ACTH level is <5 pg/mL.

Which of the following is the most appropriate next diagnostic study for this patient?

(A) CT scan of the adrenal glands
(B) Hemoglobin A_{1c}
(C) MRI of the pituitary gland
(D) Serum luteinizing hormone, prolactin, and testosterone measurements
(E) Ultrasonography of the testes

Item 30

A 38-year-old woman is evaluated in the office for a 6-kg (13.2-lb) weight gain over the preceding 2 years. She was also recently found to have fasting glucose levels of 130 mg/dL and 136 mg/dL on two separate visits. Her only medication is a multivitamin, and she has taken no prescribed medications in the past 5 years.

On physical examination, the blood pressure is 160/94 mm Hg and BMI is 32. The patient has terminal hairs over her chin, facial acne, and violaceous striae, approximately 1 cm wide, bilaterally over her lateral abdomen. Her face is full, her abdomen is prominent, and her arms and legs seem disproportionately thin.

Which of the following is the most appropriate next step in the evaluation of this patient?

(A) Measurement of 24-hour urine collection for free cortisol
(B) Measurement of serum ACTH
(C) Measurement of afternoon (4 PM) serum cortisol
(D) MRI of the head

Item 31

A 72-year-old woman is evaluated in the office for mid-thoracic back pain. She does not smoke cigarettes and drinks alcohol rarely. Her only medications are aspirin, calcium supplements, and a multivitamin. She consumes few dairy products.

On physical examination, she has mild dorsal kyphosis with mild tenderness over the middle and lower thoracic regions. Spine radiographs show compression fractures at T8, L2, and L3.

Laboratory studies:

Calcium	9.8 mg/dL
Phosphorus	3.9 mg/dL
Alkaline phosphatase	88 U/L
Urine calcium excretion	205 mg/24 h
Bone mineral density	Spine T-score : –2.6
	Total hip T-score: –1.9

Which of the following is the most likely diagnosis?

(A) Osteomalacia
(B) Osteopenia
(C) Osteoporosis
(D) Paget's disease

Item 32

A 52-year-old postmenopausal woman with a long-standing history of chronic obstructive pulmonary disease is evaluated during a follow-up office visit. She has had three acute exacerbations of her pulmonary disease in the past year. She was hospitalized on all three occasions and required high-dose methylprednisolone as part of the therapy. She continues to smoke despite requiring ipratropium bromide, salmeterol, and inhaled fluticasone. After her most recent hospital admission 3 months ago, she continued to require oral prednisone 10 mg/d. Every time a dose reduction of prednisone is attempted, there is an exacerbation of her pulmonary disease.

Which of the following should be done next as regards this patient's bone health?

(A) Calcium supplementation
(B) Calcium and vitamin D supplementation
(C) Dual-energy x-ray absorptiometry (DEXA) scan and calcium and vitamin D supplementation
(D) Dual-energy x-ray absorptiometry (DEXA) scan, calcium and vitamin D supplementation, and bisphosphonate therapy
(E) Estrogen hormone replacement therapy

Item 33

A 55-year-old woman expresses concern about osteoporosis during a routine physical examination. Her mother had a hip fracture at the age of 55 years. The patient is healthy and exercises three times a week for 45 minutes at the gym. She eats a balanced diet and attempts to consume two servings of milk or yogurt a day. She attained menopause at age 40 years. She does not drink alcohol and has a 25-pack-year smoking history. The patient has hypertension that is treated with ramipril.

On physical examination, blood pressure is 120/70 mm Hg and BMI is 26. The remainder of the examination is unremarkable. All laboratory test results are normal.

Which of the following is the most appropriate evaluation for this patient?

(A) Dual-energy x-ray absorptiometry (DEXA) scan now
(B) Dual-energy x-ray absorptiometry (DEXA) scan at age 65 years
(C) Measurement of serum osteocalcin
(D) Measurement of urine pyridinoline and deoxypyridinoline
(E) Plain radiographs of the hips and lumbosacral spine

Chapter 2

Endocrinology and Metabolism

Answers and Critiques

Item 1   Answer: D

This patient presents with classic symptoms of a prolactinoma, i.e., amenorrhea and galactorrhea. Although the differential diagnosis for hyperprolactinemia is extensive, the most likely diagnosis in this patient is a prolactin-producing pituitary adenoma. It is critical to rule out pregnancy, as this is the most common physiologic reason for an elevated prolactin level. However, this patient is unlikely to be pregnant because she has had multiple negative pregnancy tests. Additionally, since she is otherwise healthy, it is unlikely that chronic renal failure is a cause of her elevated prolactin concentration. Two key clinical features that suggest a prolactinoma include the presence of headaches and a very high prolactin level. In general, prolactin levels greater than 100 to 200 ng/mL in a nonpregnant woman usually suggest a tumor instead of another cause.

Primary hypothyroidism is also important to consider, especially in women (who have a higher incidence of hypothyroidism than men). Primary hypothyroidism causes an elevation in prolactin concentration because thyrotropin-releasing hormone stimulates both thyroid-stimulating hormone and prolactin production from the pituitary gland. However, the most likely diagnosis for hyperprolactinemia in this patient is a pituitary tumor because she has had negative pregnancy tests, does not take any medications, has no symptoms to suggest chronic renal failure or hypothyroidism, and has a prolactin level >200 ng/mL.

KEY POINTS

- The classic characteristics of prolactinoma in a woman are amenorrhea and galactorrhea.

- Serum prolactin levels >200 ng/mL in a nonpregnant woman suggest a pituitary tumor.

Bibliography
1. **Schlechte JA.** Clinical practice. Prolactinoma. N Engl J Med. 2003;349:2035-41. [PMID: 14627789]

Item 2   Answer: C

Metformin accumulates in patients with renal insufficiency, which may lead to lactic acidosis. Therefore, because of the potential nephrotoxicity of radiocontrast agents, the current prescribing guidelines for metformin include strict precautions when radiographic procedures employing an intravenous contrast agent are performed. These procedures include pyelog-raphy, arteriography, venography, and CT studies. The recommendation is that metformin be stopped on the day of the study and resumed once renal function normalizes 24 to 48 hours after the procedure.

Pioglitazone, a thiazolidinedione, can be continued, as it will not predispose the patient to hypoglycemia during fasting. However, pioglitazone could also be withheld without any untoward effects because of its long duration of action.

KEY POINT

- Metformin, which accumulates in patients with renal insufficiency, should not be administered when any radiographic procedure using an intravenous contrast agent is performed.

Bibliography
1. **Setter SM, Iltz JL, Thams J, Campbell RK.** Metformin hydrochloride in the treatment of type 2 diabetes mellitus: a clinical review with a focus on dual therapy. Clin Ther. 2003;25:2991-3026. [PMID: 14749143]

Item 3   Answer: A

This patient's glucose control will improve by switching to insulin glargine at bedtime with three premeal injections of insulin lispro during the day. Generally, more complex regimens with more frequent injections of both short/rapid–acting and long/intermediate–acting insulins result in better glucose control, as long as the patient has the required motivation and capabilities. This patient has suboptimal glucose control on premixed (intermediate plus rapid-acting) insulin administered twice daily. Premixed insulins, although convenient, lack the more precise dosing flexibility of self-mixed or individually administered insulins. High glucose levels during the morning fasting period suggest the need for greater insulin exposure to a long-acting insulin during the night. However, the overnight hypoglycemic episodes prevent increasing the patient's premixed evening insulin dose. Indeed, these episodes likely reflect the peak action of the intermediate-acting insulin protamine lispro administered before dinner.

Increasing the dose of both the morning and the evening premixed insulin may result in better glucose levels during the day but will probably increase the hypoglycemic episodes overnight. Reducing caloric consumption is an inappropriate recommendation for a normal-weight person with type 1 diabetes, although proper food choices may improve control to some degree. This patient will derive the most benefit from switching to a regimen of the long-acting insulin glargine at bedtime, providing 24 hours of basal insulin, with three adjusted doses of the rapid-acting insulin lispro at mealtimes to prevent postprandial glucose excursions.

KEY POINT

- In patients with type 1 diabetes mellitus, fasting hyperglycemia is treated with an evening injection of a long-acting basal insulin such as glargine and postprandial hyperglycemia is controlled with multiple injections of a short-acting insulin such as lispro.

Bibliography

1. **Flood TM.** Appropriate use of insulin analogs in an increasingly complex type 2 diabetes mellitus (T2DM) landscape. J Fam Pract. 2007;56:S1-S10; [PMID: 17217893]

Item 4   Answer: D

The most appropriate test for this patient is a fasting plasma glucose measurement. The current American Diabetes Association criteria for the diagnosis of diabetes mellitus are a fasting plasma glucose level ≥126 mg/dL, a 2-hour plasma glucose level ≥200 mg/dL after a 75-g oral glucose load, or a random plasma glucose level ≥200 mg/dL plus symptoms of diabetes. If any of these tests is abnormal, the diagnosis must be confirmed on a subsequent day by repeating any of the three tests. The best test for this patient, who does not have symptoms and who already has a single elevated fasting glucose level, is to repeat the fasting glucose now. If the level exceeds 125 mg/dL on repeated testing, the diagnosis of diabetes mellitus is established.

While a 2-hour plasma glucose after a 75-g oral glucose load can establish the diagnosis of diabetes, it is not currently recommended as a diagnostic choice by the American Diabetes Association because of its inconvenience, difficulty in standardization, and potential risk to patients with existing fasting hyperglycemia. There are no hemoglobin A_{1c} criteria for the diagnosis of diabetes mellitus, although this test is extremely useful in assessing the degree of glucose control over the preceding 3 months. There is no role for measuring a plasma insulin level in the diagnosis of diabetes mellitus.

KEY POINT

- The American Diabetes Association criteria for the diagnosis of diabetes mellitus are a fasting plasma glucose ≥126 mg/dL, a 2-hour plasma glucose ≥200 mg/dL after a 75-g oral glucose load, or a random plasma glucose ≥200 mg/dL plus symptoms of diabetes.

Bibliography

1. American Diabetes Association. Diagnosis and classification of diabetes mellitus. Diabetes Care. 2007;30 Suppl 1:S42-7. [PMID: 17192378]

Item 5   Answer: C

This patient has impaired fasting glucose and impaired glucose tolerance. The American Diabetes Association and World Health Organization have similar classifications of the various glycemic abnormalities that are becoming increasingly com-

mon. Diabetes mellitus is now defined by a fasting plasma glucose level of ≥126 mg/dL or by a 2-hour plasma glucose level of ≥200 mg/dL during an oral glucose tolerance test (the oral glucose tolerance test is not recommended for routine clinical use by the American Diabetes Association). Alternatively, a "casual" (without respect to meals) plasma glucose level of ≥200 mg/dL, if accompanied by classic symptoms of hyperglycemia, may also be used to make the diagnosis. Prediabetes glycemic states consist of impaired glucose tolerance, defined as a 2-hour glucose level of 140–199 mg/dL during an oral glucose tolerance test, and impaired fasting glucose, defined as a fasting glucose level of 100–125 mg/dL.

This patient therefore has both impaired glucose tolerance and impaired fasting glucose. Both of these prediabetes states predispose a patient to type 2 diabetes mellitus; impaired glucose tolerance appears to be a stronger factor than impaired fasting glucose. When both are present, as in this patient, the risk is incrementally higher.

KEY POINT

- Prediabetes glycemic states consist of impaired glucose tolerance, defined as a 2-hour glucose level of 140–199 mg/dL during an oral glucose tolerance test, and impaired fasting glucose, defined as a fasting glucose level of 100–125 mg/dL.

Bibliography

1. American Diabetes Association. Standards of medical care in diabetes—2007. Diabetes Care. 2007;30 Suppl 1:S4-S41. [PMID: 17192377]

Item 6   Answer: B

The Diabetes Prevention Program showed that patients with impaired glucose tolerance, such as this patient has, can reduce their risk of developing type 2 diabetes mellitus by 58% with a conscientious lifestyle modification program consisting of diet, exercise, and weight loss. In the same study, metformin decreased the risk by 31%, although its use was associated with frequent diarrhea and flatulence. Rosiglitazone has been shown to reduce the incidence of type 2 diabetes by 62% in middle-aged, overweight men, although its use was associated with an increased frequency of edema (6.8%) and heart failure (0.5%). Acarbose has been shown to reduce the incidence of type 2 diabetes by 25%, but 31% of patients discontinued treatment because of side effects, primarily diarrhea and flatulence. Patients treated with the anti-obesity drug orlistat had a 44% reduced risk of developing diabetes as compared with patients treated with placebo, but approximately 25% of patients experienced drug-induced gastrointestinal side effects, especially after meals high in fat. In Hispanic women with previous gestational diabetes mellitus, troglitazone was shown to reduce the risk of developing type 2 diabetes mellitus by 55%, but neither pioglitazone nor rosiglitazone has yet been shown in published data to reduce the risk of diabetes in patients such as the one presented here. Similarly, there are no published data regarding early insulin therapy in this group.

Although metformin, rosiglitazone, acarbose, and orlistat have been shown to reduce the incidence of diabetes, their side effects must be considered before initiating treatment, and the long-term health benefits of early drug treatment remain unclear.

KEY POINT

- High-risk patients with impaired glucose tolerance can most effectively reduce their risk of developing type 2 diabetes mellitus with a conscientious lifestyle modification program consisting of diet, exercise, and weight loss.

Bibliography

1. **Gillies CL, Abrams KR, Lambert PC, Cooper NJ, Sutton AJ, Hsu RT, Khunti K.** Pharmacological and lifestyle interventions to prevent or delay type 2 diabetes in people with impaired glucose tolerance: systematic review and meta-analysis. BMJ. 2007;334:299. Epub 2007 Jan 19. [PMID: 17237299]

Item 7   Answer: E

This patient needs an increase in the basal insulin glargine dose. He is consistently having fasting and preprandial hyperglycemia, while his postprandial glucose excursions, although not perfect, are close to the desired excursion of 30 to 50 mg/dL. Fasting glucose levels, which are due primarily to excessive hepatic glucose production, are controlled mainly by the basal insulin dose. Pre-lunch, pre-dinner, and bedtime glucose values are controlled by both the basal insulin and the amount of short-acting insulin taken with the previous meal. Patients on basal bolus insulin therapy often take 40% to 50% of their total daily dose as basal insulin (glargine) and 50% to 60% as meal boluses (lispro or aspart). This patient is taking 33% of his insulin as glargine with inadequate fasting and preprandial glucose control. The best choice, therefore, is to increase his morning glargine dose. Reducing the glargine dose would only make the situation worse. Increasing mealtime short-acting insulin is not necessary because his postprandial excursions are not severe, while lowering the short-acting insulin doses might result in excessive excursions. NPH insulin, which peaks in the mid-afternoon, might improve mid-afternoon and late-afternoon glucose levels but would have no effect on the other periods of time when his glucose levels are high.

KEY POINT

- In patients with type 2 diabetes mellitus, fasting blood glucose levels, which are due primarily to excessive hepatic glucose production, are controlled mainly by the basal insulin dose.

Bibliography

1. **Hirsch IB.** Intensifying insulin therapy in patients with type 2 diabetes mellitus. Am J Med. 2005;118 Suppl 5A:21S-6S. [PMID: 15850550]

Item 8   Answer: D

The current American Diabetes Association recommended goals for management of adults with diabetes mellitus are as follows: hemoglobin A_{1c} <7.0%, preprandial glucose 90–130 mg/dL, 2-hour postprandial glucose <180 mg/dL, blood pressure <130/80 mm Hg, triglycerides <150 mg/dL, HDL cholesterol >40 mg/dL, and LDL cholesterol <100 mg/dL (but <70 mg/dL may be considered). Since this patient has a hemoglobin A_{1c} of 7.4%, the most appropriate change is to increase his anti-hyperglycemic medication. His blood pressure, triglycerides, LDL cholesterol, and HDL cholesterol are all below the recommended goal and therefore adding a fibrate or niacin or increasing the doses of lisinopril or atorvastatin is not necessary at this time.

KEY POINT

- The recommended goals for management of adults with diabetes mellitus are hemoglobin A_{1c} <7.0%, preprandial glucose 90–130 mg/dL, 2-hour postprandial glucose <180 mg/dL, blood pressure <130/80 mm Hg, triglycerides <150 mg/dL, HDL cholesterol >40 mg/dL, and LDL cholesterol <100 mg/dL.

Bibliography

1. American Diabetes Association. Standards of medical care in diabetes—2007. Diabetes Care. 2007;30 Suppl 1:S4-S41. [PMID: 17192377]

Item 9   Answer: A

Insulin is the only therapeutic agent listed that will control this patient's blood glucose levels adequately. Repaglinide, an insulin secretagogue, would add no benefit in a patient who is already on the maximal dose of a sulfonylurea. Metformin should not be used in men with creatinine levels >1.5 mg/dL or in women with creatinine levels >1.4 mg/dL and is also contraindicated in patients with advanced heart failure that may be associated with tissue ischemia due to poor cardiac output. A thiazolidinedione (such as pioglitazone) should not be used in patients with New York Heart Association class III congestive heart failure and will often cause worsening edema even in patients with less severe congestive heart failure. A combination of metformin and a thiazolidinedione may lower the hemoglobin A_{1c} adequately but should not be used for the reasons stated above for the individual agents.

KEY POINTS

- Metformin should not be used in men with creatinine levels >1.5 mg/dL or in women with creatinine levels >1.4 mg/dL.

- Metformin and thiazolidinediones should not be used in patients with New York Heart Association class III congestive heart failure.

Bibliography

1. **Hirsch IB.** Intensifying insulin therapy in patients with type 2 diabetes mellitus. Am J Med. 2005;118:21S-6S. [PMID: 15850550]

Item 10   Answer: B

The correct management step is to decrease glargine at bedtime. This patient is having significantly low blood glucose levels during the night and early morning with less severe low glucose levels throughout the day. Her highest glucose values also occur on arising each morning, possibly as a result of having low glucose levels at night. She is on basal bolus insulin therapy. The average patient with type 1 diabetes mellitus who does not have coexisting insulin resistance requires a total daily dose of about 0.4 to 0.5 units of insulin per kg of body weight. Most patients take 40% to 50% of their total daily dose as basal insulin (glargine) and 50% to 60% as meal boluses (lispro or aspart). This patient weighs 60 kg (132 lb) and would therefore have an anticipated total daily insulin dose of 24 to 30 units. However, she is currently taking 28 units of basal insulin and another 12 units as boluses. Her insulin dose may therefore be excessive and imbalanced because of excessive glargine. Therefore, her frequent hypoglycemia, which is most prominent during the night and early morning but which also occurs during the daytime, is most likely due to excessive bedtime glargine. Excessive lispro at dinner most often causes hypoglycemia 2 to 5 hours after dinner, rather than at 3 AM, and would not be expected to cause hypoglycemia during the day. Reducing her bedtime glargine is the most prudent initial adjustment to make. Once the hypoglycemia is corrected by lowering the bedtime glargine dose, preprandial and postprandial glucose monitoring will help to determine if her mealtime lispro doses should be adjusted.

KEY POINT

- The average patient with type 1 diabetes mellitus who does not have coexisting insulin resistance requires a total daily dose of about 0.4 to 0.5 units of insulin per kg of body weight with 40% to 50% delivered as long-acting basal insulin.

Bibliography
1. **Hirsch IB.** Insulin analogues. N Engl J Med. 2005;352:174-83. [PMID: 15647580]

Item 11   Answer: D

The most appropriate change in this patient's medical program is to add short-acting insulin (lispro or aspart) with meals. This patient is having significant postprandial hyperglycemia. Postprandial glucose excursions should ideally be limited to 30 to 50 mg/dL above premeal glucose values. This patient should do more postprandial glucose testing, but the values she has obtained so far show excursions much greater than 50 mg/dL above premeal values. This can be best corrected by using a bolus of short-acting insulin (lispro or aspart) just before or with each meal.

Acarbose is not effective enough to reduce postprandial glucose excursions sufficiently in this situation. Bedtime NPH insulin is used mainly to lower elevated fasting glucose levels, which are not a problem in this patient. Morning NPH insulin would provide a peak in mid-afternoon, but the NPH peak would not occur at a completely reliable time and would also

not cover breakfast or dinner. Since glargine is a basal insulin, increasing the dose would still not provide the post-meal insulin peaks that are required to control postprandial hyperglycemia.

KEY POINT

- Significant postprandial hyperglycemia can be managed by using a bolus of short-acting insulin (lispro or aspart) just before or with each meal.

Bibliography
1. **Hirsch IB.** Intensifying insulin therapy in patients with type 2 diabetes mellitus. Am J Med. 2005;118 Suppl 5A:21S-6S. [PMID: 15850550]

Item 12   Answer: A

This patient will do better by adding metformin to the glimepiride. Progressive β-cell dysfunction is common in patients with type 2 diabetes mellitus. With increasing duration of disease, patients whose disease was initially well controlled with one drug ultimately require more aggressive therapy. Antihyperglycemic agents with distinct mechanisms of action have additive effects on glucose levels. As a result, when necessary, they should be used in combination.

Clinical trials have shown that increasing sulfonylurea doses beyond half the maximal dosing range has minimal further benefit on hyperglycemia. Therefore, increasing the glimepiride dose is unlikely to help this patient very much. Moreover, substituting one class of drug for another typically does not provide any long-term benefit. Therefore, stopping glimepiride and starting either metformin or a thiazolidinedione as monotherapy would not be the most appropriate action at this time. Instead, adding one class of drug to another is the current favored approach in a patient with progressive hyperglycemia despite monotherapy. Accordingly, adding either metformin or a thiazolidinedione, such as pioglitazone, is the preferred approach in this patient.

KEY POINTS

- Adding one class of drug to another is indicated for patients with type 2 diabetes mellitus and progressive hyperglycemia despite monotherapy.
- Increasing sulfonylurea doses beyond half the maximal dosing range has minimal further benefits on treating hyperglycemia.

Bibliography
1. **Chipkin SR.** How to select and combine oral agents for patients with type 2 diabetes mellitus. Am J Med. 2005;118 Suppl 5A:4S-13S. [PMID: 15850548]

Item 13   Answer: B

This patient has diabetes secondary to pancreatic disease. Diabetes may be the direct result of other underlying disease states, in which case it is referred to as "secondary diabetes." Potentiating conditions include other endocrinopathies, such as Cushing's syndrome, acromegaly, pheochromocytoma, and hyperthyroidism. Rarely, islet cell neoplasms, such as glucagonoma and somatostatinoma, lead to diabetes. Medications, such as glucocorticoids, may lead to diabetes as well. Disorders of the exocrine pancreas can also manifest as hyperglycemia as a result of, among other things, direct damage to the pancreatic islet cells. These conditions include acute or chronic pancreatitis, pancreatic malignancies, and cystic fibrosis. The patient's recent hospitalization showed convincing evidence of pancreatitis. Therefore, his condition should be classified as secondary diabetes. Treatment may be challenging. Sulfonylureas may be effective, depending on the number of functioning islet cells remaining. Insulin sensitizers have no role in treating this patient's secondary diabetes. He may eventually require insulin. Unfortunately, patients with pancreatic disease and diabetes may be quite labile regarding glycemic control, since they often lack adequate glucagon secretion for counterregulation.

Type 1 diabetes mellitus is the result of islet cell destruction due to autoimmunity. Type 2 diabetes mellitus culminates from the combination of both insulin resistance and relative insulin deficiency and comprises more than 90% of all cases of diabetes worldwide. Gestational diabetes is diagnosed during pregnancy and has a similar pathogenesis to that of type 2 diabetes. The form of diabetes recently called latent autoimmune diabetes of adulthood (LADA) occurs in patients with type 2 diabetes who develop insulin requirements later in life and exhibit labile glycemic tendencies and many of the autoimmune markers that occur in those with type 1 diabetes. LADA involves slowly progressive loss of β-cell function and usually occurs in lean, older patients.

KEY POINT

- Secondary diabetes mellitus is the direct result of other underlying disease states.

Bibliography

1. American Diabetes Association. Diagnosis and classification of diabetes mellitus. Diabetes Care. 2007;30 Suppl 1:S42-7. [PMID: 17192378]

Item 14   Answer: A

Therapy with a sulfonylurea such as glyburide is indicated for this patient. Drug treatment for type 2 diabetes mellitus is initiated when diet and exercise have failed or are likely to fail because of the degree of hyperglycemia, or when there are symptoms secondary to hyperglycemia. The goal of therapy is a hemoglobin A_{1c} value less than 7%. This patient has a value of 7.3% despite 8 months of diet and exercise. Although these lifestyle interventions should be continued, they are unlikely to lead to further reduction in blood glucose levels, and pharmacologic therapy is therefore indicated.

In the past decade, more than 12 new medications for type 2 diabetes have become available. Initial pharmacologic therapy for type 2 diabetes is generally an oral agent. There are few differences in outcomes with different drug classes, and patient characteristics and preferences help guide the initial choice of agent. For example, in obese patients the use of metformin as a first-line agent may reduce cardiovascular events and all-cause mortality, although these findings remain controversial. Stepped therapy with bedtime insulin is effective in achieving glycemic targets in patients for whom oral agents alone are ineffective; insulin also effectively controls the disease in a substantial proportion of patients for whom oral therapy is unsuccessful. In patients in whom insulin therapy is started, current oral therapy (metformin or the thiazolidinedione pioglitazone) should be continued.

For the choice of oral therapy, it is also important to understand the relative and absolute contraindications for each medication. Metformin is contraindicated in patients with renal insufficiency, defined as a serum creatinine concentration >1.6 mg/dL in men and >1.5 mg/dL in women. Metformin may increase the risk of lactic acidosis in such patients. This patient has a serum creatinine concentration of 1.9 mg/dL, precluding use of metformin. A thiazolidinedione pioglitazone is also contraindicated because of the patient's heart failure. Thiazolidinediones increase fluid retention and can lead to decompensated heart failure. Metformin is also commonly avoided in patients with advanced heart failure because of the increased risk of tissue ischemia and lactic acidosis related to decreased cardiac output.

KEY POINTS

- Metformin is contraindicated in patients with type 2 diabetes mellitus and renal insufficiency.
- Thiazolidinediones are contraindicated in patients with type 2 diabetes mellitus and heart failure.

Bibliography

1. **Nathan DM.** Clinical practice. Initial management of glycemia in type 2 diabetes mellitus. N Engl J Med. 2002;347:1342-9. [PMID: 12397193]

Item 15   Answer: D

Nausea, vomiting, and abdominal pain are common presentations of diabetic ketoacidosis and may be explained by the combination of dehydration, hyperkalemia, ketonemia, and delayed gastric emptying. Typically, the abdominal pain resolves with rehydration. Diabetic ketoacidosis may occur during superimposed acute infections, such as influenza, pneumonia, or gastroenteritis, especially in patients who do not follow "sick day" rules and inappropriately stop insulin because they are not eating; who use insulin pumps when the insulin infusion is technically interrupted; or who are noncompliant. Noncompliance is generally a problem in teenagers and in substance abusers. In almost all cases, diabetic ketoacidosis is preventable by a well-educated patient who is compliant with glucose monitoring and understands the need for increased insulin doses during stress.

Acute pancreatitis typically presents with abdominal pain, nausea, and vomiting but is unlikely in this patient based upon the normal amylase and lipase concentrations. The symptoms of alcoholic hepatitis are typical of many acute liver diseases and include jaundice, anorexia, weight loss, fever, and abdominal pain usually confined to the right upper quadrant. The absence of fever, jaundice, and localized pain and the normal aminotransferase levels make alcoholic hepatitis unlikely in this patient. Although alcoholic ketoacidosis can mimic diabetic ketoacidosis, the blood glucose concentration is the key in differentiating these disorders. If blood glucose is normal or low in the presence of ketonemia and metabolic acidosis, alcoholic ketoacidosis is likely.

KEY POINT

• Nausea, vomiting, and abdominal pain are common presentations of diabetic ketoacidosis.

Bibliography
1. Umpierrez G, Freire AX. Abdominal pain in patients with hyperglycemic crises. J Crit Care. 2002;17:63-7. [PMID: 12040551]

Item 16   Answer: A

This patient should be started on an angiotensin-converting enzyme (ACE) inhibitor. Currently, ACE inhibitors are indicated in the treatment of diabetic patients with hypertension. Randomized clinical trials have demonstrated their benefit on both cardiovascular disease endpoints and the progression of diabetic nephropathy. They are typically well tolerated. ACE inhibitors are also indicated for the treatment of albuminuria, both with and without hypertension. In this setting, ACE inhibitor therapy has been shown to reduce albuminuria and its progression. Angiotensin receptor blockers (ARBs) are likely to be effective as well, although data are lacking for patients with type 1 diabetes. The American Diabetes Association recommends either an ACE inhibitor or an ARB in the treatment of micro- and macroalbuminuria, except during pregnancy.

This patient's glucose control is already at target, and therefore improving glucose control will not likely improve urine albumin excretion. Calcium channel blockers are not recommended for the treatment of albuminuria in patients with normal blood pressure, although the nondihydropyridine calcium channel blockers (diltiazem and verapamil) may reduce proteinuria, and may be used in the management of hypertension in patients unable to tolerate an ACE inhibitor or an ARB. Continued observation without initiating an ACE inhibitor will result in more rapid progression of diabetic nephropathy.

KEY POINT

• Angiotensin-converting enzyme inhibitors reduce albuminuria and retard the progression of renal disease in diabetic patients with and without hypertension.

Bibliography
1. American Diabetes Association. Standards of medical care in diabetes—2007. Diabetes Care. 2007;30:S4-S41. [PMID: 17192377]

Item 17   Answer: C

The best initial treatment for this patient is normal saline infusion followed by intravenous insulin infusion. She has hyperglycemic hyperosmolar syndrome, previously referred to as hyperglycemic hyperosmolar nonketotic syndrome. This state develops over several days and is typically due to marked hyperglycemia in the setting of a medical stressor, such as infection. Free water and sodium losses can be dramatic, and patients are usually markedly volume contracted. This patient's physical examination, especially the hypotension and tachycardia, suggest marked volume deficits in the extracellular fluid space (i.e., sodium losses). The serum sodium concentration is an excellent marker of free water deficits. Although normal on admission, the sodium concentration belies actual free water deficit because it requires correction for the degree of hyperglycemia. Conventionally, 1.6 meq/L of sodium should be added to the measured sodium for every 100 mg/dL of glucose exceeding 100 mg/dL. Therefore, in this patient, the "corrected" serum sodium is actually 163 meq/L. Such hypernatremia is indicative of significant superimposed free water losses. Correction of this patient's deficits requires repletion with both normal saline crystalloid and free water. The preservation of vascular volume remains paramount, however. Therefore, normal saline (0.9% NaCl) should be the initial fluid of choice. After the volume deficit is corrected, the free water deficit may be corrected with administration of half-normal saline or free water. Intravenous insulin should be given to normalize this patient's blood glucose, but the most immediate concern is administration of intravenous fluids to correct hypotension. Dopamine is not an appropriate treatment of hypovolemic shock.

KEY POINT

• In patients with hyperglycemic hyperosmolar syndrome, the preservation of vascular volume is critical, and normal saline is the initial fluid of choice, even before intravenous insulin.

Bibliography
1. Kitabchi AE, Umpierrez GE, Murphy MB, Barrett EJ, Kreisberg RA, Malone JI, et al. Hyperglycemic crises in diabetes. Diabetes Care. 2004;27 Suppl 1:S94-102. [PMID: 14693938]

Item 18   Answer: B

Diabetes mellitus is a coronary artery disease equivalent in this patient. Lipid-lowering therapy is most beneficial in patients with coronary artery disease equivalents, which include clinical coronary artery disease, symptomatic carotid artery disease, peripheral artery disease, abdominal aortic aneurysm, diabetes mellitus, and a Framingham risk score >20%. These states are considered equivalent to having coronary artery disease and are associated with a high risk for future coronary events. Lipid-lowering goals in patients with one of these conditions are the same as in patients with a previous myocardial infarction. In patients with established coronary artery disease or a coronary artery disease equivalent, LDL cholesterol should be decreased to <100 mg/dL; an optional LDL cholesterol goal for the highest-risk patients is <70 mg/dL.

Cigarette smoking and hypertension are risk factors for the development of coronary events. These factors, as well as age (≥45 years for men; ≥55 years for women), HDL cholesterol levels <40 mg/dL, and a family history of premature coronary artery disease are used to estimate risk and to determine subsequent LDL cholesterol goals but are not coronary artery disease equivalents.

KEY POINTS

- Diabetes mellitus is considered a coronary artery disease equivalent for establishing LDL cholesterol treatment goals.

- In patients with coronary artery disease or a coronary artery disease equivalent, LDL cholesterol should be decreased to <100 mg/dL with an optional goal of <70 mg/dL in the highest-risk patients.

Bibliography

1. **Expert Panel on Detection, Evaluation, and Treatment of High Blood Cholesterol in Adults.** Executive Summary of The Third Report of The National Cholesterol Education Program (NCEP) Expert Panel on Detection, Evaluation, And Treatment of High Blood Cholesterol In Adults (Adult Treatment Panel III). JAMA. 2001;285:2486-97. [PMID: 11368702]

Item 19   Answer: D

This patient's thyroid-stimulating hormone level should be measured because she is experiencing symptoms consistent with hypothyroidism. Elevated cholesterol levels, which can occur in hypothyroidism, may reverse after thyroid replacement.

She is at low risk for coronary artery disease based on her risk factors. If she does not have hypothyroidism, her LDL cholesterol and triglyceride levels necessitate institution of therapeutic lifestyle changes as a first-step approach. A statin would be an option in this patient if diet and exercise were ineffective in reducing her cholesterol values to acceptable levels. Fibric acid derivatives are most effective in patients with mainly elevated triglyceride levels not responding to diet and exercise. Fish oil supplements are not recommended for treatment of hyperlipidemia because no evidence indicates that they reduce mortality or morbidity.

KEY POINT

- Hypothyroidism may be an underlying cause of elevated cholesterol levels, and thyroid replacement therapy can reverse this finding.

Bibliography

1. **Stone NJ.** Secondary causes of hyperlipidemia. Med Clin North Am. 1994;78:117-41. [PMID: 8283927]

Item 20   Answer: C

This patient should be advised to have her cholesterol levels re-measured in 5 years. The National Cholesterol Education Program (NCEP) has recommended a nine-step procedure for identifying and treating patients at risk for coronary artery disease (CAD). The first three steps are pertinent to this patient. After cholesterol numbers are checked (Step 1), the presence of CAD or CAD equivalents (Step 2) should be established. The definition of CAD includes myocardial infarction, unstable angina, coronary artery procedures, or evidence of myocardial ischemia. CAD equivalents include diabetes mellitus, symptomatic carotid artery disease, peripheral artery disease, and abdominal aortic aneurysm.

Because this patient does not have CAD or CAD equivalents, the next step (Step 3) is to determine if she has any other risk factors, other than the increased LDL cholesterol level, for CAD. These risk factors include cigarette smoking, hypertension (blood pressure >140/90 mm Hg or taking an antihypertensive medication), low HDL cholesterol levels (<40 mg/dL), family history of premature CAD (male first-degree relative <55 years; female first-degree relative <65 years), and age (men >45 years; women >55 years). This patient's only risk factor is her age. She is therefore at low risk for CAD. The Adult Treatment Panel of the NCEP does not recommend further treatment for her cholesterol, and her cholesterol levels should be followed regularly.

A diet that is rich in plant stanols or sterols, recommended among other therapeutic lifestyle changes to lower cholesterol, is indicated for patients who have a higher risk for CAD than this patient. Treatment with either a statin or niacin is also recommended for patients at higher risk for CAD than this patient.

KEY POINT

- Cholesterol monitoring is indicated once every 5 years in patients with ≤1 risk factor for coronary artery disease.

Bibliography

1. **Stone NJ, Bilek S, Rosenbaum S.** Recent National Cholesterol Education Program Adult Treatment Panel III update: adjustments and options. Am J Cardiol. 2005;96:53E-59E. [PMID: 16098845]

Item 21   Answer: B

This patient has subclinical hyperthyroidism, which is defined as having a low or undetectable thyroid-stimulating hormone (TSH) level with free T_4 and total T_3 or free T_3 values that are still within the reference ranges. Patients older than 60 years with subclinical hyperthyroidism and undetectable TSH values have been shown to have a 3-fold increased risk of developing atrial fibrillation. In this woman, who is 54 years old and asymptomatic, periodic monitoring of symptoms and thyroid function is indicated.

Thyroiditis is characterized by low TSH levels, normal or high free T_4 and T_3 levels, a nontender thyroid gland, and reduced radioiodine uptake. The disorder is due to a transient lymphocytic inflammatory process of the thyroid gland. The radioiodine uptake of 38% in this patient excludes the diagnosis of thyroiditis. Surreptitious thyroid ingestion would suppress the TSH level and would also suppress radioiodine uptake and visualization of the tracer on the thyroid scan. In response to a severe nonthyroidal illness, total T3 and free T3 levels decrease, reverse T3 levels increase, and the TSH level is variable (low, normal, or high). The absence of illness in this patient makes this diagnosis unlikely.

KEY POINT

- Subclinical hyperthyroidism is characterized by a low or undetectable thyroid-stimulating hormone level and normal free T_4 and total T_3 or free T_3 values.

Bibliography

1. Surks MI, Ortiz E, Daniels GH, Sawin CT, Col NF, Cobin RH, et al. Subclinical thyroid disease: scientific review and guidelines for diagnosis and management. JAMA. 2004;291:228-38. [PMID: 14722150]

Item 22   Answer: D

This patient has myxedema coma, a rare disorder characterized by progressive obtundation, hypothermia, hypotension, and bradycardia. A precipitating event, such as infection, trauma, cold exposure, or use of sedatives, is generally present. Most cases of myxedema coma occur in elderly women and are more likely to occur during the winter. The diagnosis is made clinically, and there are many clues in this case history, including numerous physical examination findings of hypothyroidism and a thyroidectomy scar. Since infection is a common precipitant of myxedema coma, pan-cultures and empiric antibiotic therapy with broad-spectrum antibiotics are generally recommended. Corticosteroids are given prophylactically in case of concurrent adrenal insufficiency, which might otherwise become manifest as replacement thyroid hormone therapy is begun. The diagnosis can be confirmed by serum thyroid hormone studies.

Intracerebral hemorrhage, meningitis, and hypoglycemia are all potential causes of coma, but none of these entities is likely to produce the constellation of hypothermia, hypotension, hyponatremia, and bradycardia.

KEY POINT

- Myxedema coma is a rare disorder characterized by progressive obtundation, hypothermia, hypotension, and bradycardia and is typically precipitated by infection, trauma, cold exposure, or use of sedatives.

Bibliography

1. Savage MW, Mah PM, Weetman AP, Newell-Price J. Endocrine emergencies. Postgrad Med J. 2004;80:506-15. [PMID: 15356351]

Item 23   Answer: D

This patient has central hypothyroidism, and her thyroid hormone (levothyroxine) dose should be increased to normalize the free T_4 level and alleviate signs and symptoms of hypothyroidism. The thyroid-stimulating hormone (TSH) level cannot be used to monitor thyroid hormone replacement therapy in patients with central hypothyroidism. In these patients, the pituitary thyrotropes are absent, and the TSH level is always low, regardless of the level of circulating thyroid hormone. It is not uncommon to decrease the thyroid hormone dose in such patients because the suppressed TSH appears to suggest hormone overreplacement. The goal of thyroid hormone replacement in these patients is to titrate the dose to normalize the free T_4 level (or total T_4 concentration and free T_4 index), not to normalize the TSH level.

The hydrocortisone dose does not need to be reduced because this patient does not have any clinical signs to suggest overreplacement (central obesity, hypertension, acne, hirsutism). Similarly, the desmopressin dose should not be altered because her symptoms are controlled on her current dose and she has normal electrolyte values. Finally, the patient is doing well on oral contraceptives, and there is no reason to discontinue them; in addition, they will help prevent the development of osteopenia/osteoporosis induced by hypogonadism.

KEY POINT

- The thyroid-stimulating hormone level cannot be used to monitor thyroid hormone replacement therapy in patients with central hypothyroidism.

Bibliography

1. Clarke N, Kabadi UM. Optimizing treatment of hypothyroidism. Treat Endocrinol. 2004;3:217-21. [PMID: 16026104]

Item 24   Answer: D

This patient's levothyroxine dosage should be increased. On average, a 30% to 40% increase in levothyroxine dosage is required during pregnancy to maintain a euthyroid state. This increased demand may occur early in pregnancy, often before a patient's pregnancy is confirmed. If the thyroid gland is functional, increased pituitary demand stimulates increased thyroid hormone production, and no biochemical abnormality is detected. In hypothyroid patients, the thyroid gland cannot adapt to pituitary stimulation, and the levothyroxine replacement must be increased. Normally, a 30% to 40% dosage increase is initially provided, and thyroid-stimulating hormone (TSH) testing should be repeated in 2 to 4 weeks. Frequent monitoring of thyroid function during pregnancy is important because children born to mothers with elevated TSH levels have been shown to have lower intelligence.

Levothyroxine is converted to triiodothyronine by peripheral tissues at an appropriate rate for overall metabolic needs. Levothyroxine effectively relieves symptoms and normalizes serum TSH levels in most patients with hypothyroidism and is the replacement hormone of choice. Combined levothyroxine/triiodothyronine products contain a higher ratio of tri-iodothyronine to thyroxine (1:4) than is present in normal thyroid secretions. Triiodothyronine in these preparations is rapidly absorbed into the circulation and may result in supra-physiologic serum triiodothyronine levels for several hours after administration. This action may be particularly hazardous to some patients, including those with underlying coronary artery disease, and is not recommended.

KEY POINT

• Thyroid hormone requirement increases during pregnancy by 30% to 40%.

Bibliography

1. Alexander EK, Marqusee E, Lawrence J, Jarolim P, Fischer GA, Larsen PR. Timing and magnitude of increases in levothyroxine requirements during pregnancy in women with hypothyroidism. N Engl J Med. 2004;351:241-9. [PMID: 15254282]

Item 25   Answer: C

This patient has postpartum thyroiditis, a condition that occurs following 5% to 15% of pregnancies. It is characterized by thy-rotoxicosis, a nontender thyroid gland, and reduced radioio-dine uptake (and therefore no visualization of uptake) on the thyroid scan. The disorder is due to a transient lymphocytic inflammatory process of the thyroid gland. There is typically a 2- to 4-month period of thyrotoxicosis due to leakage of preformed thyroid hormone from the damaged follicles, fol-lowed by a 2- to 4-month period of hypothyroidism due to depletion of stored thyroid hormone in the thyroid gland and continued inflammation that prevents new thyroid hormone synthesis. After 6 to 9 months, 75% of patients recover and are euthyroid, whereas about 25% develop permanent hypothy-roidism. β-Blockers to reduce thyrotoxic symptoms are the most appropriate therapy during the hyperthyroid phase.

The distinction between low and high radioactive iodine uptake (RAIU) thyrotoxicosis assists in determining the cause of thyrotoxicosis, thereby guiding the selection of appropri-ate therapy and prompting surveillance for associated condi-tions (i.e., ophthalmopathy or autoimmune disease involving other endocrine glands in patients with Graves' disease). There is a critical distinction between thyrotoxicosis due to hormone release from a damaged thyroid gland in patients with spo-radic, postpartum, or subacute thyroiditis (suppressed iodine uptake) and that due to excess thyroid hormone production due to Graves' disease, toxic multinodular goiter, or autonomous thyroid nodules (elevated iodine uptake). Graves' disease is associated with a diffusely enlarged thyroid gland, ele-vated iodine uptake, and a thyroid scan demonstrating homo-geneous uptake of the tracer. Toxic multinodular goiter is rec-ognized by a goiter that is nodular to palpation, an elevated iodine uptake, and a thyroid scan demonstrating heteroge-neous uptake of the tracer. A hyperfunctioning adenomatous thyroid nodule is palpable on thyroid examination, is associ-ated with increased iodine uptake, and a thyroid scan that localizes the adenoma as a "hot" focus.

KEY POINTS

• In patients with hyperthyroidism, a radioiodine uptake study and thyroid scan can distinguish between Graves' disease, multinodular goiter, hyperfunctioning adenoma, and thyroiditis.

• Thyroiditis is characterized by thyrotoxicosis, a nontender thy-roid gland, absent radioiodine uptake, and no visualization of tracer on the thyroid scan.

Bibliography

1. Casey BM, Leveno KJ. Thyroid disease in pregnancy. Obstet Gynecol. 2006;108:1283-92. [PMID: 17077257]

Item 26   Answer: A

The most appropriate treatment for this patient is atenolol. He has developed silent thyroiditis, an autoimmune disorder characterized by high levels of antithyroid peroxidase anti-bodies and painless enlargement of the thyroid gland. Silent thyroiditis has a triphasic course with early thyrotoxicosis (damage phase), followed by hypothyroidism (healing phase), and then a return to euthyroidism (recovery phase) in most patients. Mild thyrotoxicosis may not require treatment, but if symptoms of tachycardia or palpitations are present, β-blocker therapy may be helpful. Mild transient hypothyroidism also may not require treatment, but if the patient is sympto-matic or if the phase is prolonged or permanent, thyroid hor-mone replacement should be given.

The clinical data in this patient support thyroiditis rather than Graves' disease because the radioactive iodine uptake is low, as is typical of thyroiditis, rather than high, as in Graves' dis-ease.

β-Adrenergic blockade is indicated to control this patient's rapid pulse, but the other treatment options are not indicated or useful. Specifically, antithyroid drugs such as methimazole, which block new thyroid hormone synthesis, and radioiodine ablation, which destroys overactive thyroid tissue, will not pro-vide benefit in a patient with thyroiditis, since the responsible mechanism is leakage of thyroid hormone from a damaged gland. Prednisone therapy is useful in patients with severe thy-roiditis, particularly subacute (painful) thyroiditis, but is not generally required in patients with silent thyroiditis. Thy-roidectomy is not indicated for this disorder, as most patients have a spontaneous recovery of normal thyroid function.

KEY POINTS

• Silent thyroiditis is an autoimmune disorder characterized by high levels of antithyroid peroxidase antibodies, painless enlargement of the thyroid gland, and a triphasic course with early thyrotoxicosis followed by hypothyroidism and then a return to euthyroidism in most patients.

• The main treatment for symptomatic thyroiditis is β-adrenergic blockade.

Bibliography

1. Pearce EN. Diagnosis and management of thyrotoxicosis. BMJ. 2006;332:1369-73. [PMID: 16763249]

Item 27   Answer: A

This patient most likely has adrenal insufficiency (Addison's disease). Her hypothyroidism due to autoimmune (Hashimoto's) thyroiditis was previously well controlled on a stable dose of levothyroxine. She currently has a low-normal free T$_4$ level and a minimally elevated thyroid-stimulating hormone (TSH) level, but this degree of elevation is not sufficient to explain her malaise, fatigue, and weight loss. Patients with Hashimoto's thyroiditis are at risk for other autoimmune endocrine disorders, including adrenal insufficiency, pernicious anemia, type 1 diabetes mellitus, vitiligo, and premature ovarian failure. Adrenal insufficiency is the best explanation for this patient's hyperkalemia, mild hypercalcemia, orthostatic hypotension, and hyperpigmentation, as well as the presenting signs and symptoms of fatigue, malaise, and weight loss. The concurrence of autoimmune thyroid disease and Addison's disease is known as Schmidt's syndrome. An isolated elevation in TSH has also been described in patients with adrenal insufficiency as a result of an absence of the suppressive effect of cortisol upon TSH synthesis and release from the anterior pituitary. None of the other options sufficiently explains all of the patient's symptoms, physical findings, and laboratory values.

KEY POINT

- Patients with Hashimoto's thyroiditis are at risk for other autoimmune endocrine disorders, including adrenal insufficiency (Addison's disease), pernicious anemia, type 1 diabetes mellitus, vitiligo, and premature ovarian failure.

Bibliography
1. **Majeroni BA, Patel P.** Autoimmune polyglandular syndrome, type II. Am Fam Physician. 2007;75:667-70. [PMID: 17375512]

Item 28   Answer: A

This patient most likely has adrenal insufficiency and requires urgent corticosteroid replacement therapy. This patient's signs and symptoms (malaise and fatigue, orthostatic dizziness, and persistent hypotension following minor surgery) strongly suggest adrenal insufficiency. An abnormal cosyntropin (ACTH) stimulation test established the diagnosis of adrenal insufficiency. A rise in the serum cortisol level ≥23 µg/dL following stimulation is strong evidence against primary adrenal insufficiency; failure to rise to this level supports a diagnosis of adrenal insufficiency. A subsequent measurement of the ACTH level will indicate whether the patient has primary adrenal insufficiency (elevated ACTH [Addison's disease]) or central adrenal insufficiency (normal or low ACTH).

MRI of the head or abdominal imaging is premature until results of the ACTH measurement are known. Furthermore, the first priority is to stabilize the patient with corticosteroid replacement to prevent catastrophic cardiovascular collapse. The patient was afebrile with no evidence of sepsis as a cause of his hypotension, and empiric antibiotics are therefore not indicated.

KEY POINTS

- The cosyntropin (ACTH) stimulation test is used to establish the diagnosis of adrenal insufficiency.
- The first priority in suspected adrenal insufficiency is to stabilize the patient with corticosteroid replacement to prevent catastrophic cardiovascular collapse.

Bibliography
1. **Dorin RI, Qualls CR, Crapo LM.** Diagnosis of adrenal insufficiency. Ann Intern Med. 2003;139:194-204. Erratum in: Ann Intern Med. 2004;140:315. [PMID: 12899587]

Item 29   Answer: A

The most appropriate next diagnostic study for this patient is a CT scan of the adrenal glands. In men, excessive production of glucocorticoids causes hypogonadotropic hypogonadism with diminished libido and loss of secondary sexual characteristics, in conjunction with commonly recognized manifestations of Cushing's syndrome (truncal obesity, round facies, acne, easy bruising, purple striae). An elevated 24-hour urine free cortisol concentration with an undetectable ACTH level strongly suggests an ACTH-independent source of cortisol. Therefore, CT imaging of the adrenal glands with thin sections through the glands is most appropriate.

MRI of the pituitary gland is not indicated because suppressed ACTH concentration would suggest an autonomous adrenal source of cortisol. Serum luteinizing hormone, prolactin, and testosterone concentrations are assessed in patients with erectile dysfunction when cortisol excess is not suspected, but are not indicated in this patient at this time. Hemoglobin A$_{1c}$ indicates glycemic control but cannot explain the excess production of cortisol and suppressed ACTH level. Ultrasonography of the testes is a useful diagnostic test when assessing acute testicular pain or mass. However, this patient's genitalia examination was normal, and testicular ultrasonography is not indicated.

KEY POINTS

- In men, Cushing's syndrome can cause hypogonadotropic hypogonadism with diminished libido and loss of secondary sexual characteristics.
- In ACTH-independent Cushing's syndrome, imaging of the adrenal glands is the next diagnostic step.

Bibliography
1. **Lindsay JR, Nieman LK.** Differential diagnosis and imaging in Cushing's syndrome. Endocrinol Metab Clin North Am. 2005;34:403-21, x. [PMID: 15850850]

Item 30   Answer: A

The most appropriate diagnostic test for this patient is a 24-hour urine collection for cortisol. Clinical suspicion for Cushing's syndrome is high in this patient based upon her history of recent diabetes mellitus and weight gain and physical examination findings that include hypertension, central obesity, acne, hirsutism, and purple striae. Initial testing for Cushing's syndrome relies on demonstration of excess cortisol production. Urine collected for 24 hours contains the excreted cortisol that is not bound to cortisol binding–globulin (urine free cortisol). Patients with Cushing's syndrome produce three to four times the amount of urine free cortisol that unaffected persons produce, and this test is often the first test in patients with a strong clinical suspicion for Cushing's syndrome. Renal insufficiency may decrease excretion of free cortisol, causing a false-negative test.

Another test to screen for Cushing's syndrome is the overnight dexamethasone suppression test (not included in the options listed above), which depends on suppression of hypothalamus/pituitary function by synthetic glucocorticoid that will not cross-react with cortisol assays. Dexamethasone, 1 mg, administered orally at 11 PM, is adequate to suppress ACTH (and subsequently cortisol) production by the normal central axis, but not by corticotropin-producing pituitary adenomas or cortisol-producing adrenal adenomas. Cortisol levels measured at 8 AM will be suppressed in normal persons but not in patients with Cushing's syndrome. Drugs such as anti-epileptic agents may interfere with hepatic metabolism of dexamethasone and result in false-positive results.

Although loss of diurnal variation in cortisol secretion is one of the first manifestations of Cushing's syndrome, cortisol levels obtained at 4 PM are not sensitive or specific for the diagnosis of the condition. An ACTH concentration determined at 8 AM is useful only after excess cortisol production has been documented and helps differentiate between ACTH-dependent (pituitary or ectopic) and ACTH-independent (adrenal adenoma, carcinoma, or macronodular hyperplasia) Cushing's syndrome. An MRI of the head should be performed only after biochemical confirmation of excess cortisol secretion and an elevated ACTH concentration have been confirmed.

KEY POINT

- Two common screening tests for Cushing's syndrome are measurement of urine free cortisol and the overnight dexamethasone suppression test.

Bibliography
1. **Findling JW, Raff H.** Screening and diagnosis of Cushing's syndrome. Endocrinol Metab Clin North Am. 2005;34:385-402, ix-x. [PMID: 15850849]

Item 31   Answer: C

This patient has had recent vertebral compression fractures in response to minimal or no trauma. Osteoporosis is diagnosed by the presence of fragility fractures, whenever present, or by a bone mineral density (BMD) value <–2.5 in patients who have not experienced a fragility fracture. Osteopenia is defined as a BMD value that is between 1 and 2.5 SD below the young adult mean. In all patients, the presence of a fragility fracture takes priority over BMD results in regard to diagnosing osteoporosis. This patient has also had an evaluation for causes of secondary bone loss. The normal serum calcium, phosphorus, and alkaline phosphatase values and normal urine calcium excretion do not suggest the presence of osteomalacia. Paget's disease, which is not a cause of low bone mass, is nonetheless ruled out by the normal alkaline phosphatase measurement.

KEY POINT

- Osteoporosis is diagnosed by the presence of fragility fractures or by a bone mineral density value <–2.5 in patients who have not experienced a fragility fracture.

Bibliography
1. **Raisz LG.** Clinical practice. Screening for osteoporosis. N Engl J Med. 2005;353:164-71. [PMID: 16014886]

Item 32   Answer: D

The best management for this patient is a dual-energy x-ray absorptiometry (DEXA) scan, calcium and vitamin D supplementation, and bisphosphonate therapy. Bone loss induced by exogenous corticosteroids is the most common form of secondary osteoporosis. There is a generalized decrease of bone mineral density, and 30% to 50% of patients develop vertebral fractures. The effect is determined by the dose and duration of corticosteroid therapy. Trabecular bone loss primarily occurs and is significant in the spine. After the initiation of corticosteroid therapy, there is a rapid phase of bone loss, followed by a slow continuous decline. The decreased bone formation is due to the toxic effects of glucocorticoids on osteoblasts. There is also decreased osteoblast recruitment and increased osteoblast apoptosis.

The prevention and treatment include oral calcium supplementation, 1500 mg/d, and oral vitamin D, 800 IU/d. A DEXA scan should be performed at the initiation of corticosteroid therapy along with patient education and treatment of underlying risk factors. Bisphosphonates are recommended at the start of therapy for the prevention of bone loss if prednisone, 5 mg/d or higher (or its equivalent), is to be used for more than 3 months. Bisphosphonates should be started in patients with T scores < –1.0 who are receiving long-term corticosteroid therapy, regardless of the dose.

Hormone replacement therapy is no longer regarded as the mainstay of treatment for osteoporosis in women. In the Women's Health Initiative study, the use of conjugated estrogens and medroxyprogesterone in postmenopausal women increased the risk of cardiovascular disease, invasive breast cancer, stroke, deep venous thrombosis, and pulmonary embolism.

KEY POINT

- The prevention and treatment of corticosteroid-induced osteoporosis include calcium and vitamin D supplementation, a DEXA scan at the initiation of therapy, and bisphosphonates in patients taking prednisone, ≥5 mg/d (or its equivalent), for >3 months.

Bibliography

1. **Maricic M.** Glucocorticoid-induced osteoporosis: treatment options and guidelines. Curr Osteoporos Rep. 2005;3:25-9. [PMID: 16036098]

Item 33   Answer: A

Screening now for osteoporosis is indicated in this patient. Screening is generally recommended for all women ≥65 years of age and women <65 years of age who have one or more risk factors for osteoporosis. The large number of risk factors encountered in numerous publications and in guidelines of scientific organizations may sometimes confuse more than enlighten. The National Osteoporosis Foundation has attempted to simplify the assessment of skeletal health by identifying five major risk factors for osteoporosis and related fractures in white postmenopausal women: personal history of fracture as an adult, history of fragility fracture in a first-degree relative, low body weight (<127 lb), current smoking, and use of oral corticosteroid therapy for more than 3 months. The World Health Organization project to validate clinical risk factors in multiple large observational studies in men and women of different ethnicity and world regions has resulted in the selection of seven key risk factors: age, previous fragility fracture, parental history of hip fracture, smoking, use of systemic corticosteroids, excess alcohol intake, and rheumatoid arthritis. Since the patient has a family history of hip fracture in a first-degree relative and she smokes, a dual-energy x-ray absorptiometry (DEXA) scan should be done now to assess the bone mineral density and rule out osteopenia or osteoporosis. DEXA is the gold standard for measuring bone mass. This technique has the best correlation with fracture risk, requires a short scanning time of 5 minutes, and measures the bone mineral density of all areas of the skeleton with high accuracy and reproducibility and low exposure to radiation.

Standard radiographs are not sensitive indicators of bone loss, since 30% to 40% of bone mineral density has already been lost by the time osteoporosis appears on radiographs. The use of markers of bone formation (alkaline phosphatase, osteocalcin, and procollagen) and bone resorption (hydroxyproline, pyridinoline, and deoxypyridinoline) is controversial. Their use is limited by a wide range of normal values, their circadian rhythm, and large intra-assay and inter-assay variability.

KEY POINT

- Osteoporosis screening is generally recommended for all women ≥65 years and women <65 years who have one or more risk factors for osteoporosis.

Bibliography

1. **Geusens PP.** Review of guidelines for testing and treatment of osteoporosis. Curr Osteoporos Rep. 2003;1:59-65. [PMID: 16036066]

Chapter 3
Gastroenterology and Hepatology

Gastroenterology and Hepatology contains self-assessment items that correspond to the following chapters in the *Internal Medicine Essentials for Clerkship Students 2* textbook:

Approach to Abdominal Pain
Approach to Diarrhea
Diseases of the Gallbladder and Bile Ducts
Acute Pancreatitis
Gastroesophageal Reflux Disease
Peptic Ulcer Disease
Dyspepsia
Approach to Gastrointestinal Bleeding
Viral Hepatitis
Cirrhosis
Inflammatory Bowel Disease

Gastroenterology and Hepatology contains self assessment items that correspond to the following Training Problems in the *Core Medicine Clerkship Guide*:

Abdominal Pain
Gastrointestinal Bleeding
Liver Disease

Chapter 3
Gastroenterology and Hepatology
Questions

Item 1

A 63-year-old man with chronic alcoholism has a 2-day history of fatigue and confusion. For the past 2 weeks, he has had fever and myalgias for which he is taking acetaminophen. Last week, he felt so ill that he stopped consuming alcohol. He has no history of injection drug use, blood transfusions, or known exposure to anyone with hepatitis.

On physical examination, temperature is 37.4 °C (99.3 °F). Findings include spider angiomata, mild splenomegaly, no hepatomegaly or ascites, and disorientation with asterixis.

Laboratory studies:

Hemoglobin	15 g/dL
Platelet count	91,000/µL
Aspartate aminotransferase	8124 U/L
Alanine aminotransferase	6557 U/L
Total bilirubin	1.2 mg/dL
Direct bilirubin	0.8 mg/dL
Creatinine	1.8 mg/dL
Ammonia	103 µg/dL

A peripheral blood smear is normal.

Which of the following is the most likely diagnosis?

(A) Acetaminophen hepatotoxicity
(B) Alcoholic hepatitis
(C) Herpes simplex virus hepatitis
(D) Thrombotic thrombocytopenic purpura

Item 2

A 45-year-old man has a 2-year history of chest pain and dysphagia that was initially induced only by solid foods but has progressed over the past year to include both solids and liquids. He also describes intermittent chest pain, retrosternal burning with occasional regurgitation of undigested food, and a 4.5-kg (10-lb) weight loss over the past 2 years.

Physical examination is normal. Upper endoscopy shows a small amount of retained food in the distal esophagus but is otherwise normal. The endoscope passes easily through the esophagogastric junction and biopsy specimens are taken. An esophageal motility study demonstrates a hypertensive lower esophageal sphincter that does not relax fully with wet swallows. A film from an upper gastrointestinal series is shown.

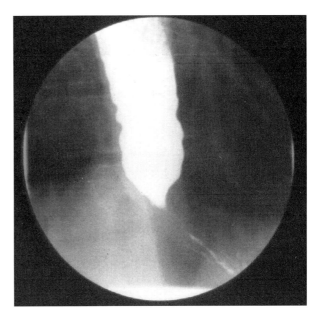

Which of the following is the most likely diagnosis?

(A) Achalasia
(B) Esophageal cancer
(C) Gastroesophageal reflux disease
(D) Scleroderma

Item 3

A 42-year-old woman has a 2-week history of jaundice, low-grade fever, and fatigue. Medical history is noncontributory. The patient lives in Honduras but was born in the United States and returned to this country when she became ill. She has consumed at least one bottle of rum daily for 15 years and has taken acetaminophen, 1 g daily, for the past 3 days. She has no history of injection drug use, blood transfusions, or known exposure to anyone with hepatitis.

On physical examination, temperature is 37.9 °C (100.2 °F), heart rate is 100/min, and blood pressure is 110/70 mm Hg. Jaundice, spider angiomata, and mild muscle wasting are noted. Abdominal examination shows mild splenomegaly, mild hepatomegaly with tenderness, and no ascites.

Laboratory studies:

Hemoglobin	12.8 g/dL
Leukocyte count	3400/µL
Platelet count	99,000/µL
Aspartate aminotransferase	124 U/L
Alanine aminotransferase	57 U/L
Total bilirubin	6.2 mg/dL
Direct bilirubin	3.8 mg/dL
Albumin	3.4 g/dL
INR	1.2
IgG antibodies to hepatitis A virus (anti-HAV IgG)	Positive

Which of the following is the most likely diagnosis?

(A) Acetaminophen hepatotoxicity
(B) Alcoholic hepatitis
(C) Autoimmune hepatitis
(D) Hepatitis A

Item 4

A 30-year-old woman is evaluated in the office because of an abnormal total bilirubin level detected when she had a life insurance examination. Medical history is unremarkable. Her only medication is an oral contraceptive agent. Physical examination is normal.

Laboratory studies:

Hemoglobin	13.9 g/dL
Mean corpuscular volume	88 fL
Red cell distribution width	10.8% (normal)
Total bilirubin	2.4 mg/dL
Direct bilirubin	0.2 mg/dL
Aspartate aminotransferase	23 U/L
Alanine aminotransferase	22 U/L

Which of the following is the most appropriate management at this time?

(A) Discontinue the oral contraceptive agent
(B) Evaluate for the presence of hemolysis
(C) Repeat the liver chemistry tests in 3 months
(D) Schedule abdominal ultrasonography

Item 5

A 26-year-old woman who is 36 weeks pregnant is evaluated in the office because of right-sided abdominal pain. The patient has had mild preeclampsia for 4 weeks. She vomited twice this morning but is able to drink liquids. She also developed a nosebleed this morning.

On physical examination, blood continues to ooze from her nostrils. Temperature is normal, heart rate is 105/min, and blood pressure is 135/85 mm Hg. Abdominal examination discloses right upper quadrant tenderness and uterine enlargement consistent with gestational age. There is 2+ bilateral lower extremity edema.

Laboratory studies:

Hemoglobin	7.7 g/dL
Leukocyte count	9500/µL
Platelet count	45,000/µL
Aspartate aminotransferase	160 U/L
Alanine aminotransferase	172 U/L
Total bilirubin	4.8 mg/dL
Direct bilirubin	0.9 mg/dL
Urinalysis	2+ protein

The peripheral blood smear shows schistocytes and diminished platelets.

Which of the following is the most likely diagnosis?

(A) Cholelithiasis
(B) HELLP syndrome
(C) Herpes simplex virus hepatitis
(D) Idiopathic thrombocytopenia

Item 6

A 78-year-old man with a history of cardiomyopathy and heart failure was hospitalized 2 days ago after a syncopal episode. He has no history of liver disease, abdominal pain, or excess alcohol use. Medications prior to admission were furosemide, digoxin, lisinopril, metoprolol, and aspirin. Admission physical examination disclosed a heart rate of 150/min and blood pressure of 80/60 mm Hg. Electrocardiogram showed atrial flutter with a rapid ventricular response, which spontaneously converted to sinus rhythm. Blood pressure after conversion was 120/80 mm Hg. Initial laboratory studies showed an aspartate aminotransferase value of 8968 U/L and an alanine aminotransferase value of 6534 U/L.

On hospital day 2, abdominal ultrasonography shows mild hepatomegaly without bile duct dilatation or gallbladder stones. Liver chemistry studies obtained 1 month ago, on the day of admission, and today (hospital day 2) are shown below:

	1 Month Ago	Day of Admission	Hospital Day 2
Aspartate amino-transferase (U/L)	34	8968	283
Alanine amino-transferase (U/L)	38	6534	264
Alkaline phosphatase (U/L)	124	132	123
Total bilirubin (mg/dL)	1.1	1.1	1.4

Which of the following is most likely causing this patient's abnormal liver chemistry values?

(A) Choledocholithiasis
(B) Drug-induced liver disease
(C) Hepatic ischemia
(D) Viral hepatitis

Item 7

A 32-year-old previously healthy woman who is 15 weeks pregnant is evaluated in the office because of hematemesis. The patient has had hyperemesis gravidarum for most of her pregnancy. This morning, she became very nauseated and began vomiting repeatedly after eating breakfast. She also vomited several hours later and noted bright red blood in the emesis. Her only medications are a prenatal multivitamin and an iron supplement. She does not drink alcohol and has no risk factors for chronic hepatitis.

On physical examination, vital signs are normal without orthostatic changes. Findings include spider angiomata, palmar erythema, and a slightly protuberant abdomen consistent with gestational age. Rectal examination shows normal-colored stool in the rectal vault.

Laboratory studies:

Hemoglobin	10.4 g/dL
Platelet count	215,000/μL
Blood urea nitrogen	44 mg/dL
Creatinine	0.9 mg/dL
Aspartate aminotransferase	23 U/L
Alanine aminotransferase	28 U/L
Alkaline phosphatase	218 U/L

Which of the following is the most likely diagnosis?

(A) Gastroesophageal varices
(B) Peptic ulcer disease
(C) Pill-induced esophagitis
(D) Mallory-Weiss tear

Item 8

A 67-year-old woman has an 8- to 10-month history of intermittent dysphagia for both solid foods and liquids. The dysphagia initially developed over the course of 10 to 14 days. She reports no abdominal symptoms but has lost 13.5 kg (30 lb) during this time.

An upper gastrointestinal barium radiograph shows a smooth narrowing in the distal esophagus. An esophageal motility study is consistent with achalasia.

Which of the following is the most appropriate next step in managing this patient?

(A) Laparoscopic Heller myotomy
(B) Pneumatic dilation of the esophagus
(C) Sublingual nifedipine before meals
(D) Upper endoscopy

Item 9

A 23-year-old woman is evaluated in the office for abdominal pain of several years' duration and a 5.4- kg (12-lb) weight loss occurring over the past few months. The pain is diffuse (although it occurs mostly in the lower abdomen), is crampy in nature, and is so severe at times that it "doubles her over." Pain is neither increased nor relieved with eating. The pain is frequently associated with diarrhea, especially when she is under stress, or intermittent constipation, although on most days she has a normal bowel movement. Currently, she reports

having up to six bowel movements daily, consisting of loose, watery, and foul-smelling stools, but without blood or mucus. She obtains some relief of pain with defecation, and the diarrhea is relieved with loperamide. She does not have fecal urgency. She has never sought care for her abdominal problems but seeks help now because the pain has become more severe and is interfering with her activities of daily living. Her family history is remarkable for irritable bowel syndrome.

On physical examination, she is a thin, fatigued woman in mild distress. Temperature is 36.9 °C (98.4 °F), respiration rate is 12/min, and blood pressure is 114/53 mm Hg. BMI is 18.9. The abdominal examination reveals normal bowel sounds and no hepatosplenomegaly, and the abdomen is diffusely tender without guarding, rebound, or rigidity. No palpable masses are noted. The remainder of the examination, including pelvic and rectal examinations, is unremarkable.

Hemoglobin is 9.5 g/dL, the leukocyte count is 4000/μL, and the platelet count is 148,000/μL.

Which of the following is the best diagnostic option for this patient?

(A) Abdominal ultrasonography
(B) Colonoscopy
(C) CT scan of the abdomen
(D) Flexible sigmoidoscopy

Item 10

A 25-year-old woman is evaluated in the office for acute abdominal pain that began 6 hours ago. Initially localized to the umbilical area, the pain has now migrated to the right lower quadrant. After the onset of pain, she developed anorexia and she vomited once. The patient has regular menstrual periods, and her most recent period ended 2 days ago. She is sexually active with one male partner and uses oral contraceptives; her partner does not use condoms.

On physical examination, the temperature is 39.0 °C (102.3 °F), blood pressure is 120/90 mm Hg, and heart rate is 100/min. Abdominal examination reveals normal bowel sounds and tenderness in the right lower quadrant. Pain is elicited with internal rotation of the hip. Pelvic examination reveals tenderness on the right side but no adnexal enlargement or masses. There is no cervical or vaginal discharge or cervical motion tenderness.

Leukocyte count is 10,000/μL. Urinalysis shows 20 to 30 leukocytes/hpf without bacteriuria. Urine pregnancy test is negative.

Which of the following is the most likely diagnosis?

(A) Acute appendicitis
(B) Pelvic inflammatory disease
(C) Pyelonephritis
(D) Ruptured ectopic pregnancy

Item 11

A 60-year-old woman is evaluated in the office for a 2-month history of diffuse, dull lower abdominal pain. She has frequent bloating but no nausea or vomiting. She has noted a recent change in bowel habits, characterized by passing hard, pellet-like stools alternating with loose stools; there is no visible blood. She has lost 2.2 kg (5 lb) over the past 2 months. Her medical history includes osteoarthritis for which she takes ibuprofen; she also takes omeprazole for heartburn. She has never undergone screening for breast cancer, cervical cancer, or colon cancer.

On physical examination, vital signs are normal. She has evidence of osteoarthritis involving the right knee and both hands. Abdominal examination reveals normal bowel sounds and no evidence of tenderness or masses. Rectal examination is normal, and the stool is negative for occult blood. Laboratory test results are pending.

Which of the following is the most appropriate next step in the management of this patient?

(A) Abdominal ultrasonography
(B) Colonoscopy
(C) Contrast-enhanced abdominal CT scan
(D) Discontinuation of ibuprofen
(E) High-fiber diet

Item 12

A 70-year-old man is evaluated in the office for a 5-day history of left lower quadrant abdominal pain and tenesmus. For the past 2 days he has had increasing pain, nausea without vomiting, and occasional hematochezia. He has a history of chronic constipation for which he takes milk of magnesia. He has no other significant medical history.

On physical examination, temperature is 38.2 °C (100.8 °F), blood pressure is 140/90 mm Hg, and heart rate is 90/min. Cardiovascular and lung examinations are normal. Bowel sounds are hypoactive but present, and there is significant tenderness in the left lower quadrant with guarding but no rebound. Hemoglobin is 12 g/dL and the leukocyte count is 12,400/µL.

Which of the following is the most appropriate next step in the management of this patient?

(A) Colonoscopy
(B) Empiric antibiotic therapy
(C) High-residue diet
(D) Left colectomy

Item 13

A 35-year-old woman is evaluated in the office for lower abdominal pain, bloating, and nausea of 7 months' duration. Her bowel habits typically alternate between constipation with the passage of hard, small-caliber stools and watery diarrhea with mucus. The abdominal pain is associated with looser stools and defecation; the pain has no relation to food intake. She has no weight loss, blood in the stool, or nocturnal symptoms or rectal bleeding. She has a history of fibromyalgia and chronic headache for which she uses acetaminophen and a

graded exercise program. She has never used alcohol or illicit drugs. She has no family history of gastrointestinal disorders.

Physical examination is normal except for mild lower abdominal tenderness to deep palpation. On pelvic examination, there is no discharge, tenderness, or adnexal masses.

Which of the following is the most likely diagnosis?

(A) Cholecystitis
(B) Crohn's disease
(C) Diverticulitis
(D) Irritable bowel syndrome
(E) Pelvic inflammatory disease

Item 14

A 27-year-old woman is evaluated in the office for a 2-year history of intermittent lower abdominal pain and discomfort. She describes the pain as crampy and diffuse, somewhat relieved with defecation, and usually associated with 3 to 5 days of loose, watery stools. Between episodes, she feels well and has normal, formed stools. She has not had fecal urgency, hematochezia, weight loss, fever, arthralgia, or rashes. She is not depressed. Her family history is negative for colon cancer and inflammatory bowel disease.

The physical examination is unremarkable. Laboratory studies obtained within the past 6 months, including complete blood count, renal function and liver chemistry tests, and thyroid-stimulating hormone, electrolyte, and calcium levels, were normal.

Which of the following treatment options is most appropriate for this patient?

(A) Alosetron
(B) Loperamide
(C) Nortriptyline
(D) Psyllium
(E) Sertraline

Item 15

A 72-year-old woman is hospitalized because of a 6-hour history of hematochezia and lower abdominal pain. She has had three bloody bowel movements during this period. Earlier this morning she had an episode of angina that was relieved after taking three nitroglycerin tablets. The patient underwent coronary artery bypass graft surgery 2 years ago. At that time her ejection fraction was 40%. Current medications are an angiotensin-converting enzyme inhibitor, metoprolol, a statin, and low-dose aspirin. Screening colonoscopy 5 months ago was normal.

On physical examination, temperature is normal, heart rate is 70/min and regular, and blood pressure is 126/72 mm Hg. Cardiac examination discloses a soft pansystolic apical murmur. The abdomen is soft with minimal left lower quadrant tenderness. There is no abdominal distention.

A CT scan of the abdomen shows diffuse left-sided colonic thickening.

Which of the following is the most likely diagnosis?

(A) Colon cancer
(B) Crohn's disease
(C) Diverticulitis
(D) Ischemic colitis
(E) Pseudomembranous colitis

Item 16

A 70-year-old man is evaluated in the emergency department for severe abdominal pain that has persisted for 12 hours. The pain was initially limited to the periumbilical area but is now diffuse. The patient also has had nausea and one episode of vomiting without hematemesis. Since the onset of pain, he has had four large, forceful bowel movements without blood. The patient has a 10-year history of type 2 diabetes mellitus, stable coronary artery disease, and hypertension; his medications are aspirin, pravastatin, atenolol, hydrochlorothiazide, and glyburide. He has never had surgery.

On physical examination, the patient is very uncomfortable. Temperature is 38.8 °C (101.8 °F), blood pressure is 100/60 mm Hg, and heart rate is 123/min and irregularly irregular. Cardiac examination reveals an irregular rhythm with varying intensity of S_1 and no extra sounds or murmurs. Abdominal examination shows absent bowel sounds, dullness to percussion, and diffuse tenderness on palpation. Rectal examination reveals a small amount of brown stool that is positive for occult blood.

Laboratory studies:

Hemoglobin	15.5 g/dL
Leukocyte count	14,500/μL
Sodium	140 meq/L
Potassium	5.6 meq/L
Chloride	108 meq/L
Bicarbonate	12 meq/L

Serum amylase and lipase concentrations and urinalysis are normal.

Which of the following is the most likely diagnosis?

(A) Acute mesenteric artery ischemia
(B) Acute pancreatitis
(C) Diverticulitis
(D) Nephrolithiasis
(E) Small bowel obstruction

Item 17

A 72-year-old man has a 6-week history of epigastric discomfort that is not relieved with over-the-counter antacids. He does not have fever, heartburn, jaundice, or change in bowel habits but believes that his clothes are becoming loose, although he has not weighed himself recently. The patient has a 15-year history of hypertension, treated with a thiazide diuretic, and a several-month history of type 2 diabetes mellitus, treated with an oral hypoglycemic agent. He also takes a statin and low-dose aspirin.

Physical examination reveals a thin, elderly man who appears uncomfortable. Vital signs and abdominal examination are normal. There is no scleral icterus.

Laboratory studies:

Hemoglobin	11.8 g/dL
Glucose	145 mg/dL
Total bilirubin	2.8 mg/dL
Aspartate aminotransferase	35 U/L
Alanine aminotransferase	48 U/L
Alkaline phosphatase	350 U/L
Amylase	140 U/L

Which of the following diagnostic studies is most appropriate at this time?

(A) Endoscopic retrograde cholangiopancreatography
(B) Endoscopic ultrasonography
(C) Helical CT scan of the abdomen
(D) Mesenteric angiography

Item 18

A 39-year-old woman is evaluated in the office for a 6-month history of foul-smelling, large-volume diarrhea, fatigue, postprandial bloating, and a 2.3-kg (5-lb) weight loss. She does not have fever, abdominal pain, hematochezia, or melena and has never traveled outside the United States. She takes no medications. Her mother has lactose intolerance, but the family history is otherwise noncontributory.

Physical examination is normal except for a rash on the extensor surfaces of the elbows, knees, and trunk (*see Figure 2 in Color Plates*).

Laboratory studies include hemoglobin, 11.2 g/dL; mean corpuscular volume, 74 fL; and ferritin, 12 ng/mL.

Which of the following studies is most likely to determine the cause of this patient's diarrhea?

(A) Colonoscopy
(B) CT scan of the abdomen
(C) IgA tissue transglutaminase antibody assay
(D) Stool culture

Item 19

A 55-year-old man has a 1-month history of increasing flatulence and loose stools with bowel movements occurring two or three times daily. He has not had weight loss, fever, or other symptoms. The patient has type 2 diabetes mellitus, managed with diet, exercise, and glyburide. His last hemoglobin A_{1c} measurement 2 months ago was 7%. He has been trying unsuccessfully to lose weight by dieting, exercising more, and using sugar-free snacks. He does not drink milk and avoids other milk-based products but does take a calcium supplement. Screening colonoscopy 1 year ago was normal.

On physical examination, blood pressure is 128/78 mm Hg, and heart rate is 76/min without orthostatic changes. The BMI is 28. The abdominal examination is normal and the stool is negative for occult blood. Stool cultures show no growth of pathogens.

An empiric trial of which of the following is most appropriate at this time?

(A) Discontinuation of calcium supplements
(B) Discontinuation of sugar-free snacks
(C) Initiation of a 2-week course of ciprofloxacin
(D) Substitution of metformin for glyburide

Item 20

A 63-year-old woman, who was on a group tour to the Yucatan Peninsula, developed abdominal cramping and flatulence on the third day of her trip. The next day, she had watery diarrhea with five or six stools daily. Five of the other 32 members of the tour had similar symptoms. The group stayed in excellent hotels and ate only in hotel restaurants. They all drank bottled water and tried to eat well-cooked foods.

The patient took loperamide and bismuth subsalicylate for her symptoms. She felt well by the sixth day of the trip and had only two formed stools daily.

Which of the following pathogens was the most likely cause of her diarrhea?

(A) *Campylobacter jejuni*
(B) *Escherichia coli*
(C) *Salmonella typhimurium*
(D) *Shigella dysenteriae*
(E) *Vibrio cholerae*

Item 21

A 78-year-old man is brought to the emergency department by family members because of increasing somnolence and "not acting normally" for several hours. The patient has hypertension and type 2 diabetes mellitus. Current medications are hydrochlorothiazide, pravastatin, low-dose aspirin, and metformin.

On physical examination, temperature is 38.3 °C (101 °F), heart rate is 100/min, and blood pressure is 110/62 mm Hg. Jaundice is present. He is lethargic and oriented to person and place but not to year. The right upper abdominal quadrant is tender to palpation without guarding. The remainder of the examination is unremarkable.

Laboratory studies:

Hemoglobin	12.8 g/dL
Leukocyte count	18,600/µL, with 86% segmented neutrophils
Aspartate aminotransferase	186 U/L
Alanine aminotransferase	230 U/L
Total bilirubin	4.1 mg/dL
Alkaline phosphatase	260 U/L

Abdominal ultrasonography shows normal liver architecture, a common bile duct caliber of 9 mm (normal <6 mm), multiple gallstones, and no evidence of gallbladder wall thickening or pericholecystic fluid. Broad-spectrum antibiotics are begun.

Which of the following is the most likely diagnosis?

(A) Acute hepatitis A
(B) Cholangitis
(C) Cholecystitis
(D) Pancreatitis

Item 22

A 20-year-old woman is evaluated in the office for acute abdominal pain and nausea of 6 hours' duration; she has also had two episodes of vomiting during that time. The pain began in the mid-epigastrium 2 hours after she ate her evening meal and is now centered in the right upper quadrant. She has had similar but less intense episodes that she attributed to heartburn. She has two children, is otherwise healthy, and her only medication is an oral contraceptive.

On physical examination, she appears uncomfortable. Temperature is 37.7 °C (99.9 °F), blood pressure is 130/80 mm Hg, heart rate is 100/min, and BMI is 32.6. Abdominal examination reveals right upper quadrant tenderness, and palpation in the right upper quadrant causes inspiratory arrest when she is asked to take a deep breath. There are no peritoneal signs, and the pelvic examination is normal.

Laboratory studies:

Hemoglobin	12 g/dL
Leukocyte count	13,000/µL
Alkaline phosphatase	300 U/L
Aspartate aminotransferase	50 U/L
Alanine aminotransferase	80 U/L
Total bilirubin	3 mg/dL

Amylase and lipase concentrations are normal.

Which of the following is the most appropriate next step in the evaluation of this patient?

(A) Abdominal ultrasonography
(B) CT scan of the abdomen and pelvis
(C) Endoscopic retrograde cholangiopancreatography (ERCP)
(D) Hepato-iminodiacetic acid (HIDA) scan

Item 23

A 52-year-old woman is evaluated in the emergency department for acute abdominal pain of 8 hours' duration. She has had 3 to 4 weeks of intermittent, sharp right upper quadrant abdominal pain lasting 30 minutes to 1 hour occasionally associated with nausea but not with fever or diarrhea. The pain is precipitated by meals. Last night after dinner the pain recurred and has persisted despite treatment with acetaminophen. She is otherwise healthy, has never had surgery, and takes no other medications.

On physical examination, she is overweight (BMI 28) and appears uncomfortable. Temperature is 38.1 °C (100.5 °F), blood pressure is 122/68 mm Hg, and heart rate is 76/min. There is scleral icterus. Bowel sounds are normal; there is right upper quadrant abdominal tenderness to palpation, particularly with inspiration, but no masses.

Laboratory studies:

Leukocyte count	12,400/µL
Aspartate aminotransferase	12 U/l
Alanine aminotransferase	18 U/L
Alkaline phosphatase	218 U/L
Total bilirubin	2.6 mg/dL

Which of the following is the most appropriate next step in the management of this patient?

(A) Abdominal ultrasonography
(B) CT scan of the abdomen
(C) Endoscopic retrograde cholangiopancreatography (ERCP)
(D) Low-fat diet and diclofenac
(E) Magnetic resonance cholangiopancreatography (MRCP)

Item 24

A 58-year-old man has a 1-week history of jaundice, dark urine, and vague upper abdominal pain. He has lost 4.5 kg (10 lb) over the past month despite having a good appetite. The patient has a 25-year history of ulcerative colitis that has been in remission since he began taking daily mesalamine 8 years ago. He has had no increase in stool frequency and no rectal bleeding. He has a 3-year history of abnormal liver chemistry test results that have never been evaluated but are attributed to fatty liver. The patient drinks 4 to 6 cans of beer daily.

On physical examination, he is obese and has mild jaundice. Abdominal examination shows only scars from a cholecystectomy.

Laboratory studies:

Aspartate aminotransferase	190 U/L
Alanine aminotransferase	212 U/L
Alkaline phosphatase	586 U/L
Total bilirubin	3.9 mg/dL

A CT scan of the abdomen shows mildly dilated peripheral intrahepatic ducts, mild dilatation of the common hepatic duct, and a normal common bile duct.

Which of the following is the most likely diagnosis?

(A) Acute hepatitis B infection
(B) Choledocholithiasis
(C) Primary biliary cirrhosis
(D) Sclerosing cholangitis

Item 25

A 51-year-old woman is hospitalized because of the acute onset of severe, constant upper abdominal pain associated with nausea and vomiting. She has type 2 diabetes mellitus controlled with metformin and glyburide. Other medications are a statin and low-dose aspirin.

On physical examination, the patient is obese. Temperature is normal. There is bilateral upper abdominal tenderness without rebound.

Laboratory studies:

Aspartate aminotransferase	180 U/L
Alanine aminotransferase	285 U/L
Amylase	1010 U/L

Symptomatic treatment for pancreatitis is begun with intravenous fluids and pain management as needed. On evaluation 12 hours later, she has minimal symptoms.

Repeated laboratory studies:

Aspartate aminotransferase	82 U/L
Alanine aminotransferase	100 U/L
Amylase	580 U/L

Which of the following is the most appropriate next step in managing this patient?

(A) Abdominal ultrasonography
(B) Cholescintigraphy (HIDA scan)
(C) Endoscopic retrograde cholangiopancreatography (ERCP)
(D) Laparoscopic cholecystectomy

Item 26

A 48-year-old man is hospitalized because of acute severe upper abdominal pain associated with nausea and vomiting. The patient has mild hypertension and poorly controlled type 2 diabetes mellitus (his most recent hemoglobin A_{1c} measurement was 10%). Medications are glyburide, hydrochlorothiazide, an angiotensin-converting enzyme inhibitor, a statin, and low-dose aspirin, all of which he has been taking for 3 years. He does not drink alcoholic beverages and has no recent history of abdominal trauma. There is no family history of pancreatic disease.

Physical examination discloses only epigastric tenderness to palpation without rebound.

Laboratory studies:

Total bilirubin	0.1 mg/dL
Aspartate aminotransferase	48 U/L
Alanine aminotransferase	61 U/L
Alkaline phosphatase	128 U/L
Lipase	390 U/L

Transabdominal ultrasonography shows a normal gallbladder without stones, mild fatty liver disease, and normal bile duct diameter. The pancreas is not well visualized. A CT scan of the abdomen shows marked peripancreatic stranding with a small amount of fluid around the tail of the pancreas, consistent with acute pancreatitis.

Which of the following diagnostic studies should be done next?

(A) Endoscopic ultrasonography
(B) Repeated transabdominal ultrasonography
(C) Triglyceride measurement
(D) Thyroid function tests

Item 27

A 55-year-old man is evaluated in the emergency department for 2 days of constant and progressively severe upper abdominal pain and vomiting. The patient has a history of alcohol abuse and had been drinking steadily for 1 week before the onset of the abdominal pain. He has noticed streaking of blood in the vomitus today. He has had previous episodes of hematemesis for which he had undergone upper endoscopy. He does not recall the cause of bleeding.

On physical examination, the patient is in significant pain and is curled up on his left side. Temperature is 37.5 °C (99.6 °F), heart rate is 120/min, and blood pressure is 90/60 mm Hg. Spider angiomata are present, and ecchymotic discoloration of the skin is noted over the left flank. There is no jaundice. The heart rate is rapid, with no murmurs or extra sounds. The abdomen is diffusely tender to palpation with no guarding. Laboratory test results are pending. An upright chest radiograph is normal, with no air seen beneath the diaphragms; a supine abdominal radiograph is nondiagnostic. An abdominal CT scan is shown.

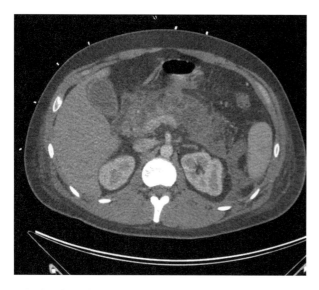

Which of the following is the most likely diagnosis?

(A) Acute cholecystitis
(B) Acute necrotizing pancreatitis
(C) Alcoholic hepatitis
(D) Perforated peptic ulcer
(E) Small bowel obstruction

Item 28

A 42-year-old woman is hospitalized because of pancreatitis. On physical examination, the patient appears ill and dehydrated. Temperature is 37.6 °C (99.6 °F), heart rate is 118/min, respiration rate is 19/min, and blood pressure is 110/60 mm Hg. Abdominal examination discloses diffuse tenderness without rebound.

Laboratory studies:

Hematocrit	54%
Triglycerides	1482 mg/dL
Total bilirubin	0.9 mg/dL
Aspartate aminotransferase	220 U/L
Amylase	62 U/L
Lipase	250 U/L

The patient is given narcotics as needed for pain control. A CT scan of the abdomen performed in the emergency department showed marked pancreatic edema and diffuse peripancreatic stranding.

In addition to continuing pain relief as needed, which of the following is the most essential next step in managing this patient?

(A) Endoscopic retrograde cholangiopancreatography
(B) Endoscopic ultrasonography
(C) Intravenous hyperalimentation
(D) Vigorous intravenous hydration

Item 29

A 62-year-old man is hospitalized for epigastric pain, nausea, and vomiting of 3 days' duration. His symptoms worsen when he eats and are alleviated when he lies in the fetal position; acetaminophen and ibuprofen have been ineffective. He has a history of occasional colicky, postprandial upper abdominal pain and hypertension treated with hydrochlorothiazide. He has a 23-pack-year history of cigarette smoking and drinks approximately two beers daily.

On physical examination, temperature is 37.2 °C (99.0 °F), heart rate is 100/min, and blood pressure is 150/90 mm Hg. The abdomen is distended, and bowel sounds are present but infrequent. There is tenderness without guarding in the midabdomen and epigastrium.

Laboratory studies:

Aspartate aminotransferase	Normal
Alanine aminotransferase	Normal
Alkaline phosphatase	187 U/L
Amylase	418 U/L
Lipase	198 U/L
Triglycerides	321 mg/dL

Abdominal ultrasonography shows stones in the gallbladder and a dilated common bile duct.

Which of the following is the most appropriate immediate next step in the management of this patient?

(A) Abstinence from alcohol
(B) Endoscopic retrograde cholangiopancreatography (ERCP)
(C) Gemfibrozil
(D) Low-fat diet
(E) Smoking cessation

Item 30

A 55-year-old man has a several-year history of epigastric pain and daily heartburn without dysphagia or weight loss. He has tried over-the-counter antacids and, more recently, intermittent over-the-counter proton pump inhibitors but still has breakthrough symptoms.

Physical examination is normal. Upper endoscopy is performed; findings from the distal esophagus are shown (*see Figure 3 in Color Plates*). Esophageal biopsy specimens show intestinal metaplasia.

Which of the following is the most likely diagnosis?

(A) Achalasia
(B) Barrett's esophagus
(C) Esophageal adenocarcinoma
(D) Esophageal candidiasis

Item 31

A 69-year-old man is brought to the emergency department because of a 3-week history of gnawing epigastric pain that is slightly improved with meals and antacids. He also reports early satiety, nausea without vomiting, and a 3.6-kg (8-lb) weight loss over the past 4 weeks. There is no melena, fever, or chills. He has degenerative joint disease of both knees, treated with ibuprofen.

On physical examination, temperature is normal, heart rate is 102/min, respiration rate is 13/min, and blood pressure is 110/90 mm Hg. There is temporal wasting. Abdominal examination discloses epigastric tenderness to palpation. Hemoglobin is 11 g/dL, and the leukocyte count and platelet count are normal.

Which of the following is the most appropriate next step in managing this patient?

(A) Abdominal ultrasonography
(B) Proton pump inhibitor and re-evaluation in 2 weeks
(C) Therapy to eradicate *Helicobacter pylori*
(D) Upper endoscopy

Item 32

A 33-year-old woman has a 3-week history of burning epigastric pain, nausea, and early satiety. The pain improves slightly with antacids. Medical history includes two previous duodenal and gastric ulcers that were treated with an H_2-receptor antagonist; all studies for *Helicobacter pylori* have been negative. She is otherwise healthy, takes no medications, and does not drink alcohol.

Physical examination is normal except for mid-epigastric tenderness to palpation. Upper endoscopy shows several gastric antral ulcers, ulcers at the gastroesophageal junction, esophageal ulcers, and ulcers distal to the duodenum with some narrowing of the pyloric channel.

Which of the following is the most likely diagnosis?

(A) Gastric cancer
(B) Gastrinoma
(C) Glucagonoma
(D) *Helicobacter pylori* infection

Item 33

A 33-year-old woman is evaluated in the office for a 2-month history of epigastric pain. She usually feels the pain early in the morning and before her evening meal. Eating often relieves the pain. She describes the pain as gnawing and burning. She does not have reflux, heartburn, nausea or vomiting, weight loss, early satiety, change in bowel habits, or blood in the stool. Her medical history includes only a 3-month history of headache for which she takes daily ibuprofen.

Physical examination is normal except for mild epigastric tenderness. The results of serologic tests for *Helicobacter pylori* are pending.

Which of the following is the most appropriate next step in the management of this patient?

(A) Abdominal ultrasonography
(B) Begin a proton pump inhibitor
(C) Stop ibuprofen
(D) Stop ibuprofen and begin a proton pump inhibitor
(E) Upper endoscopy

Item 34

A 59-year-old man has a 3-month history of epigastric discomfort and nausea without weight loss, melena, or vomiting. Over-the-counter H_2-receptor antagonists have been ineffective. The patient is otherwise healthy and takes no other medications. Physical examination reveals mild epigastric tenderness to palpation. Upper endoscopy shows a 1-cm duodenal ulcer, and antral biopsy specimens demonstrate chronic gastritis and *Helicobacter pylori* infection.

Which of the following is the most appropriate therapy for this patient?

(A) An H_2-receptor antagonist
(B) A proton pump inhibitor
(C) A proton pump inhibitor and two antibiotics
(D) Bismuth subsalicylate and a proton pump inhibitor

Item 35

A 27-year-old man has a 3-month history of intermittent burning epigastric pain that is made worse by fasting and improves with meals. Antacids provide temporary relief. He is otherwise healthy and has no other symptoms. His only medication is occasional acetaminophen for knee discomfort. Physical examination discloses only mild epigastric tenderness to palpation; vital signs are normal.

Which of the following diagnostic studies should be done next?

(A) Abdominal ultrasonography
(B) Serologic testing for *Helicobacter pylori*
(C) Upper endoscopy
(D) Upper gastrointestinal barium study

Item 36

A 64-year-old woman is evaluated because of a 4-month history of iron deficiency anemia and positive fecal occult blood tests. She does not have hematochezia. Her hemoglobin level has ranged from 9 g/dL to 11 g/dL, and she has not required blood transfusions.

Extended upper endoscopy and complete colonoscopy, obtained 2 months ago, showed only left-sided colonic diverticula. Small bowel biopsy specimens obtained at the time of upper endoscopy were normal. A CT scan of the abdomen was also normal. Physical examination today is unremarkable.

Which of the following is the most likely diagnosis?

(A) Angiodysplasia
(B) Aortoenteric fistula
(C) Celiac sprue
(D) Colonic diverticula
(E) Meckel's diverticulum

Item 37

A 42-year-old man is hospitalized because of hematemesis and melena. The patient takes ibuprofen for management of arthritis. He is otherwise healthy and takes no other medications. The patient is hypotensive on admission, and intravenous fluids are begun. No blood transfusions are needed. Upper endoscopy shows a bleeding duodenal ulcer that is treated with injectable epinephrine and clipping. Biopsy specimens for *Helicobacter pylori* are negative. Ibuprofen is discontinued, and a proton pump inhibitor is begun.

On hospital day 3, review of the patient's laboratory studies shows a hemoglobin level of 13.5 g/dL on admission, 12.7 g/dL on day 2, and 11.4 g/dL on day 3. He has not had recurrent hematemesis, melena, dizziness, pain, nausea, or orthostatic hypotension. His last bowel movement, 24 hours ago, was a formed, normal-appearing stool.

Which of the following is the most appropriate next step in managing this patient?

(A) Blood transfusion
(B) Colonoscopy
(C) Fecal occult blood testing
(D) Repeat upper endoscopy
(E) Hospital discharge with outpatient follow-up

Item 38

A 63-year-old man is evaluated in the emergency department for two large, bloody bowel movements and dizziness upon standing that occurred 1 hour ago. He has a 10-year history of hypertension controlled with hydrochlorothiazide. A colonoscopy performed 3 years ago was normal.

On physical examination, heart rate is 96/min supine and 126/min standing and blood pressure is 128/88 mm Hg supine and 102/84 mm Hg standing. There are no stigmata of chronic liver disease. On abdominal examination, bowel sounds are active and there is no tenderness to palpation or hepatosplenomegaly. Digital rectal examination reveals bright red blood. Initial laboratory studies show: hematocrit, 38%;

blood urea nitrogen, 16 mg/dL; and serum creatinine, 1.2 mg/dL.

Which of the following is the most appropriate next step in this patient's management?

(A) Colonoscopy
(B) Intravenous octreotide
(C) Intravenous omeprazole
(D) Upper endoscopy
(E) Volume replacement with normal saline

Item 39

A 20-year-old woman has a 1-week history of jaundice and somnolence. She has no history of liver disease. The patient traveled to Nicaragua 4 weeks ago.

On physical examination, she is somnolent but is arousable and oriented. Vital signs are normal. Jaundice and asterixis are present. Abdominal examination is normal. There are no focal neurologic findings.

Laboratory studies:

Aspartate aminotransferase	3936 U/L
Alanine aminotransferase	4183 U/L
Alkaline phosphatase	284 U/L
Total bilirubin	10.2 mg/dL
Ammonia	253 µg/dL
IgM antibodies to hepatitis A virus (anti-HAV IgM)	Positive
Hepatitis B surface antigen (HBsAg)	Negative
IgM antibodies to hepatitis B core antigen (anti-HBc IgM)	Negative
Prothrombin time	20 s

Abdominal ultrasonography shows a normal-appearing liver and no ascites.

Which of the following is the most appropriate next step in managing this patient?

(A) CT scan of the abdomen
(B) CT scan of the head
(C) Evaluation for liver transplantation
(D) Liver biopsy

Item 40

A 22-year-old male daycare employee has a 2-week history of fatigue and nausea with occasional vomiting and a 2-day history of jaundice. He was previously well, takes no medications, and has no history of liver disease, injection drug use, blood transfusions, sexual exposures, or known exposure to anyone with hepatitis. Several children in the daycare center have recently been ill, but none had jaundice.

Physical examination is significant only for jaundice and a slightly enlarged, nontender liver. There are no spider angiomata or signs of encephalopathy.

Laboratory studies:

Aspartate aminotransferase	1586 U/L
Alanine aminotransferase	1897 U/L
Total bilirubin	6.2 mg/dL

Which of the following is the most likely diagnosis?

(A) Hepatitis A
(B) Hepatitis B
(C) Hepatitis C
(D) Hepatitis D
(E) Hepatitis E

Item 41

A 25-year-old man is evaluated in the office for a 3-week history of fatigue, weakness, myalgias, and anorexia. Two days ago, he noticed that his eyes appeared yellow. The patient takes no medications or illicit drugs and drinks six to eight alcohol-containing beverages per week. Three weeks ago, he took acetaminophen, 4 g daily for 3 days, for diffuse arthralgias and myalgias but stopped when it proved to be ineffective. He has a history of multiple same-sex encounters and had unprotected sex with a man 2 months ago. His past immunizations include polio, diphtheria, pertussis, and tetanus.

On physical examination, he is afebrile, blood pressure is 120/70 mm Hg, and heart rate is 70/min. His soft palate and sclerae are icteric. The liver edge is palpable and moderately tender. There is no rash or lymphadenopathy.

Laboratory studies:

Hemoglobin	12 g/dL
Leukocyte count	8000/µL
Alkaline phosphatase	120 U/L
Aspartate aminotransferase	1200 U/L
Alanine aminotransferase	1450 U/L
Total bilirubin	5 mg/dL

Which of the following is the most likely cause of this patient's findings?

(A) Acetaminophen hepatotoxicity
(B) Acute alcoholic hepatitis
(C) Acute hepatitis B infection
(D) Acute hepatitis C infection
(E) Acute retroviral infection

Item 42

A 44-year-old man was recently found to have abnormal serologic test results for viral hepatitis when he attempted to donate blood. The patient is asymptomatic. He used injection drugs and drank alcohol excessively for 2 years 25 years ago but has not used either drugs or alcohol since. Medical history is otherwise unremarkable, and he takes no medications.

Physical examination discloses a BMI of 23, no stigmata of chronic liver disease, and a normal-sized liver.

Laboratory studies:

Aspartate aminotransferase	53 U/L
Alanine aminotransferase	64 U/L
Total bilirubin	0.9 mg/dL
Hepatitis B surface antigen (HbsAg)	Negative
Antibodies to hepatitis B surface antigen (anti-HBs)	Positive
IgG antibodies to hepatitis B core antigen (anti-HBc IgG)	Positive
IgM antibodies to hepatitis B core antigen (anti-HBc IgM)	Negative
Antibodies to hepatitis C virus (anti-HCV)	Positive

Which of the following diagnostic studies should be done next?

(A) Hepatitis B e antigen (HBeAg)
(B) Hepatitis B virus DNA (HBV DNA)
(C) Hepatitis C virus RNA (HCV RNA)
(D) IgM antibodies to hepatitis A virus (anti-HAV IgM)

Item 43

A 63-year-old woman has a 3-month history of gradually increasing abdominal distention and fatigue. She has no other symptoms, and medical history is noncontributory.

On physical examination, the patient has jaundice and evidence of mild muscle wasting. Xanthelasma and spider angiomata are present. Abdominal examination discloses hepatosplenomegaly and moderate ascites.

Laboratory studies:

Aspartate aminotransferase	53 U/L
Alanine aminotransferase	47 U/L
Alkaline phosphatase	123 U/L
Total bilirubin	3.2 mg/dL
Albumin	2.9 g/dL

Abdominal ultrasonography shows hepatomegaly, a coarse echotexture of the liver, patent portal and hepatic veins, mild splenomegaly, moderate ascites, and no bile duct dilatation. Paracentesis is performed. The ascitic fluid leukocyte count is 80/µL, protein is 1.4 g/dL, and albumin is 0.7 g/dL.

Which of the following is the most likely cause of the ascites?

(A) Budd-Chiari syndrome
(B) Cirrhosis
(C) Heart failure
(D) Peritoneal carcinomatosis

Item 44

A 37-year-old woman has a 1-week history of fatigue, jaundice, and fever. The patient has hypothyroidism for which she has taken levothyroxine for the past 10 years. She has no other medical problems, does not drink alcohol, and takes no other medications. She traveled to Mexico 7 months ago and had hepatitis A vaccine before her trip. Her sister has systemic lupus erythematosus and her mother has rheumatoid arthritis.

Physical examination discloses normal vital signs, mild jaundice, and nontender hepatomegaly.

Laboratory studies:

Aspartate aminotransferase	310 U/L
Alanine aminotransferase	455 U/L
Alkaline phosphatase	180 U/L
Total bilirubin	2.3 mg/dL
γ-Globulin	5.0 g/dL
Anti–smooth muscle antibodies	1:160
Anti-LKM antibodies	1:160

Which of the following is the most likely diagnosis?

(A) Acetaminophen hepatotoxicity
(B) Acute hepatitis A
(C) Autoimmune hepatitis
(D) Primary biliary cirrhosis

Item 45

A 42-year-old man is evaluated in the office for a progressive increase in abdominal girth and a 4.5-kg (10-lb) weight gain over the past 2 months. He has no pain or fever or hematemesis, melena, or hematochezia but has noted dark urine. His only medication is occasional acetaminophen for headache. He has not used illicit drugs or alcohol for the past 20 years, but he did use injection drugs and abused alcohol from age 20 to 22 years. His father has type 2 diabetes mellitus and his mother has hypertension. One aunt died of colon cancer at age 68 years.

On physical examination, he appears jaundiced but is in no distress. Temperature is 37.2 °C (99.0 °F), blood pressure is 138/80 mm Hg, and heart rate is 80/min. The abdomen is distended, with bulging flanks and shifting dullness. Bowel sounds are present, and there is no tenderness to palpation. The liver edge cannot be palpated, but the tip of the spleen is palpable during normal respiration. Stool is negative for occult blood. There is pitting edema of the ankles.

Laboratory studies:

Hematocrit	43%
Platelet count	80,000/µL
Aspartate aminotransferase	50 U/L
Alanine aminotransferase	55 U/L
Total bilirubin	3.0 mg/dL
Direct bilirubin	1.0 mg/dL
Prothrombin time	14 s (control, 10 s)
INR	1.4

Which of the following is the most likely cause of this patient's findings?

(A) Acetaminophen hepatotoxicity
(B) Alcoholic cirrhosis
(C) Hemochromatosis
(D) Hepatitis C infection
(E) Metastatic colon cancer

Item 46

A 66-year-old woman comes for her annual physical examination. She reports only mild fatigue. The patient has prediabetes that is managed by diet alone. She takes no medications and drinks one glass of wine each day.

On physical examination, she is afebrile, blood pressure is 132/86 mm Hg, heart rate is 70/min, and BMI is 32. The remainder of the examination is normal.

Laboratory studies:

Hemoglobin	13.1 g/dL
Platelet count	85,000/µL
Glucose (fasting)	119 mg/dL
Lipid profile	Normal
Aspartate aminotransferase	138 U/L
Alanine aminotransferase	124 U/L
Alkaline phosphatase	50 U/L
Total bilirubin	0.8 mg/dL
Albumin	3.1 g/dL
Serologic studies for hepatitis A, B, and C	Negative
Transferrin saturation	Normal

Abdominal ultrasonography shows evidence of mild fatty infiltration of the liver.

Which of the following is the most likely diagnosis?

(A) Acute viral hepatitis
(B) Alcoholic liver disease
(C) Hemochromatosis
(D) Nonalcoholic fatty liver disease

Item 47

A 51-year-old woman has a 3-week history of pruritus that interferes with her sleep and increases when she exercises or bathes. Her only medication is atorvastatin, which was begun 5 months ago for management of hyperlipidemia. Medical history is otherwise noncontributory, and she has no risk factors for viral hepatitis. Physical examination is remarkable only for linear excoriations of the upper back, arms, and legs.

Laboratory studies:

Aspartate aminotransferase	40 U/L
Alanine aminotransferase	45 U/L
Alkaline phosphatase	650 U/L
Total bilirubin	2.7 mg/dL
Direct bilirubin	2.1 mg/dL
γ-Globulin	Normal
Antinuclear antibodies	1:20
Anti–smooth muscle antibodies	Negative
Antimitochondrial antibodies	1:80 (positive)
Serologic studies for hepatitis A, B, and C	Negative

Which of the following is the most likely diagnosis?

(A) Atorvastatin hepatotoxicity
(B) Autoimmune hepatitis
(C) Primary biliary cirrhosis
(D) Primary sclerosing cholangitis

Item 48

A 73-year-old man is brought to the office by his wife after she found him trying to put his shoes in the refrigerator. The patient has cirrhosis due to α_1-antitrypsin deficiency and has been taking diuretics for ascites. There is no history of head trauma or gastrointestinal bleeding.

On physical examination, temperature is 38.4 °C (101.1 °F). The patient is disoriented to time and place and has asterixis. Abdominal examination discloses moderate ascites, and rectal examination demonstrates brown stool. There are no focal neurologic findings.

Laboratory studies:

Sodium	128 meq/L
Potassium	4.0 meq/L
Creatinine	1.3 mg/dL
Aspartate aminotransferase	63 U/L
Alanine aminotransferase	71 U/L
Total bilirubin	3.2 mg/dL
Albumin	2.8 g/dL

Which of the following is most appropriate for managing this patient at this time?

(A) CT scan of the head
(B) Fluid restriction
(C) Fresh frozen plasma
(D) Paracentesis

Item 49

A 53-year-old man with cirrhosis due to nonalcoholic steatohepatitis undergoes upper endoscopy. Large esophageal varices are found. The patient is otherwise well, has had no esophageal variceal bleeding, and does not have ascites, peripheral edema, encephalopathy, or gastrointestinal bleeding.

Which of the following is the most appropriate primary prophylaxis for this patient?

(A) Esophageal variceal sclerotherapy
(B) Norfloxacin
(C) Propranolol
(D) Transjugular intrahepatic portosystemic shunt

Item 50

A 35-year-old man with a 10-year history of ulcerative colitis involving the entire colon comes for a follow-up office visit. A small-bowel follow-through radiographic series obtained at the time of diagnosis was normal.

The patient is doing well on mesalamine maintenance therapy. He has only occasional diarrhea and bleeding and has rarely required corticosteroids.

Which of the following surveillance options is most appropriate for this patient?

(A) Barium enema examination now
(B) Colonoscopy with biopsies now
(C) Colonoscopy with biopsies starting at age 50 years
(D) Virtual colonoscopy (CT colonography) now

Item 51

A 26-year-old man has a 4-week history of increasingly severe bloody diarrhea, urgency, tenesmus, and abdominal pain without fever, chills, or sweating. The patient has an 8-pack-year smoking history.

On physical examination, he appears well. Vital signs are normal. The abdomen is mildly tender without guarding or rebound. Rectal examination is normal. Hemoglobin is 12 g/dL, the leukocyte count is 11,300/µL, and the erythrocyte sedimentation rate is 38 mm/h.

Colonoscopy shows areas of inflammation throughout the colon associated with friability, granularity, and deep ulcerations. The inflamed areas are separated by relatively normal-appearing mucosa, including normal rectal mucosa. The ileum appears normal.

Which of the following is the most likely diagnosis?

(A) Crohn's disease
(B) Ischemic colitis
(C) Microscopic colitis
(D) Ulcerative colitis
(E) *Yersinia* enterocolitis

Item 52

A 75-year-old asymptomatic man undergoes an annual physical examination. He is obese and has a long history of smoking, hypertension, and chronic kidney disease (creatinine concentration 2.7 mg/dL). His medications are furosemide, ramipril, atorvastatin, and aspirin.

On physical examination, the blood pressure is 170/78 mm Hg bilaterally, and heart rate is 70/min and regular. There is a grade 2/6 holosystolic murmur heard at the apex with radiation to the axilla. Examination of the abdomen discloses a soft systolic bruit and a tender midline pulsatile mass. There are bilateral femoral bruits with absent distal pulses. Laboratory studies show a total cholesterol level of 250 mg/dL and LDL cholesterol level of 162 mg/dL.

Which of the following diagnostic studies should be done next?

(A) Abdominal CT scan with contrast
(B) Abdominal plain radiograph
(C) Abdominal ultrasonography
(D) Contrast aortography

Item 53

A 19-year-old woman is evaluated in the office for a 2-year history of lower abdominal pain. She is particularly bothered by the pain during the first few days of her menstrual period. She has tried acetaminophen and cimetidine without benefit. The patient has mild constipation but no diarrhea or genitourinary symptoms and is currently not sexually active.

On physical examination, there is mild lower abdominal tenderness but no hepatosplenomegaly, masses, or guarding. Pelvic examination is normal except for bilateral lower abdominal tenderness.

Laboratory studies, including hemoglobin and urinalysis, are normal. A pregnancy test is negative. Results of abdominal-pelvic ultrasonography are normal.

Which of the following is the most appropriate treatment for alleviating this patient's pain?

(A) Anesthetic/corticosteroid injection
(B) Naproxen
(C) Polyethylene glycol laxative
(D) Psyllium

Chapter 3

Gastroenterology and Hepatology
Answers and Critiques

Item 1   **Answer: A**

The most common causes of aminotransferase values >5000 U/L are acetaminophen hepatotoxicity, hepatic ischemia, and hepatitis due to unusual viruses such as herpes simplex virus. Because of depleted glutathione stores, patients with chronic alcoholism are at risk for developing acetaminophen hepatotoxicity when taking acetaminophen at lower doses than those necessary to cause liver damage in patients who drink alcohol moderately or not at all. Given this patient's clinical history, acetaminophen hepatotoxicity is the most likely diagnosis, and *N*-acetylcysteine is the most appropriate treatment. Although *N*-acetylcysteine is most effective if administered within 24 hours of acetaminophen ingestion, it can generally be given to patients who later develop hepatotoxicity.

This patient does not have alcoholic hepatitis, since this disease rarely causes aminotransferase values >400 U/L. Herpes simplex virus hepatitis is very unlikely because it occurs most often in pregnant or immunosuppressed patients and causes fever, aminotransferase values >5000 U/L, and often skin lesions. Thrombotic thrombocytopenic purpura (TTP) could account for this patient's fever, thrombocytopenia, mental status changes, and renal insufficiency. However, this patient has no evidence of the microangiopathic hemolytic anemia that is characteristic of TTP.

KEY POINTS

- The most common causes of aminotransferase values >5000 U/L are acetaminophen hepatotoxicity, hepatic ischemia, and hepatitis due to unusual viruses.

- Persons with alcoholism can develop acetaminophen hepatotoxicity when taking therapeutic doses of acetaminophen.

Bibliography
1. **Lee WM.** Drug-induced hepatotoxicity N Engl J Med. 2003;349:474-85 [PMID: 12890847]

Item 2   **Answer: A**

This patient has typical symptoms and radiographic findings (dilated esophageal lumen and smooth narrowing at the esophageal outlet) of achalasia. All, or nearly all, patients with achalasia report dysphagia, over 80% report regurgitation, two thirds report weight loss, and one third report chest discomfort. All patients with suspected achalasia require upper endoscopy to rule out pseudoachalasia due to adenocarcinoma. Pneumatic dilation is appropriate therapy for a patient of this age with achalasia, as 60% to 80% of patients will experience marked improvement that may last for several years following this procedure.

Symptoms of dysphagia, regurgitation, and weight loss can also be due to esophageal adenocarcinoma; such symptoms are indistinguishable from those of idiopathic achalasia. Physical examination may rarely show findings suggestive of the presence of a neoplasm (lymphadenopathy, abdominal mass, and hepatomegaly). Pseudoachalasia may result from tumor invasion of the myenteric plexus or as a paraneoplastic phenomenon. Patients typically are older, have shorter symptom duration, and have greater weight loss than patients with idiopathic achalasia, but these are not reliable features. Radiography and manometry cannot reliably discriminate between pseudoachalasia and idiopathic achalasia. In patients with adenocarcinoma, there is resistance to passage of the endoscope through the gastroesophageal junction even if a tumor mass is not readily apparent. Biopsy is therefore essential to rule out adenocarcinoma in patients presenting with apparent achalasia.

Heartburn and acid regurgitation are the most common symptoms of gastroesophageal reflux disease. Dysphagia is less common and often associated with complications of peptic stricture and/or peristaltic dysfunction. The esophageal lumen is not dilated and upper endoscopy may show erosions and/or Barrett's esophagus, both of which are absent in this patient.

Patients with scleroderma esophagus usually have other clinical features typical of progressive systemic sclerosis or CREST syndrome (calcinosis, Raynaud's phenomenon, esophageal motility disorders, sclerodactyly, and telangiectasia). Manometry in these patients may show low-amplitude peristaltic waves or even absence of peristalsis as a result of fibrosis of the esophageal circular muscle. However, unlike patients with achalasia, the basal lower esophageal sphincter pressure is typically reduced in patients with scleroderma and also relaxes with deglutition.

KEY POINTS

- Patients with achalasia report dysphagia, regurgitation, weight loss, and chest discomfort.

- Upper endoscopy is required to differentiate achalasia from esophageal adenocarcinoma.

Bibliography
1. **Mittal RK, Bhalla V.** Oesophageal motor functions and its disorders. Gut. 2004;53:1536-42. [PMID: 15361508]

Item 3   Answer: B

Fatigue, a history of excessive alcohol consumption, low-grade fever, jaundice, tender hepatomegaly, examination findings consistent with chronic liver disease, and an aspartate aminotransferase to alanine aminotransferase ratio (AST:ALT) >2 are most consistent with alcoholic hepatitis.

Hepatitis A is associated with both AST and ALT values >500 U/L, often >1000 U/L, with the ALT greater than the AST. In addition, positive IgG antibodies to hepatitis A virus (anti-HAV IgG) are consistent with a remote prior infection with current immunity and not with acute hepatitis A. Patients who consume excess alcohol are at greater risk for developing acetaminophen hepatotoxicity than those who drink alcohol moderately or not at all. However, acetaminophen doses of >3 g/d are probably needed to cause hepatotoxicity, even for patients with alcoholism. In addition, acetaminophen toxicity typically results in AST and ALT values >5000 U/L. A patient with autoimmune hepatitis would generally have AST and ALT values similar to those of a patient with acute viral hepatitis and the AST:ALT ratio would be < 2.

KEY POINT

• Fever, a history of alcoholism, tender hepatomegaly, examination findings consistent with chronic liver disease, and an aspartate aminotransferase to alanine aminotransferase ratio (AST:ALT) >2 are associated with alcoholic hepatitis.

Bibliography

1. **Green RM, Flamm S.** AGA technical review on the evaluation of liver chemistry tests. Gastroenterology. 2002;123:1367-84. [PMID: 12360498]

Item 4   Answer: C

This patient has indirect (unconjugated) hyperbilirubinemia, which in an asymptomatic patient with a normal hemoglobin level and otherwise normal liver chemistry tests is suggestive of Gilbert's syndrome. Gilbert's syndrome is the most common inherited disorder of bilirubin metabolism. In adults, it is a benign disorder, and a presumptive diagnosis can be made based on repeated testing showing only mildly elevated indirect bilirubin.

Cholestasis due to an oral contraceptive agent will cause conjugated (direct) hyperbilirubinemia, which is not present in this patient. Patients with hemolysis significant enough to cause unconjugated hyperbilirubinemia generally have a low hemoglobin level and abnormal values for mean corpuscular volume and red cell distribution width as a result of reticulocytosis. Abdominal ultrasonography may be a helpful study for patients with direct hyperbilirubinemia, which is usually associated with hepatobiliary disease, but is not indicated in this patient who has indirect hyperbilirubinemia.

KEY POINT

• The incidental finding of indirect (unconjugated) hyperbilirubinemia in an asymptomatic patient with a normal hemoglobin

level and otherwise normal liver chemistry tests is indicative of Gilbert's syndrome.

Bibliography

1. **Roche SP, Kobos R.** Jaundice in the adult patient. Am Fam Physician. 2004;69:299-304. [PMID: 14765767]

Item 5   Answer: B

This patient has HELLP syndrome (hemolysis, elevated liver enzymes, low platelets). The treatment of choice is prompt delivery of the infant. Following delivery, the mother's condition often resolves within 48 hours. Since the patient is in her 36th gestational week, delivery would most likely be safe for both the mother and the infant.

Gallstones often form during pregnancy and are associated with right upper quadrant abdominal pain and aminotransferase elevations. However, a common bile duct stone would not explain the hemolysis (indicated by the indirect hyperbilirubinemia and peripheral blood smear showing schistocytes) and thrombocytopenia.

Herpes hepatitis should always be considered in a pregnant woman with an acute elevation in aminotransferase values. However, patients with herpes hepatitis usually have fever and marked aminotransferase elevations (>5000 U/L). This patient is afebrile and has only mildly increased aminotransferase values. Herpes hepatitis would also not explain the anemia or thrombocytopenia. Patients with idiopathic (immune) thrombocytopenia present with isolated thrombocytopenia without elevated liver enzymes or hemolysis, findings that are not compatible with this patient's clinical presentation.

KEY POINT

• HELLP syndrome is characterized by microangiopathic hemolytic anemia, elevated liver enzymes, and low platelets.

Bibliography

1. **Guntupalli SR, Steingrub J.** Hepatic disease and pregnancy: an overview of diagnosis and management. Crit Care Med. 2005;33:S332-9. [PMID: 16215356]

Item 6   Answer: C

Hepatic ischemia is characterized by marked elevations in aminotransferase values that rapidly improve over the course of several days. Because of the dual blood supply of the liver, a hypotensive episode is usually required to cause hepatic ischemia. Improvements in the total bilirubin level may lag behind improvements in aminotransferase values.

Choledocholithiasis may also induce transient elevations of aminotransferase values (up to 1000 U/L) but is usually associated with significant abdominal pain. Viral hepatitis generally causes jaundice and other systemic symptoms such as fatigue. In addition, the abnormal aminotransferase values in patients with viral hepatitis improve over a period of weeks rather than days. Drug-induced liver disease (other than acetaminophen hepatotoxicity) does not usually cause such markedly increased aminotransferase values (usually <500 U/L), and the abnormal values that do occur do not improve after only 2 days.

KEY POINT

- Hepatic ischemia is characterized by marked elevations in aminotransferase values that rapidly improve within several days.

Bibliography

1. Seeto RK, Fenn B, Rockey DC. Ischemic hepatitis: clinical presentation and pathogenesis. Am J Med. 2000;109:109-13. [PMID: 10967151]

Item 7 Answer: D

This patient's hematemesis is most likely due to a Mallory-Weiss tear as a result of her pregnancy-related vomiting. A Mallory-Weiss tear refers to a laceration near the gastro-esophageal junction that is often caused by forceful retching. The bleeding stops spontaneously in >90% of patients, and endoscopic therapy is reserved for those with continued active bleeding or an underlying bleeding diathesis.

Although the patient takes an iron supplement that could cause pill-induced esophagitis, this rarely is associated with hematemesis. Peptic ulcer disease accounts for approximately 50% of cases of upper gastrointestinal bleeding and can occur without pain. However, the patient's history of repeated vomiting followed by a bleeding episode is not typical for peptic ulcer disease. Spider angiomata, palmar erythema, and an elevated alkaline phosphatase value are physiologic changes associated with pregnancy and do not indicate cirrhosis. Therefore, without known cirrhosis, this patient is unlikely to have gastroesophageal varices.

KEY POINT

- A Mallory-Weiss tear is a laceration near the gastroesophageal junction that often results from forceful retching.

Bibliography

1. Wu JC, Chan FK. Esophageal bleeding disorders. Curr Opin Gastroenterol. 2004;20:386-90. [PMID: 15703670]

Item 8 Answer: D

This patient requires an upper endoscopy despite a normal barium radiograph and an esophageal motility study that is consistent with achalasia. Symptoms of pseudoachalasia, an esophageal motility disorder that is associated with malignancy, may mimic those of idiopathic (benign) achalasia. Patients with pseudoachalasia are usually 60 years of age or older and have profound weight loss, although they can have typical manometric findings of achalasia. Elderly patients with symptoms of achalasia should therefore be evaluated for the presence of a malignant lesion, as a tumor is often found in the distal esophagus. Some tumors may cause aperistalsis by

a paraneoplastic phenomenon. Upper endoscopy is the most appropriate study for detecting these tumors.

Because treatment of pseudoachalasia involves management of the underlying tumor, neither pneumatic dilation nor a Heller myotomy is appropriate, although either procedure may be reasonable for patients with idiopathic achalasia. Although calcium channel blockers have a role in the non-surgical management of achalasia, establishing the diagnosis is the next management step.

KEY POINT

- Patients with achalasia should undergo upper endoscopy to rule out pseudoachalasia.

Bibliography

1. Portale G, Costantini M, Zaninotto G, Ruol A, Guirroli E, Rampado S, Ancona E. Pseudoachalasia: not only esophago-gastric cancer. Dis Esophagus. 2007;20:168-72. [PMID: 17439602]

Item 9 Answer: B

Irritable bowel syndrome (IBS) occurs very commonly in patients in this age group and many features of this patient's presentation suggest this syndrome (including the chronicity of the problem, its association with stress, and the pattern of alternating diarrhea and constipation). However, she also has two alarm symptoms, weight loss and anemia. Therefore, she should undergo colonoscopy. Rome II criteria for IBS require the presence of 3 (not necessarily consecutive) months of pain relieved with defecation and onset associated with change in stool frequency or consistency. In clinical practice, these criteria have a positive predictive value of 98%. However, this diagnostic rule should be applied only to patients who have no alarm symptoms suggesting a potentially serious underlying condition, such as hematochezia, weight loss, family history of colon cancer, recurring fever, anemia, or chronic severe diarrhea. These alarm symptoms require careful evaluation.

Patients with tenesmus or hematochezia likely have disease in the distal bowel, and flexible sigmoidoscopy may be sufficient for diagnosis. Crohn's disease is frequently characterized by skip areas (that is, areas of normal-appearing bowel interrupted by large areas of diseased bowel) and often is associated with terminal ileitis and is usually diagnosed by colonoscopy. However, a small-bowel follow-through is sometimes required to find disease that does not extend to the colon. If the patient were febrile, a CT scan of the abdomen might be necessary to identify fistulas and abscesses, which can occur in association with Crohn's disease.

KEY POINT

- Alarm symptoms in patients with abdominal pain include hematochezia, weight loss, family history of colon cancer, fever, anemia, or chronic severe diarrhea and require careful evaluation.

Bibliography

1. Mertz HR. Irritable bowel syndrome. N Engl J Med. 2003;349:2136-46. [PMID: 14645642]

Item 10   Answer: A

This patient has acute appendicitis. Initial symptoms usually include pain in the epigastrium or periumbilical region, which usually is mild, constant, and difficult to localize precisely. Pain eventually localizes to the right lower quadrant. Nausea and vomiting, if present, follow the onset of pain; if they precede the onset of pain, a diagnosis other than appendicitis is likely. Leukocytosis and low-grade fever are common. Urine leukocytosis, as seen in this patient, is probably due to the proximity of the inflamed appendix to the bladder and can cause a delay in diagnosis. Physical examination usually reveals localized tenderness in the right lower quadrant; tenderness in the right lower quadrant during rectal and pelvic examination may also be present. Pain with internal rotation of the hip (obturator sign) is associated with a pelvic appendix, whereas pain in the right lower quadrant with extension of the right hip (iliopsoas sign) is associated with a retrocecal appendix.

Ruptured ectopic pregnancy and acute pelvic inflammatory disease should always be considered in the differential diagnosis of women presenting with lower abdominal pain. A pregnancy test should always be done in a woman of reproductive age evaluated for abdominal or pelvic pain; the negative test in this patient makes an ectopic pregnancy unlikely. No single symptom or test is pathognomonic for pelvic inflammatory disease, but combinations of symptoms, signs, and other findings can provide a diagnosis with reasonable accuracy. Numerous leukocytes on a wet mount of vaginal discharge, lower abdominal pain, and pelvic tenderness on physical examination have reasonable sensitivity and specificity for pelvic inflammatory disease. The absence of a discharge and pelvic pain with cervical movement makes pelvic inflammatory disease unlikely in this patient. Acute uncomplicated pyelonephritis is suggested by the abrupt onset of fever, chills, and flank pain and costovertebral angle tenderness on physical examination. Pyuria, particularly if associated with bacteriuria or leukocyte casts, provides strong support for the presence of pyelonephritis. This patient's primarily abdominal and pelvic pain in the absence of flank pain or tenderness makes pyelonephritis unlikely.

KEY POINTS

- Initial symptoms of acute appendicitis usually include pain in the epigastrium or periumbilical region, which eventually localizes to the right lower quadrant.
- Nausea and vomiting follow the onset of pain in acute appendicitis.

Bibliography
1. Paulson EK, Kalady MF, Pappas TN. Clinical practice. Suspected appendicitis. N Engl J Med. 2003;348:236-42. [PMID: 12529465]

Item 11   Answer: B

This patient requires a colonoscopy. Signs and symptoms of colorectal cancer are usually nonspecific but when present may indicate locally advanced or metastatic disease. The possibility of colon cancer should be considered when any of the following "red flags" are present: rectal bleeding, change in bowel habits, hypogastric pain, abdominal distention, nausea or vomiting, pelvic pain or tenesmus, weight loss, or fatigue. Physical examination findings that should prompt investigation for colon cancer include a rectal or abdominal mass, hepatomegaly, abdominal tenderness, or iron deficiency anemia. If one or more such findings are present, a full colorectal examination with colonoscopy should be done. However, the examination may be limited to sigmoidoscopy for rectal bleeding in most persons younger than 40 years of age because colorectal cancer is uncommon in such patients (except those with hereditary colorectal cancer syndromes), and in most young patients with hematochezia, a rectosigmoid lesion, usually hemorrhoids, is the cause of rectal bleeding. This patient is older than 40 years of age and has weight loss, change in bowel habits, and abdominal pain, and therefore an immediate colonoscopy is indicated. With appropriate health care maintenance and screening, colorectal cancer can usually be prevented or at least detected before any signs or symptoms occur.

A contrast-enhanced CT scan of the abdomen is not sensitive for diagnosing colon cancer. Abdominal ultrasonography is useful for diagnosing hepatobiliary disease but not colon cancer. Stopping the ibuprofen or initiating a high-fiber diet may ultimately be useful therapeutic interventions but cannot replace the immediate need to investigate possible colon cancer.

KEY POINTS

- Colon cancer should be considered when any of the following "red flags" are present: rectal bleeding, change in bowel habits, hypogastric pain, abdominal distention, nausea or vomiting, pelvic pain or tenesmus, weight loss, and fatigue.
- Colonoscopy is the preferred test to diagnose possible colon cancer.

Bibliography
1. Regula J, Rupinski M, Kraszewska E, Polkowski M, Pachlewski J, Orlowska J, Nowacki MP, Butruk E. Colonoscopy in colorectal-cancer screening for detection of advanced neoplasia. N Engl J Med. 20062;355:1863-72. [PMID: 17079760]

Item 12   Answer: B

This patient has acute diverticulitis and should be treated empirically with antibiotics. Patients with uncomplicated diverticulitis present with left lower quadrant abdominal pain and fever. Physical examination discloses left lower quadrant abdominal tenderness. Leukocytosis is present. Uncomplicated diverticulitis can often be diagnosed based on clinical findings alone, although a CT scan of the abdomen and pelvis is indicated if the diagnosis is uncertain or a complication is suspected. Uncomplicated mild diverticulitis can be treated in the outpatient setting using broad-spectrum antibiotics such as ciprofloxacin and metronidazole for 7 to 10 days and a soft, low-residue diet. Patients who cannot maintain oral intake require hospitalization. If fever and pain persist for several days after initiation of antibiotics, a CT scan of the abdomen and pelvis should be performed to exclude the formation of an abscess that may require drainage. As symptoms improve, a full diet can be resumed. The role of diet in preventing recurrence is not well documented, although patients are often asked to follow a high-fiber diet after recovering from acute uncomplicated diverticulitis. Patients have also been asked to avoid popcorn, nuts, and seeds, although this recommendation is not evidence-based. Several weeks after resolution, patients should undergo colonoscopy to exclude other disorders that may mimic diverticulitis, such as a malignancy.

Colectomy is not indicated in the absence of a complication such as abscess, obstruction, or fistula formation. Colonoscopy should not be performed during the acute phase of diverticulitis because the risk of perforation is increased; colonoscopy is appropriate after the patient recovers from the acute episode. A high-residue diet is often recommended following recovery from acute diverticulitis in an attempt to prevent further recurrences. During the acute stage, a soft, low-residue diet is preferred.

KEY POINTS

- Patients with uncomplicated diverticulitis present with left lower quadrant abdominal pain and fever.

- Uncomplicated mild diverticulitis can be treated in the outpatient setting using broad-spectrum antibiotics such as ciprofloxacin and metronidazole.

Bibliography
1. **Janes SE, Meagher A, Frizelle FA.** Management of diverticulitis. BMJ. 2006;332:271-5. [PMID: 16455722]

Item 13   Answer: D

This patient has irritable bowel syndrome (IBS). There are now validated symptom-based diagnostic criteria that discriminate IBS from other disorders; the most common such criteria are the Rome II and Manning symptom criteria. The Rome criteria include at least 12 weeks (which need not be consecutive) in the preceding 12 months of abdominal discomfort or pain that has two of the following three features: relieved with defecation; onset associated with a change in the frequency of stool; and onset associated with a change in the form (appearance) of stool. Symptoms that support the diagnosis are abnormal stool frequency (>3 bowel movements/day or <3 bowel movements/week), abnormal stool form, abnormal stool passage, presence of mucus, and bloating or feeling of abdominal distention.

The Manning criteria include the following: pain relief with defecation, often; looser stools at pain onset, often; more frequent stools at pain onset, often; visible abdominal distention; mucus per rectum; feeling of incomplete evacuation, often. The diagnostic accuracy of the Manning criteria is even

better than that of the Rome criteria in women, younger patients, and when more criteria are positive. This patient fulfills the Rome and Manning criteria for the diagnosis. She does not have any "red flags" to suggest an alternative diagnosis (weight loss, nocturnal awakening with symptoms, fever, blood mixed in stool, new progressive symptoms, symptom onset after age 50 years, recent antibiotic use, or family history of colon cancer or inflammatory bowel disease). Fibromyalgia, depression, chronic pelvic pain, and tension headaches are often associated with IBS.

Crohn's disease may affect any segment of the gastrointestinal tract, is often discontinuous, and may cause transmural inflammation. Patients with Crohn's disease commonly present with abdominal pain, diarrhea, and weight loss. Disease involving the small intestine often causes nonbloody diarrhea, whereas hematochezia is more likely when the colon is involved. Abdominal examination may demonstrate tenderness or a mass that most often occurs in the right lower quadrant. High fever suggests an abscess or peritonitis. Perianal examination may reveal skin tags, inflammation, induration, or fistulas. In the absence of these "red flags," the patient is unlikely to have Crohn's disease.

The pain of chronic cholelithiasis is typically located in the right upper quadrant and is usually associated with fever, mild hyperbilirubinemia, and mild elevations of aminotransferase levels. Diverticulitis usually occurs in older patients with a history of change in bowel habits, fever, and left lower or suprapubic abdominal pain. The patient's normal pelvic examination makes pelvic inflammatory disease unlikely.

KEY POINTS

- Recent clinical and epidemiologic studies have led to the development of symptom-based diagnostic criteria (Rome and Manning criteria) that can accurately discriminate irritable bowel syndrome from other disorders.

- "Red flags" to suggest an alternative diagnosis to irritable bowel syndrome include the following: weight loss, nocturnal awakening with symptoms, fever, blood mixed in stool, new progressive symptoms, symptom onset after age 50 years, recent antibiotic use, or family history of colon cancer or inflammatory bowel disease.

Bibliography
1. **Horwitz BJ, Fisher RS.** The irritable bowel syndrome. N Engl J Med. 2001;344:1846-50. [PMID: 11407347]

Item 14   Answer: B

This patient meets Rome II criteria for irritable bowel syndrome (IBS) and will most likely respond to loperamide. Treatment for IBS is largely symptomatic, and loperamide has been found to be effective for diarrhea-predominant IBS.

Both tricyclic antidepressants and selective serotonin reuptake inhibitors have been shown to improve overall well-being and pain levels in patients with IBS but have no impact on other symptoms such as diarrhea. Alosetron is approved by the Food and Drug Administration for diarrhea-predominant IBS. However, its use should be restricted to patients with severe, diarrhea-predominant IBS who have not responded to other symptomatic measures because this drug has been associated with ischemic colitis in approximately 1 in 700 patients. Physicians who prescribe alosetron must register with the manufacturer, and patients must sign a consent form before beginning therapy. Adding fiber to the diet is a common approach to treating IBS. Although safe, fiber was found to be no more beneficial in treating global IBS symptoms than placebo in a recent meta-analysis. Although clinical trials suggest that antispasmodic agents, such as dicyclomine and hyoscyamine, may be helpful in managing pain in patients with IBS, a recent meta-analysis suggests that the benefit is weak.

KEY POINTS

- For diarrhea-predominant irritable bowel syndrome (IBS), loperamide has been found to be effective.

- Although safe, fiber is no more beneficial in treating global IBS symptoms than placebo.

Bibliography

1. Wilson JF. In the clinic. Irritable bowel syndrome. Ann Intern Med. 2007;147:ITC7-1-ITC7-16. [PMID: 17606954]

Item 15   Answer: D

This patient has ischemic colitis, which is a frequent cause of self-limited, relatively painless hematochezia in elderly patients. Systemic signs and symptoms do not usually occur, although patients may have had a hypotensive episode associated with another disorder such as underlying coronary artery disease. It is possible that this patient's use of nitroglycerin tablets earlier in the day, coupled with her low cardiac output, resulted in decreased blood flow at the site of mesenteric artery collateral vessels that led to the ischemia. Most episodes are self-limited and resolve following supportive therapy. Other than endoscopic evaluation of the colon, additional studies or medical interventions are usually not needed.

In Crohn's disease, the abdominal pain is frequently in the right lower quadrant and is associated with diarrhea and weight loss with or without associated nausea and vomiting or rapid bleeding. In diverticulitis, abdominal pain is more typically confined to the left lower quadrant and is associated with fever, not bleeding. Diverticulosis is a common cause of gastrointestinal bleeding in the elderly, but is painless. Colon cancer must always be considered in the differential diagnosis of elderly patients with bowel symptoms, but colonic neoplasms more typically cause progressive symptoms of colonic obstruction, such as intermittent abdominal pain, nausea, and vomiting followed by obstipation and distention. Patients with colon cancer may also present with gastrointestinal bleeding. However, this patient is unlikely to have colon cancer because of her normal colonoscopy 5 months ago. Pseudomembra-

nous colitis is associated with abdominal pain and cramping, diarrhea, nausea, vomiting, and fever, but not with rapid gastrointestinal bleeding. Pseudomembranous colitis is also associated with recent antibiotic use or hospital-acquired infection, both absent in this patient.

KEY POINT

- Ischemic colitis is a common cause of self-limited hematochezia and mild to moderate abdominal pain in elderly patients.

Bibliography

1. Green BT, Tendler DA. Ischemic colitis: a clinical review. South Med J. 2005;98:217-22. [PMID: 15759953]

Item 16   Answer: A

This patient has acute mesenteric artery ischemia, an uncommon disorder that accounts for less than 0.5% of all hospital admissions in the United States. Causes include emboli, arterial or venous thrombosis, vasoconstriction from hypoperfusion, and, rarely, vasculitis. The most common cause is a mesenteric arterial embolism originating from the heart (50% of patients) most often due to atrial fibrillation (as in this patient), followed by mesenteric arterial thrombosis due to atherosclerotic lesions (25% of patients), and mesenteric venous thrombosis, predominantly in the superior mesenteric vein (10% of patients). The clinical manifestations of acute mesenteric artery ischemia are nonspecific. Patients present with acute diffuse abdominal pain that is more severe than the findings suggested by abdominal palpation. Signs of peritonitis (such as fever, abdominal pain, rebound tenderness, and preferential flexion of the hips and knees) are ominous because they may signify intestinal infarction. Associated laboratory abnormalities include leukocytosis, hyperkalemia, and metabolic acidosis.

Acute pancreatitis may present similarly to acute mesenteric artery ischemia, but the normal serum amylase and lipase values eliminate this diagnosis in this patient. Patients with uncomplicated diverticulitis present with abdominal pain and fever; hyperkalemia and a metabolic acidosis (present in this patient) are not associated with uncomplicated diverticulitis. Physical examination reveals left lower quadrant abdominal tenderness. Leukocytosis is present, and sterile pyuria may occur due to bowel inflammation close to the bladder. Pain due to nephrolithiasis is paroxysmal and usually located in the flank, although it may radiate to the groin. Hematuria is common in patients with renal colic; hyperkalemia and acidosis are not found. Small bowel obstruction tends to be more insidious in onset, and patients usually have predisposing factors such as multiple surgical procedures. The abdomen is often distended and tympanitic to percussion in obstruction, and the rectal vault is often empty.

KEY POINTS

- Patients with acute mesenteric artery ischemia present with sudden, severe generalized abdominal pain.

- The most common cause of acute mesenteric artery ischemia is arterial embolism originating from the heart, most often due to atrial fibrillation.

Bibliography

1. **Oldenburg WA, Lau LL, Rodenberg TJ, Edmonds HJ, Burger CD.** Acute mesenteric ischemia: a clinical review. Arch Intern Med. 2004;164:1054-62. [PMID: 15159262]

Item 17   Answer: C

This patient's clinical presentation of abdominal pain, weight loss indicated by loose-fitting clothes, new-onset diabetes mellitus, and liver chemistry tests indicating cholestasis is suggestive of pancreatic carcinoma. A helical CT scan of the abdomen is the most sensitive and specific initial imaging study for this patient, as it can identify a pancreatic mass, determine the presence of biliary obstruction, and stage the disease, if present.

Endoscopic retrograde cholangiopancreatography may be appropriate to treat obstructive jaundice and obtain tissue for histologic studies but should only be done after a cross-sectional imaging study, such as a CT scan, has been obtained. Mesenteric angiography is appropriate if ischemic bowel disease is being considered as a cause of symptoms and weight loss, but this more invasive study should be done only after a normal CT scan is obtained. In addition, ischemic bowel disease would not cause cholestasis. Endoscopic ultrasonography is very sensitive for detecting pancreatic tumors and can also provide tissue for histologic study. However, endoscopic ultrasonography is also more invasive than CT scanning and should be performed only if a CT scan is normal, additional tissue is needed, or further staging is indicated.

KEY POINT

- A helical CT scan of the abdomen is the most sensitive and specific initial imaging study for a patient with possible pancreatic adenocarcinoma.

Bibliography

1. **Freelove R, Walling AD.** Pancreatic cancer: diagnosis and management. Am Fam Physician. 2006;73:485-92. [PMID: 16477897]

Item 18   Answer: C

Celiac sprue is the most likely cause of this patient's chronic diarrhea with associated weight loss, iron deficiency anemia, and rash consistent with dermatitis herpetiformis. IgA tissue transglutaminase antibody testing has a high sensitivity and specificity for this relatively common condition and is the most appropriate first step in pursuing a diagnosis in this patient. Celiac sprue is a chronic disease that can cause various symptoms and syndromes, most of which can also be caused by more common conditions. Irritable bowel syndrome may cause chronic diarrhea and abdominal pain; however, as many as 5% of patients with these symptoms may instead have celiac sprue. A high index of suspicion is needed to determine whether testing for celiac sprue is warranted. In affected patients, dermatitis herpetiformis is an uncommon but highly characteristic itchy vesicobullous rash that predominantly involves the extensor surfaces, particularly the elbows and knees, interscapular region, and buttocks. Typical symptoms of malabsorption may be absent in patients with skin involvement.

Colonoscopy may be useful in evaluating chronic diarrhea, particularly when there is suspicion for malignancy (weight loss, blood in stool, change in stool) or inflammatory bowel disease (fever, weight loss, pain, blood in stool), but is not helpful in diagnosing celiac sprue. If IgA tissue transglutaminase antibody testing is positive, an upper endoscopy with small-bowel biopsy will establish a diagnosis of celiac sprue. CT scanning of the abdomen can help to identify other causes of chronic diarrhea, such as pancreatic cancer, chronic pancreatitis, inflammatory bowel disease, chronic infections, or intestinal lymphoma. However, this test is not the most appropriate first diagnostic study for a patient with a high likelihood of celiac sprue. Stool cultures are useful for evaluation of acute infectious causes of diarrhea but are unlikely to be helpful in a patient with a 6-month history of diarrhea along with dermatitis herpetiformis.

KEY POINT

- IgA tissue transglutaminase antibody testing has a high sensitivity and specificity for diagnosing celiac sprue.

Bibliography

1. **Ciclitira PJ, King AL, Fraser JS.** AGA technical review on Celiac Sprue. American Gastroenterological Association. Gastroenterology. 2001;120:1526-40. [PMID: 11313324]

Item 19   Answer: B

Candies and other products using artificial sweeteners often contain poorly absorbed carbohydrates (e.g., sorbitol, mannitol) that may cause flatulence and diarrhea. Discontinuing these products is the most appropriate empiric management of a patient with these findings.

Calcium supplements may cause constipation or reduced frequency of bowel movements. Therefore, discontinuing this patient's calcium is unlikely to improve his symptoms. Although metformin is used for patients with diabetes mellitus, this agent is associated with the development of diarrhea and may therefore increase stool frequency even more. Because he has diabetes mellitus, this patient is at risk for small-bowel bacterial overgrowth for which an empiric trial of antibiotics might be considered. However, this diagnosis should be considered only after excluding a dietary source for his symptoms.

KEY POINT

- Artificial sweeteners that contain poorly absorbed carbohydrates (e.g., sorbitol, mannitol) may cause flatulence and diarrhea.

Bibliography
1. **Sibley E.** Carbohydrate intolerance. Curr Opin Gastroenterol. 2004;20:162-7. [PMID: 15703639]

Item 20   Answer: B

Although all of the pathogens listed are possible causes of this patient's illness, enterotoxigenic *Escherichia coli* diarrhea occurs most often in travelers. This patient's presentation is fairly typical of *E. coli* infection experienced by travelers to developing countries. Although the disease can be quite severe (fever, nausea, vomiting, abdominal pain, and malaise), it is usually relatively benign and self-limited. Antibiotics are generally not required for mild traveler's diarrhea and may even exacerbate certain types of diarrheal illness.

Vibrio cholerae is an unusual cause of diarrhea in travelers except in areas where cholera is highly endemic. Although *Campylobacter jejuni* is the most common bacterial cause of diarrhea in the United States, it occurs much less often than enterotoxigenic *E. coli* diarrhea in other countries. *Shigella dysenteriae* is a much less frequent cause of diarrhea than *E. coli* and is associated with a more severe illness that persists longer without treatment. *Salmonella typhimurium* is also a possible cause of diarrhea in travelers but occurs much less frequently than *E. coli* infection.

KEY POINT
• Enterotoxigenic *Escherichia coli* is the most common cause of diarrhea in travelers to developing countries.

Bibliography
1. **Riddle MS, Sanders JW, Putnam SD, Tribble DR.** Incidence, etiology, and impact of diarrhea among long-term travelers (US military and similar populations): a systematic review. Am J Trop Med Hyg. 2006;74:891-900. [PMID: 16687698]

Item 21   Answer: B

This elderly man has features suggestive of severe cholangitis, including fever, abdominal pain, altered mental status, and jaundice. Results of liver chemistry tests support a diagnosis of bile duct obstruction (elevated serum alkaline phosphatase and total bilirubin concentrations), and gallstones are seen on ultrasonography. The common bile duct is also minimally dilated, which may indicate ductal obstruction caused by stones with resultant secondary cholangitis. Even when broad-spectrum antibiotics are administered, the mortality rate for cholangitis is high unless ductal decompression is performed. Urgent endoscopic retrograde cholangiopancreatography (ERCP) is therefore warranted to document choledo-cholithiasis (common bile duct stones) and perform endoscopic therapy, if indicated.

Symptoms of acute hepatitis A usually include malaise, fatigue, nausea and vomiting, and the aminotransferase levels are generally >1000 U/L. In addition, acute hepatitis A cannot explain the dilated common bile duct or the gallstones. Acute

cholecystitis is not supported by the ultrasound findings (absence of gallbladder wall thickening and pericholecystic fluid) and cannot explain the dilated common bile duct. Acute pancreatitis does not typically cause right upper quadrant pain and is unlikely to cause a septic state (fever, tachycardia, hypotension, and altered mental status) over just a few hours.

KEY POINT
• Patients with severe cholangitis generally present with fever, jaundice, and altered mental status; abdominal pain is usually, but not invariably, present.

Bibliography
1. **Flasar MH, Goldberg E.** Acute abdominal pain. Med Clin North Am. 2006;90:481-503. [PMID: 16473101]

Item 22   Answer: A

The patient has acute cholecystitis and the next diagnostic step is abdominal ultrasonography. The typical history for acute cholecystitis includes prior episodes of biliary colic, midepigastric pain radiating to the right upper quadrant, fever, chills, nausea, and vomiting. Physical examination findings usually include right upper quadrant or midepigastric tenderness and pain and arrest of respiration on palpation of the right upper quadrant (Murphy's sign). Leukocytosis, mild elevations in aminotransferase concentrations and mild hyperbilirubinemia are common in acute cholecystitis.

Both abdominal ultrasonography and hepato-iminodiacetic acid (HIDA) scans are accurate for the diagnosis of acute cholecystitis. The general recommendation has been to obtain ultrasonography first, followed by a HIDA scan, if necessary. Despite most organizations recommending ultrasonography as the primary diagnostic tool for acute cholecystitis, the literature shows that a HIDA scan has equal or better sensitivity and specificity; however, cost and ease of access favor the use of ultrasonography. The classic findings of acute cholecystitis on ultrasonography are pericholecystic fluid and a thickened gallbladder wall of 3 to 4 mm. The presence of a sonographic Murphy's sign (Murphy's sign elicited during palpation by the ultrasound transducer) further confirms the diagnosis. The classic finding of acute cholecystitis on a HIDA scan is nonvisualization of the gallbladder.

A contrast-enhanced CT scan can show gallstones, gallbladder wall thickening, gallbladder distention, pericholecystic fluid, and inflammation of the pericholecystic fat. An unenhanced CT scan can show gallstones and a hyperdense gallbladder wall, which can suggest the presence of gangrenous cholecystitis. CT scanning is expensive and is generally reserved for diagnostic dilemmas and to detect possible complications of acute cholecystitis. Endoscopic retrograde cholangiopancreatography (ERCP) is an invasive procedure used to remove common duct stones and facilitate biliary drainage and is indicated for patients with cholangitis or for those with gallstone pancreatitis complicated by cholangitis but is not used in the diagnosis of cholecystitis.

- Abdominal ultrasonography is the initial test of choice for the diagnosis of acute cholecystitis.

Bibliography
1. **Trowbridge RL, Rutkowski NK, Shojania KG.** Does this patient have acute cholecystitis? JAMA. 2003;289:80-6. [PMID: 12503981]

Item 23   Answer: A

Prolonged right upper quadrant abdominal pain, fever, leukocytosis, and hyperbilirubinemia suggest the diagnosis of acute cholecystitis. The patient requires urgent abdominal imaging to confirm the diagnosis. Abdominal ultrasonography has a sensitivity of 81% to 98% and a specificity of 70% to 98% for diagnosing acute cholecystitis, and it is also readily available, inexpensive, and safe. The classic findings of acute cholecystitis on ultrasonography are pericholecystic fluid and a thickened gallbladder wall of 3 to 4 mm. A sonographic Murphy's sign (maximal tenderness directly over the visualized gallbladder when palpated with the ultrasound transducer) further confirms the diagnosis.

Abdominal CT scanning may be helpful if the diagnosis is not confirmed by ultrasonography or if cholangitis is suspected (total bilirubin >4.0 mg/dL, elevated aminotransferase levels, diminished consciousness or shock). However, the diagnosis of acute cholecystitis should not be delayed by waiting for a CT scan. Endoscopic retrograde cholangiopancreatography (ERCP) with sphincterotomy is reserved for patients with common bile duct stones or cholangitis and should not be considered until a diagnosis is confirmed. Magnetic resonance cholangiopancreatography (MRCP) may be slightly more sensitive than ultrasonography in detecting gallstones, but it is very expensive and not universally available.

Patients with uncomplicated cholecystitis should be hospitalized and treated with antimicrobial therapy and cholecystectomy. A low-fat diet may decrease the incidence of gallstones but is not useful in treating acute cholecystitis. Nonsteroidal anti-inflammatory agents, such as diclofenac, provide pain relief in biliary colic and may decrease the risk of progression to acute cholecystitis but are not adequate therapy once cholecystitis has developed.

- Prolonged right upper quadrant abdominal pain, fever, leukocytosis, and hyperbilirubinemia suggest the diagnosis of acute cholecystitis.
- Patients with suspected cholecystitis require abdominal imaging with ultrasonography to confirm the diagnosis.

Bibliography
1. **Trowbridge RL, Rutkowski NK, Shojania KG.** Does this patient have acute cholecystitis? JAMA. 2003;289:80-6. [PMID: 12503981]

Item 24   Answer: D

This patient with long-standing ulcerative colitis and abnormal liver chemistry test results is at risk for developing primary sclerosing cholangitis, which is a well-recognized complication of inflammatory bowel disease. The key to the diagnosis is the recognition of laboratory results compatible with cholestatic liver disease, including high alkaline phosphatase concentration, normal or minimally elevated bilirubin level, and modestly elevated aminotransferase values. Another important diagnostic clue is the presence of dilated peripheral bile ducts on the CT scan without evidence of apparent obstruction in the common bile duct. Endoscopic retrograde cholangiopancreatography (ERCP) is warranted to confirm the diagnosis of sclerosing cholangitis. ERCP can also be used to perform endoscopic stenting, if indicated.

Choledocholithiasis is associated with abdominal pain and fever and evidence of common bile duct dilatation, which is absent in this patient. Primary biliary cirrhosis is a progressive cholestatic liver disease of unknown cause. It is an autoimmune disorder that occurs predominantly in women (80% to 90%) between 40 and 60 years of age. The most common symptoms are fatigue and pruritus. Primary biliary cirrhosis is not associated with inflammatory bowel disease. Patients with acute viral hepatitis most commonly have fatigue, nausea, mild right upper quadrant abdominal pain, and jaundice. The hepatocellular injury primarily results in elevated aminotransferase concentrations, usually >1000 U/L, which is not seen in this patient.

- Patients with inflammatory bowel disease have an increased risk for developing primary sclerosing cholangitis.

Bibliography
1. **Cullen SN, Chapman RW.** Review article: current management of primary sclerosing cholangitis. Aliment Pharmacol Ther. 2005;21:933-48. [PMID: 15813829]

Item 25   Answer: A

This patient has the classic presentation of acute gallstone pancreatitis with markedly abnormal aminotransferase and amylase values that rapidly return toward normal with relief of symptoms. Abdominal ultrasonography is used to exclude cholelithiasis because a CT scan may not detect gallstones or sludge. Cholescintigraphy (HIDA scan) may demonstrate cystic duct obstruction indicative of chronic cholecystitis but will not show gallstones. Endoscopic retrograde cholangiopancreatography (ERCP) is indicated if the patient's liver chemistry test results become significantly abnormal, especially if jaundice develops and abdominal ultrasonography shows ductal dilatation, but is not the initial diagnostic study for suspected gallstone pancreatitis. Since the relapse rate for gallstone pancreatitis is high, laparoscopic cholecystectomy should be performed before hospital discharge but should not be done until diagnostic studies are obtained.

- Patients with acute gallstone pancreatitis present with elevated aminotransferase and pancreatic enzyme values that rapidly return toward normal.

Bibliography
1. **Kingsnorth A, O'Reilly D.** Acute pancreatitis. BMJ. 2006;332: 1072-6. [PMID: 16675814]

Item 26   Answer: C

This patient presents with acute pancreatitis of undetermined cause and may have hypertriglyceridemia because of his poorly controlled diabetes mellitus. However, his triglyceride level was not assessed initially and should be done now. Triglyceride values should be checked in all patients with acute pancreatitis of unclear etiology because hypertriglyceridemia can be the underlying cause. Mild hypertriglyceridemia (triglyceride value ≤400 mg/dL) occurs in up to 75% of patients with acute pancreatitis. However, marked hypertriglyceridemia (triglyceride value >400 mg/dL) develops in approximately 20% of patients, and in this setting is most likely due to an antecedent disorder of lipoprotein metabolism. Patients whose triglyceride level exceeds 1000 mg/dL most likely have hypertriglyceridemic pancreatitis.

Hyper- or hypothyroidism is not a cause of acute pancreatitis, and thyroid function tests are therefore not indicated. The initial abdominal ultrasound examination showed no gallstones or sludge; a second examination is not indicated at this time. Although endoscopic ultrasonography is more sensitive than transabdominal ultrasonography for detecting gallbladder stones and sludge, hyperlipidemia should be excluded before more invasive studies are done.

- A patient with acute pancreatitis of undetermined cause should be evaluated for hypertriglyceridemia.

Bibliography
1. **Whitcomb DC.** Clinical practice. Acute pancreatitis. N Engl J Med. 2006;354:2142-50. [PMID: 16707751]

Item 27   Answer: B

This patient has acute necrotizing pancreatitis. Abdominal pain is the most common symptom of acute pancreatitis and occurs in 95% of patients. The pain is usually epigastric or diffuse throughout the entire upper abdomen, is moderate to severe and constant, radiates to the back, and occasionally decreases when the patient sits or leans forward or assumes the fetal position. The physical examination commonly reveals abdominal tenderness without peritoneal signs (the pancreas is a retroperitoneal organ). Signs of hypovolemia indicate severe pancreatitis and portend a poor prognosis. Ecchymosis of the flanks (Grey-Turner's sign) suggests pancreatic hemorrhage due to necrosis; pancreatic necrosis is very rare, occurring in less than 1% of patients and is an ominous finding.

Abdominal and chest radiographs should be obtained in patients with suspected acute pancreatitis to exclude intraabdominal or intrathoracic processes (for example, bowel perforation or obstruction) that can mimic acute pancreatitis. In patients with severe pancreatitis, a contrast-enhanced CT scan can exclude conditions that present similarly to acute pancreatitis, confirm the diagnosis of pancreatitis by showing an abnormal appearance of the pancreas, and grade the severity of pancreatitis by determining the presence or absence of local complications, such as necrosis, abscess, or pseudocyst. This patient's CT scan shows diffuse hypoperfusion of the entire pancreas, which is consistent with necrotizing pancreatitis.

The essential features of acute cholecystitis include previous episodes of biliary colic, midepigastric pain radiating to the right upper quadrant, fever, chills, nausea, and vomiting; the absence of these findings in this patient makes acute cholecystitis unlikely. Alcoholic hepatitis is associated with symptoms typical of many acute liver diseases. The most common symptoms are jaundice (60%), anorexia (49%), weight loss (28%), fever (22%), and abdominal pain (18%). Diffuse abdominal tenderness and signs of hypovolemia are not consistent with alcoholic hepatitis. A perforated peptic ulcer may present with diffuse abdominal pain and hypotension, but peritoneal signs are frequently present and air should be detected beneath the diaphragms on the upright chest radiograph. Bowel obstruction is unlikely based upon the nondiagnostic supine radiograph and evidence of necrotizing pancreatitis on the abdominal CT scan.

- Patients with acute pancreatitis have abdominal pain that is epigastric or diffuse throughout the entire upper abdomen, is moderate to severe and constant, and radiates to the back.
- Ecchymosis of the flanks (Grey-Turner's sign) suggests pancreatic hemorrhage due to pancreatic necrosis, which is a very rare presentation of acute pancreatitis.

Bibliography
1. **Whitcomb DC.** Clinical practice. Acute pancreatitis. N Engl J Med. 2006;354:2142-50. [PMID: 16707751]

Item 28   Answer: D

This patient has hypertriglyceridemic pancreatitis. She is markedly volume depleted, as indicated by the elevated hematocrit value, tachycardia, and low blood pressure. Vigorous hydration is critical in order to maximize pancreatic perfusion and thus possibly reduce the number of subsequent complications.

Intravenous hyperalimentation is inappropriate because a patient with severe pancreatitis requires enteral, rather than parenteral, nutritional supplementation. Endoscopic ultrasonography is usually done to exclude common bile ducts stones in a patient with acute pancreatitis. However, stones are unlikely to be present in someone with hypertriglyceridemic pancreatitis. Likewise, endoscopic retrograde cholangiopancreatography is appropriate for diagnosing suspected common bile duct stones and cholangitis in a patient with severe biliary pancreatitis but not with hypertriglyceridemic pancreatitis. Even if these diagnostic tests were indicated, fluid resuscitation is the first and most critical management step in patients with acute pancreatitis.

KEY POINT

• Vigorous hydration is critical in a patient with acute pancreatitis and marked volume depletion in order to maximize pancreatic perfusion and reduce subsequent complications.

Bibliography

1. **Whitcomb DC.** Clinical practice. Acute pancreatitis. N Engl J Med. 2006;354:2142-50. [PMID: 16707751]

Item 29   Answer: B

This patient has gallstone pancreatitis, and urgent endoscopic retrograde cholangiopancreatography (ERCP) with biliary sphincterotomy is indicated to relieve the obstruction and minimize complications and recurrences. Alcohol abuse and gallstones are the leading causes of pancreatitis in the United States. This patient's previous episodes of colicky abdominal pain, evidence of cholelithiasis and common bile duct obstruction (dilated bile duct) on ultrasonography, and elevated amylase and lipase levels are supportive of biliary pancreatitis. Although the association between gallstones and acute pancreatitis is well established, the pathophysiology is unknown. Use of ERCP to extract the stones and to perform biliary sphincterotomy improves patient outcomes and prevents future acute attacks.

In patients with alcoholic pancreatitis, abstinence from alcohol is the most important measure in preventing recurrences. Although this patient's amount of alcohol consumption may be deleterious, abstinence from alcohol will not resolve this attack of gallstone pancreatitis. Gemfibrozil is an option to treat hypertriglyceridemia, which may cause pancreatitis; however, pancreatitis is uncommon in such patients with triglyceride levels less than 500 mg/dL. A low-fat diet may be useful for treating hypertriglyceridemia and preventing future gallstones but would not decrease complications and recurrences of pancreatitis. Cigarette smoking increases the risk for pancreatic cancer but not acute pancreatitis. Smoking cessation, although important for all patients' overall health, will not alleviate this patient's pancreatitis.

KEY POINT

• Urgent endoscopic retrograde cholangiopancreatography (ERCP) with biliary sphincterotomy is indicated for gallstone pancreatitis to relieve the obstruction and minimize complications and recurrences.

Bibliography

1. **Whitcomb DC.** Clinical practice. Acute pancreatitis. N Engl J Med. 2006;354:2142-50. [PMID: 16707751]

Item 30   Answer: B

This patient with long-standing symptoms of gastroesophageal reflux disease has upper endoscopy findings consistent with Barrett's esophagus. The figure shows displacement of the squamocolumnar junction proximal to the anatomic esophageal junction and is recognized as a zone of salmon-pink tissue. Esophageal biopsy specimens show the presence of intestinal metaplasia, which confirms the diagnosis. Barrett's esophagus is a risk factor for development of adenocarcinoma of the esophagus. Because this patient has no dysplasia on initial endoscopy, current recommendations call for repeated endoscopies with biopsies to exclude dysplasia followed by surveillance endoscopy with esophageal biopsies every 3 years.

Achalasia causes a dilated esophagus with a narrowed gastroesophageal junction in a patient with regurgitation and weight loss. No intestinal metaplasia is seen on biopsy specimens. Patients with achalasia are at risk for squamous cell carcinoma. Patients with esophageal adenocarcinoma will have a nodular or a flat region within a segment of Barrett's esophagus or a mass lesion with or without stricture. Biopsy specimens show adenocarcinoma. Esophageal candidiasis is manifested by diffuse, plaque-like lesions in a linear configuration. The salmon-colored mucosa in the distal esophagus typical of Barrett's esophagus is not present, and biopsy specimens of esophageal ulcerations will show hyphae.

KEY POINT

• Chronic and severe symptoms of gastrointestinal reflux disease predispose to the development of Barrett's esophagus, which is a risk factor for esophageal adenocarcinoma.

Bibliography

1. **Grover M, Strickland C, Kesler E, Crawford P.** How should patients with Barrett's esophagus be monitored? J Fam Pract. 2006;55:243-7. [PMID: 16510060]

Item 31   Answer: D

This patient requires upper endoscopy. Determining the specific diagnosis in this elderly patient is essential. His age, weight loss, nausea, anemia, and use of ibuprofen are highly suggestive of a structural lesion in the upper gastrointestinal tract. The differential diagnosis includes a complication of peptic ulcer disease or a malignancy. Upper endoscopy is the most appropriate diagnostic study at this time because it allows direct visualization of the upper gastrointestinal tract and can also provide therapy if arterial bleeding or gastric outlet obstruction is found.

Because the patient's pain does not suggest biliary tract disease, abdominal ultrasonography should not be the first study done. However, if results of upper endoscopy are normal, additional evaluation for pancreatic or biliary tract disease is required. Because of his advanced age and clinical presentation suggestive of structural disease, empiric therapy with acid-suppressive agents or antibiotics to eradicate *Helicobacter pylori* is unacceptable without first establishing a diagnosis.

KEY POINT

- Upper endoscopy is indicated for patients with suspected peptic ulcer disease and alarm features (vomiting, weight loss, and anemia).

Bibliography

1. **Cappell MS, Friedel D.** The role of esophagogastroduodenoscopy in the diagnosis and management of upper gastrointestinal disorders. Med Clin North Am. 2002;86:1165-216. [PMID: 12510452]

Item 32   Answer: B

This patient's clinical presentation is consistent with gastrinoma (Zollinger-Ellison syndrome), including multiple ulcers, ulcers in unusual locations, and ulcers that recur frequently. Other "red flags" include ulcers in the absence of nonsteroidal anti-inflammatory drug ingestion or *Helicobacter pylori* infection. Patients with these findings require serum gastrin measurement because virtually all patients with gastrinoma will have an increased serum gastrin concentration.

Glucagonoma, like gastrinoma, is a functional endocrine tumor of the pancreas or duodenum. Glucagonomas are recognized by the "4-D syndrome" consisting of: diabetes mellitus, dermatitis (necrolytic migratory erythema), deep venous thrombosis, and depression. Recurrent and recalcitrant peptic ulcer disease is not part of this syndrome. Patients with gastric cancer may present with abdominal pain, nausea, and weight loss, but multiple ulcers, esophageal ulcers, and ulcers distal to the pyloric channel are not consistent with the diagnosis of gastric cancer. *H. pylori* infection is the most common cause of peptic ulcer disease and is found in up to 80% of patients with duodenal ulcers and 50% of those with gastric ulcers. However, multiple ulcers, particularly esophageal ulcers and those distal to the duodenum, are uncharacteristic for *H. pylori* infection. Furthermore, previous negative tests for *H. pylori* in this patient make *H. pylori* peptic ulcer disease unlikely.

KEY POINT

- Gastrinoma (Zollinger-Ellison syndrome) should be suspected in patients with multiple ulcers, ulcers in unusual locations, and ulcers that recur frequently, particularly in the absence of nonsteroidal anti-inflammatory drug use or *Helicobacter pylori* infection.

Bibliography

1. **Gibril F, Schumann M, Pace A, Jensen RT.** Multiple endocrine neoplasia type 1 and Zollinger-Ellison syndrome: a prospective study of 107 cases and comparison with 1009 cases from the literature. Medicine (Baltimore). 2004;83:43-83.[PMID: 14747767]

Item 33   Answer: D

Up to 50% of patients who take a nonsteroidal anti-inflammatory drug (NSAID) develop dyspepsia, nausea, and abdominal pain. However, the incidence of ulcer disease is low in such patients, and these findings are not highly predictive of ulcer. The best management option for this patient is to stop the ibuprofen and begin therapy with a proton pump inhibitor.

Most patients with uncomplicated peptic ulcer disease present with dyspepsia (chronic pain or discomfort in the upper abdomen) or other upper gastrointestinal symptoms. The differential diagnosis of dyspepsia also includes gastroesophageal reflux disease (GERD), biliary tract disease, pancreatitis, cancer, and nonulcer dyspepsia. The classic symptoms of GERD are substernal heartburn and acid regurgitation. If GERD is suspected and the patient has no other significant findings or alarm features (weight loss, bleeding, early satiety, vomiting, or anemia), acid suppression therapy is indicated. If biliary tract or pancreatic disease may be present, serologic tests for hepatic and pancreatic diseases plus abdominal ultrasonography should be obtained first. If alarm features are present, upper endoscopy is indicated. A patient with dyspepsia but no alarm features should stop taking all NSAIDs and begin empiric acid suppression therapy. Expert opinion varies on the efficacy of serologic testing for *Helicobacter pylori* in such patients, but it should probably be performed, and a patient with a positive test result should receive *H. pylori* eradication therapy. Patients whose symptoms persist after completing a course of empiric therapy should undergo upper endoscopy.

Starting a proton pump inhibitor without discontinuing the NSAID or simply stopping the NSAID is less likely to relieve the patient's symptoms. Abdominal ultrasonography may be useful if cholecystitis is being considered as the cause of the pain. However, most patients with acute cholecystitis have had discrete prior episodes of biliary colic, midepigastric pain radiating to the right upper quadrant, fever, chills, nausea, and vomiting. Upper endoscopy is typically reserved for patients with alarm features or whose symptoms do not respond to empiric therapy.

KEY POINTS

- Symptoms and physical findings have poor positive or negative predictive value for *H. pylori*– or NSAID–associated peptic ulcer disease.
- Patients with dyspepsia and alarm features for gastric malignancy or an ulcer complication (weight loss, bleeding, early satiety, vomiting, or anemia) require upper endoscopy.

Bibliography

1. **Yeomans ND.** Management of peptic ulcer disease not related to Helicobacter. J Gastroenterol Hepatol. 2002;17:488-94. [PMID: 11982732]

Item 34   Answer: C

Treatment of *Helicobacter pylori* infection requires the combination of two antibiotics and an acid-suppressive agent. Triple therapy including a proton pump inhibitor plus clarithromycin and either amoxicillin or metronidazole is associated with eradication rates of greater than 85%. Amoxicillin should be used if the patient has previously been treated with metronidazole, and metronidazole should be used if the patient is allergic to penicillin.

The standard of care for patients with duodenal ulcers was formerly acid suppression with either a proton pump inhibitor or an H_2-receptor antagonist for 2 months. However, documenting the presence of *H. pylori* requires adding two antibiotics to the regimen, as eradication of this organism significantly decreases the likelihood of ulcer recurrence. Despite initial encouraging results using dual therapy (amoxicillin plus a proton pump inhibitor), subsequent experience in the United States has determined that this is less effective than triple therapy. Triple therapy should be given for 10 to 14 days. Bismuth-based triple therapy (bismuth subsalicylate plus two antibiotics) is also effective for treating *H. pylori* infection, but bismuth subsalicylate plus a proton pump inhibitor is not effective.

KEY POINT

• Triple therapy (a proton pump inhibitor or bismuth subsalicylate and two antibiotics) is the most effective regimen for eradication of *Helicobacter pylori.*

Bibliography
1. Ables AZ, Simon I, Melton ER. Update on Helicobacter pylori treatment. Am Fam Physician. 2007;75:351-8. [PMID: 17304866]

Item 35   Answer: B

Approximately 80% of patients with gastric or duodenal ulcer disease have *Helicobacter pylori* infection. The patient's clinical presentation is consistent with dyspepsia (epigastric discomfort following meals), and his young age and absence of alarm features (vomiting, weight loss, anemia, bleeding, early satiety) suggestive of ulcer complications support a "test and treat" approach for *H. pylori* infection rather than an immediate evaluation for other disorders. Blood, serum, and saliva can be analyzed for the presence of IgG antibody to *H. pylori*, but because antibody results may remain positive for months after successful eradication of infection, such tests are not recommended for determining whether active infection is still present after treatment is completed.

Abdominal ultrasonography is not indicated because it cannot diagnose gastric or duodenal ulcer disease and there are no biliary symptoms that would otherwise prompt its use. The absence of alarm features in a young person supports an empiric management approach without the need for structural studies (upper endoscopy, upper gastrointestinal barium study) until a therapeutic intervention for *H. pylori* eradication is attempted and has failed.

KEY POINT

• Patients with dyspepsia without alarm features (vomiting, weight loss, anemia, bleeding, early satiety) can usually be tested for *Helicobacter pylori*, and if positive, treated empirically for *H. pylori* infection.

Bibliography
1. Malfertheiner P, Megraud F, O'Morain C, Bazzoli F, El-Omar E, Graham D, Hunt R, Rokkas T, Vakil N, Kuipers EJ. Current concepts in the management of Helicobacter pylori infection: the Maastricht III Consensus Report.Gut. 2007;56:772-81. Epub 2006 Dec 14. [PMID: 17170018]

Item 36   Answer: A

Given this patient's age, the most likely cause of her chronic gastrointestinal bleeding is angiodysplasia (vascular malformations). In patients with this disorder, obscure occult bleeding is generally believed to develop in the small intestine, but lesions in the esophagus (esophagitis, Cameron's erosions), stomach (gastric antral vascular ectasia, portal hypertensive gastropathy), and colon (proximal angiodysplasia) may be overlooked during initial upper endoscopy or colonoscopy. Small bowel causes include tumors (which are typically benign in younger patients and either benign or malignant in older patients), vascular lesions (particularly in older patients), and ulcerating lesions (nonsteroidal anti-inflammatory drug–induced enteropathy, Crohn's disease). The differential diagnosis should also include occult bleeding due to less common disorders such as von Willebrand's disease, celiac sprue, and atrophic gastritis. These lesions may develop anywhere in the gastrointestinal tract and may be beyond the reach of standard upper endoscopes and colonoscopes. Vascular malformations may cause either occult bleeding (as in this patient) or active bleeding. Vascular malformations are the most common cause of occult gastrointestinal bleeding in patients over 60 years of age.

Meckel's diverticulum is much more common in younger patients and usually causes overt bleeding. Colonic diverticula usually cause hematochezia (or occasionally melena if right-sided) and are not associated with ongoing iron deficiency anemia. Patients with an aortoenteric fistula typically present with acute, often massive, bleeding rather than with chronic low-grade bleeding. In addition, this patient's normal abdominal CT scan makes an aortoenteric fistula unlikely. Celiac sprue should always be considered in a patient with iron deficiency anemia, but the normal small bowel biopsy specimens exclude this diagnosis, as do the positive fecal occult blood tests.

KEY POINT

• Angiodysplasia (vascular malformations) is most often diagnosed in elderly patients with chronic occult gastrointestinal bleeding.

Bibliography
1. Lin S, Rockey DC. Obscure gastrointestinal bleeding. Gastroenterol Clin North Am. 2005;34:679-98. [PMID: 16303577]

Item 37   Answer: E

This patient can be discharged from the hospital and followed as an outpatient. He presented with a bleeding duodenal ulcer and was treated appropriately with injectable and mechanical therapy. His young age, lack of comorbid disorders, and absence of transfusion requirements make hospital discharge with outpatient follow-up the most reasonable management option. Although his hemoglobin level has decreased, this likely represents redistribution of fluid into the vascular space, especially since he has no clinical features to suggest new or ongoing bleeding or clinical evidence of hypovolemia.

Repeating the upper endoscopy or performing colonoscopy is unnecessary at this time because he is clinically stable and the most likely site of the bleeding has been discovered and treated. Fecal occult blood testing is inappropriate, as the result may be positive because of residual blood in the gastrointestinal tract, and the positive result may lead to unnecessary testing. Given his age and absence of cardiovascular disease, the patient does not require a transfusion at this time, since his hemoglobin is still at an acceptable level.

KEY POINT

- A decreasing hemoglobin level in a stable patient with a recent episode of upper gastrointestinal bleeding may be due to redistribution of fluid into the vascular space rather than to continuing bleeding.

Bibliography

1. Wassef W. Upper gastrointestinal bleeding. Curr Opin Gastroenterol. 2004;20:538-45. [PMID: 15703679]

Item 38   Answer: E

In this patient with gastrointestinal bleeding and hypovolemia, urgent volume replacement with normal saline is indicated to achieve hemodynamic stability before diagnostic testing or therapeutic interventions are initiated. Orthostatic changes in blood pressure ($\geq$10 mm Hg) or heart rate ($\geq$120/min) indicate a loss of 20% to 25% of intravascular volume. Volume replacement with crystalloid therapy is indicated until these measurements normalize and should not be deferred until blood products are available. Hemoglobin and hematocrit levels are unreliable indicators of the volume of the bleeding and should not be used to determine the need for volume replacement.

After hemodynamic stability is achieved, colonoscopy is indicated for diagnosis and treatment for lower gastrointestinal bleeding. For upper gastrointestinal bleeding, upper endoscopy is indicated to identify the location and cause of the bleeding, achieve hemostasis, and provide prognostic information. Although hematochezia more often is a sign of lower gastrointestinal bleeding, as many as 10% to15% of patients with hematochezia may have an upper gastrointestinal source.

Octreotide is a long-acting somatostatin analogue that inhibits the release of vasodilatory hormones and therefore indirectly causes splanchnic vasoconstriction and reduced portal inflow. In acute esophageal variceal bleeding, this agent is a useful adjunct to endoscopic treatment in achieving hemostasis and preventing early rebleeding. Octreotide therapy also may decrease the rate of nonvariceal bleeding. Because gastric acid reduction may improve hemostasis and facilitate healing, therapy with a proton pump inhibitor may help stop acute bleeding from a peptic ulcer. Intravenous proton pump inhibitors (omeprazole and pantoprazole) are available in the United States, but the U.S. Food and Drug Administration has not yet approved these agents for management of acute upper gastrointestinal bleeding.

KEY POINT

- In patients presenting with gastrointestinal bleeding, hemodynamic stability should be achieved before diagnostic testing or specific therapeutic interventions are initiated.

Bibliography

1. Zuccaro G Jr. Management of the adult patient with acute lower gastrointestinal bleeding. American College of Gastroenterology. Practice Parameters Committee. Am J Gastroenterol. 1998;93:1202-8. [PMID: 9707037]

Item 39   Answer: C

Fulminant hepatic failure is the clinical syndrome of severe acute liver failure and hepatic encephalopathy (asterixis and depressed consciousness) in a patient without pre-existing liver disease. This patient has fulminant hepatic failure due to hepatitis A (most likely as a result of her trip to Nicaragua) and should be evaluated for liver transplantation immediately. Fulminant hepatic failure is associated with a high mortality rate in many patients, and liver transplantation can be a lifesaving therapy. For obvious ethical reasons, no controlled trials of liver transplantation have been carried out in patients with fulminant hepatic failure. The decision to offer liver transplantation is based on an assessment of the patients' prognosis and an evaluation of their suitability for transplantation. The most important indication for liver transplantation is declining mental status despite maximal medical management. Frequent reassessment of mental status is the single most important element in determining immediate prognosis. Unequivocal deterioration in mental status despite maximal medical management should prompt consideration for liver transplantation.

A CT scan of the head is unlikely to be helpful in the absence of focal neurologic findings, and a CT scan of the abdomen is unlikely to provide additional findings not already noted on the physical examination and ultrasonography. Liver biopsy is seldom helpful in establishing the diagnosis or prognosis in a patient with acute hepatic failure and places the patient at risk for bleeding.

KEY POINTS

- Fulminant hepatic failure is the clinical syndrome of severe acute liver failure and encephalopathy in a patient without pre-existing liver disease.

- Patients with fulminant hepatic failure require immediate evaluation for liver transplantation.

Bibliography

1. **Sass DA, Shakil AO**. Fulminant hepatic failure. Liver Transpl. 2005;11:594-605. [PMID: 15915484]

Item 40   Answer: A

The patient has clinical symptoms and laboratory findings consistent with acute hepatitis (fatigue, jaundice, aminotransferase concentrations >1000 U/L). Patients with acute hepatitis are generally more symptomatic, more likely to be jaundiced, and have higher aminotransferase values than those with chronic hepatitis. Although any of the hepatitis viruses can cause symptomatic acute hepatitis, hepatitis A is the most likely infection in a daycare employee without other risk factors. Adults with acute hepatitis A usually have jaundice; however, many infants and children with this infection are not jaundiced, and their illness is therefore not recognized as hepatitis.

Hepatitis B, C, and D are less likely without a history of parenteral exposure. In addition, acute hepatitis C rarely causes symptoms. Hepatitis E causes findings similar to those of hepatitis A, but hepatitis E is rare in the United States.

KEY POINT

- Patients with acute hepatitis generally have fatigue, nausea, sometimes vomiting, jaundice and aminotransferase values >1000 U/L.

Bibliography

1. **Brundage SC, Fitzpatrick AN.** Hepatitis A. Am Fam Physician. 2006;73:2162-8. [PMID: 16848078]

Item 41   Answer: C

Hepatitis B virus (HBV) causes 20% to 30% of cases of acute viral hepatitis and 15% of cases of chronic viral hepatitis in the United States. Multiple sex partners and injection drug use are the major risk factors for hepatitis B virus infection, accounting for 80% of cases in the United States, Canada, and Western Europe. Many infected persons in the United States are immigrants from highly endemic areas in Asia and Africa where HBV is acquired perinatally or during early childhood. The incubation period for hepatitis B infection is 1 to 4 months. Although some patients with acute disease may develop anorexia, nausea, and abdominal pain, most children and some adults with acute hepatitis B infection have subclinical or anicteric hepatitis. Aminotransferase levels are variably increased in patients with acute hepatitis B infection, but do not correlate with prognosis. About 1% of infected patients develop a hyperreactive immune response to infected hepatocytes, leading to a rapid loss in functioning liver mass and resultant acute liver failure characterized by rapidly progressive coagulopathy and encephalopathy. A diagnosis of acute hepatitis B infection is based upon the detection of circulating hepatitis B surface antigen (HBsAg) and IgM hepatitis B core antibodies (anti-HBc [IgM]). Treatment is supportive.

Acute retroviral syndrome is most commonly recognized as a "viral syndrome" approximately 2 to 12 weeks after a high-risk sexual or parenteral exposure to HIV. There are no sensitive and specific signs and symptoms for the diagnosis, but the most consistently reported findings include fever (97%), fatigue (90%), lymphadenopathy (50% to 77%), pharyngitis (73%), transient rash (40% to 70%), and headache (30% to 60%). A primarily hepatic syndrome (tender hepatomegaly, jaundice, and markedly elevated aminotransferase levels) is not characteristic of acute retroviral syndrome.

Clinically relevant alcoholic hepatitis is characterized by the presence of jaundice, fever, and hepatomegaly. The disease may be accompanied by other features and complications of decompensated chronic liver disease such as ascites, encephalopathy, and gastrointestinal hemorrhage. For men, the relative risk of alcoholic liver disease becomes significant at more than 14 drinks per week; for women, it becomes significant at more than 7 drinks per week. Alcoholic hepatitis is distinguishable from other forms of liver disease by relatively mild absolute elevations in aspartate and alanine aminotransferase (AST and ALT) levels and an AST/ALT ratio >2.0. This patient's current level of alcohol consumption and liver chemistry profile do not support the diagnosis of acute alcoholic hepatitis.

Acetaminophen-induced fulminant hepatic failure is usually due to ingestion of more than 4 g/d, but occasionally less in patients with alcoholic cirrhosis. Sudden onset of elevated AST and ALT levels, typically up to 20 times the upper limit of normal, is characteristic. The interval from ingestion to manifestations of liver injury is usually 12 to 36 hours. The patient's acetaminophen dose, time course, and aminotransferase levels argue against acetaminophen hepatotoxicity as the cause of his clinical presentation.

Patients with acute hepatitis C infection are usually asymptomatic and therefore rarely present clinically, but 60% to 85% of persons who acquire acute hepatitis C develop chronic infection. Hepatitis C is a primarily a blood-borne infection and is not typically acquired through sexual contact. The precise risk of hepatitis C transmission among long-term sex partners and the importance of sexual transmission remain controversial, as does the importance of tattooing and body piercing in causing this infection.

KEY POINTS

- Multiple sex partners and injection drug use are the major risk factors for hepatitis B infection, accounting for 80% of cases in the United States, Canada, and Western Europe.

- A diagnosis of acute hepatitis B infection is based upon the detection of circulating HBsAg and anti-HBc (IgM).

Bibliography
1. Lin KW, Kirchner JT. Hepatitis B. Am Fam Physician. 2004;69:75-82. Erratum in: Am Fam Physician. 2004;69:1863. [PMID: 14727820]

Item 42   Answer: C

This patient requires an HCV RNA assay. He has elevated aminotransferase values and positive antibodies to hepatitis C virus (anti-HCV). In a patient with a history of injection drug use, these findings are highly suggestive of hepatitis C, and an HCV RNA assay should be done to confirm the presence of viremia.

Positive tests for antibodies to hepatitis B surface antigen (anti-HBs) and IgG antibodies to hepatitis B core antigen (anti-HBc IgG) are consistent with immunity from prior infection, and determination of hepatitis B e antigen (HBeAg) and HBV DNA is therefore not necessary. Testing for IgM antibodies to hepatitis A virus (anti-HAV IgM) is not indicated because acute hepatitis A tends to cause systemic symptoms, jaundice, and more marked elevations in aminotransferase values. Furthermore, hepatitis A does not cause chronic hepatitis and cannot explain the finding of anti-HCV.

KEY POINT
• Patients with a positive assay for antibodies to hepatitis C virus (anti-HCV) should be tested for HCV RNA to determine if viremia is present.

Bibliography
1. Patel K, Muir AJ, McHutchison JG. Diagnosis and treatment of chronic hepatitis C infection. BMJ. 200629;332:1013-7. [PMID: 16644828]

Item 43   Answer: B

This patient has cirrhosis with ascites. Patients with new-onset ascites should undergo diagnostic paracentesis to confirm the cause. Paracentesis is a safe procedure even in patients with coagulopathy. Because cirrhosis is the cause of ascites in 85% of patients, measurement of the serum–ascites albumin gradient (SAAG) and ascitic fluid protein and cell count is recommended at the time of the initial paracentesis. A SAAG of >1.1 g/dL supports a diagnosis of cirrhosis, right-sided heart failure, or Budd–Chiari syndrome; a gradient of <1.1 g/dL supports a diagnosis of nephrotic syndrome, malignancy, or tuberculosis. Measurement of ascitic fluid protein further differentiates causes of ascites. A result <2.5 g/dL indicates a diagnosis of cirrhosis or nephrotic syndrome; a result >2.5 g/dL supports a diagnosis of right-sided heart failure, Budd–Chiari syndrome, malignancy, or tuberculosis. Analysis of this patient's ascitic fluid shows a protein concentration of 1.4 g/dL and a SAAG of 2.2 g/dL, which are most consistent with ascites due to sinusoidal hypertension from a chronic liver disease such as cirrhosis.

KEY POINT
• Ascitic fluid analysis showing a protein concentration of <2.5 g/dL and a serum–ascites albumin gradient (SAAG) >1.1 g/dL is consistent with ascites due to chronic liver disease, such as cirrhosis.

Bibliography
1. Gines P, Cardenas A, Arroyo V, Rodes J. Management of cirrhosis and ascites. N Engl J Med. 2004 15;350:1646-54. [PMID: 15084697]

Item 44   Answer: C

This patient most likely has autoimmune hepatitis because of her concomitant autoimmune thyroid disease, family history of autoimmune diseases, and abnormal liver test results. Autoimmune hepatitis is an inflammatory condition of the liver of unknown cause. It primarily develops in women 20 to 40 years of age, but all age groups and most ethnic groups are affected. Certain viruses (e.g., hepatitis A virus) and drugs (e.g., minocycline) have been implicated; however, most patients have no recognizable risk factors or triggers. Although most patients have features of chronic liver disease, up to 40% have an acute or fulminant presentation. Fatigue, which occurs in 85% of patients, is the most common presenting symptom, followed by jaundice (46%), anorexia (30%), myalgias (30%), and diarrhea (28%). On physical examination, 78% of patients have an enlarged liver. Others have a normal examination despite the presence of advanced disease. Laboratory findings in patients with autoimmune hepatitis include elevated aminotransferase values, hypergammaglobulinemia, mild hyperbilirubinemia, elevated alkaline phosphatase values, and the presence of autoantibodies. Aminotransferase values range from 150 U/L to >1000 U/L, but are typically <500 U/L at presentation, and γ-globulin values ≥1.5 times the upper limit of normal are common. Mild hyperbilirubinemia (values <3 mg/dL) is present in 83% of patients. Viral hepatitis serologic test results are typically negative, and there is a high prevalence of autoantibodies, including antinuclear antibodies, anti–smooth muscle antibodies, and anti-LKM antibodies; titers ≥1:80 support a diagnosis of autoimmune hepatitis.

Primary biliary cirrhosis is a cholestatic liver disease. Patients with primary biliary cirrhosis tend to have higher alkaline phosphatase and total bilirubin levels and lower aminotransferase values than patients with autoimmune hepatitis. Although this patient traveled to Mexico 7 months ago, hepatitis A is unlikely because the incubation period for this virus is typically within 2 to 6 weeks of exposure. She also received hepatitis A vaccine before travel, which protects most people from infection. Acetaminophen hepatotoxicity tends to cause significantly elevated aminotransferase values (≥5000 U/L) and is not associated with the week-long prodrome that this patient has.

- Autoimmune hepatitis can manifest as acute hepatitis with elevated aminotransferase values and jaundice; the AST:ALT ratio is typically <2.0.

- Antinuclear antibody and anti–smooth muscle antibody titers ≥1:80 support a diagnosis of autoimmune hepatitis.

Bibliography

1. **Krawitt EL.** Autoimmune hepatitis. N Engl J Med. 2006;354:54-66. [PMID: 16394302]

Item 45   Answer: D

In this patient with a remote history of injection drug use and without a history of chronic alcohol abuse, cirrhosis due to chronic hepatitis C infection is the most likely explanation for the symptoms, clinical findings, and laboratory abnormalities. The patient's jaundice and elevated aminotransferase and bilirubin levels indicate hepatocellular disease. The bulging flanks with shifting dullness suggest ascites, and the palpable spleen and thrombocytopenia suggest hypersplenism from portal hypertension. Approximately 40% of cases of chronic liver disease in the United States are attributable to chronic hepatitis C virus (HCV) infection. Cirrhosis is a well-documented complication that may lead to end-stage liver disease or hepatocellular carcinoma. The diagnosis of active HCV infection is based on the presence of circulating HCV RNA.

Acetaminophen hepatotoxicity should not occur with the patient's reported intake and produces acute hepatotoxicity and fulminant hepatic failure, but not cirrhosis. Alcoholic cirrhosis is very unlikely with this patient's remote history of alcohol use. Hemochromatosis is a multi-organ systemic disease and may affect one or more organs as it progresses. In a retrospective study of affected patients, hepatomegaly (83%), hyperpigmentation (75%), and clinical diabetes mellitus (55%) were common initial findings. In the era of screening iron studies, less than 20% of newly identified patients with hemochromatosis have an abnormal physical finding. Hemochromatosis may present with cirrhosis, but it is very unlikely, and hemochromatosis is a much less common cause of cirrhosis than HCV infection. New-onset ascites is an uncommon presentation of metastatic colon cancer, and the patient's age argues against this diagnosis. The patient's normal hematocrit and negative stool specimen also make metastatic colon cancer unlikely.

- Injection drug use, even in the remote past, is a major risk factor for hepatitis C infection.

- Hepatitis C infection is often asymptomatic until sequelae such as cirrhosis develop.

Bibliography

1. **Liang TJ, Rehermann B, Seeff LB, Hoofnagle JH.** Pathogenesis, natural history, treatment, and prevention of hepatitis C. Ann Intern Med. 2000;132:296-305. [PMID: 10681285]

Item 46   Answer: D

This patient most likely has nonalcoholic fatty liver disease (NAFLD). NAFLD refers to a spectrum of histologic changes in the liver initiated by steatosis in the absence of excess alcohol consumption. NAFLD is common in the United States, with a prevalence of 15% to 39%. A liver biopsy is indicated to determine whether nonalcoholic steatohepatitis (NASH) or fibrosis is also present. This distinction is important, as a patient with evidence of cirrhosis should be screened for complications of end-stage liver disease, such as esophageal varices and hepatocellular carcinoma. Although a liver biopsy is not required for all patients with NAFLD, biopsy should be considered for those who are older than 45 years of age, are obese, have diabetes mellitus, or have an aspartate aminotransferase to alanine aminotransferase ratio (AST/ALT) >1, as these may be predictors of fibrosis. This patient has several predictors of fibrosis, including her age, obesity, and increased AST/ALT ratio. She also has a low albumin level, making synthetic hepatic dysfunction of the liver likely. Her low platelet count may also be a marker for hypersplenism due to portal hypertension.

Patients with hemochromatosis are typically asymptomatic until after age 40 years in men and age 50 years in women. Clinical symptoms are vague but can include abdominal pain and features of cirrhosis (jaundice, ascites). Typically the transferrin saturation is ≥45% and liver biopsy results show iron accumulation in hepatocytes. Patients with NAFLD have a normal fasting transferrin saturation. Patients with alcoholic liver disease have a history of excessive alcohol consumption and an AST/ALT ratio >2; neither condition is present in this patient. Acute viral hepatitis can present with abdominal pain, anorexia, nausea, vomiting, fever, and jaundice. Typically, tender hepatomegaly is present along with aminotransferase values >500 U/L and positive serologic studies for hepatitis A virus (anti-HAV IgM) or hepatitis B virus (HBsAg and anti-HBc IgM). The diagnosis of acute viral hepatitis is not supported by either this patient's clinical picture or her serologic studies.

- Nonalcoholic fatty liver disease (NAFLD) refers to a spectrum of histologic changes in the liver initiated by steatosis in the absence of excess alcohol consumption.

Bibliography

1. **Adams LA, Angulo P, Lindor KD.** Nonalcoholic fatty liver disease. CMAJ. 2005;172:899-905. [PMID: 15795412]

Item 47   Answer: C

The findings of pruritus, hypercholesterolemia, cholestatic liver disease, and a positive antimitochondrial antibody titer strongly favor the diagnosis of primary biliary cirrhosis. Although fatigue and pruritus used to be the most common presenting symptoms of primary biliary cirrhosis, the disease is now more widely recognized and many patients are diagnosed at earlier stages when they are asymptomatic. Patients with certain findings in their history and physical examination may be more likely to have primary biliary cirrhosis. For example, pruritus, hyperpigmentation of the skin, hepatomegaly and a cholestatic pattern of liver chemistry tests are common in women with primary biliary cirrhosis but unusual in those with other liver disorders, such as acute and chronic hepatitis and alcoholic liver disease. Antimitochondrial antibodies are found in 95% of patients with primary biliary cirrhosis and have a specificity of 98% for this disorder. The most appropriate therapy for primary biliary cirrhosis is ursodeoxycholic acid, which improves pruritus and abnormal liver chemistry findings and helps decrease the progression to cirrhosis.

Although atorvastatin can be associated with elevated liver chemistry values, increases occur primarily in aminotransferase values rather than in the bilirubin and alkaline phosphatase levels. Autoimmune hepatitis is associated with an antinuclear antibody titer ≥1:80 and a γ-globulin level ≥1.5 times the upper limit of normal and is not associated with a cholestatic liver injury pattern. Primary sclerosing cholangitis is more common in men and is frequently associated with inflammatory bowel disease.

KEY POINT

• Pruritus, hypercholesterolemia, laboratory evidence of cholestatic liver disease, and a positive antimitochondrial antibody titer suggest primary biliary cirrhosis.

Bibliography

1. Kaplan MM, Gershwin ME. Primary biliary cirrhosis. N Engl J Med. 2005;353:1261-73. Erratum in: N Engl J Med. 2006;354:313. [PMID: 16177252]

Item 48   Answer: D

This patient requires a paracentesis. Spontaneous bacterial peritonitis, or primary peritonitis, is a bacterial infection of ascitic fluid without an intra-abdominal source for infection. This diagnosis should be considered in any patient with cirrhotic ascites and clinical deterioration. Risk factors include prior episodes of spontaneous bacterial peritonitis, hospitalization for gastrointestinal bleeding, and an ascitic fluid protein value <1 g/dL. Patients suspected of having spontaneous bacterial peritonitis should undergo diagnostic paracentesis with cell counts and culture of the ascitic fluid. Because spontaneous bacterial peritonitis is almost always caused by only one pathogen, polymicrobial infection of the ascitic fluid should prompt a search for an intra-abdominal focus of infection. Clinical evidence suggests that patients with spontaneous bacterial peritonitis who are given cefotaxime and albumin have improved survival and a decreased risk of hepatorenal syndrome compared with patients given cefotaxime alone.

Hyponatremia is common in patients who are taking diuretics for cirrhosis, and fluid restriction is only necessary when hyponatremia is severe (sodium <120 meq/L). A CT scan of the head is not likely to be helpful in the absence of focal neu-

rologic findings. Fresh frozen plasma has no role in the treatment of worsening hepatic encephalopathy.

KEY POINT

• Spontaneous bacterial peritonitis should be suspected in any patient with cirrhosis and new or worsening decompensation.

Bibliography

1. Han MK, Hyzy R. Advances in critical care management of hepatic failure and insufficiency. Crit Care Med. 2006;34:S225-31. [PMID: 16917427]

Item 49   Answer: C

This patient should be started on propranolol. Patients with cirrhosis should undergo upper endoscopy to determine the presence of esophageal varices. Because of the risk of bleeding associated with large esophageal varices, prophylaxis is recommended for patients with this finding. Nonselective β-blockers such as propranolol or nadolol decrease splanchnic blood flow and are recommended for initial prophylaxis.

Transjugular intrahepatic portosystemic shunt is used only for patients with refractory bleeding or ascites. Norfloxacin is used as prophylaxis against spontaneous bacterial peritonitis in patients who have cirrhosis and gastrointestinal bleeding or a history of spontaneous bacterial peritonitis. Esophageal variceal sclerotherapy is not recommended for prophylaxis because of the adverse effects associated with this procedure, such as ulcerations, pleural effusions, and esophageal strictures.

KEY POINTS

• Patients with cirrhosis should undergo upper endoscopy to determine the presence of esophageal varices.

• Patients with large esophageal varices should receive a nonselective β-blocker for prophylaxis against variceal bleeding.

Bibliography

1. Mathews RE Jr, McGuire BM, Estrada CA. Outpatient management of cirrhosis: a narrative review. South Med J. 2006;99:600-6. [PMID: 16800415]

Item 50   Answer: B

This patient requires a colonoscopy with biopsies now. Chronic inflammatory bowel disease, such as ulcerative colitis, is a risk factor for the development of colorectal cancer. The risk increases with the duration and extent of the disease, early age of onset, and presence of primary sclerosing cholangitis. Patients with inflammatory bowel disease should regularly undergo surveillance colonoscopy with biopsies obtained from throughout the colon to detect dysplasia, which is a marker for possible colorectal cancer. Current guidelines recommend colonoscopy every 1 to 2 years for patients with pancolitis of 10 years or more duration.

Barium enema examination and virtual colonoscopy (CT colonography) do not allow biopsies for detection of early cancer or dysplasia and therefore are inappropriate for colorectal cancer surveillance in patients with pancolitis. Colonoscopy beginning at the age of 50 years is appropriate for patients at average risk for colon cancer, but not for this individual who is at high risk.

KEY POINT

• Patients with pancolitis for 10 or more years should undergo colonoscopy with biopsies every 1 to 2 years for cancer surveillance.

Bibliography
1. **Baumgart DC, Sandborn WJ.** Inflammatory bowel disease: clinical aspects and established and evolving therapies. Lancet. 2007;369:1641-57. [PMID: 17499606]

Item 51   Answer: A

This patient has Crohn's colitis. Because his colonoscopic examination shows areas of deep ulceration separated by areas of normal mucosa (skip lesions) and rectal sparing, his findings are more consistent with Crohn's disease than with ulcerative colitis. In addition, the patient is a smoker, which increases the risk for Crohn's disease.

Patients with ulcerative colitis have continuous inflammation, typically including the rectum, and usually do not have deep ulcers or skip lesions. Ulcerative colitis is more common in former smokers or nonsmokers. Microscopic colitis is typically found in middle-aged women, is often associated with other autoimmune diseases, does not cause abdominal pain, and is not associated with the changes on colonoscopy found on this patient's examination. Finally, the patient's history and biopsy findings are not consistent with infectious colitis (no fever, chills, or sweating) or ischemic colitis (young age and no history of a preceding hypotensive or embolic event predisposing to bowel ischemia).

KEY POINTS

• Colonoscopic findings in Crohn's disease include deep ulcerations separated by areas of normal mucosa (skip lesions) and rectal sparing.

• Colonoscopic findings in ulcerative colitis include continuous inflammation, typically including the rectum, but without deep ulcerations or skip lesions.

Bibliography
1. **Baumgart DC, Sandborn WJ.** Inflammatory bowel disease: clinical aspects and established and evolving therapies. Lancet. 2007;369:1641-57. [PMID: 17499606]

Item 52   Answer: C

This man is at high risk for abdominal aortic aneurysm, which should be suspected in patients with an abdominal bruit and a tender pulsatile abdominal mass. Smoking, hypertension, advanced age, and male sex are risk factors for abdominal aortic aneurysm. Abdominal ultrasonography is the preferred initial evaluation for patients with suspected abdominal aortic

aneurysm. Abdominal magnetic resonance angiography would also be an acceptable alternative for this patient, but is a more expensive study. Because of the patient's renal insufficiency, abdominal CT with contrast and contrast angiography should be avoided. An abdominal radiograph may show aortic calcification but is not sensitive for diagnosing an aneurysm. The 3rd National Cholesterol Education Program considers abdominal aortic aneurysm to be a coronary heart disease equivalent with target LDL cholesterol level <100 mg/dL.

KEY POINT

• Abdominal aortic aneurysm should be suspected in patients with an abdominal bruit and a tender, pulsatile abdominal mass.

Bibliography
1. **Upchurch GR Jr, Schaub TA.** Abdominal aortic aneurysm. Am Fam Physician. 2006;73:1198-204. Summary for patients in: Am Fam Physician. 2006;73:1205-6. [PMID: 16623206]

Item 53   Answer: B

The leading diagnosis in this patient is primary dysmenorrhea, a common cause of lower abdominal pain that often begins in women in their late teens or early 20s. A key feature of dysmenorrhea is the onset of pain during the menstrual cycle. Pain is believed to be hormonally related, and anatomic abnormalities are typically not found on pelvic examination and ultrasonography. Nonsteroidal anti-inflammatory drugs (NSAIDs) are generally safe and often effective initial treatment for these symptoms. Oral contraceptives may also be helpful in treating the symptoms of primary dysmenorrhea. However, in a woman who has no other indications for oral contraceptives, an empiric trial of NSAIDs may be preferable as initial treatment.

Constipation associated with lower abdominal pain could also denote irritable bowel syndrome (IBS). However, the occurrence of pain principally during menstruation is not characteristic of IBS. Although psyllium and low-dose daily administration of polyethylene glycol laxatives are first- and second-line treatments for IBS-related constipation, their benefits for the abdominal pain of IBS are not well-established. Local anesthetic/corticosteroid injections may be beneficial in patients with abdominal wall pain. However, abdominal wall pain is characterized by very localized pain in which the most intense component can be covered by a fingertip and/or increased point tenderness with abdominal wall muscle tensing.

KEY POINTS

• Dysmenorrhea is characterized by onset of pain during the menstrual cycle and the absence of anatomic abnormalities on pelvic examination and ultrasonography.

• Nonsteroidal anti-inflammatory drugs are a generally safe and often effective initial treatment for dysmenorrhea.

Bibliography
1. **Dawood MY.** Primary dysmenorrhea: advances in pathogenesis and management. Obstet Gynecol. 2006;108:428-41. [PMID: 16880317]

Chapter 4
General Internal Medicine

General Internal Medicine contains self-assessment items that correspond to the following chapters in the *Internal Medicine Essentials for Clerkship Students 2* textbook:

Test Interpretation
Health Promotion, Screening, and Prevention
Approach to Syncope
Depression
Substance Abuse
Approach to Low Back Pain
Approach to Cough
Smoking Cessation
Obesity
Approach to Involuntary Weight Loss
Disorders of Menstruation and Menopause
Common Dermatologic Disorders
Comprehensive Geriatric Assessment
Hypertension

General Internal Medicine contains self assessment items that correspond to the following Training Problems in the *Core Medicine Clerkship Guide*:

The Healthy Patient: Health Promotion, Disease Prevention, and Screening
Back Pain
Cough
Rash
Hypertension
Major Depression
Obesity
Smoking Cessation
Substance Abuse

Chapter 4

General Internal Medicine
Questions

Item 1

A 50-year-old man is evaluated in the office for substernal chest pain. The pain is not consistently associated with exertion, nor is it always relieved by rest; it sometimes occurs when he is eating or when he is anxious. The patient has a history of hypertension treated with hydrochlorothiazide and a 15-pack-year history of cigarette smoking.

On physical examination, blood pressure is 148/92 mm Hg and heart rate is 78/min. The cardiac rhythm is regular; heart sounds are normal with no murmurs, gallops, or rubs. The lungs are clear.

The patient's probability of having coronary artery disease is estimated from these findings to be 40%. A nuclear stress test is scheduled to evaluate the chest pain further. This test has a positive likelihood ratio of 5.0 and a negative likelihood ratio of 0.1. The patient's nuclear stress test is positive.

Which of the following values best approximates the patient's post-test probability of having coronary artery disease?

(A) 5%
(B) 25%
(C) 50%
(D) 60%
(E) 75%

Item 2

A 67-year-old asymptomatic man is evaluated in the office during a routine physical examination. He quit smoking 3 years ago, watches his diet, and exercises 60 minutes every day. He wears his seatbelt while driving and consumes fewer than four alcoholic drinks per week. He takes no medications other than an occasional ibuprofen for muscle-related symptoms.

At age 63 years, he had a negative colonoscopy, a booster tetanus and diphtheria vaccination, and pneumococcal vaccination. This fall, he received herpes zoster and influenza vaccinations. He had a normal fasting lipid panel and blood glucose level 6 months ago.

On physical examination, blood pressure is 130/78 mm Hg, pulse rate is 60/min, and BMI is 24. General examination is normal.

Which of the following screening or preventive measures is recommended for this patient at this time?

(A) Abdominal ultrasonography
(B) Colonoscopy
(C) Electrocardiography
(D) Pneumococcal vaccine
(E) Tetanus and diphtheria vaccine

Item 3

A 43-year-old woman is evaluated in the office for an annual clinical breast examination. A careful visual inspection of each breast is completed. She is then carefully draped and positioned on the table to flatten the breast tissue evenly over the chest wall and is examined using an overlapping vertical-strip search pattern to systematically palpate the breast tissue, for a total of 3 minutes of examination time per breast.

Which of the following single clinical breast examination components is most likely to increase the accuracy of this patient's examination?

(A) Duration of the examination
(B) Movement and location of the examining fingers
(C) Positioning of the patient
(D) Type of search pattern used
(E) Visual inspection of the breasts

Item 4

A 22-year-old woman is evaluated in the office during a routine physical examination. She does not smoke, does not have risk factors for diabetes mellitus or cardiovascular disease, and does not use alcohol or illicit drugs. She has had a total of four sexual partners and currently is in a monogamous relationship with her boyfriend. She has no history of sexually transmitted infections and takes an oral contraceptive. A recent Pap smear and HIV test were negative.

Which of the following is most appropriate evidence-based screening/prevention recommendation for this patient?

(A) Daily multivitamin with folic acid
(B) Fasting blood glucose
(C) Screening for *Chlamydia* infection
(D) Sunscreen use

Item 5

A 50-year-old man comes to the office for an annual health maintenance visit. He feels well, and medical history is unremarkable. There is no family history of colorectal cancer. Physical examination and routine laboratory studies are normal.

Which of the following is the most appropriate recommendation for colorectal cancer screening for this patient?

(A) Barium enema examination now; repeat every 2 to 3 years
(B) Colonoscopy now; repeat every 10 years
(C) Fecal occult blood testing now; repeat every 2 to 3 years
(D) Flexible sigmoidoscopy now; repeat every 2 to 3 years
(E) Virtual colonoscopy (CT colonography) now; repeat every 10 years

Item 6

A 45-year-old man is evaluated during a routine office visit. The patient is healthy and asymptomatic. His father was diagnosed with colon cancer at the age of 49 years. Physical examination is normal.

Which of the following is the most appropriate next step in the management of this patient?

(A) Colonoscopy
(B) Flexible sigmoidoscopy
(C) Measurement of carcinoembryonic antigen
(D) Single-contrast barium enema examination
(E) Virtual colonoscopy (CT colonography)

Item 7

A 45-year-old married premenopausal woman is evaluated in the office during a routine examination. She has no medical problems, and her family and medical history are noncontributory. Her most recent laboratory studies 2 years ago were normal, including cholesterol level. She does not drink or smoke, have any risk factors for HIV infection, or have any depressive symptoms.

On physical examination, blood pressure is 120/80 mm Hg, and BMI is 26. The breast and pelvic examinations are normal. The most recent Pap smear and mammogram performed 1 year ago were also normal.

In addition to the evaluations performed above, which of the following screening maneuvers is most likely to reduce this patient's 10-year mortality?

(A) Cardiac auscultation
(B) Complete skin examination
(C) Dilated funduscopy
(D) Pulmonary auscultation
(E) No other physical examination maneuvers

Item 8

An 87-year-old wheelchair-bound woman is evaluated in the office during a routine examination. She is accompanied by her son. The patient resides in a residential living setting in her own apartment and has recently become socially isolated. She no longer visits with friends, eats in the common dining room, or enjoys watching television. Her medical history includes hypertension, coronary artery disease, and osteoporosis, for which she takes hydrochlorothiazide, metoprolol, pravastatin, aspirin, calcium carbonate, and alendronate.

On physical examination, the patient appears well-groomed and has a friendly demeanor. The heart rate is 70/min, and the blood pressure is 125/75 mm Hg. The BMI is 18.3. She is oriented to person, place, and time and is able to ambulate with assistance. Neurologic examination shows no focal findings. Laboratory studies, including complete blood count, basic serum chemistry studies, and thyroid-stimulating hormone level, are normal. The score on the Five-Item Geriatric Depression Screen is 1/5.

Which of the following is the most appropriate management option in addressing this patient's social isolation?

(A) Assess hearing and vision
(B) Discontinue hydrochlorothiazide
(C) Initiate sertraline
(D) Schedule neuropsychologic testing

Item 9

A 50-year-old man is evaluated during a routine office visit. He received a heart transplant 2 months ago. Current medications are prednisone, mycophenolate mofetil, and cyclosporine. Influenza A and B are now occurring in the community. The patient has no signs or symptoms of infection. His wife and three teen-aged children are well and have been immunized against influenza.

Which of the following is most appropriate for preventing influenza in this patient?

(A) Immune globulin
(B) Live attenuated influenza vaccine
(C) Oseltamivir
(D) Rimantadine

Item 10

A 52-year-old woman with atrial fibrillation and heart failure requests a flu shot. She takes warfarin for atrial fibrillation. She reports a milk allergy.

Which of the following is the most appropriate management of this patient?

(A) Inactivated influenza vaccine
(B) Live intranasal influenza vaccine
(C) Neuraminidase inhibitor therapy
(D) No influenza vaccine

Item 11

A 30-year-old woman asks for advice about lung cancer screening. She has read that several celebrities recently developed lung cancer, and she is worried that she may have this disease. She smoked cigarettes for a short time as a teenager, but quit smoking when she found that smoking caused her to cough and wheeze.

Which of the following is the most appropriate management for this patient?

(A) Order a plain chest radiograph
(B) Order a spiral CT scan of the chest
(C) Obtain sputum cytology
(D) Reassure her that no screening is needed

Item 12

A 24-year-old woman who is 28 weeks pregnant is evaluated in the office because of shortness of breath after climbing 4 flights of stairs. She also has palpitations, described as a pause followed by a forceful heart beat occurring once or twice per day. Her medical history prior to pregnancy is unremarkable with no previous surgical procedures or hospitalizations.

On physical examination, blood pressure is 124/62 mm Hg, heart rate is 94/min and regular, and respiration rate is 14/min. Jugular venous pressure is 8 cm H_2O, carotid upstrokes are normal, and the lungs are clear. There is a grade 2/6 systolic murmur that is heard best at the upper left sternal border and does not radiate. An S_3 gallop is also heard. She has 1+ bilateral lower extremity edema. Urinalysis shows no protein or glucose.

Which of the following is most appropriate at this time?

(A) Echocardiogram
(B) Exercise electrocardiographic stress test
(C) 24-Hour ambulatory electrocardiographic monitoring
(D) Ventilation/perfusion lung scan
(E) Reassurance

Item 13

A 72-year-old woman is seen during a routine office evaluation to establish care. Medical history includes hypertension and hyperlipidemia. There is a family history of coronary artery disease. The patient does not smoke, is active, and walks daily. She does not have angina, dyspnea, fatigue, or edema.

On physical examination, blood pressure is 128/70 mm Hg. There are no carotid bruits. Cardiac examination shows a normal S_1, a physiologically split S_2, and a grade 2/6 midsystolic murmur that does not radiate and is best heard at the second right intercostal space. The remainder of the physical examination is normal.

Which of the following diagnostic tests is most appropriate at this time?

(A) Electron-beam cardiovascular CT scanning
(B) 24-Hour ambulatory electrocardiographic monitoring
(C) Transthoracic echocardiography
(D) Treadmill stress echocardiography
(E) No further testing at this time

Item 14

A 59-year-old woman is evaluated in the office during a routine examination. Her family history includes a sister who was recently diagnosed with advanced-stage ovarian cancer. The remainder of her medical and family history is noncontributory. The physical examination is normal.

The patient asks whether there are any routine screening methods to decrease her risk for ovarian cancer.

Which of the following is the most appropriate recommendation for ovarian cancer screening in this patient?

(A) CA-125 measurement
(B) Color Doppler ovarian imaging
(C) Transvaginal ultrasonography
(D) No screening test

Item 15

A 45-year-old man is evaluated for concerns about prostate cancer. A friend was recently diagnosed with extensive disease and has a poor prognosis. The patient asks if he should have a screening test for this disease. He reports once-nightly nocturia but has no hesitancy, urinary frequency, or dribbling.

Which of the following is the most appropriate first course of action for this patient?

(A) Prostate-specific antigen (PSA) testing
(B) PSA testing and digital rectal examination
(C) Transrectal ultrasonography
(D) Transrectal ultrasonography with random biopsies
(E) Discussion of benefits and harms of PSA testing

Item 16

A 76-year-old man is evaluated in the office for a syncopal episode that occurred last night after a coughing paroxysm following a fit of laughter. The patient is accompanied by his wife, who found him unconscious and slumped against the wall in the bathroom but reported that he regained consciousness quickly when she laid him fully on the floor and raised his legs. On regaining consciousness, he was fully oriented, spoke clearly, and had no difficulty standing up or walking. He reports having felt lightheaded and faint several times recently while trying to urinate but had not passed out before. His history includes coronary artery disease, stable angina, hypertension, chronic obstructive pulmonary disease with paroxysmal coughing, and benign prostatic hyperplasia with increasing difficulty urinating. Physical examination, including complete neurologic evaluation, is normal.

Which of the following is the most likely diagnosis?

(A) Carotid sinus syncope
(B) Generalized seizure
(C) Situational syncope
(D) Vertebrobasilar transient ischemic attack

Item 17

A 29-year-old man is evaluated in the office following a syncopal episode. He was seated in his office typing and lost consciousness for approximately 60 seconds. There was no prodrome of dizziness, palpitations, nausea, chest pain, or visual impairment. There was no confusion following the episode. He has had no previous known medical illnesses. He has noticed exertional dyspnea and occasional palpitations for the last 5 years. He takes no medications.

On physical examination, heart rate is 50/min and blood pressure is 125/75 mm Hg. There are no orthostatic changes when he goes from a supine to a standing position. There is no jugular venous distention, and carotid pulses are 2+ with normal upstrokes. Lungs are clear. Cardiac examination shows a grade 3/6 systolic murmur at the left sternal border that increases with the Valsalva maneuver. A soft S_4 gallop is present. Electrocardiogram shows sinus bradycardia, first-degree atrioventricular block, left ventricular hypertrophy, and secondary ST- and T-wave changes.

Which of the following is the most likely cardiac diagnosis in this patient?

(A) Dilated cardiomyopathy
(B) Hypertrophic cardiomyopathy
(C) Hypertensive cardiomyopathy
(D) Restrictive cardiomyopathy

Item 18

A 42-year-old man with idiopathic cardiomyopathy is hospitalized after an episode of syncope 1 hour ago. The event occurred while he was sitting in a chair; he did not have any symptoms before the episode, and he was alert and had no incontinence afterward. He had previously been well and exercises regularly without difficulty. Idiopathic cardiomyopathy was diagnosed 6 months ago. Echocardiography at that time showed left ventricular enlargement and a left ventricular ejection fraction of 30%. Coronary angiography showed normal coronary arteries and decreased left ventricular systolic function. His medications are furosemide, carvedilol, and lisinopril.

On physical examination, heart rate is 60/min and blood pressure is 100/60 mm Hg when supine, and heart rate is 66/min and blood pressure is 95/58 mm Hg when standing. Cardiac examination reveals an enlarged point of maximal impulse that is laterally displaced and regular cardiac rhythm. Results of the neurologic examination are normal. Electrocardiogram shows normal sinus rhythm without significant change compared with his last tracing

Which of the following is the most likely cause of his syncope?

(A) Complete heart block
(B) Generalized seizure
(C) Neurocardiogenic syncope
(D) Orthostatic hypotension
(E) Ventricular arrhythmia

Item 19

A 48-year-old woman is evaluated in the office after fainting 30 minutes ago. She states that she was at church and while standing and singing a hymn, she started feeling warm, then "got sweaty and woozy." The next thing she remembers is waking up on the floor with people standing around her. She is unclear how long she was unconscious but was immediately alert and oriented after the event. She has never had such an episode before. She did not have chest pain, palpitations, or loss of bowel or bladder control. She had not been feeling ill before this event. She has no medical problems and takes no medications.

On physical examination, she is in no distress. Her blood pressure is 122/76 mm Hg and heart rate is 84/min. Her cardiopulmonary and neurologic examinations are normal.

An electrocardiogram shows only normal sinus rhythm and is unchanged from a tracing performed 1 year ago for a life insurance examination.

Which of the following is the most appropriate management for this patient?

(A) CT scan of the head
(B) Duplex ultrasonography of the carotid arteries
(C) Echocardiography
(D) Exercise electrocardiography stress test
(E) Reassurance

Item 20

A 19-year-old man is evaluated for depression of 6 weeks' duration. He enrolled in college as a freshman 5 months ago and began participating in extramural basketball, football, and soccer in addition to carrying a full academic load and having a part-time job. He smokes cigarettes and marijuana and consumes more than 12 alcoholic drinks on weekends and at parties. He is sexually active with four different partners. However, during the past 6 weeks he has seldom left his room and has stopped attending classes because he cannot concentrate; he is in danger of failing all of his classes. He feels restless, cannot sleep, has a poor appetite, and feels depressed. He can identify no precipitating event related to his change in mood, although he had a similar episode once before at age 16 years. There is no family history of mood disorders.

Which of the following is the most likely diagnosis?

(A) Bipolar disorder
(B) Dysthymia
(C) Major depressive disorder
(D) Seasonal affective disorder
(E) Situational adjustment reaction with depressed mood

Item 21

A 47-year-old man is evaluated in the office for difficulty falling asleep for the past several months. He does not have snoring or sleepwalking, shortness of breath, or chest pain. He is employed as an accountant and recently went through a divorce. The divorce has caused some personal and financial stress in his life. He has a 15-pack-year smoking history.

On physical examination, heart rate is 72/min and blood pressure is 138/85 mm Hg. The BMI is 26. The remainder of the examination is normal.

Laboratory studies:

Hematocrit	42%
Leukocyte count	4200/µL
Fasting glucose	100 mg/dL
Thyroid-stimulating hormone	2.5 µU/mL

Which of the following is the most appropriate next diagnostic step?

(A) Cardiac stress testing
(B) Depression screening
(C) Polysomnography
(D) Spirometry

Item 22

A 52-year-old man is evaluated in the office because of difficulty concentrating and performing his work as a department manager over the past 6 months. The patient's wife reports that he has always had memory lapses and that he does not seem particularly different lately. The patient's history includes depression, for which he has been treated with antidepressants in the past for as long as 6 months. He currently takes no medications.

On physical examination, he replies slowly to questions and has a Mini–Mental State Examination score of 26/30. On neuropsychological examination, he has impairments of attention and speed of processing, but normal recent memory and visuospatial function.

Which of the following is the most appropriate next step in evaluating this patient?

(A) Assay for presenilin-1 mutation
(B) Electroencephalography
(C) MRI of the head
(D) Positron emission tomography
(E) Screening for depression

Item 23

A 22-year-old woman is evaluated in the office for feelings of sadness and guilt 6 weeks after an uncomplicated delivery of twins. Her symptoms have been present for 3 weeks but have worsened over the past week, and she cannot sleep, is preoccupied about the babies' health, and has discontinued all social activities. She says that her husband is supportive and that they have no marital problems. She is willing to start treatment for her disorder but is concerned about taking medication because she is breastfeeding.

Which of the following is the best treatment for this patient's disorder?

(A) Electroconvulsive therapy
(B) Exercise
(C) Fluoxetine
(D) Psychotherapy

Item 24

A 37-year-old woman is evaluated in the office for major depression that was diagnosed 1 month ago and treated with fluoxetine. Two weeks after treatment, she had no suicidal ideation, and her depressive symptoms had improved, with a 5-point decrease in her Patient Health Questionnaire-9 (PHQ-9) score. During today's visit, she reports that her depressive symptoms have continued to improve, although she has experienced sexual dysfunction manifested by anorgasmia. She is also overweight and is worried about gaining more weight.

On physical examination, the BMI is 29, and blood pressure is 140/80 mm Hg. The remainder of the examination is normal.

Which of the following is the most appropriate alternative treatment option for this patient's depression?

(A) Bupropion
(B) Citalopram
(C) Mirtazapine
(D) Sertraline

Item 25

An 18-year-old man is evaluated during a routine follow-up office visit for depression. He was diagnosed with major depression 2 weeks ago and therapy with a selective serotonin reuptake inhibitor (SSRI) was begun; however, he still has daily sadness, lack of interest in all activities, and a sense of lack of meaning in his life. He immigrated to the United States less than 1 year ago, leaving behind his family and friends. He admits to having constant suicidal thoughts and has plans to purchase a gun tomorrow.

Which of the following is the most appropriate next step in the management of this patient?

(A) Add psychotherapy
(B) Electroconvulsive therapy
(C) Immediate hospitalization
(D) Stop the SSRI and start a dopamine uptake inhibitor

Item 26

A 35-year-old man is evaluated in the office for a swollen wrist 2 days after having fallen on the sidewalk on his way home from a local bar. He indicates that he "may have had one too many" that evening. He has a stable marriage and has not missed work or received any citations for driving under the influence of alcohol. This is the first time he has presented with an alcohol-related injury.

Which of the following is the most appropriate initial step in managing this patient?

(A) Ask the CAGE questions
(B) Assess the average frequency and quantity of alcohol intake
(C) Deliver a clear, personalized message about the hazards of excess alcohol intake
(D) Recommend that he attend an Alcoholics Anonymous meeting

Item 27

A 26-year-old man is evaluated in the emergency department for anterior chest pain that began 1 hour ago. The pain is a dull substernal pressure with associated dyspnea and diaphoresis. He has never had a similar episode. The patient is otherwise healthy and takes no medications, but he admits to smoking cocaine 1 hour before the onset of the chest pain.

On physical examination, the patient is diaphoretic and appears anxious. The skin is cool and clammy, but there is no cyanosis. The blood pressure is 200/90 mm Hg, heart rate 110/min, respiration rate 12/min, and oxygen saturation is 98% on oxygen, 2 L/min by nasal cannula. There is no jugular venous distention. Heart sounds are loud, and an S_4 is present at the cardiac apex. There are no murmurs or rubs. The lungs are clear. The peripheral pulses are equal but somewhat diminished.

The electrocardiogram shows 0.02-mV ST-segment elevations in leads V_1-V_3. Results of serum troponin levels are pending.

What of the following medications is contraindicated in this patient?

(A) Aspirin
(B) β-Blockers
(C) Benzodiazepines
(D) Calcium channel blockers
(E) Nitroglycerin

Item 28

A 22-year-old man is evaluated in the office for a 12-month history of gradually worsening low back stiffness that is present for 2 hours after awakening in the morning. He has significant fatigue but no fever, chills, night sweats, or weight loss. He does not have pains in the peripheral joints but does have bilateral buttock pains throughout the day on sitting. One year ago, he also had a 2-week episode of uveitis of the right eye, which responded to corticosteroid eye drops.

On physical examination, vital signs are normal. He appears healthy but walks with a mild forward bending of his spine. Deep pressure and palpation of the lumbar spine in the midline and both sacroiliac joints elicits tenderness. Chest expansion in the fourth intercostal space is 2 cm (normal ≥5 cm), and he can only reach the midcalf region when attempting to touch his fingers to the floor.

On laboratory studies, hemoglobin is 12.5 g/dL, erythrocyte sedimentation rate is 85 mm/h, and C-reactive protein is 5 mg/dL. Anteroposterior radiograph of the pelvis and sacroiliac joints is shown.

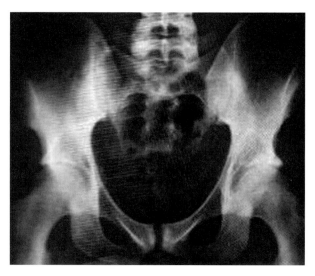

Which of the following is the most likely diagnosis?

(A) Ankylosing spondylitis
(B) Metastatic cancer
(C) Osteoarthritis
(D) Sacral fracture

Item 29

A 48-year-old man is evaluated in the office for back pain of 1 month's duration. He describes the pain as an ache that has been slowly worsening and is only partially relieved with acetaminophen. He is most comfortable lying down and least comfortable sitting or moving. He has not had any recent trauma or previous back pain. He has not had weight loss, fever, chills, numbness or weakness in his legs, or problems with bowel or bladder function. His only other medical problems are hypertension and osteoarthritis of the knees, for which he takes hydrochlorothiazide and acetaminophen, with occasional ibuprofen.

On physical examination, vital signs, including temperature, are normal. He has mild lumbar paravertebral tenderness and spasm. Neurologic examination, including muscle strength, deep tendon reflexes, and sensation, is normal. The straight-leg-raising test is normal.

Complete blood count and metabolic panel performed in the office 3 months ago were normal.

Which of the following is the best initial management plan for this patient?

(A) Analgesics and strict bed rest
(B) CT scan of the lumbosacral spine
(C) MRI of the lumbosacral spine
(D) Physical therapy
(E) Symptomatic treatment

Item 30

A 64-year-old woman is evaluated in the emergency department for a 4-day history of progressive bilateral leg weakness and numbness and a 1-day history of urinary incontinence. She has also had increasingly severe midback pain for the past 2 months. She has a history of breast cancer diagnosed 2 years ago and treated with surgery and local radiation therapy. Her only current medication is tamoxifen.

Physical examination shows normal mental status and cranial nerves. Strength in the arms is normal. The legs are diffusely weak, 3/5 proximally and 4/5 distally. Sensory examination shows diminished pinprick sensation from the nipples downward; vibratory sense is severely diminished in the feet. Reflexes are 2+ in the biceps and triceps and 3+ in the knees and ankles. An extensor plantar response is present bilaterally. Anal sphincter tone is diminished.

Which of the following is the most appropriate diagnostic study at this time?

(A) CT scan of the lumbar spine
(B) Electromyography and nerve conduction studies
(C) MRI of the brain
(D) MRI of the entire spine
(E) Plain radiographs of the entire spine

Item 31

A 51-year-old woman with chronic low back pain is evaluated in the office for a 2-week history of worsening low back pain radiating down her right leg to her right foot following a paroxysm of sneezing. She has no leg weakness or numbness. She takes no prescription medications.

On physical examination, the temperature is 36.9 °C (98.5 °F). The lumbar paraspinal muscles are tender to palpation. A straight-leg-raising test is positive on the right. Perineal sensation and anal sphincter tone are intact. She has difficulty extending her right great toe against resistance, but lower-extremity strength, sensation, and reflexes are otherwise normal.

Plain radiographs of the spine show some degenerative changes in the lower lumbar spine but no disk narrowing or vertebral collapse.

Which of the following is the most appropriate initial management for this patient?

(A) Bed rest for 7 days
(B) MRI of the lumbar spine
(C) Referral to an orthopedic surgeon
(D) Symptomatic treatment

Item 32

A 64-year-old man is evaluated in the office for right buttock pain of 1 month's duration. The pain occurs when he is standing and walking and is relieved by learning forward or sitting. The patient has a history of hypertension and coronary artery disease. He stopped smoking 5 years ago. He had an anterior myocardial infarction 3 years ago that was treated with stenting of the left anterior descending coronary artery; he has not had angina since that time. His medications are lisinopril, metoprolol, simvastatin, and low-dose aspirin.

On physical examination, he is thin and in no distress. The blood pressure is 130/80 mm Hg, and the heart rate is 70/min and regular. There is a grade 2/6 early systolic murmur at the right upper sternal border and a soft abdominal bruit but no pulsatile mass. Femoral pulses are 2+ with bilateral bruits, and distal pulses are 1+ bilaterally. Ankle-brachial index is 1.0 and does not decline with exercise.

Which of the following is the most likely cause of the patient's symptoms?

(A) Abdominal aortic aneurysm
(B) Common femoral artery stenosis
(C) Common iliac artery stenosis
(D) Spinal stenosis

Item 33

A 28-year-old woman is evaluated in the office for a 2-week history of cough productive of yellowish sputum, sneezing, tearing and gritty sensation in the eyes, nasal and sinus congestion, and postnasal drainage. Her medical history includes seasonal allergies. She has not had any recent contacts with sick or febrile persons. She is requesting antibiotics because her previous physician prescribed them during allergy season to prevent bacterial sinusitis.

On physical examination, temperature is 37.0 °C (98.6 °F). The conjunctivae are mildly injected without drainage, and the oropharynx is clear except for the presence of clear postnasal discharge. Sinus examination by transillumination and percussion is negative. There is no cervical lymphadenopathy, and the lungs are clear except for end-expiratory wheezes.

Which of the following is the most appropriate management?

(A) Oral antibiotics, nasal decongestant, and cough suppressant
(B) Oral antibiotics, nasal decongestant, and inhaled β-agonist
(C) Oral antihistamine, nasal corticosteroid, and inhaled β-agonist
(D) Oral antihistamine, cough suppressant, and inhaled β-agonist

Item 34

A 60-year-old man is evaluated in the office during a routine examination. He has been attempting to quit smoking cigarettes for several months but has been unsuccessful despite numerous office-based counseling interventions, participation in smoking-cessation support groups, nicotine-replacement therapy, and bupropion therapy. His medical history is noncontributory, and his family history is unremarkable. The physical examination is normal.

Which of the following interventions is most likely to reduce this patient's risk of dying from lung cancer?

(A) Annual chest radiograph
(B) Annual spiral CT scan of the chest
(C) Annual sputum cytology
(D) Repeated smoking-cessation attempts

Item 35

A 66-year-old woman is evaluated in the office for pain and cramping of her right leg while vacuuming and shopping. She has no nocturnal pain. She is a long-time smoker (140 pack-year history) and has hypertension and heart failure. Her medications are lisinopril, hydrochlorothiazide, and atenolol.

On physical examination, the blood pressure is 146/68 mm Hg and heart rate is 74/min and regular. The lungs are clear. Cardiac examination reveals an S_4. There is a right femoral artery bruit with absent right foot pulses but no pedal edema.

Which of the following interventions would be most effective for limb preservation in this patient?

(A) Discontinuation of atenolol
(B) Exercise training
(C) Initiation of cilostazol
(D) Initiation of warfarin
(E) Smoking cessation

Item 36

A 55-year-old man is evaluated in the office for cough, scant clear-to-yellow sputum, and malaise of 3 days' duration. He has not had fever, chills, wheezing, or pleuritic chest pain or recent contact with anyone who has been ill. He has a 40-pack-year smoking history. The patient has had similar symptoms three times in the past 6 months and feels well in the intervals between episodes.

On physical examination, temperature is 37.2 °C (99.0 °F), and heart rate, respiration rate, and blood pressure are normal. The cardiopulmonary examination is normal, including clear lungs with no signs of consolidation.

Which of the following is the most appropriate initial smoking-cessation management step during this visit?

(A) Prescribe bupropion
(B) Provide a clear, personalized message about smoking cessation
(C) Recommend nicotine gum
(D) Refer the patient to a behavioral-modification program

Item 37

A 32-year-old woman is evaluated in the office for concerns about her weight. She was thinner when she was younger, but gained weight with both of her pregnancies and has had trouble losing it. Her father and sister are overweight. She is a medical technician but now works at home raising her children. She is otherwise healthy and takes no medications.

On physical examination, the blood pressure is 130/78 mm Hg and heart rate is 76/min; the BMI is 26. The results of screening blood tests are pending.

Which of the following is the best initial management approach for this patient?

(A) Bariatric surgery
(B) Diet and exercise
(C) Diet and exercise and therapy with sibutramine
(D) Therapy with orlistat
(E) Reassurance and observation

Item 38

A 55-year-old man is evaluated in the office for consideration of gastric bypass surgery. The patient has been obese all his life. He has tried a balanced calorie-restricted diet for the past 6 months and has increased his exercise to include walking for 20 minutes three times weekly. Although he was initially successful in losing weight, he has not been able to maintain the weight loss. He works as a high school teacher and believes that his weight has interfered with his success in being asked to take leadership positions in his field. He does not smoke, and he drinks alcohol occasionally. His medical history is significant for hyperlipidemia and hypertension, both controlled with medications.

On physical examination, the heart rate is 65/min, and the blood pressure is 142/88 mm Hg. The BMI is 40. Fasting plasma glucose is 116 mg/dL, and LDL cholesterol is 120 mg/dL. A chest radiograph shows borderline cardiomegaly, and the electrocardiogram is normal.

Which of the following treatments is most appropriate for this patient?

(A) A low-carbohydrate diet
(B) A restricted-fat diet
(C) Gastric bypass surgery
(D) Orlistat
(E) Sibutramine

Item 39

A 55-year-old woman is evaluated during a routine office visit and seeks help losing weight. The patient had begun to put on weight after menopause at age 49 years. She has tried multiple diets but has failed to maintain the weight loss she initially achieves with each diet. She does not smoke or drink alcohol. Her medical history is significant for hypertension, for which she takes three medications.

On physical examination, the heart rate is 65/min, and the blood pressure is 158/98 mm Hg. The BMI is 33. The remainder of the physical examination is normal.

In addition to a low-calorie diet and regular exercise, which of the following is the most appropriate treatment for this patient?

(A) Gastric bypass surgery
(B) Mirtazapine
(C) Orlistat
(D) Sibutramine

Item 40

An 82-year-old woman is evaluated in the office for a 4.5-kg (10-lb) weight loss from baseline over the past 6 months. Her medical history includes hypertension, depression, and osteoarthritis of the knees, treated with hydrochlorothiazide, sertraline, and ibuprofen as needed. She has never smoked. She states that her mood is good and has a score of 1/5 on the Five-Item Geriatric Depression Scale. She shops on her own at the grocery store but finds it a difficult task and has trouble doing it weekly. She does not have anorexia, abdominal pain, or change in bowel habits.

On physical examination, vital signs are normal. The BMI is 18.6. The lungs are clear, and the cardiac, abdominal, and rectal examinations are normal. There is no pedal edema.

Laboratory studies, including complete blood count and thyroid-stimulating hormone level, are normal. Results of a recent fecal occult blood test and chest radiograph were normal. Colonoscopy 5 years ago was normal.

Which of the following is the most appropriate next step in the management of this patient?

(A) Colonoscopy
(B) CT scan of the abdomen
(C) Discontinuation of ibuprofen
(D) Shopping or meal preparation assistance
(E) Substitution of mirtazapine for sertraline

Item 41

A 79-year-old woman is evaluated in the office for anorexia and involuntary weight loss of 15 kg (33 lb) over the past 3 months. She also has hoarseness and a depressed mood. She does not have abdominal pain, dysphagia, nausea, vomiting, diarrhea, change in bowel movements, or difficulty chewing food. She lives with her daughter who prepares her meals. She has a history of anxiety, depression, and agoraphobia, and her only medication is a benzodiazepine, which she has been taking in increasing doses over the past few months. She is otherwise healthy. She has never smoked and does not use alcohol.

On physical examination, she is mildly obese (BMI 31). Vital signs are normal, and except for hoarseness, the physical examination is normal. The mental status examination is also normal, but her responses are slow, and she is occasionally tearful.

Complete blood count, comprehensive metabolic panel, urinalysis, and chest radiograph are normal, as are tests for thyroid-stimulating hormone and C-reactive protein. Direct laryngoscopy is normal.

Which of the following is the most appropriate next step in this patient's management?

(A) CT scan of the chest, abdomen, and pelvis
(B) Reassurance and reassessment in 4 to 6 months
(C) Screening test for major depression
(D) Therapy with an appetite stimulant

Item 42

A 48-year-old woman is evaluated in the office for frequent hot flushes and night sweats that interfere with her work and sleep. She has not menstruated for 8 months. She is speaking at a conference in 3 weeks and desires immediate resolution to the embarrassing sweats associated with her hot flushes. Her medical history is noncontributory, and she takes no medications. Physical examination, including vital signs, is normal.

Which of the following is the most appropriate next step in the treatment of this patient's symptoms?

(A) Cognitive behavioral therapy
(B) Imipramine
(C) Red clover
(D) Short-term, low-dose hormone replacement therapy

Item 43

A 25-year-old woman is evaluated for a 3-month history of amenorrhea. She underwent menarche at the age of 14 years and has always had irregular periods. At the age of 21 years, her periods became increasingly irregular, and over the past year, she has had several episodes of very heavy bleeding, interspersed by several months without menstrual bleeding, resulting in a total of five periods. She has not had headaches, visual changes, or intolerance to heat or cold. She is otherwise healthy and takes no medications.

On physical examination, the patient is overweight (BMI 29). The blood pressure is 120/75 mm Hg, and heart rate is 70/min. She has a few terminal hairs on her chin but no acne. Pelvic examination reveals a normal-sized and regularly shaped uterus. Speculum examination is normal. Urine pregnancy test is negative.

Which of the following is the most likely diagnosis?

(A) Cushing's syndrome
(B) Hyperprolactinemia
(C) Hypothyroidism
(D) Polycystic ovary syndrome
(E) Uterine fibroids (leiomyomas)

Item 44

A 22-year-old woman is evaluated in the office for acne on her face that has worsened over the past few weeks and includes inflammatory and small nodular lesions. The patient has a history of moderate-to-severe acne outbreaks occurring since she was 14 years old. Her parents and siblings also had acne. She has been using a topical retinoid and topical antibiotic preparations with no improvement. She is otherwise healthy. She takes combined (estrogen-progestin) oral contraceptives for birth control and has regular menses.

On physical examination, she has several papulonodular lesions on the face. The lesions are tender, and some have pustules.

Which of the following is the most appropriate next step in the management of this patient?

(A) Discontinue oral contraceptive
(B) Prescribe a course of oral corticosteroids
(C) Prescribe oral isotretinoin
(D) Prescribe oral tetracycline

Item 45

An 18-year-old woman is evaluated in the office for acne. She has had intermittent outbreaks of acne over the past 5 years. She is a college student who experiences stress associated with her studies. Because of her busy schedule, she often eats fast food and snacks on chocolate bars. She has tried over-the-counter topical salicylic acid and antibiotic medications to treat her acne without benefit. She is sexually active and uses barrier contraception.

On physical examination, she has comedonal acne with open (blackheads) and closed (whiteheads) comedones on her face. There are no nodular lesions.

Which of the following is the most appropriate management strategy for this patient's acne?

(A) Avoidance of fast foods and chocolate
(B) Oral corticosteroids
(C) Oral tetracycline
(D) Topical retinoid medications

Item 46

A 21-year-old man is evaluated in the office for painful sores in his mouth. Episodes of these sores have occurred two to three times yearly since he was 16 years old, and he believes they are associated with stress. They usually appear on the inside of his mouth as a single, round, painful lesion, lasting for 5 to 10 days and resolving without scarring.

He has had no fever, chills, arthralgias, genital ulcers, rashes, eye problems, diarrhea, abdominal pain, or weight loss. He is sexually active, has had only a few sexual partners, and has been in a monogamous relationship for the last 12 months. All of his sexual interactions have been heterosexual. He does not use illicit drugs. Results of HIV testing for his sexual partner and him from 3 months ago were negative. The remainder of the history is noncontributory.

On physical examination, the vital signs are normal. The oral examination is significant for the lesion shown (*see Figure 4 in Color Plates*). The remainder of the physical examination is unremarkable.

Which of the following is the most likely diagnosis?

(A) Aphthous ulcer
(B) Behçet's disease
(C) *Candida* infection
(D) Herpes simplex virus infection
(E) HIV infection

Item 47

A 20-year-old male college student is having trouble sleeping because of an itchy rash on the inner aspect of his arms, elbow creases, and behind the knees. This rash and itching have been recurring for several years, becoming more severe in the winter despite his use of a daily moisturizer. His history is remarkable for seasonal allergies, and the only medication he uses is a nasal corticosteroid in the fall.

The physical examination, including vital signs, is normal, with the exception of the skin findings, as shown (*see Figure 5 in Color Plates*).

Which of the following is the most likely diagnosis?

(A) Atopic dermatitis
(B) Cellulitis
(C) Contact dermatitis
(D) Seborrheic dermatitis

Item 48

A 32-year-old man comes to the office because of a 1-week history of worsening erythema and pruritus of both axillae. He is otherwise asymptomatic, his appetite is unchanged, and his weight is stable.

On physical examination, temperature is 37.1 °C (98.8 °F), heart rate is 72/min, respiration rate is 16/min, and blood pressure is 128/62 mm Hg. Both axillae show marked erythema, minimal tenderness, several small nonpustular vesicles, and a small amount of serous exudate coming from ruptured vesicles. There is no erythema adjacent to the axillae and no palpable lymphadenopathy.

Leukocyte count is 5300/μL with 72% neutrophils, 18% lymphocytes, 2% monocytes, and 8% eosinophils.

Which of the following is the most likely diagnosis?

(A) Contact dermatitis
(B) *Pasteurella multocida* cellulitis
(C) Staphylococcal cellulitis
(D) Streptococcal cellulitis

Item 49

A 35-year-old farmer is evaluated in the office for an extremely itchy rash on his face, arms, and legs that keeps him awake at night. He noticed the rash several days after raking and burning brush along his driveway. The rash on the forearm is shown (*see Figure 6 in Color Plates*). Some involved parts have extensive edema and bullae formation. The remainder of the physical examination, including vital signs, is normal.

Which of the following is the first-line treatment for this condition?

(A) Oral corticosteroids
(B) Topical corticosteroids
(C) Topical mupirocin
(D) Topical pimecrolimus

Item 50

A 22-year-old woman living in Massachusetts is evaluated in the office for a 4-day history of multiple "bug bites" and left ankle pain. She initially developed painful, nonpruritic nodules on her legs and severe left ankle pain 4 days after mowing her lawn. She has been walking with a limp.

On physical examination, temperature is 38.2 °C (100.8 °F). The left ankle is slightly swollen. On musculoskeletal examination, passive motion of the left ankle elicits pain. The skin lesions are shown (*see Figure 7 in Color Plates*) and are tender to palpation.

On laboratory studies, complete blood count, serum chemistry studies, and urinalysis are normal. Arthrocentesis of the left ankle yields 1.5 mL of fluid (leukocyte count, 4000/μL; 45% neutrophils). Examination using polarized light microscopy shows no crystals. Culture results are pending.

Which of the following is the most likely diagnosis for the skin lesions?

(A) Disseminated gonorrhea
(B) Erythema nodosum
(C) Psoriasis
(D) Systemic lupus erythematosus

Item 51

A 75-year-old man is evaluated in the office because of increasingly severe pain and a rash on the left side of his chest. The pain began 3 days ago, and the rash developed 2 days ago. The patient has never had similar symptoms. His only medication is a nonsteroidal anti-inflammatory drug for the pain.

On physical examination, vital signs are normal. The rash is shown (*see Figure 8 in Color Plates*).

Which of the following antiviral agents is most appropriate at this time?

(A) Famciclovir
(B) Ganciclovir
(C) Penciclovir
(D) Valganciclovir

Item 52

A 55-year-old woman is evaluated in the office for what she believes is toenail fungus. She is interested in treatment. She is otherwise healthy and takes no medications.

On physical examination, thickened and dystrophic nails are noted on each of her largest toes. The remainder of the examination is normal.

Which of the following is the most appropriate next step in management?

(A) Aggressive nail débridement
(B) Culture of debris under the nail
(C) Oral terbinafine
(D) Topical ciclopirox

Item 53

A 40-year-old emergency medicine physician is evaluated in the office for a rash on the back of her elbows and anterior knees. Similar rashes have occurred in the past; the first episode occurred when she was a young adult. Typically the rash develops in the winter and improves with exposure to sunlight in the summer. She has used over-the-counter hydrocortisone cream without relief. She is otherwise healthy.

The skin findings on the back of the patient's elbows are shown (*see Figure 9 in Color Plates*). Laboratory studies, including complete blood count and differential, serum chemistry studies, and urinalysis, are normal.

Which of the following is the most likely diagnosis?

(A) Dermatophyte infection
(B) Eczema
(C) Pityriasis rosea
(D) Psoriasis
(E) Subacute cutaneous lupus erythematosus

Item 54

A 45-year-old woman is evaluated in the office for a facial rash of 6 months' duration that involves the cheeks and nose. She is unsure whether sun exposure worsens the rash. She does not have rash elsewhere, fatigue, ulcers, or joint pain. She has a history of autoimmune hypothyroidism with positive antimicrosomal and antinuclear antibody assays.

Physical examination reveals a rash limited to the cheeks, nasolabial folds, and nose (*see Figure 10 in Color Plates*). The remainder of the examination is unremarkable. Current laboratory studies, including complete blood count, serum chemistry studies, and thyroid-stimulating hormone, are normal.

Which of the following is the most likely diagnosis?

(A) Dermatomyositis
(B) Psoriasis
(C) Rosacea
(D) Seborrheic dermatitis
(E) Systemic lupus erythematosus

Item 55

A 30-year-old woman is evaluated in the office for pruritus that interferes with her sleep and has persisted for at least 1 week. She had recently visited her grandfather who resides in a nursing home and who also complained of itching. The patient is otherwise healthy, takes no medications, and has not had any new exposures to household chemicals.

Physical examination reveals multiple small papules, some excoriated, distributed predominantly on her hands (*see Figure 11 in Color Plates*), feet, and areolae.

Which of the following is the most appropriate treatment for this patient?

(A) Bacitracin, topically
(B) Ivermectin, orally
(C) Permethrin 5%, topically
(D) Triamcinolone 0.1%, topically

Item 56

A 42-year-old man is evaluated in the office for a nonpruritic, nonpainful spreading rash on his thorax that he has noticed over the past several weeks. The patient has been outdoors more often over the past few weeks, and his skin is beginning to tan. He has used an over-the-counter corticosteroid cream without success.

The findings of the skin examination are shown (*see Figure 12 in Color Plates*). Direct microscopic examination of scale with 10% potassium hydroxide shows large, blunt hyphae and thick-walled budding spores in a "spaghetti and meatballs" pattern.

Which of the following is the most likely diagnosis?

(A) Pityriasis rosea
(B) Psoriasis
(C) Tinea corporis
(D) Tinea versicolor

Item 57

A 30-year-old woman is evaluated in the office for a wart on her right thumb that she first noticed 6 months ago. She began treating the wart with over-the-counter salicylic acid 1 month ago when writing with the affected hand became painful. She has noticed a reduction in the size and pain of the wart, but she wants a more effective treatment. The medical history is noncontributory.

On physical examination, a common wart is found to be directly adjacent to the thumb nail bed and is 4 × 4 mm in size. The remainder of the examination is unremarkable.

Which of the following is the most appropriate next step in management?

(A) *Candida* antigen injection
(B) Continuation of salicylic acid therapy
(C) Cryotherapy
(D) Topical imiquimod

Item 58

A 78-year-old man is evaluated in the office for a 4-month history of difficulty managing his finances and shopping for products to care for his home and prepare his meals. However, if food is available in the house, he can prepare it for himself. He has been widowed for 5 years and prefers living alone but does engage in activities outside of the home and enjoys visiting with his friends, playing checkers, and watching television. He has no other medical problems and takes no medications. He does not smoke cigarettes or drink alcohol. He is well groomed, clean, and neatly dressed and denies feeling sad or unhappy. He was driven to the office by a friend.

Which of the following screening tests is most likely to be useful in managing this patient?

(A) Activities of Daily Living (ADL)
(B) Confusion Assessment Method
(C) Geriatric Depression Scale
(D) Instrumental Activities of Daily Living (IADL)

Item 59

A 22-year-old man was discovered to have atrial fibrillation following an episode of palpitations while playing soccer 2 hours ago. He is currently in sinus rhythm and asymptomatic.

Physical examination demonstrates blood pressure of 148/96 mm Hg in both upper extremities. The lungs are clear. The apical impulse is prominent and laterally displaced. An ejection click and a grade 2/6 early systolic murmur are noted at the left sternal border. An apical S_4 is present. A systolic murmur can be heard over the posterior left side of the chest. The

femoral pulses are reduced, and there is a delay between the radial and femoral arterial pulses. A chest radiograph is shown.

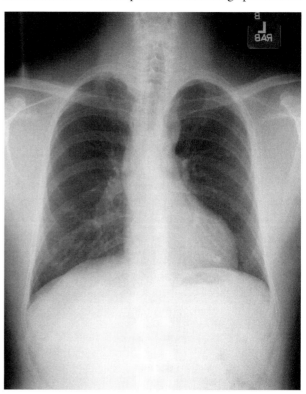

This constellation of findings suggests which of the following diagnoses?

(A) Atrial septal defect
(B) Coarctation of the aorta
(C) Mitral valve regurgitation
(D) Patent ductus arteriosus
(E) Ventricular septal defect

Item 60

A 59-year-old woman who has had type 2 diabetes mellitus for 8 years is evaluated in the office during a routine examination. She has no significant symptoms at this time. Her current medications are glyburide, metformin, and low-dose aspirin. She previously took lisinopril but developed a chronic cough, resulting in discontinuation of the medication.

On physical examination, the blood pressure is 135/90 mm Hg, heart rate is 84/min, and BMI is 31.3. She has no evidence of retinopathy or peripheral neuropathy.

Laboratory studies:

Fasting glucose	103 mg/dL
Hemoglobin A1c	6.1%
Creatinine	0.9 mg/dL
Total cholesterol	198 mg/dL
Triglycerides	166 mg/dL
HDL cholesterol	53 mg/dL
LDL cholesterol	112 mg/dL
Urine albumin–creatinine ratio	62 mg/g

Which of the following would most likely reduce proteinuria and preserve renal function in this patient?

(A) An angiotensin receptor blocker
(B) A β-adrenergic blocker
(C) Insulin
(D) A statin
(E) A thiazolidinedione

Item 61

A 62-year-old woman is evaluated in the office for mild hypercalcemia. She has a history of hypertension, type 2 diabetes mellitus, dyslipidemia, and hypothyroidism. She does not have polyuria, polydipsia, polyphagia, constipation, fatigue, or neurocognitive impairment. Medications are glipizide, metformin, atorvastatin, ramipril, hydrochlorothiazide, low-dose aspirin, and levothyroxine.

Physical examination reveals a blood pressure of 130/90 mm Hg, heart rate of 70/min, a goiter, and a normal relaxation of the deep tendon reflexes.

Laboratory studies:

Blood urea nitrogen	25 mg/dL
Creatinine	1.2 mg/dL
Hemoglobin A1c	7.5%
Albumin	4.0 g/dL
Calcium	11.0 mg/dL
Alkaline phosphatase	110 U/L
Alanine aminotransferase	25 U/L
Aspartate aminotransferase	28 U/L

Review of old medical records shows that the calcium level has been intermittently elevated over the past 2 years.

Which of the following is the most appropriate next step in the management of this patient's hypercalcemia?

(A) Measure thyroid-stimulating hormone
(B) Measure parathyroid hormone
(C) Stop atorvastatin
(D) Stop hydrochlorothiazide
(E) Stop ramipril

Item 62

A 39-year-old man is evaluated in the office for a 6-year history of difficult-to-control hypertension. Initially, he was treated with hydrochlorothiazide, but within 1 week, he developed profound muscle weakness; follow-up potassium concentration was 2.1 meq/L. Hydrochlorothiazide was discontinued, and he has not been on a diuretic for 6 years. He has struggled with obesity throughout his life and has a 7-year history of type 2 diabetes mellitus. His current medications are lisinopril, diltiazem, pravastatin, metformin, glipizide, and aspirin.

On physical examination, his blood pressure is 189/92 mm Hg, heart rate is 87/min, and BMI is 32.8. There is no jugular venous distention, and his lungs are clear. Cardiac examination reveals an S_4. He has no edema.

Laboratory studies:

Sodium	141 meq/L
Potassium	3.1 meq/L
Chloride	104 meq/L
Bicarbonate	33 meq/L
BUN	11 mg/dL
Creatinine	0.9 mg/dL
24 hour urine:	
Sodium	90 meq
Potassium	57 meq
Free cortisol	36 µg/24 h (normal <55 µg/24 h)

Which of the following is the most likely cause of this patient's hypertension?

(A) Cushing's syndrome
(B) Essential hypertension
(C) Hyperaldosteronism
(D) Pheochromocytoma
(E) Renovascular hypertension

Item 63

An 80-year-old man is evaluated in the office during a routine examination. He has a history of hypertension, and chronic osteoarthritis was diagnosed 20 years ago. His hypertension has been well controlled on submaximal dosages of both atenolol and hydrochlorothiazide. Three months ago, he began taking ibuprofen.

On physical examination, heart rate is 60/min and blood pressure is 180/90 mm Hg without orthostatic changes. There is trace peripheral edema.

Laboratory studies:

Blood urea nitrogen	40 mg/dL
Creatinine	1.5 mg/dL
Sodium	134 meq/L
Potassium	4.9 meq/L

Which of the following treatment strategies is indicated for this patient?

(A) Add lisinopril
(B) Discontinue ibuprofen
(C) Increase the atenolol dose
(D) Increase the hydrochlorothiazide dose

Item 64

A 65-year-old man is admitted to the intensive care unit for a 3-month history of frequent headache and progressive shortness of breath. Over the last 3 days, he has developed 2-pillow orthopnea and paroxysmal nocturnal dyspnea. He does not have chest pain. He has a 25-year history of hypertension that has become more difficult to control over the past several months, hyperlipidemia, and multiple transient ischemic attacks. He also has a history of coronary artery bypass and aorto-bifemoral bypass surgery. His current daily medications are metoprolol, lisinopril, amlodipine, hydrochlorothiazide, low-dose aspirin, and pravastatin; he has been compliant about taking his medications.

On physical examination, he is a thin man without acne or abdominal striae. The blood pressure is 210/130 mm Hg, with a heart rate of 60/min and respiration rate of 14/min. The jugular venous pressure is elevated, and there is a right carotid artery bruit. Bibasilar crackles are present. Cardiac examination shows a summation (S_3 and S_4) gallop. Routine laboratory studies are normal.

The patient is treated with intravenous diuretics, and his dyspnea improves. His diastolic blood pressure remains between 110 and 130 mm Hg, and he continues to have headache but no focal neurologic deficits. Serum electrolytes are normal.

Which of the following is the most appropriate next step in the evaluation of this patient?

(A) Measurement of 24-hour urine for cortisol
(B) Measurement of 24-hour urine for potassium excretion
(C) Renal ultrasonography with renal artery Doppler examination
(D) Spot urine for metanephrines

Item 65

A 48-year-old man is evaluated in the office for poorly controlled hypertension. His blood pressure has been elevated for 12 years and remains between 150/105 mm Hg and 170/105 mm Hg despite the use of multiple medications. He also has poor exercise tolerance and fatigue and often falls asleep in the afternoon. Medications are atenolol, amlodipine, and hydrochlorothiazide.

On physical examination, blood pressure is 168/110 mm Hg. He is obese (BMI 35) and appears plethoric. The remainder of the examination is normal.

Laboratory studies:

Creatinine	1.4 mg/dL
Sodium	140 meq/L
Potassium	3.9 meq/L
Bicarbonate	25 meq/L

Which of the following is the most likely cause of this patient's resistant hypertension?

(A) Pheochromocytoma
(B) Primary hyperaldosteronism
(C) Renovascular hypertension
(D) Sleep apnea syndrome

Item 66

An 85-year-old woman is evaluated in the office for resistant hypertension. She has a long-standing history of hypertension that had been well controlled with β-blocker therapy. Her physician recently died, and results of blood pressure measurement performed in a new office have been high. Records from her previous physician show that office blood pressure measurements were always normal. She also has fatigue, weakness, and dizziness, particularly after standing up. She has been unable to tolerate angiotensin-converting enzyme inhibitor, angiotensin receptor blocker, and dihydropyridine calcium antagonist therapy. Current medications are metoprolol, 50 mg/d, and hydrochlorothiazide, 25 mg/d.

On physical examination, heart rate is 60/min and blood pressure in the supine and standing positions is 170/70 mm Hg. The remainder of the examination is normal.

Serum creatinine is 0.8 mg/dL, blood urea nitrogen is 18 mg/dL, and serum potassium is 3.6 meq/L.

Which of the following is the most appropriate next step in this patient's management?

(A) Ambulatory blood pressure monitoring
(B) Discontinuation of metoprolol
(C) Increase in the hydrochlorothiazide dose to 50 mg/d
(D) Magnetic resonance angiography of the renal arteries

Item 67

A 52-year-old woman with type 2 diabetes mellitus, hyperlipidemia, and hypertension is evaluated during a routine office visit. She has a 30-pack-year smoking history. Her mother had diabetes and required hemodialysis. Medications are insulin, metoprolol, fosinopril, hydrochlorothiazide, atorvastatin, and low-dose aspirin.

On physical examination, blood pressure is 165/95 mm Hg. Retinal microaneurysms are noted on funduscopic examination. There is no jugular venous distention. The lungs are clear. Cardiac examination reveals a regular rhythm with an S_4. There is bilateral pedal edema. The distal pulses are absent in both feet.

Laboratory studies:

Hemoglobin A1c	7.2%
Glucose	180 mg/dL
Creatinine	1.2 mg/dL
24-Hour urine protein excretion	1.8 g/24 h

Which of the following factors is most likely to cause this patient's chronic kidney disease to rapidly progress to end-stage renal disease?

(A) Cigarette smoking
(B) Poorly controlled diabetes mellitus
(C) Poorly controlled hypertension
(D) Proteinuria

Item 68

A 60-year-old man with type 2 diabetes mellitus, hypertension, and coronary artery disease is evaluated during a routine office visit. Medications are metformin, a β-blocker, an angiotensin-converting enzyme inhibitor, aspirin, and a statin.

On physical examination, blood pressure is repeatedly 160/90 mm Hg. There is evidence of early diabetic retinopathy.

Laboratory studies:

Blood urea nitrogen	15 mg/dL
Creatinine	1.1 mg/dL
Potassium	5.4 meq/L
Spot urine albumin–creatinine ratio	175 mg/g

Addition of which of the following agents is indicated to treat this patient's hypertension?

(A) An angiotensin receptor blocker
(B) An α-blocker
(C) A potassium-sparing diuretic
(D) A thiazide diuretic

Item 69

A 57-year-old woman is evaluated in the office for intermittent claudication of the left calf that she has had for 5 years. The symptoms reproducibly occur after she walks 100 yards and resolve after 5 minutes of rest. The patient has an 80-pack-year smoking history but no longer smokes; she also has hypertension, type 2 diabetes mellitus, hypercholesterolemia, and chronic stable angina. Her medications are atenolol, atorvastatin, lisinopril, low-dose aspirin, and glyburide.

On physical examination, the blood pressure is 142/94 mm Hg in both upper extremities, and heart rate is 66/min. Carotid artery pulsations are brisk, with a right carotid artery bruit. The lungs are clear. Cardiac examination discloses an S_4. There is a left femoral artery bruit with absent pulses in the left foot and trace pulses in the right foot.

Which of the following is the maximum acceptable blood pressure limit in this patient?

(A) <140/90 mm Hg
(B) <140/85 mm Hg
(C) <130/90 mm Hg
(D) <130/80 mm Hg

Item 70

A 59-year-old black man is evaluated during a routine follow-up office visit. He has occasional headaches but has otherwise been well. He had an anterior myocardial infarction 18 months ago and has hypertension, compensated congestive heart failure, type 2 diabetes mellitus, dyslipidemia, and mild chronic renal insufficiency. He is compliant with therapy, which includes metoprolol, lisinopril, amlodipine, metformin, atorvastatin, and aspirin.

On physical examination, heart rate is 62/min and blood pressure is 142/88 mm Hg. BMI is 24. Jugular venous pressure is 6 cm H_2O. Cardiac examination reveals a regular rhythm; normal S_1 and S_2; and no S_3, S_4, or murmurs. The lungs are clear. There is no edema.

Laboratory studies: serum creatinine, 1.3 mg/dL; LDL cholesterol, 68 mg/dL; and spot urine albumin–creatinine ratio, 45 mg/g.

Which of the following is the most appropriate next step in this patient's management?

(A) Add clonidine
(B) Add hydrochlorothiazide
(C) Discontinue metoprolol; add hydralazine and isosorbide mononitrate
(D) Measure 24-hour urine catecholamines
(E) Reevaluate blood pressure in 2 to 3 months

Item 71

A 35-year-old woman who is 15 weeks pregnant is referred for evaluation of chronic hypertension. She discontinued her antihypertensive regimen when she learned that she was pregnant.

On physical examination, heart rate is 90/min and blood pressure is 160/98 mm Hg. Cardiac and pulmonary examinations are normal.

Laboratory studies:

Blood urea nitrogen	6 mg/dL
Creatinine	0.6 mg/dL
Sodium	136 meq/L
Potassium	3.7 meq/L
Bicarbonate	23 meq/L

Treatment with which of the following agents is most appropriate for this patient?

(A) Hydrochlorothiazide
(B) Labetalol
(C) Lisinopril
(D) Losartan

Item 72

A 67-year-old man is evaluated in the emergency department 8 hours after the onset of headache, nausea, vomiting, and chest pain that radiates to his back. He has a history of hypertension, hyperlipidemia, peripheral vascular disease, and coronary artery disease. He had stenting of his left anterior descending coronary artery 1 year ago. Routine stress testing performed 1 month ago was normal. Medications are metoprolol, atorvastatin, and aspirin.

On physical examination, he appears anxious and diaphoretic. Blood pressure is 250/128 mm Hg, heart rate is 76/min, and respiration rate is 22/min. There are no carotid bruits. On chest auscultation, rhonchi are heard at both bases. An S_1, S_2, and S_4 are heard. There is a grade 2/6 systolic ejection murmur in the aortic area and a grade 2/6 early diastolic murmur heard along the left sternal border. Bounding femoral pulses are palpated bilaterally. The remainder of the physical examination is normal. An electrocardiogram shows sinus rhythm with left ventricular hypertrophy with a strain pattern and ST-segment depression in the lateral leads. An urgent CT scan of the chest is ordered.

Which of the following is the most appropriate next step in this patient's management?

(A) Intravenous heparin
(B) Intravenous labetalol and sodium nitroprusside
(C) Intravenous thrombolytic therapy
(D) Oral nifedipine and furosemide

Item 73

A 46-year-old black man is evaluated in the office for hypertension. He was told several years ago at an employee health fair that his blood pressure was elevated. Therapy was initiated at that time but was discontinued after 3 months because of side effects. He has since been checking his blood pressure at the pharmacy; his blood pressure typically is 160/90 mm Hg. He currently takes no medications.

On physical examination, heart rate is 64/min and resting blood pressure is 158/88 mm Hg. Funduscopic examination reveals hypertensive retinopathy.

Laboratory studies:

Blood urea nitrogen	34 mg/dL
Creatinine	1.9 mg/dL
Sodium	142 meq/L
Potassium	3.9 meq/L
Chloride	110 meq/L
Bicarbonate	22 meq/L
Urinalysis	2+ protein, no blood
Urine protein–creatinine ratio	0.45 mg/g

Renal ultrasonography reveals a right kidney 9.2 cm in diameter and a left kidney 9.1 cm in diameter with two simple cysts.

Which of the following is the most appropriate treatment of this patient's hypertension?

(A) Amlodipine
(B) Metoprolol
(C) Ramipril
(D) Terazosin

Item 74

A 36-year-old man is evaluated in the emergency department for headache and palpitations. He has been hypertensive for the past 2 years, but his blood pressure has been suboptimally controlled with a combination of hydrochlorothiazide, diltiazem, and lisinopril. He frequently experiences similar episodic headache and diaphoresis, during which his blood pressure is alarmingly high. These episodes had been attributed to migraine headaches, but the addition of propranolol for prophylaxis worsened their frequency and severity.

On physical examination, he is anxious, tremulous, and diaphoretic. Blood pressure is 198/106 mm Hg, and heart rate is 110/min. Baseline laboratory studies, including hemoglobin, serum creatinine, blood urea nitrogen, and electrolytes, are normal.

Which of the following is the most likely diagnosis?

(A) Carcinoid syndrome
(B) Cushing's syndrome
(C) Pheochromocytoma
(D) Primary aldosteronism

Item 75

A 38-year-old man who was recently diagnosed with pheochromocytoma comes to the office for evaluation in anticipation of surgery. On physical examination, his blood pressure is 190/105 mm Hg. The remainder of the examination is unremarkable.

Therapy with which of the following drugs is indicated in preparation for surgery in this patient?

(A) Atenolol
(B) Hydrochlorothiazide
(C) Nifedipine
(D) Phenoxybenzamine

Item 76

A 64-year-old man with a history of coronary artery disease, peripheral vascular disease, chronic cigarette smoking, chronic kidney disease, and uncontrolled hypertension is evaluated during a routine office visit. He was recently hospitalized for acute pulmonary edema. His estimated glomerular filtration rate is 45 mL/min. Renal ultrasonography performed during his hospitalization revealed a left kidney of 8.5 cm and a right kidney of 11 cm and increased echogenicity of both kidneys. He has been compliant with his diet restrictions. Medications are aspirin, simvastatin, carvedilol, furosemide, digoxin, and maximal doses of losartan, amlodipine, and clonidine.

On physical examination, the patient is thin. Heart rate is 62/min and blood pressure is 186/72 mm Hg. Cardiac examination reveals an S_4 gallop. An abdominal bruit is heard. There is bilateral lower-extremity edema.

Which of the following is the most likely diagnosis?

(A) Cushing's syndrome
(B) Hyperthyroidism
(C) Renal artery stenosis
(D) Sleep apnea syndrome

Item 77

A 41-year-old woman is evaluated in the office for a 1-week history of increasing frequency of headaches. Within the past year, scleroderma was diagnosed when she developed Raynaud's phenomenon, gastroesophageal reflux, and skin thickening. She does not have dyspnea or chest pain. She takes only omeprazole.

On physical examination, temperature is normal, heart rate is 95/min, respiration rate is 18/min, and blood pressure is 189/106 mm Hg (blood pressure 3 months ago was 128/70 mm Hg). Conjunctivae are pale, and funduscopic examination is normal. The lungs are clear, and cardiac examination reveals a normal S_1 and a physiologically split S_2. Skin examination reveals digital pitting and skin thickening over her face, trunk, and extremities. Neurologic examination is normal. There is lower-extremity edema.

The hemoglobin is 10 g/dL, platelet count is 84,000 μL, serum creatinine is 1.9 mg/dL, and serum electrolytes are normal. Previous studies 3 months ago were all normal.

In addition to admitting the patient to the hospital, which of the following medications should be started?

(A) Captopril
(B) Hydrochlorothiazide
(C) Labetalol
(D) Nifedipine

Chapter 4

General Internal Medicine
Answers and Critiques

Item 1   Answer: E

The patient's post-test probability of having coronary artery disease is 77%. The patient's pretest probability, which is based on his chest pain, age, and sex, is estimated to be 40%. To calculate the patient's post-test probability of disease, the pretest probability is first converted to pretest odds as follows:

Pretest probability / (1 – pretest probability) = pretest odds
= 0.4/0.6 = 0.67

Because the nuclear stress test had a positive result, the pretest odds value is then multiplied by the test's positive likelihood ratio to obtain the post-test odds as follows:

Pretest odds × positive likelihood ratio = post-test odds = 0.67 × 5.0 = 3.35

The post-test odds is then used to calculate the post-test probability as follows:

Post-test odds / (post-test odds +1) = post-test probability = 3.35/4.35 = 0.77 or 77%

If the result of the nuclear stress test had been negative, the test's negative likelihood ratio would be used with the pretest odds to calculate the post-test probability of disease as follows:

0.67 × 0.1 = .067

.067 / 1.067 = .06 or 6%

KEY POINT

- Post-test probability is calculated from the patient's pretest probability of disease and the diagnostic test's likelihood ratio as follows: convert pretest probability to pretest odds (pretest probability / 1 – pretest probability); then multiply pretest odds by the likelihood ratio (positive if the test result is positive; negative, if negative) to obtain the post-test odds; then convert post-test odds to probability (post-test odds / post-test odds +1).

Bibliography

1. **Jaeschke R, Guyatt GH, Sackett DL.** Users' guides to the medical literature. III. How to use an article about a diagnostic test. B. What are the results and will they help me in caring for my patients? The Evidence-Based Medicine Working Group. JAMA. 1994;271:703-7. [PMID: 8309035]

Item 2   Answer: A

The most appropriate screening or preventive measure for this patient is abdominal ultrasonography. One-time screening for abdominal aortic aneurysm with ultrasonography is recommended for men ages 65 to 79 years who are, or have ever been, smokers. Data from randomized clinical trials indicate that ultrasound screening reduces abdominal aortic aneurysm–related mortality in older men with a smoking history. The U.S. Preventive Services Task Force makes no recommendation regarding screening for men who have never smoked because of insufficient evidence and recommends against screening for women because the harms outweigh the benefits.

All adults older than 50 years should be screened for adenomatous colon polyps, and removal of detected polyps significantly decreases the incidence of colorectal cancer. Colonoscopy every 10 years is a recommended screening technique. Some studies have found that colonoscopy is the most effective screening tool. Other recommended screening methods include annual fecal occult blood testing, flexible sigmoidoscopy every 5 years, annual fecal occult blood testing with flexible sigmoidoscopy every 5 years, and double-contrast barium enema examination every 5 to 10 years. This patient's most recent colonoscopy was 4 years ago, and therefore repeat screening is not indicated.

Routine screening for coronary artery disease in asymptomatic persons without cardiovascular risk factors is not recommended. Screening electrocardiograms are not recommended because abnormalities of the resting electrocardiogram are rare, not specific for coronary artery disease, and do not predict subsequent mortality from coronary disease. Because this patient has no cardiovascular risk factors other than his age, an electrocardiogram is not indicated.

The pneumococcal vaccine is associated with substantial reductions in morbidity and mortality among the elderly and high-risk adults and is therefore recommended for all adults age 65 years or older or with other risk factors (for example, asplenia). Patients who receive their initial vaccine at younger than 65 years should receive a second dose after 5 years. Because this patient was vaccinated at age 63 years, a second vaccination is not indicated at this time.

Booster tetanus and diphtheria vaccinations are recommended every 10 years; because this patient's vaccination is up to date, a repeat booster is not necessary at this time. If he were in the 19- to 64-year-old age range, the new tetanus, diphtheria, and acellular pertussis vaccine would be appropriate. A single dose of the new vaccine can replace a single dose of tetanus and diphtheria vaccine for active booster vaccination against tetanus, diphtheria, and pertussis.

KEY POINT

- One-time ultrasonographic screening for abdominal aortic aneurysm is recommended for men ages 65 to 79 years, if current or former smokers.

Bibliography

1. **U.S. Preventive Services Task Force.** Screening for abdominal aortic aneurysm: recommendation statement. Ann Intern Med. 2005;142:198-202. [PMID: 15684208]

Item 3   Answer: A

A careful examination should take approximately 3 minutes per breast. The duration of the examination correlates significantly with lump detection and accuracy in experimental models, which also has shown that the sensitivity of the examination increases, as does the number of proper techniques used.

Evidence supporting the role of careful inspection in breast cancer detection is lacking. Many physical examination textbooks recommend inspecting the patient's breasts while she is in various sitting positions, including arms at the side, arms above the head, hands pressed against the hips, and leaning forward to allow the breasts to hang from the chest wall. These maneuvers are performed to emphasize skin dimpling that may be associated with an underlying neoplasm. In one series of patients with breast cancer, 96% of cancers were discovered by palpation, 1% by skin retraction or dimpling, and 3% by visible nipple abnormalities. The study did not indicate whether special patient positioning was performed to elicit these signs. Based on these results, and because positioning the patient in three or four different positions takes time and has a relatively low yield of inspection, one authority has suggested that practitioners should concentrate on breast palpation as the primary means of cancer detection. During palpation, the practitioner can inspect the breasts for dimpling and nipple abnormalities.

The first step in the breast examination is to properly position the patient to spread the breast tissue over the chest wall. To examine the right breast, the patient should be shifted onto her left hip but with her shoulders rotated back to a supine position. Placing the right hand on the forehead completes the maneuver to flatten the lateral aspect of the breast. After examining the lateral right breast, asking the patient to resume a completely supine position and to move her right elbow level with her shoulder can flatten the medial portion of the breast. This process can be repeated for the left breast.

The breast examination should extend to an area bounded by the clavicles (top), midsternum and midaxillary line (sides),

and the inframammary fold or bra line (bottom). Palpation is best accomplished with the finger pads of the middle three fingers, using a small circular motion. At each spot, the examiner should palpate three times, using different pressures to detect potential lumps located at superficial, intermediate, and deep levels of breast tissue. The preferred search technique begins in the axilla and extends down the midaxillary line to the inframammary fold. Then, the examiner should palpate along a vertical line upward, just medially to the first downward search line, until the clavicle is reached. The up-and-down pattern is repeated with overlapping rows until the entire rectangular search area is palpated thoroughly. This technique has been found to result in a more thorough examination than a radial or circular search pattern. The supraclavicular and axillary regions are then palpated to detect lymphadenopathy. Isolated lymphadenopathy in association with a normal clinical breast examination is an unusual but important presentation of breast cancer.

KEY POINT

- A careful clinical breast examination should take approximately 3 minutes per breast and correlates significantly with lump detection and accuracy.

Bibliography

1. **Barton MB, Harris R, Fletcher SW.** The rational clinical examination. Does this patient have breast cancer? The screening clinical breast examination: should it be done? How? JAMA. 1999;282:1270-80. [PMID: 10517431]

Item 4   Answer: C

Based on current guidelines, the best intervention for this patient is screening for chlamydial infection. The Centers for Disease Control and Prevention recommend annual screening for sexually active women aged 24 years and younger and for other women at increased risk for *Chlamydia* infection (women with new or multiple sex partners, history or current symptoms of sexually transmitted disease, or history of unprotected intercourse). Age younger than 25 years is the strongest predictor of chlamydial infection in both men and women. Untreated chlamydial infection can lead to pelvic inflammatory disease (PID) and subsequent infertility. Randomized controlled trials have shown that routine screening for *Chlamydia trachomatis* prevents PID. In Sweden, screening has been associated with decreases in both gonorrheal and chlamydial infection rates and with a dramatic decline in PID.

Patients with high cumulative levels of sun exposure and those with prior skin cancers should be encouraged to wear sunscreen and protective clothing, although the benefit of sunscreen is unknown. A multivitamin with a folic acid supplement is recommended for pregnant women to prevent neural tube birth defects; it is unnecessary for this patient since she is not pregnant and has adequate birth control measures. A fasting blood glucose level is not recommended for routine screening in adults without risk factors for cardiovascular disease or type 2 diabetes mellitus.

- Annual chlamydial screening for sexually active women aged 24 years and younger and for other women at increased risk for *Chlamydia trachomatis* infection prevents pelvic inflammatory disease.

Bibliography

1. U.S. Preventive Services Task Force. Screening for chlamydial infection: U.S. Preventive Services Task Force recommendation statement. Ann Intern Med. 2007;147:128-34. Epub 2007 Jun 18. Summary for patients in: Ann Intern Med. 2007;147:I44. [PMID: 17576996]

Item 5   Answer: B

This person is at average risk for developing colorectal cancer because he is asymptomatic and has no personal or family history of colorectal neoplasia. Current guidelines recommend screening average-risk individuals beginning at age 50 years using any of the following studies: fecal occult blood testing annually, flexible sigmoidoscopy every 5 years, annual fecal occult blood testing plus flexible sigmoidoscopy every 5 years, barium enema examination every 5 years, or colonoscopy every 10 years. Of the options listed, the patient should undergo colonoscopy now and every 10 years thereafter.

Although fecal occult blood testing, flexible sigmoidoscopy, and barium enema examination may also be used for colorectal cancer screening, the time periods listed in the options are incorrect. Virtual colonoscopy (CT colonography) is a promising screening technique, but this study has not yet been incorporated into colorectal cancer screening guidelines.

- Recommended colorectal cancer screening studies for average-risk persons include fecal occult blood testing, flexible sigmoidoscopy, barium enema examination, and colonoscopy.

Bibliography

1. Pignone M, Rich M, Teutsch SM, Berg AO, Lohr KN. Screening for colorectal cancer in adults at average risk: a summary of the evidence for the U.S. Preventive Services Task Force. Ann Intern Med. 2002;137:132-41. [PMID: 12118972]

Item 6   Answer: A

This patient has a strong familial risk for colorectal cancer and should be screened with colonoscopy at this time. A strong familial risk is defined as having multiple first-degree relatives with colorectal cancer or a first-degree relative diagnosed with colon polyps or colon cancer at age 60 years or younger. For persons with a strong familial risk for colon cancer, the recommended screening strategy is colonoscopy every 5 years starting at age 40 years or at an age 10 years younger than the earliest diagnosis in the family. If a colonoscopy cannot be done in this patient, a double-contrast barium enema examination is the procedure of choice.

Patients with an average risk for colon cancer are screened beginning at the age of 50 years. Screening modalities for average-risk patients include annual fecal occult blood testing, flexible sigmoidoscopy every 5 years, annual fecal occult blood testing with flexible sigmoidoscopy every 5 years, colonoscopy every 10 years, or double-contrast barium enema examination every 5 to 10 years. Single-contrast barium enema examination is not sufficiently sensitive for colon cancer screening. In high-risk patients, sigmoidoscopy alone does not allow evaluation of the entire colon and is therefore inadequate. Carcinoembryonic antigen (CEA) is a tumor marker used for following response to treatment, but it is not sensitive or specific enough for screening. Also, CEA may be absent in poorly differentiated adenocarcinoma of the colon, and it may be present in other tumor types such as lung cancer. Virtual colonoscopy, using CT scanning or MRI with three-dimensional reconstruction, is not currently recommended for screening.

- For persons with strong familial risk for colon cancer, the recommended screening strategy is colonoscopy every 5 years starting at age 40 years or at an age 10 years younger than the earliest diagnosis in the family.

Bibliography

1. Smith RA, Cokkinides V, Eyre HJ; American Cancer Society. American Cancer Society guidelines for the early detection of cancer, 2003. CA Cancer J Clin. 2003;53:27-43. [PMID: 12568442]

Item 7   Answer: E

This patient with no apparent health problems requires no additional physical examination maneuvers. The value of the periodic health examination is unclear, and little evidence exists for its effectiveness as measured by important clinical outcomes such as morbidity and mortality. However, a recent review demonstrated that periodic evaluation provides better than usual care in the delivery of some recommended preventive services and may decrease patient worry. Conditions or lifestyle factors that do warrant periodic evaluation in all asymptomatic patients of appropriate age and sex include hypertension, hyperlipidemia, smoking, cervical cancer, breast cancer, colon cancer, and alcoholism. No other conditions or lifestyle factors have received general endorsement as targets for screening in asymptomatic individuals who do not have specific risk factors.

- Periodic health screening should be performed for hypertension; hyperlipidemia; cervical, breast, and colon cancer; smoking; and alcoholism in age- and sex-appropriate asymptomatic populations.

Bibliography

1. Boulware LE, Marinopoulos S, Phillips KA, Hwang CW, Maynor K, Merenstein D, Wilson RF, Barnes GJ, Bass EB, Powe NR, Daumit GL. Systematic review: the value of the periodic health evaluation. Ann Intern Med. 2007;146:289-300. [PMID: 17310053]

Item 8   Answer: A

A common reason for social isolation in the elderly is functional decrease in vision and/or hearing. Hearing and vision assessments are simple to conduct in the office and are helpful prior to performing assessments requiring the patient to respond to oral or written questions or prompts.

Elderly patients who take more than four prescription medications are at increased risk for falls and may need to receive fewer medications, but reducing medications at this time is unlikely to address this patient's current symptoms. Depression is a possible explanation for her increasing social isolation, but a score of less than 2 on the Five-Item Geriatric Depression Screen is considered a negative depression screening result and does not necessitate initiation of antidepressant therapy. Neuropsychologic testing may be indicated, but a clinical cognitive assessment could first be conducted in the office with a tool such as the Mini–Mental State Examination.

KEY POINT

- A common reason for social isolation in the elderly is functional decrease in vision and/or hearing.

Bibliography

1. Ensberg M, Gerstenlauer C. Incremental geriatric assessment. Prim Care. 2005;32:619-43. [PMID: 16140119]

Item 9   Answer: C

This patient should receive oseltamivir, which is active against both influenza A and B. In addition, all family members of an immunosuppressed patient should be immunized against influenza to decrease the patient's risk of exposure to this virus. Although chemoprophylaxis is not a substitute for vaccination, the Centers for Disease Control and Prevention recommend that it should be considered in those individuals at high risk and expected to have an inadequate response to vaccine. Chemoprophylaxis should be continued throughout the influenza epidemic because this patient is immunosuppressed and cannot respond to either live or inactivated vaccine.

Rimantadine is only active against influenza A and is no longer recommended by the Centers for Disease Control and Prevention as adequate prophylaxis against influenza because of the emergence of resistant influenza A virus strains. Because the patient is immunosuppressed, a live attenuated vaccine is contraindicated. Immune globulin will not provide protection against influenza A or B.

KEY POINTS

- Live attenuated influenza vaccine is contraindicated in an immunosuppressed patient.

- All family members of an immunosuppressed patient should be immunized against influenza to decrease the patient's risk of exposure to this virus.

Bibliography

1. Fiore AE, Shay DK, Haber P, Iskander JK, Uyeki TM, Mootrey G, Bresee JS, Cox NJ; Advisory Committee on Immunization Practices (ACIP), Centers for Disease Control and Prevention (CDC). Prevention and control of influenza. Recommendations of the Advisory Committee on Immunization Practices (ACIP), 2007. MMWR Recomm Rep. 2007;56(RR-6):1-54. [PMID: 17625497]

Item 10   Answer: A

The inactivated influenza vaccine is recommended for patients with chronic medical conditions, including heart failure, kidney disease, lung disease, diabetes mellitus, asthma, HIV/AIDS, and cancer, as well as for patients requiring chronic corticosteroid therapy. It is also recommended for infants 6 to 23 months old, persons 65 years or older, residents of long-term care facilities, women who will be pregnant during flu season, and household contacts or caretakers of infants and people at serious risk from influenza. The vaccine is provided as an intramuscular injection every fall.

Chronic warfarin therapy is not a contraindication to the inactivated influenza vaccine, but attention to strong compression at the injection site is warranted. In general, warfarin therapy does not complicate skin or dental procedures, lumbar punctures, or ophthalmologic interventions. A milk allergy is also not a contraindication to the inactivated influenza vaccine, but persons with an egg allergy should avoid the inactivated vaccine because it contains eggs.

The live intranasal formulation of the influenza vaccine is approved for persons aged 5 to 49 years, but should be avoided in persons over 50 years and in all those with chronic medical conditions. Although there has not been a head-to-head trial of the live intranasal formulation versus the inactivated influenza vaccine in chronically ill persons, animal models and immunologic studies are inconclusive about whether the formulations are equally effective. For now, the Centers for Disease Control and Prevention recommend limiting live intranasal vaccination to nonpregnant persons between 5 and 49 years who do not have a chronic medical condition.

Prevention of influenza with vaccination is more effective than treatment with neuraminidase inhibitors. If given within 48 hours of onset of symptoms, a 5-day course of neuraminidase inhibitors can decrease duration of symptoms by 1 day as compared with placebo. Cost-effectiveness studies support limiting use of neuraminidase inhibitors to those individuals most likely to have significant benefit from avoiding pneumonia or hospitalization, including unvaccinated individuals at high risk for complications or residents in a long-term care facility during an outbreak of influenza.

KEY POINT

- The inactivated influenza vaccine is recommended for patients with chronic medical conditions, including heart failure, kidney disease, lung disease, diabetes, asthma, HIV/AIDS, and cancer, as well as for patients requiring chronic corticosteroid therapy.

Bibliography

1. Fiore AE, Shay DK, Haber P, Iskander JK, Uyeki TM, Mootrey G, Bresee JS, Cox NJ; Advisory Committee on Immunization Practices (ACIP), Centers for Disease Control and Prevention (CDC). Prevention and control of influenza. Recommendations of the Advisory Committee on Immunization Practices (ACIP), 2007. MMWR Recomm Rep. 2007;56(RR-6):1-54. [PMID: 17625497]

Item 11 Answer: D

Screening for lung cancer is not indicated. Lung cancer is the most common cause of cancer death in women in the United States. However, lung cancer is uncommon at age 30 years, and smoking a few cigarettes is not an important lung cancer risk. Screening for lung cancer remains very controversial, but there is substantial evidence that screening with chest radiography or sputum cytology does not decrease lung cancer mortality in the screened population. Interest in screening has recently been reawakened by the advent of spiral CT scans that can detect tumors at an earlier stage. No test is currently recommended by the American Cancer Society, the American Thoracic Society, or the U.S. Preventive Services Task Force for lung cancer screening.

KEY POINT

- Screening for lung cancer with chest radiography or sputum cytology does not decrease lung cancer mortality in the screened population and is not indicated.

Bibliography

1. Mulshine JL, Sullivan DC. Clinical practice. Lung cancer screening. N Engl J Med. 2005;352:2714-20. [PMID: 15987920]

Item 12 Answer: E

In this woman with normal symptoms and signs of pregnancy, reassurance is appropriate. A basal systolic murmur is present in 80% of pregnant women owing to increased flow across the pulmonic and aortic valves. The resting heart rate increases by 20% to 30% during pregnancy, and an S_3 gallop is common because of increased early diastolic ventricular filling.

An echocardiogram is needed only if there are additional abnormal findings or if there is a history of cardiac disease. A 24-hour electrocardiographic monitoring study is not needed because occasional premature atrial and ventricular contractions (as described by this patient) are common and do not signify underlying cardiac disease. Most pregnant women develop mild dyspnea on exertion, and stress testing is not needed. Mild peripheral edema is common during pregnancy, and evaluation for deep venous thrombosis or pulmonary embolism is not needed unless unilateral lower extremity swelling or more typical symptoms of thrombosis or embolism are present.

KEY POINT

- A systolic murmur, an S_3 gallop, and mild peripheral edema are normal findings during pregnancy.

Bibliography

1. Mishra M, Chambers JB, Jackson G. Murmurs in pregnancy: an audit of echocardiography. BMJ. 1992;304:1413-4. [PMID: 1628016]

Item 13 Answer: E

This elderly patient has a benign midsystolic murmur that is grade 2/6 in intensity. In the absence of any cardiac symptoms, further diagnostic testing is not warranted. The most common cause of this type of murmur in persons older than 65 years is minor valvular abnormalities due to aortic sclerosis. Aortic sclerosis is characterized by focal areas of valve thickening leading to mild valvular turbulence, producing the murmur that is heard on auscultation. Aortic sclerosis is present in approximately 25% of persons between the ages of 65 and 74 years and in 48% of persons older than 84 years. A hyperdynamic circulation (e.g., from severe anemia, thyrotoxicosis, or pregnancy) may also produce an innocent midsystolic pulmonary or aortic flow murmur.

Transthoracic echocardiography is indicated when a grade 3/6 systolic murmur or greater is heard on examination, in the presence of any diastolic murmur, or if a new murmur is diagnosed in the interval since a normal previous physical examination. Midsystolic murmurs grade 2/6 intensity or less are considered benign (innocent) flow murmurs, especially when they are short in duration, heard best at the left sternal border, associated with a normal S_2, are not accompanied by any other abnormal cardiac sounds or murmurs, and do not change in intensity following a Valsalva maneuver. These murmurs fall into the low risk category for endocarditis prophylaxis and do not warrant routine antibiotic prophylaxis prior to dental procedures.

The role of electron-beam CT as a diagnostic tool is not clear, and current clinical guidelines do not advocate routine use of electron-beam CT as a screening tool to identify asymptomatic coronary artery disease. A screening cardiac stress test is not warranted in this asymptomatic patient. However, her treatable cardiovascular risk factors, hypertension and hyperlipidemia, should be addressed and managed according to current guideline recommendations. Continuous 24-hour ambulatory electrocardiographic monitoring is useful to identify the cardiac rhythm during symptoms of palpitations, syncope, or presyncope and can diagnose associated arrhythmias such as atrial fibrillation, supraventricular arrhythmias, or ventricular ectopy. However, this patient is asymptomatic from a cardiovascular standpoint, and such testing is not indicated.

KEY POINTS

- Midsystolic murmurs in the elderly are usually benign and due to minor, age-related changes of the aortic valve (aortic sclerosis).

- An echocardiogram is warranted in patients with cardiac symptoms, with systolic murmurs that are continuous or >3/6 in intensity, or when any diastolic murmur is present.

Bibliography
1. **Otto CM, Lind BK, Kitzman DW, Gersh BJ, Siscovick DS.** Association of aortic-valve sclerosis with cardiovascular mortality and morbidity in the elderly. N Engl J Med. 1999;341:142-7. [PMID: 10403851]

Item 14   Answer: D

To date, no cancer screening tool has been shown to decrease ovarian cancer mortality, whether in general or high-risk populations. Mathematical models predict that available screening tools would have at most a small benefit. Pending the outcome of randomized ovarian cancer screening trials, no organizations recommend routine screening for this disease in asymptomatic women, including the U.S. Preventive Services Task Force, which has concluded that routine screening could lead to important harms considering the infrequency with which the disease occurs and the invasiveness of the associated procedures and their potential for morbidity. They recommend that women with increased-risk family histories for developing *BRCA1* or *BRCA2* tumors be referred for genetic counseling and evaluation for *BRCA* testing. CA-125 measurement, transvaginal ultrasonography, and color Doppler imaging do not have adequate specificity to obviate their potential harms for routine use, except within the investigational setting. None of these tests is approved by the Food and Drug Administration for screening purposes.

KEY POINT

• The infrequency of ovarian cancer occurrence and invasiveness of the associated diagnostic procedures make routine ovarian cancer screening inappropriate.

Bibliography
1. **Jacobs IJ, Menon U.** Progress and challenges in screening for early detection of ovarian cancer. Mol Cellular Proteomics. 2004;3:355-66. [PMID: 14764655]

Item 15   Answer: E

This patient is asymptomatic and needs to be told the benefits and harms of prostate-specific antigen (PSA) testing before any other diagnostic tests are performed. Screening for prostate cancer continues to be controversial owing to the poor sensitivity and specificity of serum PSA testing. With a cutoff of 4 ng/mL, a single PSA assay has a sensitivity of 70% to 80% and a specificity of 60% to 70% for diagnosing prostate cancer. In asymptomatic patients, it has a positive predictive value of 30%, meaning that less than one in three men with an elevated PSA level actually has prostate cancer. Levels can be normal in the presence of prostate cancer or elevated without cancer present. There are age and racial differences in normal PSA values, although use of these values is not recommended for clinical use. The U.S. Preventive Services Task Force cites the level of evidence for screening with PSA as insufficient for determining whether the benefits outweigh the harms because of mixed and inconclusive evidence that early detection improves health outcomes. Screening is asso-

ciated with frequent false-positive results, unnecessary anxiety, risks of biopsies, and complications associated with the treatment of some cancers that may never have affected the patient's health.

Digital rectal examination is unreliable, because physicians have relatively low inter-rater agreement on findings. The combination of PSA assay and digital rectal examination provides an overall rate of cancer detection that is higher than either test alone. However, this strategy should be preceded by adequate discussion with the patient about its benefits and harms. Transrectal ultrasonography with biopsy is an invasive test used in the evaluation of an abnormal screening result, such as a palpable nodule or elevated or rising PSA level. Given its low sensitivity and low positive predictive value, it is a poor screening test and not feasible in most clinical practices.

KEY POINTS

• Asymptomatic patients need to be told the benefits and harms of prostate-specific antigen testing before any other diagnostic tests are performed.

• In patients with no symptoms of prostate disease, prostate-specific antigen testing has a positive predictive value of only 30%.

Bibliography
1. **Thompson IM, Ankerst DP.** Prostate-specific antigen in the early detection of prostate cancer. CMAJ. 2007;176:1853-8. [PMID: 17576986]

Item 16   Answer: C

True syncope is an abrupt, transient loss of consciousness due to global cerebral hypoperfusion without focal neurologic deficit and with spontaneous recovery. This patient experienced situational syncope, in which syncope is associated with a particular situation. It includes syncope associated with vagal stimulation, such as straining at micturition, defecation, cough, and, occasionally, swallowing, especially very cold liquids.

Vertebrobasilar transient ischemic attacks (TIAs) may cause transient loss of consciousness but usually involve focal neurologic deficits, such as hemianopsia or ataxia; carotid TIAs involve focal neurologic deficits without loss of consciousness. Carotid sinus syncope, which is also vagally mediated, is caused by pressure on the carotid sinus due to turning the head, a tight collar, shaving, a tumor, or vascular dissection. Prodromal aura, secondary incontinence, slowness in regaining full consciousness (>5 minutes), and postictal disorientation are characteristic of a generalized seizure, although syncope may be associated with brief prodromal nausea or sweating.

KEY POINT

• Situational syncope is associated with a particular situation and includes syncope associated with vagal stimulation, such as straining at micturition, defecation, cough, and, occasionally, swallowing, especially very cold liquids.

Bibliography
1. **Strickberger SA, Benson DW, Biaggioni I, Callans DJ, Cohen MI, Ellenbogen KA, Epstein AE, Friedman P, Goldberger J, Heidenreich PA, Klein GJ, Knight BP, Morillo CA, Myerburg RJ, Sila CA; American Heart Association Councils on Clinical Cardiology, Cardiovascular Nursing, Cardiovascular Disease in the Young, and Stroke; Quality of Care and Outcomes Research Interdisciplinary Working Group; American College of Cardiology Foundation; Heart Rhythm Society.** AHA/ACCF scientific statement on the evaluation of syncope: from the American Heart Association Councils on Clinical Cardiology, Cardiovascular Nursing, Cardiovascular Disease in the Young, and Stroke, and the Quality of Care and Outcomes Research Interdisciplinary Working Group; and the American College of Cardiology Foundation In Collaboration With the Heart Rhythm Society. J Am Coll Cardiol. 2006;47:473-84. [PMID: 16412888]

Item 17   Answer: B

This patient's clinical presentation and diagnostic findings are indicative of hypertrophic cardiomyopathy. Although most patients with hypertrophic cardiomyopathy are asymptomatic, symptoms of pulmonary congestion, chest pain, fatigue, palpitations, dizziness, and syncope may develop. In patients with hypertrophic cardiomyopathy, syncope sometimes results from left ventricular outflow tract obstruction, but in patients without such obstruction syncope may be caused by arrhythmias secondary to arrhythmogenic ventricular muscle. In this patient, an arrhythmogenic cause of syncope is likely because the event occurred with the patient sitting. Although the electrocardiogram shows evidence of left ventricular hypertrophy, the clinical absence of hypertension is not compatible with hypertensive cardiomyopathy. Hypertensive, dilated, and restrictive cardiomyopathy are not associated with a heart murmur that increases in intensity with the Valsalva maneuver and are therefore unlikely in this patient.

KEY POINT

• Hypertrophic cardiomyopathy is an important potential cause of syncope and is suspected in the presence of a systolic heart murmur that increases in intensity with the Valsalva maneuver.

Bibliography
1. **Nishimura RA, Holmes DR Jr.** Clinical practice. Hypertrophic obstructive cardiomyopathy. N Engl J Med. 2004;350:1320-7. [PMID: 15044643]

Item 18   Answer: E

This patient's syncopal episode is strongly suggestive of ventricular arrhythmia. Syncope of any cause is an ominous prognostic sign in patients with systolic heart failure, indicating high risk for sudden death. This patient's syncope was of sudden onset, with no or few prodromal or post-event symptoms (some patients have palpitations or signs or symptoms related to hypotension), and he has an underlying cardiac structural abnormality. A patient with a hemodynamically significant ventricular arrhythmia (i.e., causing syncope, near-syncope, or cardiac arrest) and left ventricular dysfunction should receive an implantable cardioverter-defibrillator.

This patient's symptoms (sudden-onset syncope, no history of syncope with exercise) do not suggest heart block, and this diagnosis is not supported by the electrocardiogram demonstrating normal sinus rhythm. Generalized seizure is an unlikely cause of the patient's syncope because of its brief duration and lack of postictal confusion following the event. Orthostatic hypotension is not supported by the history (patient was sitting at the onset) or by the physical examination that failed to demonstrate any changes in the vital signs with standing. Neurocardiogenic syncope is typically preceded by symptoms of lightheadedness, nausea, warmth, diaphoresis, or blurred vision. These presyncopal warning symptoms are highly sensitive for the diagnosis of neurocardiogenic syncope, and their absence makes the diagnosis unlikely.

KEY POINT

• Syncope in a patient with cardiomyopathy may be due to potentially fatal ventricular arrhythmia.

Bibliography
1. **Ezekowitz JA, Rowe BH, Dryden DM, Hooton N, Vandermeer B, Spooner C, McAlister FA.** Systematic review: implantable cardioverter defibrillators for adults with left ventricular systolic dysfunction. Ann Intern Med. 2007;147:251-62. [PMID: 17709759]

Item 19   Answer: E

This patient has neurocardiogenic syncope, and reassurance is the best management option. Neurocardiogenic syncope is characterized by a reflex withdrawal of sympathetic tone accompanied by an increase in vagal tone (vasovagal syncope), producing hypotension and bradycardia. When the increase in vagal tone does not occur, the bradycardia is absent, and the syncope is termed vasodepressor syncope. Venous pooling upon standing decreases ventricular filling, leading to a surge in sympathetic nerve activity. The sympathetic stimulation of the relatively empty ventricles results in excessive mechanical stimulation of vagal afferent C fibers and initiation of the reflex. The diagnosis of syncope is made principally by the patient's history and physical examination. In this patient, the description of feeling warm, sweaty, and woozy before loss of consciousness is consistent with neurocardiogenic syncope. In prospective studies of patients presenting to an emergency department with syncope, presyncopal warning symptoms of more than 10 seconds predicted neurocardiogenic syncope rather than a cardiac cause. Tilt-table testing has the highest sensitivity for diagnosing neurocardiogenic syncope and may be appropriate in some patients, particularly if the diagnosis is in doubt.

In the absence of trauma, a CT scan of the head has a low diagnostic utility and should not be performed to evaluate syncope. Duplex ultrasonography of the carotid arteries has no utility unless the patient had a concomitant transient ischemic attack; unilateral carotid artery disease does not cause syncope. In the absence of cardiac risk factors, structural heart disease, or syncope related to exertion, both exercise testing and echocardiography have low utility and are not indicated in this patient.

KEY POINT

• Presyncopal symptoms of warmth, diaphoresis, and lightheadedness are consistent with neurocardiogenic syncope.

Bibliography

1. **Brignole M.** Diagnosis and treatment of syncope. Heart. 2007;93:130-6. [PMID: 17170354]

Item 20   Answer: A

This patient most likely has bipolar disorder. Among young depressed adults, the presence of prior hypomanic symptoms is indicative of a bipolar disorder. Social and psychomotor hyperactivity are more frequent than increased disturbed mood. As in this patient, comorbid alcohol and substance abuse are widespread among patients with bipolar disorder. Another common characteristic is poor or deteriorated social role or occupational functioning. One study of patients with bipolar disorder found that a total of 62% reported moderate to severe impact of the illness on occupational functioning. Although a family history of affective disorders is absent in this patient, in one study almost two thirds of patients reported a family history of a mood disorder, and nearly half reported bipolar disorder in first-degree relatives.

The characteristics of a major depressive disorder include depressed mood most of the day nearly every day for at least 2 weeks; loss of all interest and pleasure; disturbances of appetite, weight, sleep, or activity; fatigue or loss of energy; self-reproach or inappropriate guilt; poor concentration or indecisiveness; morbid thoughts of death (not just fear of dying) or suicide; or all of these. Although this patient meets many of these clinical criteria, his episodes of hypomania and current episode of depression are more compatible with bipolar disorder than major depressive disorder.

Dysthymia is a chronic mood disorder characterized by depressed mood or anhedonia at least half the time for at least 2 years accompanied by two or more vegetative or psychological symptoms and functional impairment. The patient's 6-week course of depressed mood is not compatible with dysthymia, which also cannot account for his hypomanic episodes or substance abuse. Situational adjustment reaction with depressed mood is a subsyndromal depression with a clear precipitant; it usually resolves with resolution of the acute stressor without medication. The patient cannot identify a precipitating event for his altered mood, making this diagnosis unlikely. Seasonal affective disorder is a subtype of major depression, occurring with seasonal change, typically fall or winter onset and seasonal remission; rarely onset is in the spring with remission in the fall or winter. The disorder must have occurred in the two previous years without nonseasonal depression in order to make the diagnosis. Although the patient has had mood cycles, they have been separated by years, not months, making seasonal affective disorder unlikely.

KEY POINT

• Among young depressed adults, the presence of prior hypomanic symptoms is indicative of a bipolar disorder.

Bibliography

1. **Akiskal HS, Benazzi F.** Optimizing the detection of bipolar II disorder in outpatient private practice: toward a systematization of clinical diagnostic wisdom. J Clin Psychiatry. 2005;66:914-21. [PMID: 16013908]

Item 21   Answer: B

Depression can be a treatable cause of insomnia, and this patient has some risks for depression, including a recent divorce and other life stressors. Screening for depression is indicated prior to treatment of primary insomnia. The diagnosis of chronic insomnia can be established clinically. It is generally defined as a complaint of insufficient or inadequate sleep when one has the opportunity to sleep. The American Psychiatric Association Diagnostic and Statistical Manual 4th Edition (DSM-IV) defines primary insomnia as difficulty initiating or maintaining sleep or nonrestorative sleep for at least 1 month. The sleep disturbance must cause clinically significant distress or impairment of functioning and not be caused by another diagnosable sleep or mental disorder.

Polysomnography is needed only in patients with insomnia who have symptoms of a sleep-related breathing disorder, narcolepsy, or sleepwalking or who are employed as pilots or truck drivers. None of these criteria apply to this patient He does have risk factors for pulmonary disorders (smoking and being overweight) and cardiac disease (smoking, being overweight, sex, and age); however, he does not have symptoms or findings indicative of chronic obstructive pulmonary disease, obstructive sleep apnea, or coronary artery disease. Therefore, further evaluation of chronic obstructive pulmonary disease with spirometry or coronary artery disease with stress testing is not indicated. Sleep hygiene recommendations, including avoidance of strenuous exercise or alcohol within a few hours of bedtime, developing a relaxing evening routine, and avoidance of afternoon caffeine, are appropriate first steps in intervention once a diagnosis of primary insomnia is established.

KEY POINT

• Depression is a treatable underlying cause for insomnia.

Bibliography

1. **Silber MH**. Clinical practice. Chronic insomnia. N Engl J Med. 2005;353:803-10. [PMID: 16120860]

Item 22   Answer: E

This patient has a history of depression and a cognitive profile suggestive of primary impairment of concentration and attention, as opposed to memory. The most likely cause of the cognitive impairment is depression. Although degenerative conditions are possible, depression is most likely based upon his medical history and mental status examination and should be excluded before a more intense and costly work-up is undertaken.

Brain imaging in the setting of cognitive impairment is most useful for detecting evidence of cerebrovascular disease, disproportionate frontotemporal atrophy, or structural abnormalities such as hydrocephalus. This patient has no focal or abnormal neurological signs suggestive of these conditions.

Electroencephalography could be helpful if it showed slowing (suggesting a diffuse structural or metabolic process); this finding, however, is nonspecific. Electroencephalography would also be indicated if the patient had discrete episodes suggestive of complex partial seizures.

Positron emission tomography has very specific indications in the evaluation of memory and cognitive impairment, notably distinguishing between Alzheimer's disease and frontotemporal dementia in patients meeting criteria for both. This patient's cognitive profile, which does not include amnesia, is not consistent with dementia, and positron emission tomography is not indicated.

The assay for the presenilin-1 mutation is indicated for patients with dementia with presenile onset and/or a family history of presenile onset of dementia. This patient does not have a family history of dementia or a cognitive profile suggestive of dementia, and screening is not indicated.

KEY POINT

- Primary impairment of concentration and attention, as opposed to memory, is likely the result of depression rather than dementia.

Bibliography

1. **Barrett AM.** Is it Alzheimer's disease or something else? 10 disorders that may feature impaired memory and cognition. Postgrad Med. 2005;117:47-53. [PMID: 15948369]

Item 23   Answer: D

This patient has postpartum depression, and psychotherapy alone is an effective nonpharmacologic treatment. Prevalence studies estimate that up to 20% of women have a nonpsychotic major depression within the first 6 months after parturition. In addition to meeting criteria for major depressive disorder according to the American Psychiatric Association Diagnostic and Statistical Manual-IV (DSM-IV) guidelines, women with a postpartum depression may have predominant symptoms of anxiety and upsetting and unwanted thoughts of harming their infant. Because of the risks associated with untreated postpartum depression, non-drug treatments are a first-line choice for breastfeeding women who do not wish to take antidepressant medication because of concerns about exposure of the infant.

Pharmacotherapy with sertraline or paroxetine is equally beneficial, and because they are secreted less in breast milk, these drugs are the preferred agents in moderate to severe postpartum depression in breastfeeding mothers who require drug therapy. Fluoxetine is secreted in higher concentration in breast milk and is discouraged in this situation. Electroconvulsive therapy is reserved for situations warranting immediate change, for example, in patients who are profoundly suicidal or extremely malnourished. Exercise has not proven beneficial for treatment of depression.

KEY POINT

- Psychotherapy alone is an effective nonpharmacologic therapy for postpartum depression.

Bibliography

1. **Shaw E, Levitt C, Wong S, Kaczorowski J; The McMaster University Postpartum Research Group.** Systematic review of the literature on postpartum care: effectiveness of postpartum support to improve maternal parenting, mental health, quality of life, and physical health. Birth. 2006;33:210-20. [PMID: 16948721]

Item 24   Answer: A

Bupropion is the best treatment option for this patient because it has the least proclivity toward sexual dysfunction and does not cause weight gain. Anorgasmia is a common side effect of selective serotonin reuptake inhibitors (SSRIs), including citalopram and sertraline, and there is no good evidence suggesting one SSRI has fewer sexual side effects than another SSRI. Although mirtazapine is associated with fewer sexual side effects than are SSRIs, it stimulates the appetite, resulting in weight gain; therefore, although mirtazapine might be a good treatment choice in a thin patient with anorexia, it is not appropriate in this patient.

KEY POINTS

- Bupropion has the least proclivity toward sexual dysfunction and does not cause weight gain.

- Anorgasmia is a common side effect of all selective serotonin reuptake inhibitors (SSRIs).

Bibliography

1. **Kroenke K, West SL, Swindle R, Gilsenan A, Eckert GJ, Dolor R, et al**. Similar effectiveness of paroxetine, fluoxetine, and sertraline in primary care: a randomized trial. JAMA. 2001;286:2947-55. [PMID: 11743835]

Item 25   Answer: C

Patients who have an intent or plan for suicide are at the highest risk for actually committing suicide and should be hospitalized if they have poor social support, are intoxicated, are actively delusional, or are likely to be noncompliant with medication. If these features are absent and the patient is deemed able to make a contract for safety, outpatient therapy can proceed with psychiatry consultation and close follow-up. Electroconvulsive therapy is preferred in patients with severe depression who are psychotic or refractory to pharmacotherapy. In patients at high risk for suicide, multimodal inpatient treatment with addition of psychotherapy and changes in pharmacotherapy should be performed after hospitalization.

KEY POINT

• Patients who have identified a suicidal plan or intent are at the highest risk for committing suicide and should be hospitalized if they have poor social support, are intoxicated, are actively delusional, or if noncompliance is considered high.

Bibliography

1. **Hintikka U, Marttunen M, Pelkonen M, Laukkanen E, Viinamaki H, Lehtonen J.** Improvement in cognitive and psychosocial functioning and self image among adolescent inpatient suicide attempters. BMC Psychiatry. 2006;6:58. [PMID: 17196100]

Item 26   Answer: B

This patient's isolated alcohol-related incident in the context of a stable marital relationship and no other alcohol-associated problems necessitates assessment of the frequency and quantity of his alcohol intake. Such an assessment will help to determine his drinking patterns and whether he is at risk for hazardous drinking. Advising him to abstain from drinking or referring the patient to Alcoholics Anonymous would be premature before quantifying the amount and frequency of his drinking and establishing his level of alcohol abuse or dependence, if any. Similarly, although the CAGE questions have a sensitivity of 77% to 94% and a specificity of 79% to 97% for detecting alcohol abuse or dependence, they are not designed to detect hazardous drinking. Men younger than age 65 years who have more than 4 drinks on any given day or more than 14 drinks per week are considered hazardous drinkers. Women of any age and men older than age 65 years who have more than 3 drinks on any given day or more than 7 drinks per week are also considered hazardous drinkers. Once a patient reports this degree of alcohol intake, screening for abuse and dependence with the CAGE questionnaire is appropriate. If hazardous drinking is present, it is appropriate for the physician to encourage this patient to reduce his drinking by providing a clear, personalized message about the implications of his hazardous drinking patterns and the potential for alcohol-related problems.

KEY POINT

• Alcohol screening should not only focus on abuse and dependence but also on at-risk drinking patterns.

Bibliography

1. **Fiellin DA, Reid MC, O'Connor PG.** Outpatient management of patients with alcohol problems. Ann Intern Med. 2000;133:815-27. [PMID: 11085845]

Item 27   Answer: B

β-Blocker therapy is contraindicated in patients using cocaine. This patient shows the signs and symptoms that typically occur in patients who use cocaine: hypertension, tachycardia, and chest pain. Myocardial infarction is a well-known complication of cocaine use and may account for up to 25% of infarc-

tions in patients under the age of 45 years. Most infarctions occur within 3 hours of using cocaine, with the highest risk in the first hour, which is consistent with this patient's history. Cocaine's sympathomimetic actions are due to stimulation of both α- and β-adrenergic receptors. The use of β-blockers alone can result in unopposed α-receptor stimulation, further increasing vascular tone and worsening the cardiovascular effects. Combined α- and β-blocker therapy (i.e., labetalol) is both safe and effective for cocaine-induced myocardial ischemia. The patient should be hospitalized for further evaluation and treatment.

The use of aspirin is standard in the care of patients with acute coronary syndrome, including cocaine users, to prevent coronary artery thrombus formation. Both nitroglycerin and calcium channel blockers can be safely used to treat the hypertension and coronary artery vasospasm. The benzodiazepines are used to reduce blood pressure and heart rate and will help alleviate acute agitation and other effects of withdrawal from the cocaine.

KEY POINT

• The use of β-blockers alone to treat cocaine-induced myocardial ischemia can result in unopposed α-receptor stimulation, further increasing vascular tone and worsening the cardiovascular effects.

Bibliography

1. **Egred M, Davis GK.** Cocaine and the heart. Postgrad Med J. 2005;81:568-71. [PMID: 16143686]

Item 28   Answer: A

This patient most likely has ankylosing spondylitis, a systemic inflammatory disorder that most commonly occurs in men and primarily involves the spine and sacroiliac joints. Ankylosing spondylitis should be considered in the following : patients <40 years of age, patients with insidious onset of chronic low-back pain and stiffness of >3 months' duration; and those with low-back pain and stiffness that worsen at night or after prolonged rest or physical inactivity and are alleviated with physical activity or a hot shower. Within 6 to 12 months after disease onset, sacroiliac joint damage occurs and is manifested by narrowing and erosions, as seen on this patient's radiograph. The earliest finding is fuzziness and irregularity of the sacroiliac articular surface. Ankylosing spondylitis is later associated with subchondral sclerosis. These findings are first detected and are more marked on the iliac side of the joint. The erosion of the joint surface can cause erosions in and irregularity (serration) of the subchondral bone. The concomitant pseudo-widening of the joint space later leads to gradual joint space narrowing. The inflammatory process results in healing and bone formation that ultimately bring about fusion of the sacroiliac joints. Inflammatory changes also begin in the T12–L1 region of the spine and eventually lead to ossification of the outer fibers of the annulus fibrosis and the development of syndesmophytes. In the most severe cases of ankylosing spondylitis, "bamboo spine" develops, which is associated with soft tissue and bony changes that reflect this condition's inflammatory and calcifying nature.

Sacral fracture usually occurs in patients with osteoporosis and is triggered by seemingly minor episodes of trauma. Osteoarthritis of the spine or sacroiliac joints is common in older patients and is manifested by spur formation originating in the corners of the vertebrae and disk-space narrowing. In addition, pain in osteoarthritis, as well as mechanical back pain, is alleviated by a night of rest and worsens as the day progresses; conversely, low back pain in ankylosing spondylitis occurs because of inflammation and is therefore worse in the morning and is alleviated as the day progresses. Cancer of the spine or pelvis most often occurs in older patients because of metastatic disease and would be unusual in an otherwise healthy 22-year-old man. Furthermore, metastatic disease is associated with severe pain during the day and night. Imaging studies in this setting typically reveal lytic or blastic lesions.

KEY POINT

• Consider ankylosing spondylitis in patients <40 years with insidious onset of chronic low-back pain and stiffness of >3 months' duration and low-back pain and stiffness that worsen at night or after prolonged rest or physical inactivity.

Bibliography
1. Braun J, Sieper J. Ankylosing spondylitis. Lancet. 2007;369:1379-90. [PMID: 17448825]

Item 29   Answer: E

This patient should do well with symptomatic treatment alone. Most acute nonspecific pain resolves over time without the need for treatment, and controlling pain while symptoms diminish on their own is the goal for most persons. A patient with back pain but at low risk for serious disease by history and physical examination does not need anything other than simple analgesics and continued activity. Some patients may benefit from the addition of moist heat.

Strict bed rest is associated with prolongation of symptoms and higher morbidity. A systematic review of bed rest for low back pain and sciatica showed that advice to continue normal activities was more beneficial than bed rest. The need for obtaining plain radiographs of the spine can be determined on the basis of the history and physical examination. More sophisticated imaging is most useful when the pretest probability of underlying serious disease is high. Diagnostic imaging techniques are indicated in individuals with "red flags" for serious underlying disease, including fever, chills, weight loss, history of malignancy, injection drug use, trauma, or indolent course. Some authorities recommend radiographic imaging of patients >50 years of age with low back pain because of the increased incidence of malignancy, compression fractures, and spinal stenosis in this age group. Physical therapy is an appropriate adjuvant but is not an appropriate initial treatment. Clinical trial evidence has shown that beginning back exercises immediately actually delays recovery.

KEY POINTS

• Most acute nonspecific low back pain resolves over time without the need for treatment.

• Diagnostic imaging is indicated for individuals with "red flag" signs or symptoms for serious disease, including fever, chills, weight loss, history of malignancy, injection drug use, trauma, or indolent course.

Bibliography
1. Chou R, Qaseem A, Snow V, Casey D, Cross JT Jr, Shekelle P, Owens DK; Clinical Efficacy Assessment Subcommittee of the American College of Physicians; American College of Physicians; American Pain Society Low Back Pain Guidelines Panel. Diagnosis and treatment of low back pain: a joint clinical practice guideline from the American College of Physicians and the American Pain Society. Ann Intern Med. 2007;147:478-91. [PMID: 17909209]

Item 30   Answer: D

This patient has bilateral weakness and upper motor neuron signs in the legs, sensory loss below the T4 level, and sphincter dysfunction; there are no signs or symptoms of brain or brainstem dysfunction. These findings are consistent with a spinal cord process. Given her history of breast cancer, metastatic spinal cord compression from an epidural metastasis is most likely and represents a neurologic emergency that must be excluded by urgent imaging. Although the distribution of pain and the sensory level suggest that the lesion is at the thoracic level, MRI of her entire spine is most appropriate because sensory levels can be unreliable for localizing the site of an epidural tumor. In addition, patients with a metastatic epidural tumor can have multiple sites of disease in the spine. MRI gives excellent images of both the spinal cord and the vertebrae, whereas CT does not adequately show the substance of the spinal cord and epidural region, making MRI the modality of choice in this patient.

CT scan of the lumbar spine is not an appropriate imaging choice in this patient. Because the spinal cord ends at around the L1 vertebral body, the spinal cord would not be visualized if imaging of the lumbar spine alone is performed. Plain radiographs of the spine can visualize some bony metastases and fractures but are not sensitive for the site of cord compression and do not image the spinal cord. Electromyography and nerve conduction studies are helpful in diagnosing peripheral nerve and muscle diseases but have no role in the evaluation of spinal cord disorders. MRI of the brain may be needed to assess for asymptomatic brain metastases but is not as urgent as spine imaging.

KEY POINT

• Spinal cord compression due to epidural metastasis is a neurologic emergency for which urgent MRI of the entire spine is appropriate.

Bibliography
1. Winters ME, Kluetz P, Zilberstein J. Back pain emergencies. Med Clin North Am. 2006;90:505-23. [PMID: 16473102]

Item 31   Answer: D

The patient has acute sciatica with likely L5–S1 nerve-root involvement. Symptomatic, nonsurgical treatment with non-steroidal anti-inflammatory drugs (NSAIDs) is appropriate initial management because she has no evidence of spinal cord compression or cauda equina syndrome. Controlled trials demonstrate that NSAIDs provide effective short-term symptomatic relief for patients with acute low back pain with or without sciatica. Narcotic analgesics should be reserved for patients with severe pain and prescribed for only a limited time. Spinal manipulation, physical therapy, and muscle relaxants also demonstrate modest benefit in treating patients with acute back pain.

Surgical intervention should be considered only if symptoms persist for more than 6 weeks or she develops progressive neurologic deficits. Two or 3 days of bed rest may be appropriate for patients with severe pain and disability. Available evidence shows no difference in pain relief or functional status between bed rest and symptom-limited activity for patients with sciatica, although activity is more beneficial for patients without sciatica. Prolonged bed rest (≥7 days) can lead to cardiovascular deconditioning, bone demineralization, and increased subsequent absenteeism from work. MRI of the lumbar spine early in the course of low back pain is not helpful because the false-positive rate is high. Patients undergoing early MRI are more likely to undergo surgery—and incur higher health care costs—than patients evaluated with only plain radiography, but clinical outcomes are similar for both groups. However, routine plain films are appropriate in patients older than 50 years because they are at increased risk for malignancy and osteoporotic fractures and also in patients who have sustained trauma or have signs of an infection.

KEY POINTS

- Nonsteroidal anti-inflammatory drugs provide effective short-term symptom relief for patients with acute low back pain with or without sciatica.
- Surgical intervention should be considered for patients with low back pain only if symptoms persist for more than 6 weeks or if progressive neurologic deficits develop.

Bibliography
1. **Koes BW, van Tulder MW, Thomas S**. Diagnosis and treatment of low back pain. BMJ. 2006;332:1430-4. [PMID: 16777886]

Item 32   Answer: D

Although this patient is at high risk for peripheral vascular disease, he has the classic symptoms of spinal stenosis (pseudoclaudication): pain upon standing that also occurs with walking and is relieved with sitting or bending forward and a normal ankle-brachial index. Leg ischemia/claudication pain would not occur with simple standing, but would rather be progressive with walking or exercise, and the ankle-brachial index is often <0.9 and associated with a 20% or greater decline with exercise. The abdominal bruit increases suspicion for an abdominal aortic aneurysm (or renal artery stenosis) for which this patient is at increased risk, but physical examination in this thin man does not suggest an abdominal aortic aneurysm, and his buttock/extremity pain with rising and walking would not be attributable to this condition.

KEY POINTS

- Spinal stenosis is characterized by pain with standing or walking that is relieved by sitting or bending forward and is further supported by a normal ankle-brachial index.
- Leg ischemia is characterized by pain with exertion and with an ankle-brachial index <0.9 that decreases at least 20% with exercise.

Bibliography
1. **Hazard RG.** Low-back and neck pain diagnosis and treatment. Am J Phys Med Rehabil. 2007;86:S59-68. [PMID: 17370372]

Item 33   Answer: C

The most likely diagnosis in this patient is allergic rhinitis with associated bronchospasm; therefore, treatment with oral antihistamine and nasal corticosteroids is appropriate. In addition, inhaled β-agonists are also appropriate in this patient, as they appear beneficial in patients with wheezing or airflow limitation with end-expiratory wheezes.

Antibiotics are not indicated for allergic rhinitis or viral upper respiratory tract infection. Although the patient has yellowish sputum, the absence of fever, chills, and progressive illness argues against a current bacterial infection. Nasal decongestants may be of some symptomatic benefit, but direct treatment of the underlying allergic disorder with a nasal corticosteroid and an oral antihistamine is the indicated treatment. In general, antitussives or cough suppressants are indicated only for cough that is painful, causes sleep disruption, or is debilitating in frail, elderly patients. Recent systematic reviews concluded that no antitussive is clearly superior to another for cough in adults, and elderly patients are most vulnerable to adverse effects of antitussive agents, such as confusion, nausea, and constipation.

KEY POINTS

- Inhaled β-agonists for acute cough appear beneficial in patients with wheezing or airflow limitation with end-expiratory wheezes on examination.
- Antibiotics are not indicated for allergic rhinitis or viral upper respiratory tract infection.

Bibliography
1. **Bahls C.** In the clinic. Allergic rhinitis. Ann Intern Med. 2007;146:ITC4-1-ITC4-16. [PMID: 17404348]

Item 34   Answer: D

This patient should be encouraged to quit smoking once again, which is the only way to reduce his risk for lung cancer. No evidence-based screening interventions for lung cancer exist; therefore, participation by this patient in a lung cancer screening program cannot be recommended. Effective screening must detect cancer or pre-cancerous lesions early, and their therapy must be more effective than treatment of cancer or pre-cancerous lesions found at the usual time of diagnosis.

Most studies of spiral CT scanning for lung cancer screening have generally only recruited current and former cigarette smokers and detected earlier-stage cancers, but have not demonstrated decreased lung cancer mortality, although randomized trials are ongoing. Likewise, a decrease in lung cancer mortality has not been found in randomized studies of patients who were screened with chest radiography and sputum cytology. A randomized controlled trial of chest radiography and sputum cytology found that although these screening methods could detect early-stage lung cancer that is not potentially significantly lethal, they did not have an effect on lung cancer mortality. In a Japanese cohort study of spiral CT for lung cancer in smokers and never-smokers, the rates of lung cancer detected by spiral CT were similar in both groups, also suggesting the possibility of over-diagnosis.

KEY POINT

- Lung cancer screening does not decrease mortality and is not supported by evidence.

Bibliography
1. Mulshine JL, Sullivan DC. Clinical practice. Lung cancer screening. N Engl J Med. 2005;352:2714-20. [PMID: 15987920]

Item 35   Answer: E

Smoking cessation is the most important intervention in patients with peripheral vascular disease and may reduce the progression of disease. Although β-blockade may inhibit peripheral vasodilatation and thereby be detrimental to peripheral blood flow, clinical studies demonstrate no adverse effect on peripheral vascular disease. Therefore, atenolol does not need to be discontinued. Warfarin is relatively contraindicated because of increased bleeding risk without added benefit compared with aspirin. Cilostazol, a phosphodiesterase inhibitor, suppresses platelet aggregation and is a direct arterial vasodilator. Cilostazol is associated with increased maximal and pain-free walking distances, but there is no evidence that it improves limb salvage rates. Phosphodiesterase inhibitors have been associated with increased mortality in patients with heart failure and are therefore contraindicated in this patient. Although exercise training is beneficial in improving symptoms, its long-term benefits are inferior to smoking cessation.

KEY POINT

- Smoking cessation is the single most effective intervention for patients with peripheral vascular disease.

Bibliography
1. Sontheimer DL. Peripheral vascular disease: diagnosis and treatment. Am Fam Physician. 2006;73:1971-6. [PMID: 16770929]

Item 36   Answer: B

This patient's recurrent upper respiratory tract symptoms and cigarette-smoking history necessitate a smoking-cessation intervention consisting of a clear, personalized message provided by the physician during this visit. Brief interventions lasting as little as 1 to 3 minutes have been shown to result in an increase in the number of patients who quit and abstain from cigarette smoking at 1 year. Clinicians can use the 5As model (Ask, Advise, Assess, Assist, and Arrange) to frame such an intervention, providing a message that 1) summarizes the clinical findings, 2) expresses a concern that these recurrent symptoms relate to cigarette smoking, 3) strongly recommends smoking cessation, and 4) offers support in achieving this goal.

Although nicotine replacement therapy, bupropion, and behavioral therapy are appropriate adjunct interventions for smoking cessation, using these approaches would be premature before first determining the patient's readiness for behavioral change and outlining a more comprehensive plan for smoking cessation.

KEY POINTS

- Brief interventions are associated with a significant increase in the number of patients who quit and abstain from smoking at 1 year.
- Advising a patient to stop smoking through a clear, personalized message is an important component of a brief intervention.

Bibliography
1. NIH State-of-the-Science Panel. National Institutes of Health State-of-the-Science conference statement: tobacco use: prevention, cessation, and control. Ann Intern Med. 2006;145:839-44. [PMID: 16954353]

Item 37   Answer: B

This patient is overweight, and the most appropriate initial management step is diet and exercise. Obesity affects more than 30% of Americans and is the second leading cause of preventable deaths. BMI should be calculated at each visit [(BMI = weight (kg)/height (m^2)]. A BMI of 18.5 to 24.9 is normal for most people; overweight is 25 to 29; and obesity is 30 or greater. BMI is correlated with risks associated with obesity and excess body fat, such as diabetes mellitus, heart disease, osteoarthritis, gallbladder disease, gastroesophageal reflux disease, and certain types of cancer.

Patients identified as overweight or obese are assessed for obesity-associated conditions such as hypertension, metabolic syndrome, endocrinopathies, and, if appropriate, reproductive disorders such as polycystic ovary syndrome. In all patients with a BMI greater than 25, a fasting blood glucose, serum creatinine, and lipid profile (HDL cholesterol, triglycerides, and LDL cholesterol) should be determined to assess comorbidities. A sleep study may be indicated to evaluate possible sleep apnea in patients with somnolence, facial plethora, or a history of snoring. Patients with a high BMI and/or increased central adiposity should be helped to develop a plan to prevent further weight gain and ultimately reduce body weight. Initial steps include addressing modifiable risk factors for obesity and setting goals for gradual, sustainable weight loss. A reasonable goal is to lose 10% of body weight, an amount associated with significant risk reduction. Rates for weight loss vary, but 0.5 to 1 lb (0.2 to 0.45 kg) per week is a reasonable goal. Weight loss can be achieved through alterations in both diet and exercise.

When lifestyle treatments are ineffective or the patient is unable to lose excess weight, drug therapy may be helpful. Drug therapy is generally considered only for patients with a BMI of 30 or greater, or 27 or greater with comorbidities. Drug therapy is generally tried before surgical intervention. Sibutramine, which is an appetite suppressant, and orlistat, which blocks lipase and fat absorption in the intestine, are drugs that produce dose-related weight loss. Surgical treatment should be consider for patients with a BMI of at least 35 with comorbidities (as above) or a BMI of at least 40 without comorbidities in whom attempts at weight loss, including drug therapy, were unsuccessful.

KEY POINTS

- Initial treatment for overweight patients includes diet and exercise.

- Drug therapy for weight loss is considered for patients with a BMI ≥30 or ≥27 with comorbidities.

- Surgical treatment for weight loss is considered for patients with a BMI ≥35 with comorbidities or ≥40 without comorbidities in whom attempts at weight loss, including drug therapy, were unsuccessful.

Bibliography

1. Snow V, Barry P, Fitterman N, Qaseem A, Weiss K; Clinical Efficacy Assessment Subcommittee of the American College of Physicians. Pharmacologic and surgical management of obesity in primary care: a clinical practice guideline from the American College of Physicians. Ann Intern Med. 2005;142:525-31. Summary for patients in: Ann Intern Med. 20055;142:I55. [PMID: 15809464]

Item 38 Answer: C

Surgery is recommended as a treatment option for patients with class III obesity, defined as those who have a BMI of ≥40, have been unable to maintain weight loss with exercise and diet with or without drug therapy, and have obesity-related comorbid conditions, such as hypertension, impaired glucose tolerance, diabetes mellitus, hyperlipidemia, and obstructive sleep apnea. This patient meets these criteria. Gastric bypass surgery has proven efficacy in weight loss, with one meta-analysis demonstrating a 61% loss of excess weight. More recent studies have demonstrated decreased overall

mortality following bariatric surgery. Other benefits of gastric bypass surgery include improved social and economic status and improved control of chronic diseases. Patients considering gastric bypass surgery should receive counseling about the long-term side effects of this procedure, including the possibility for re-operation, gallbladder disease, and malabsorption. In addition, surgical risks include a 30-day postoperative mortality rate of 2%.

The effects of sibutramine and orlistat are significantly more modest than gastric bypass surgery, resulting in a <5-kg (11-lb) weight loss at 1 year in clinical trials. Low-carbohydrate and fat-restricted diets have limited evidence to support long-term efficacy and safety.

KEY POINT

- Surgery is a recommended treatment option for patients with class III obesity, defined as those with a BMI of ≥40 who cannot maintain weight loss with exercise and diet with or without drug therapy and who have obesity-related comorbid conditions.

Bibliography

1. Snow V, Barry P, Fitterman N, Qaseem A, Weiss K; Clinical Efficacy Assessment Subcommittee of the American College of Physicians. Pharmacologic and surgical management of obesity in primary care: a clinical practice guideline from the American College of Physicians. Ann Intern Med. 2005;142:525-31. [PMID: 15809464]

Item 39 Answer: C

Orlistat, a lipase inhibitor that increases fecal fat loss, would be an appropriate treatment for this patient to aid in her attempts at modest weight loss. Orlistat is approved by the Food and Drug Administration for weight loss in obese patients, and meta-analysis has demonstrated a mean weight loss of 2.8 kg (6.3 lb) at 12 months. Side effects of orlistat are related to malabsorption of fat in the gastrointestinal tract and include steatorrhea, bloating, and oily discharge.

In addition to lipase inhibitors, medications for weight loss consist of appetite suppressants. Sibutramine is an appetite suppressant that works through combined norepinephrine and serotonin reuptake inhibition. The side effects include a modest increase in heart rate and blood pressure, nervousness, dry mouth, headache, and insomnia. A meta-analysis of sibutramine reported a mean difference in weight loss of 4.4 kg (9.8 lb) at 12 months compared with placebo groups. Sibutramine is not recommended for patients with poorly controlled hypertension. Mirtazapine is a tetracyclic atypical antidepressant medication that has some serotonin 5-HT$_2$ and 5-HT$_3$ receptor antagonist properties. Although there is some evidence to support the use of the selective serotonin reuptake inhibitor fluoxetine in achieving modest weight loss, mirtazapine is associated with weight gain and increased appetite and is not an appropriate pharmacologic treatment for obesity. Surgery is recommended as a treatment option for patients with class III obesity, defined as patients who have a BMI of ≥40, have been unable to maintain weight loss with exercise and diet with or without drug therapy, and have obesity-related comorbid conditions, such as hypertension, impaired glucose tolerance, diabetes mellitus, hyperlipidemia, and obstructive sleep apnea. This patient does not meet these criteria.

KEY POINTS

- Orlistat is associated with a mean weight loss of 2.8 kg (6.3 lb) at 12 months.

- Sibutramine is not recommended for weight loss in patients with poorly controlled hypertension.

Bibliography

1. Li Z, Maglione M, Tu W, Mojica W, Arterburn D, Shugarman LR, et al. Meta-analysis: pharmacologic treatment of obesity. Ann Intern Med. 2005;142:532-46. [PMID: 15809465]

Item 40   Answer: D

Causes of unexplained weight loss in the elderly include depression, cancer, benign gastrointestinal conditions, medication toxicities, cognitive difficulties, and socioeconomic concerns. Elderly patients may be at nutritional risk because of difficulties with grocery shopping, meal preparation, or social isolation. In this case, the patient has difficulty grocery shopping, and the reasons for this must be explored. Arranging for assistance in shopping and/or meal preparation would an appropriate intervention.

The most common malignancies characterized by weight loss in the elderly are lung and gastrointestinal malignancies. Because this patient's physical examination, laboratory studies, and recent fecal occult blood test and chest radiograph were normal, no further workup for malignancy, including CT scan of the abdomen or colonoscopy, is required at this time. Depression can cause weight loss in the elderly, but this patient takes antidepressant medication, states that her mood is good, and has a low score on the Five-Item Geriatric Depression Scale, indicating a negative depression screening result; only patients with scores of 2 or more (of a possible 5) require further evaluation for depression. Therefore, a change in antidepressant medication is not indicated. Benign gastrointestinal problems such as gastroesophageal reflux are common causes of weight loss in the elderly, but this patient has no abdominal symptoms and takes ibuprofen only intermittently. Therefore, it is not necessary to discontinue this drug at this time.

KEY POINTS

- Causes of unexplained weight loss in the elderly include depression, cancer, benign gastrointestinal conditions, medication toxicities, and socioeconomic concerns.

- The most common malignancies characterized by weight loss in the elderly are lung and gastrointestinal malignancies.

Bibliography

1. Ensberg M, Gerstenlauer C. Incremental geriatric assessment. Prim Care. 2005;32:619-43. [PMID: 16140119]

Item 41   Answer: C

This patient should be screened for a major depressive disorder. Her history of depression, depressed mood, and tearfulness suggest a major depressive disorder. Depression accounts for 9% to 15% of all cases of involuntary weight loss and is the most common psychiatric cause. Depression is also the second most common chronic disorder in primary care medicine. Screening for depression is the first step in the diagnosis of mood disorders in all adults. There is little evidence to recommend one screening method over another, so physicians can choose the method that best suits their patient population and practice setting. Once screening verifies the clinical impression of depression, treatment should be prescribed.

Initial diagnostic testing for the evaluation of involuntary weight loss is limited to basic studies unless the history and physical examination suggest a specific cause. Occult malignancy is uncommon, and imaging of the thorax and abdomen for cancer in the absence of specific historical information or physical examination findings has not been shown to help determine the cause of involuntary weight loss. Beginning an appetite stimulant does not address the cause of the weight loss and is not indicated. Reassurance is not reasonable for a patient with a likely major mood disorder that requires treatment.

KEY POINTS

- Depression accounts for 9% to 15% of all cases of involuntary weight loss and is the most common psychiatric cause of involuntary weight loss.

- Imaging with CT or MRI scanning in the absence of historical information or physical examination findings suggesting disorders of the thorax or abdomen has not been shown to help determine the cause of involuntary weight loss.

Bibliography

1. Reife CM. Involuntary weight loss. Med Clin North Am. 1995;79:299-313. [PMID: 7877392]

Item 42   Answer: D

Because this patient is experiencing significant symptoms of hot flushes and is interested in rapid and effective treatment, she can benefit from short-term hormone replacement therapy after a discussion of its risks and benefits. The effectiveness of hormone replacement therapy to improve menopause-related vasomotor symptoms is clearly documented in studies that confirm a reduction of 6 to 22 hot flushes per week. The Food and Drug Administration recommends using the smallest effective dose of hormone replacement therapy for the shortest duration possible to treat menopausal symptoms only. Estrogen can be given orally or via a transdermal patch with progestin in women with an intact uterus to reduce the risk for endometrial cancer. Low-dose therapy that can reduce hot flushes includes conjugated equine estrogen (0.3 mg), estradiol (0.5 mg), and transdermal estradiol (2.5 µg).

Although the antidepressants venlafaxine, paroxetine, and fluoxetine have been shown to be helpful, tricyclic antidepressants such as imipramine are not effective treatment for hot flushes. Cognitive behavioral therapy may be helpful to this patient for other reasons, but no evidence supports its use to resolve hot flushes. The botanical agent red clover has been commercially promoted as a treatment for reducing hot flushes, but studies do not support its effectiveness.

There is no clear benefit of one estrogen product over another. Atypical vaginal bleeding and breast tenderness are the most common adverse effects of hormone replacement therapy. Contraindications to estrogen use include undiagnosed vaginal bleeding, breast cancer, other estrogen-sensitive cancers, current or previous history of venous or arterial thrombosis, or liver dysfunction or disease. With long-term use, the Women's Health Initiative studies indicate estrogen therapy is associated with an increased risk for breast cancer, coronary artery disease, stroke, venous thromboembolism, dementia and cognitive decline, and urinary incontinence. Quality-of-life measures are not clinically improved by hormone use.

KEY POINT

- The Food and Drug Administration recommends using the smallest effective dose of hormone replacement therapy for the shortest duration possible to treat menopausal symptoms only.

Bibliography
1. **Roberts H**. Managing the menopause. BMJ. 2007;334:736-41. [PMID: 17413174]

Item 43   Answer: D

The patient's irregular menstrual bleeding interspersed with amenorrhea, obesity, and signs of hyperandrogenism are consistent with a diagnosis of polycystic ovary syndrome (PCOS). It is the most common cause of irregular menstrual bleeding in premenopausal patients. The early onset of symptoms is the most important part of the history for differentiating PCOS from other causes of anovulatory menstrual irregularities. Most girls develop regular menses within 1 year of menarche, and failure to do so suggests the diagnosis of PCOS. If symptoms begin years after puberty or have suddenly worsened, other causes must be considered. Diagnosis requires two of following three criteria: ovulatory dysfunction, laboratory or clinical evidence of hyperandrogenism, and ultrasound evidence of polycystic ovaries. Signs of ovulatory dysfunction include amenorrhea, oligomenorrhea, and infertility. Typical signs of androgen excess include hirsutism, acne, and occasionally alopecia. Laboratory abnormalities in PCOS may include a ratio of luteinizing hormone to follicle-stimulating hormone (LH/FSH) >2 and mild elevations in serum testosterone and dehydroepiandrosterone sulfate (DHEAS)

levels; these findings, however, are not diagnostic. Insulin resistance is an important feature, as is obesity, although only 50% of affected women are obese.

Hypothyroidism can cause irregular menstrual cycles and often periods of heavy bleeding. Cold intolerance is common, as is coarsening of hair and nails. Physical examination may reveal an enlarged thyroid gland and often delayed reflexes. Signs of hyperandrogenism are not present. Cushing's syndrome is often associated with both hyperandrogenism and amenorrhea but is also typically associated with hypertension, wide purple abdominal striae, and easy bruising. Affected patients frequently have central obesity, and physical examination may reveal a prominent dorsal cervical fat pad. It is important to exclude Cushing's syndrome when a diagnosis of PCOS is being considered, but onset of Cushing's syndrome during adolescence is rare. Hyperprolactinemia is a frequent cause of amenorrhea that is often associated with medications such as tricyclic antidepressants, phenothiazines, and metoclopramide. Pituitary tumors or tumors that compress the pituitary stalk may also lead to hyperprolactinemia, often with associated visual changes and headache. Obesity and signs of androgen excess are typically absent. Uterine fibroids are a common cause of irregular and often heavy menstrual bleeding. Depending on size and location, they can often be palpated on physical examination. They are not associated with oligomenorrhea, amenorrhea, or signs of androgen excess.

KEY POINTS

- Polycystic ovary syndrome should be considered in the differential diagnosis of patients with oligomenorrhea, amenorrhea, and abnormal uterine bleeding.

- Diagnostic criteria for polycystic ovary syndrome include ovulatory dysfunction, laboratory or clinical evidence of androgen excess, and polycystic ovaries on ultrasonography.

Bibliography
1. **Ehrmann DA**. Polycystic ovary syndrome. N Engl J Med. 2005;352:1223-36. [PMID: 15788499]

Item 44   Answer: D

This patient's skin examination findings are consistent with moderate-to-severe inflammatory acne. The combination of a topical comedolytic agent (a retinoid) and a topical antibiotic has not been effective. The next step in management would be concomitant use of an oral antibiotic with a topical antibiotic. Oral antibiotics, particularly in the tetracycline group, are effective and relatively safe for treating moderate-to-severe acne. Oral antibiotic treatment generally requires 6 to 8 weeks before efficacy can be determined, but consensus is lacking on the appropriate length of oral antibiotic treatment courses. Prolonged use of topical or oral antibiotics can lead to bacterial resistance.

Combined oral contraceptives can be used as a treatment for women with acne; ethinyl estradiol and norgestimate (Ortho Tri-Cyclen®) and ethinyl estradiol and norethindrone (Estrostep®) are approved by the Food and Drug Administration (FDA) for this indication. Discontinuing oral contraceptives would not improve, and may worsen, acne. Oral isotretinoin is FDA approved only for recalcitrant nodular acne and is associated with an 80% remission rate. However, this agent is also frequently associated with mucocutaneous side effects and teratogenicity. Physicians who prescribe isotretinoin must have evidence of a recent negative pregnancy test, provide counseling regarding pregnancy prevention, and obtain informed patient consent. Oral isotretinoin has also been linked with depression, suicidal ideation, suicide attempts, and suicide, but there is no clear causal relationship between these events and isotretinoin. A rare adverse effect of oral isotretinoin is acne fulminans, which requires treatment with systemic corticosteroids. Oral corticosteroids are not a treatment for, and may cause, acne.

KEY POINTS

- Oral antibiotics, particularly in the tetracycline group, are efficacious and relatively safe for treating moderate-to-severe acne.
- Oral isotretinoin is Food and Drug Administration approved only for treating recalcitrant nodular acne and is associated with an 80% remission rate.

Bibliography
1. Purdy S, de Berker D. Acne. BMJ. 2006;333:949-53. [PMID: 17082546]

Item 45   Answer: D

This patient has mild, comedonal acne with an absence of inflammatory lesions. For comedonal-only acne, topical retinoids are the mainstay of treatment. Retinoids are derivatives of vitamin A and prevent comedone formation by normalizing desquamation of follicular epithelium. Topical retinoid therapies may be combined with other topical agents, including antibiotics or keratolytic agents, but there is no evidence that combined-agent topical therapy is better than single-agent topical therapy for treating comedonal-only acne. Combined-agent therapy with a topical antibiotic may be helpful if there are inflammatory lesions (pustules) in addition to comedonal lesions.

There is no evidence that avoidance of certain foods, including fried foods or chocolate, will prevent or treat acne. Oral corticosteroids are not a treatment for, and may cause, acne. Oral antibiotics are indicated for moderate-to-severe inflammatory acne and are not required in this patient. Topical isotretinoin is not teratogenic. In contrast, oral isotretinoin is teratogenic and requires registration in a Food and Drug Administration iPLEDGE program by prescribing physicians. The iPLEDGE program requires a recent negative pregnancy test, counseling regarding pregnancy prevention, and informed patient consent.

KEY POINT

- For comedonal-only acne, topical retinoids are the mainstay of treatment.

Bibliography
1. Rao S, Malik MA, Wilder L, Mott T. Clinical inquiries. What is the best treatment for mild to moderate acne? J Fam Pract. 2006;55:994-6. [PMID: 17090362]

Item 46   Answer: A

This patient has recurrent aphthous ulcers. Aphthous ulcers are painful lesions that are localized, shallow, and round, often with a whitish appearance. They are among the most common ulcers in persons in North America. Recurrent aphthous ulcers usually begin to occur in the teenage years and recur intermittently, and their cause is unknown.

Behçet's disease is a connective-tissue disease characterized by recurrent oral and genital ulcers. Although patients with recurrent aphthous ulcers are healthy, patients with Behçet's disease have other systemic manifestations, including genital aphthae, ocular disease, skin lesions, neurologic disease, vascular disease, or arthritis. HIV infection can also cause recurrent, often severe, aphthous ulcers, but the patient's recent negative HIV test and absence of other symptoms make this diagnosis unlikely. Patients with oropharyngeal candidiasis often describe a "cottony" sensation in the mouth, loss of taste, and, occasionally, pain induced by eating and swallowing, symptoms not present in this patient. Herpes simplex virus (HSV) labialis infection (cold sores, fever blisters) in an immunocompetent patient is usually a self-limited disease that lasts for 7 to 10 days; recurrent lesions tend to occur on the lips at the vermilion border, not inside the mouth.

KEY POINT

- Recurrent aphthous ulcers usually begin to occur in the teenage years and recur intermittently, and their cause is unknown.

Bibliography
1. Scully C. Clinical practice. Aphthous ulceration. N Engl J Med. 2006;355:165-72. [PMID: 16837680]

Item 47   Answer: A

This patient has atopic dermatitis, most commonly associated with a rash in the creases of the skin and on the hands. Atopic dermatitis is an allergic disorder with genetic and immunologic components characterized by intense itching, leading to excoriation, lichenification (epidermal thickening), hyperpigmentation, and papulosquamous eruptions. Acute eruptions are often accompanied by erythema, vesiculation, and oozing. The criteria for the diagnosis of atopic dermatitis include evidence of itchy skin plus three or more of the following: 1) involvement of the skin creases, including areas around the neck or eyes, elbows, knees, and ankles; 2) history of asthma or hay fever; 3) history of dry skin during the past year; 4) onset in a child younger than 2 years of age; and 5) visible dermatitis of skin flexures.

Contact dermatitis is precipitated by local absorption of an allergen or irritant through the stratum corneum. The location of the eruptions may help to identify the causative agents (e.g., neck rash due to necklace). Acute eruptions are characterized by erythema, edema, and vesiculation. The configuration of the rash is often geometric (e.g., linear, localized polygons) and is rarely diffuse unless there is a corresponding id reaction (generalization of the rash caused by an immunologic mechanism). Seborrheic dermatitis is characterized by erythematous plaques with a dry or oily scale occurring in hair-bearing parts of the body, including the scalp, eyelashes, eyebrows, beard, chest, external ear canal, and behind the ear. Cellulitis is an acute eruption that is characterized by a well-demarcated area of warmth, swelling, tenderness, and erythema. It is not associated with vesicles or pruritus.

KEY POINT

- Atopic dermatitis is an allergic disorder with genetic and immunologic components characterized by intense itching, leading to excoriation, lichenification (epidermal thickening), hyperpigmentation, and papulosquamous eruptions.

Bibliography

1. **Boguniewicz M, Schmid-Grendelmeier P, Leung DY.** Atopic dermatitis. J Allergy Clin Immunol. 2006;118:40-3. Epub 2006 Jun 6. [PMID: 16815136]

Item 48   Answer: A

The patient most likely has contact dermatitis, as he has no systemic signs of infection such as fever, leukocytosis, or malaise. The pruritic rash with erythema and vesicles with minimal tenderness are typical of contact dermatitis, although impetigo and some dermatophyte infections are also possible. Eosinophilia may be present but is not a necessary component of contact dermatitis. The patient's rash was presumably due to hypersensitivity to his deodorant.

Staphylococcal, streptococcal, and *Pasteurella multocida* cellulitis are highly unlikely because there are no signs or symptoms of acute bacterial infection, no signs of spreading, and no lymphadenopathy. In addition, the rash is symmetrical bilaterally (which is an unusual distribution for cellulitis) and is accompanied by pruritus (which is not commonly associated with cellulitis).

KEY POINT

- Noninfectious skin lesions are not associated with fever and other systemic signs and symptoms or abnormal laboratory studies.

Bibliography

1. **Falagas ME, Vergidis PI.** Narrative review: diseases that masquerade as infectious cellulitis. Ann Intern Med. 2005;142:47-55. [PMID: 15630108]

Item 49   Answer: A

This patient has poison ivy contact dermatitis. Severe poison ivy dermatitis, including cases with extensive involvement and edema, can be treated with oral prednisone, tapering the dosage slowly over 2 to 3 weeks. No studies support length of treatment with oral corticosteroids. However, clinical experience has shown that rapid tapering often results in rebound dermatitis.

Although high-potency topical corticosteroids may reduce the erythema that sometimes surrounds vesicles, this treatment is not recommended on the face, neck, or intertriginous areas, where corticosteroid-induced atrophy is more likely to occur. When these areas are involved with blisters, topical treatment is ineffective and oral treatment is more appropriate. Furthermore, the practical concern of applying topical medication to a large body surface area must be considered; this is often difficult for the patient to manage and consumes large quantities of the topical product. Pimecrolimus is a biologic response modifier that is used as a second-line topical treatment for atopic dermatitis and certain other forms of eczema; treatment of poison ivy dermatitis with pimecrolimus is not helpful. Topical mupirocin is an antibacterial agent and is an appropriate treatment for superficial bacterial infections such as impetigo. There is no evidence that this patient's skin is infected (absence of crusting); therefore, topical antibiotics are not indicated.

KEY POINT

- Severe cases of contact dermatitis, including those with extensive involvement and associated edema, can be treated with oral prednisone.

Bibliography

1. **Mark BJ, Slavin RG.** Allergic contact dermatitis. Med Clin North Am. 2006;90:169-85. [PMID: 16310529]

Item 50   Answer: B

This patient's skin lesions are characteristic of erythema nodosum, consisting of painful, erythematous nodules on the anterior surfaces of both legs that evolve into bruise-like lesions that resolve in several weeks. The nodules are more easily palpated than visualized. An acute presentation of erythema nodosum accompanied by arthritis or periarthritis of the ankle raises high clinical suspicion for acute sarcoidosis. These features, accompanied by fever and hilar lymphadenopathy, strongly suggest the diagnosis of Löfgren's syndrome, which is a variant of sarcoidosis. Lymphomas, fungal or streptococcal infections, inflammatory bowel disease, and some medications, including estrogen, may cause erythema nodosum. Lymphoma rarely causes acute erythema nodosum and concomitant arthritis. Histoplasmosis may mimic this acute sarcoidosis presentation in endemic areas.

Psoriasis consists of well-demarcated, symmetrically distributed, erythematous plaques affecting extensor surfaces with an overlying silvery scale. Psoriatic arthritis has multiple presentations, including monoarthritis, oligoarthritis (asymmetric), polyarthritis (symmetric), arthritis mutilans, and axial disease. The key to the diagnosis is often the presence of skin and nail changes consistent with psoriasis, which are absent in this patient.

The rash of systemic lupus erythematosus is a photosensitivity rash most commonly involving the face in a central malar pattern that spares the nasolabial folds and the areas beneath the nose and lower lip. Discoid lupus is characterized by sharply demarcated violaceous atrophic plaques with adherent scale with telangiectasias and follicular plugging. Chronic lesions produce scarring and alopecia. The arthritis associated with systemic lupus erythematosus symmetrically affects small joints of the hands, wrists and knees and is not found in this patient.

The finding of acute, nontraumatic, monoarticular arthritis, particularly in a sexually active young woman, should always prompt consideration of disseminated gonorrhea infection. However, the rash of disseminated gonorrhea classically consists of tender necrotic pustules on an erythematous base (usually <30 lesions), especially on the distal extremities, rather than the deep nodules seen in this patient. The arthritis typically involves the wrists, metacarpophalangeal joints, ankles, and knees most commonly, but any joint may be affected.

KEY POINT
- The skin lesions of erythema nodosum consist of painful, erythematous nodules on the anterior surfaces of both legs.

Bibliography
1. **Schwartz RA, Nervi SJ.** Erythema nodosum: a sign of systemic disease. Am Fam Physician. 2007;75:695-700. [PMID: 17375516]

Item 51   Answer: A

This patient has herpes zoster (shingles), which occurs with increasing frequency as people age, and should be treated with famciclovir. The most common distribution is a unilateral rash in a dermatomal distribution in the thoracic region. Famciclovir has replaced acyclovir as the treatment of choice for patients with herpes zoster because of its superior pharmacokinetics, simplified dosing schedule, and improved efficacy. Although not listed, valacyclovir would be an acceptable alternative agent. Based on reports from controlled clinical trials, both drugs are effective when initiated within 72 hours of disease onset. Antiviral therapy can be considered optional for younger patients with mild pain and limited cutaneous involvement because these patients are at relatively low risk for developing severe or protracted pain. Consider prescribing a course of antiviral therapy in elderly patients with severe pain and large areas of cutaneous involvement, even when these patients present more than 72 hours after lesion onset. Despite lack of evidence, many experts prescribe antiviral therapy for patients presenting more than 72 hours after rash onset with continued new vesicle formation or when there are cutaneous,

motor, neurologic, or ocular complications. The effectiveness of therapy begun after 72 hours is not known.

Topical antiviral therapy with penciclovir is not recommended for patients with herpes zoster because of lack of efficacy. Ganciclovir and valganciclovir are most frequently used to treat cytomegalovirus infections in immunocompromised patients. These drugs have not been evaluated for the treatment of herpes zoster and their side-effect profiles make them much less desirable than famciclovir, valacyclovir, or acyclovir.

KEY POINTS
- The most common distribution of herpes zoster (shingles) is a unilateral rash in the thoracic region.
- Famciclovir and valacyclovir are the treatments of choice for patients with herpes zoster.

Bibliography
1. **Wareham DW, Breuer J.** Herpes zoster. BMJ. 2007;334:1211-5. [PMID: 17556477]

Item 52   Answer: B

This patient may have onychomycosis. Obtaining cultures to confirm an infection is recommended before treatment because thickened and dystrophic nails can be caused by other conditions, such as psoriasis, peripheral vascular disease, lichen planus, or atopic dermatitis. It is best to culture the nail bed debris from the most proximal part of the infection. Treatment of onychomycosis is recommended for patients with peripheral vascular disease, diabetes mellitus, or other conditions that increase the risk of morbidity. Onychomycosis may also require treatment when it is a risk factor for recurrent cellulitis. A case–control study indicated that patients evaluated for cellulitis of the leg were more likely to have onychomycosis and tinea infections of the feet than the control population.

Besides terbinafine, additional approved oral treatments for onychomycosis include griseofulvin and itraconazole. Ciclopirox is a topical lacquer that is also approved for treatment of onychomycosis. The cure rate is low, and recurrence after discontinuation of treatment is common. However, topical treatment is recommended as initial therapy when superficial invasion of the nailbed is noted without nail thickening. Although nail débridement helps relieve pressure that footwear exerts on toes, this intervention does not provide a diagnosis or cure onychomycosis.

KEY POINT
- It is best to confirm the presence of an infection with a culture of debris under the nail in patients with suspected onychomycosis to rule out other conditions.

Bibliography
1. **Roberts DT, Taylor WD, Boyle J.** Guidelines for treatment of onychomycosis. Br J Dermatol. 2003;148:402-10. [PMID: 12653730]

Item 53   Answer: D

The diagnosis of psoriasis is established primarily based on clinical presentation. The most common form of psoriasis is plaque psoriasis, which occurs in more than 80% of patients. The skin lesions of this disorder are sharply demarcated erythematous plaques covered by silvery-white scales that affect the scalp and extensor surfaces (elbows and knees) as well as nails. Inverse psoriasis is characterized by the presence of lesions in flexural sites, such as the axillae and antecubital fossae. Guttate psoriasis is manifested by the sudden development of erythematous scaling papules on the trunk and extremities, usually affecting children and young adults, and often developing after infection with β-hemolytic streptococci. Erythrodermic psoriasis is characterized by generalized inflammation, erythema, and widespread scaling of the skin, affecting up to 100% of the body surface. Generalized pustular psoriasis of von Zumbusch is characterized by sterile pustules over large portions of the trunk. Erythrodermic psoriasis and generalized pustular psoriasis are rare and severe variants of psoriasis in which the skin can lose its protective function, causing susceptibility to infection and sepsis. Patients receiving systemic corticosteroids or cyclosporine are at risk for acute erythrodermic or pustular psoriasis flares following sudden cessation of medication.

Eczema is characterized by erythematous papules and plaques that lack a silvery scale and in the acute stage may be vesicular and weeping. Chronic lesions, especially on the hands and feet, may be lichenified and hyperkeratotic (difficult to distinguish from psoriasis). Eczema usually involves the flexures, whereas plaque psoriasis involves the extensor surfaces. Eczema is usually more pruritic than psoriasis. A dermatophyte infection presents with solitary or many erythematous lesions with central clearing and peripheral scale. Occasionally, deep inflammatory nodules may be present.

Subacute cutaneous lupus erythematosus (SCLE) involves predominantly sun-exposed areas, particularly the face and upper chest. SCLE lesions begin as small, red, minimally scaly papules that evolve into either a psoriasis-like rash or a round (annular) lesion. Annular lesions tend to coalesce to form larger polygonal lesions. Psoriasis improves with sun exposure, whereas lupus worsens.

Pityriasis rosea begins 1 to 2 weeks after a vague "viral" episode, presenting as a single "ringworm-like" patch on the trunk (known as the "herald patch"). Smaller lesions with collarettes of scale follow over a few days. The lesions are most commonly on the trunk and follow skin cleavage lines. Epidemics of this viral exanthem (human herpesvirus 6) occur in the spring and fall. Pityriasis rosea is usually a self-limiting, nonrecurring disease that lasts 8 to 12 weeks and requires therapy with topical cortisones and antihistamines. Rarely, phototherapy may be required if lesions are pruritic.

- The most common form of psoriasis, plaque psoriasis, is characterized by sharply demarcated erythematous plaques covered by silvery-white scales that affect the scalp and extensor surfaces as well as the nails.

Bibliography

1. **Luba KM, Stulberg DL.** Chronic plaque psoriasis. Am Fam Physician. 2006;73:636-44. [PMID: 16506705]

Item 54   Answer: C

This patient has rosacea, an inflammatory dermatitis characterized by erythema, telangiectasias, papules, pustules, and sebaceous hyperplasia that develops on the central face, including the nasolabial folds. Rhinophyma, or the presence of a bulbous, red nose, is a variant of this condition.

Dermatomyositis may be associated with various skin manifestations. Periungual erythema and malar erythema, consisting of a light purple (heliotrope) edematous discoloration of the upper eyelids and periorbital tissues, are the most common presentations. Dermatomyositis also may cause an erythematous, papular eruption that develops in a V-shaped pattern along the neck and upper torso; in a shawl-shaped pattern along the upper arms; and on the elbows, knees, ankles, and other sun-exposed areas. Involvement of the hands may include scaly, slightly raised purplish papules and plaques that develop in periarticular areas of the metacarpal and interphalangeal joints and other bony prominences (Gottron's sign) and scaly, rough, dry, darkened, cracked horizontal lines on the palmar and lateral aspects of the fingers (mechanic's hands).

Systemic lupus erythematosus may be excluded because the malar rash associated with this condition is often photosensitive and spares the nasolabial folds and the areas below the nares and lower lip (areas relatively protected from the sun). Rosacea is therefore an important finding when trying to establish a differential diagnosis of systemic lupus erythematosus. Frequently, patients may have a positive antinuclear antibody assay for reasons other than systemic lupus erythematosus. This patient's antinuclear antibody positivity is most likely associated with her thyroid disorder.

Psoriasis usually involves the scalp, elbows, or other areas but does not typically manifest as an isolated facial rash. Characteristic findings of psoriasis include an erythematous plaque with an adherent, variably thick, silvery scale. Seborrheic dermatitis causes white, scaling macules and papules that are sharply demarcated on yellowish-red skin and may be greasy or dry. Sticky crusts and fissures often develop behind the ears, and significant dandruff or scaling of the scalp frequently occurs. Seborrheic dermatitis may develop in a "butterfly"-shaped pattern but also may involve the nasolabial folds, eyebrows, and forehead. This condition usually improves during the summer and worsens in the fall and winter.

- The malar rash of systemic lupus erythematosus is often photosensitive and spares the nasolabial folds and areas below the nares and lower lip.

- Rosacea is an inflammatory dermatitis characterized by erythema, telangiectasias, papules, pustules, and sebaceous hyperplasia that affects the central face, including the nasolabial folds.

Bibliography
1. **Powell FC.** Clinical practice. Rosacea. N Engl J Med. 2005;352:793-803. [PMID: 15728812]

Item 55   Answer: C

This patient likely has scabies, an infestation of the parasitic mite *Sarcoptes scabiei* var *hominis*, and requires treatment with topical permethrin. Sudden onset of pruritus, severe enough to interrupt sleep, in a patient with papules and excoriations on the hands (especially finger webs), feet, and areolae is consistent with scabies. Burrows, which may occur on the hands as 3- to 5-mm thread-like lines, are pathognomonic of scabies but occur in fewer than 20% of cases. Scabies occurs most commonly in school children, nursing-home residents, and institutionalized patients. Scabies is usually transmitted by close physical contact with an infested person, such as hand-holding or sharing a bed, or by fomites. The patient's recent visit to a nursing home is the likely source of infection.

Skin biopsy may be useful if the diagnosis of scabies is not apparent clinically. The yield of biopsy is high only if the specimen is taken from a burrow. Epiluminescence light microscopy is another diagnostic technique that permits visualization of the mites in the skin but is not readily available in practice.

Patients with scabies are usually treated with topical permethrin 5% applied from head to toe for 8 to 14 hours (overnight) with a second application in 1 to 2 weeks. Topical 1% lindane can also be used for treatment but is more toxic. Asymptomatic household contacts should be treated with one application of topical permethrin.

Oral ivermectin may be used safely in patients who fail to respond to initial treatment with topical permethrin. Topical corticosteroids such as triamcinolone are helpful in some patients for symptomatic management of pruritus but will not eradicate the underlying infection and are not first-line therapy. Topical bacitracin is a polypeptide antibiotic active mainly against gram-positive bacteria. Bacitracin most commonly is used topically to prevent superficial skin and eye infections after minor injuries. The clinical presentation of pruritic papules in the finger webs and around the areolae is not consistent with a bacterial infection, and a topical antibiotic is not indicted for this patient.

- The earliest and most common symptom of scabies is itching, particularly at night.

- Scabies is usually transmitted by close physical contact such as hand-holding or sharing of a bed or by fomites that have been in contact with infested persons.

Bibliography
1. **Chouela E, Abeldano A, Pellerano G, Hernandez MI.** Diagnosis and treatment of scabies: a practical guide. Am J Clin Dermatol. 2002;3:9-18. [PMID: 11817965]

Item 56   Answer: D

This patient has tinea versicolor, otherwise known as pityriasis versicolor. This is a superficial mycotic (or fungal) infection of young and middle-aged adults caused by the lipophilic yeast *Malassezia furfur*. The infection is usually noticed because involved areas do not tan, and there is resulting hypopigmentation. There is also a hyperpigmented form of tinea versicolor. In patients with tinea versicolor, large, blunt hyphae and thick-walled budding spores in a "spaghetti and meatballs" pattern are evident on examination of scale with 10% potassium hydroxide. Topical ketoconazole cream or shampoo is an effective therapy for these patients. Ketoconazole is also effective as a systemic treatment.

Tinea corporis ("ringworm") involves the face, trunk, and extremities, and the size of the lesions and degree of inflammation can vary. It typically presents as an annular lesion with an active advancing border of scale and occasionally with small vesicles. Segmented, branched dermatophyte hyphae are characteristically found with 10% potassium hydroxide examination of the scale, and this finding is distinctly different from the "spaghetti and meatballs" pattern associated with tinea versicolor. Pityriasis rosea is the most important differential diagnosis of tinea corporis. Pityriasis rosea begins 1 to 2 weeks after a vague "viral" episode, presenting as a single "ringworm-like" patch on the trunk (herald patch). Smaller lesions with collarettes of scale follow over a few days. The lesions are most commonly on the trunk and follow skin cleavage lines. Unlike tinea corporis, pityriasis rosea does not have an active advancing edge or central clearing and does not exhibit hyphae on potassium hydroxide examination of the scale. The skin lesions of plaque psoriasis, the most common form of psoriasis, are sharply demarcated erythematous plaques covered by silvery-white scales that affect the scalp and extensor surfaces (elbows and knees) as well as the nails.

- In patients with tinea versicolor, large, blunt hyphae and thick-walled budding spores in a "spaghetti and meatballs" pattern are evident on examination of scale with 10% potassium hydroxide.

- Topical ketoconazole cream is an effective therapy for patients with tinea versicolor.

Bibliography

1. **Schwartz RA**. Superficial fungal infections. Lancet. 2004;364:1173-82. [PMID: 15451228]

Item 57   Answer: B

Simple topical formulations containing salicylic acid appear to be effective and safe for treating common warts. This patient's wart is responding to the treatment, indicating that it should continue. Six to 12 weeks of therapy may be necessary to completely eradicate the wart. Reassurance that the treatment is working is indicated.

No clear evidence has shown that cryotherapy is more effective than topical salicylic acid therapy. This patient has a periungual wart, which can be quite resistant to therapy, especially if it is under a fingernail. Periungual cryotherapy should be used with extreme caution because of possible complications, including matrix destruction and nail distortion. Other treatments that have not been approved by the Food and Drug Administration may be considered for resistant and recurrent warts, including topical imiquimod and intralesional injection of mumps or *Candida* antigens. In small open-label studies, these treatments have resulted in 70% to 80% cure rates. These treatments would not be appropriate for this patient at this time because salicylic acid therapy is reducing the size and pain of the common wart.

KEY POINT

- Simple topical treatment containing salicylic acid is an effective and safe initial therapy for common warts.

Bibliography

1. **Micali G, Dall'Oglio F, Nasca MR, Tedeschi A**. Management of cutaneous warts: an evidence-based approach. Am J Clin Dermatol. 2004;5:311-7. [PMID: 15554732]

Item 58   Answer: D

The most helpful screening test for this patient is the Instrumental Activities of Daily Living (IADL). Geriatric functional assessment can help to identify and address previously unrecognized problems to improve quality of life in older persons. The Katz Index of Activities of Daily Living (ADL) and the Barthel Index are functional assessment tools that assess basic ADLs, such as toileting, bathing, eating, and dressing. Patients who need help with basic ADLs are unlikely to be able to live alone safely. This patient seems to be managing these activities well both by history and clinical observation; therefore, screening with ADL is not likely to be helpful in discovering functional impairment. The Lawton & Brody Instrumental Activities of Daily Living (IADL) Scale assesses functions, such as using the telephone, checkbook, or shopping. Patients who have loss of independence for performing IADLs may have significant cognitive or physical illnesses that require further evaluation. This patient has acknowledged deficiencies in these areas, and further investigation is appropriate to learn the extent and nature of the difficulties and to help plan treatment and/or assistance.

Delirium in older persons is manifested by lethargy and decreased response to stimuli. Criteria for the diagnosis of delirium include a disturbance of consciousness or change in cognition that develops over a short period (hours or days) and often fluctuates during the course of a day. Assessment for delirium in the hospital setting can be done with the Confusion Assessment Method; however, this patient has no manifestations of delirium and this screening test is not indicated. Depression can be assessed by asking a single screening question: "Do you often feel sad or depressed?" The sensitivity and specificity of this screening method are 85% and 65%, respectively. The Five-Item Geriatric Depression Scale can be administered to patients who respond positively to this question. The Geriatric Depression Scale has a positive predictive value of 85% and a negative predictive value of 97% for the diagnosis of depression. Since this patient denies feeling sad or depressed, further screening with the Geriatric Depression Scale is not indicated.

KEY POINT

- Patients who have loss of independence for performing Instrumental Activities of Daily Living (IADL) may have significant cognitive or physical illnesses that require further evaluation.

Bibliography

1. **Sherman FT**. Functional assessment. Easy-to-use screening tools speed initial office work-up. Geriatrics. 2001;56:36-40.[PMID: 11505859]

Item 59   Answer: B

This patient has coarctation of the aorta based upon the findings of systemic hypertension together with reduced and delayed pulses in the lower extremities compared with the upper extremities (radial-femoral pulse delay). An ejection click and an aortic systolic murmur suggest the presence of a bicuspid aortic valve, which is present in more than 50% of persons with aortic coarctation. A systolic murmur over the left posterior chest may be related to the gradient through a narrowed coarctation segment or collateral vessels. The chest radiograph suggests a "figure 3 sign" denoting dilatation of the aorta both above and below the area of coarctation. Rib notching is also apparent on the chest radiograph. Notching of the posterior one-third of the upper ribs is due to erosion by the large collateral arteries formed as a result of increased resistance to flow through the aorta. All of these features are consistent with severe coarctation of the aorta.

Although a systolic murmur would be expected in patients with a small ventricular septal defect, an atrial septal defect, or mitral valve regurgitation, neither the ejection click, the radial-femoral pulse delay, nor the radiographic features seen in this patient would be expected. A patent ductus arteriosus causes a continuous murmur without an ejection click, and the pulse delay would not be expected.

- Hypertension and a radial-femoral pulse delay are characteristic physical findings in coarctation of the aorta.

Bibliography
1. **Aboulhosn J, Child JS** Left ventricular outflow obstruction: subaortic stenosis, bicuspid aortic valve, supravalvar aortic stenosis, and coarctation of the aorta. Circulation. 2006;114:2412-22. [PMID: 17130357]

Item 60   Answer: A

This patient should be started on an angiotensin receptor blocker (ARB). Inhibition of the renin–angiotensin axis has been shown to be effective in reducing proteinuria and preserving renal function in patients with diabetes mellitus. Angiotensin-converting enzyme (ACE) inhibitors and ARBs have both been shown to have benefit. However, this patient developed a cough on an ACE inhibitor. Since there are robust data supporting the use of an ARB in patients with type 2 diabetes mellitus and since cough is a far less common side effect with these agents, adding an ARB at this time is the most appropriate choice in this patient.

β-Adrenergic blockers may be indicated for patients with coronary artery disease but do not have a known beneficial effect on renal function in these patients. Good blood glucose control has beneficial renal effects in patients with diabetes, but in a patient whose glycemic control is good, the addition of insulin or a thiazolidinedione has not been shown to be as effective as ACE inhibitor or ARB therapy in reducing proteinuria. Similarly, aggressive LDL cholesterol lowering has beneficial cardiovascular effects and may also have beneficial renal effects, but adding a statin in this patient would not be expected to affect renal function as potently as would ARB therapy.

- Inhibition of the renin–angiotensin axis with an angiotensin-converting enzyme inhibitor or angiotensin receptor blocker reduces proteinuria and preserves renal function in patients with diabetes mellitus.

Bibliography
1. **Marshall SM, Flyvbjerg A.** Prevention and early detection of vascular complications of diabetes. BMJ. 2006;333:475-80. [PMID: 16946335]

Item 61   Answer: D

Use of thiazide diuretics (but not loop diuretics) has been associated with mild hypercalcemia. Cessation of thiazide therapy reverses the hypercalcemia in many patients, although it may persist in some patients. Thiazide diuretics stimulate renal tubular calcium reabsorption, a finding that has led to their use in the treatment of "renal leak" hypercalciuria and hypoparathyroidism. However, the kidney is not likely to be the only organ involved in thiazide-mediated hypercalcemia because hypercalcemia may develop in anephric patients treated with chlorthalidone. The diagnosis is confirmed by the reversal of hypercalcemia after cessation of thiazide therapy. If hypercalcemia persists, the parathyroid hormone level should be measured to assess for the presence of a parathyroid-mediated cause of hypercalcemia.

Measurement of thyroid-stimulating hormone is used to assess whether a patient is biochemically euthyroid and to rule out over-replacement with levothyroxine. Overt thyrotoxicosis can be associated with hypercalcemia, but this patient has no clinical stigmata of hyperthyroidism and testing is not indicated. Neither ramipril nor atorvastatin has been associated with hypercalcemia.

- Thiazide diuretics stimulate renal tubular calcium reabsorption and may lead to a mild hypercalcemia.

Bibliography
1. **Ramsay LE, Yeo WW, Jackson PR.** Metabolic effects of diuretics. Cardiology. 1994;84:48-56. [PMID: 7954546]

Item 62   Answer: C

This hypertensive patient has unprovoked hypokalemia, and his high urine potassium level indicates excessive renal potassium losses (in the presence of ongoing hypokalemia, a urine potassium concentration >30 meq/24 h identifies excessive renal potassium loss). These findings make hyperaldosteronism the most likely diagnosis listed. Hyperaldosteronism is included in the differential diagnosis of hypertension and hypokalemia. Unprovoked hypokalemia is highly suggestive of hyperaldosteronism—primary hyperaldosteronism has been identified in as many as 50% of patients with unprovoked hypokalemia. Severe hypokalemia following administration of a non–potassium sparing diuretic also is suggestive of hyperaldosteronism. Some patients with primary hyperaldosteronism are persistently normokalemic; thus, screening is also indicated in patients with early-onset, severe hypertension or resistant hypertension.

The diagnosis of primary hyperaldosteronism is made by showing increased autonomous aldosterone synthesis with suppression of the renin-angiotensin system. Although this test can be performed under random conditions, accuracy is increased if the sample is obtained after hypokalemia has been corrected and, preferably, in the absence of drugs that alter the renin-aldosterone axis, such as spironolactone (the effects of spironolactone can last 2 to 3 weeks), other diuretics, β-blockers, angiotensin-converting enzyme (ACE) inhibitors, and angiotensin receptor blockers (ARBs). For a diagnosis of primary hyperaldosteronism, the plasma aldosterone concentration should be >15 ng/dL and plasma renin activity should be <1.0 ng/mL/h.

Cushing's syndrome is a reasonable consideration for a patient with difficult-to-control hypertension, obesity, and diabetes. However, this patient's 24-hour urine free cortisol is normal, ruling out Cushing's syndrome. Essential hypertension is not associated with hypokalemia, renal potassium wasting, or metabolic alkalosis. These findings more strongly suggest hyperaldosteronism. Pheochromocytoma is a very rare neoplasm that is associated with paroxysmal or sustained hypertension; however, pheochromocytoma is not associated with hypokalemia, renal potassium wasting, or metabolic alkalosis, making pheochromocytoma unlikely in this patient. Renovascular hypertension is often associated with older age and signs of other peripheral vascular disease, such as carotid bruits, claudication, diminished pulses, and coronary artery disease. Although the physical examination may be normal in patients with renovascular hypertension, the presence of abdominal, femoral, or carotid bruits increases its pretest probability. Atherosclerotic renovascular disease may be associated with renal impairment (which may worsen with ACE inhibitor or ARB therapy), which is absent in this patient. Finally, renovascular hypertension is not associated with hypokalemia, renal potassium wasting, or metabolic alkalosis.

KEY POINTS

- The diagnosis of primary hyperaldosteronism is made by showing increased autonomous aldosterone synthesis with suppression of the renin-angiotensin system.

- Primary hyperaldosteronism is diagnosed in as many as 50% of patients with unprovoked hypokalemia.

Bibliography
1. **Bornstein SR, Stratakis CA, Chrousos GP.** Adrenocortical tumors: recent advances in basic concepts and clinical management. Ann Intern Med. 1999;130:759-71. [PMID: 10357696]

Item 63   Answer: B

Discontinuation of ibuprofen is indicated for this patient. Nonsteroidal anti-inflammatory drugs (NSAIDs) frequently affect sodium excretion. However, these agents are routinely used by elderly patients, who are particularly vulnerable to the blood pressure–raising effects of these drugs because of the change in sodium excretion. Most elderly patients have musculoskeletal conditions that warrant some form of therapy, but long-term daily treatment with NSAIDs may not be necessary. Alternative treatment strategies, such as physical therapy or therapy with acetaminophen, are indicated in this setting.

Discontinuing this patient's NSAID therapy is an appropriate next step to try to decrease his blood pressure. This strategy should be attempted before increasing his current medications or adding new medications, particularly because NSAIDs may contribute to renal and electrolyte disorders when used concomitantly with angiotensin-converting enzyme inhibitors or when taken by volume-depleted patients.

KEY POINT

- Nonsteroidal anti-inflammatory drug use is a common cause of resistance to antihypertensive therapy.

Bibliography
1. **Gaziano JM.** Nonnarcotic analgesics and hypertension. Am J Cardiol. 2006;97:10-6. Epub 2006 Mar 30. [PMID: 16675317]

Item 64   Answer: C

Renovascular hypertension is one of the most common types of secondary hypertension, accounting for up to 5% of cases. It occurs in patients younger than 30 years or older than 50 years. Two thirds of cases are caused by atherosclerotic disease. The initial increase in blood pressure is a direct consequence of hyperreninemia. Renal ultrasonography with renal artery Doppler examination provides anatomic and functional assessment of the renal arteries. Direct visualization of the main renal arteries (B-mode imaging) combined with measurement (via Doppler) of intrarenal pressures and velocities (by waveform) has a sensitivity of 72% to 92% for diagnosing renovascular hypertension. This technique potentially can detect both unilateral and bilateral renal disease.

A 24-hour urine collection for cortisol is useful if Cushing's syndrome is suspected, but this patient has no physical signs of cortisol excess or diabetes mellitus, making this diagnosis unlikely. Spot urine measurement for metanephrines is used to screen for pheochromocytoma. This is a much less frequent cause of secondary hypertension than renovascular hypertension and is often associated with other evidence of catecholamine excess such as tachycardia. A 24-hour urine collection for potassium excretion is a useful screening test for hyperaldosteronism, particularly in the presence of unprovoked hypokalemia (i.e., when a patient is not taking diuretics). The patient's normal potassium level while taking hydrochlorothiazide makes this diagnosis unlikely.

KEY POINT

- Renal ultrasonography with renal artery Doppler examination provides anatomic and functional assessment of the renal arteries, and has a sensitivity of 72% to 92% for diagnosing renovascular hypertension.

Bibliography
1. **Bloch MJ, Basile J.** Clinical insights into the diagnosis and management of renovascular disease. An evidence-based review. Minerva Med. 2004;95:357-73. [PMID: 15467512]

Item 65   Answer: D

Sleep apnea syndrome may contribute to resistant hypertension as well as to increased cardiovascular and cerebrovascular disease risk. Patients may have excessive fatigue and may fall asleep while driving or working. This condition has a higher prevalence in overweight men. The pathogenesis of sleep apnea syndrome is complex and linked to obesity, insulin resistance, and increased sodium retention. Several studies have shown that patients with sleep apnea syndrome have increased activity of the sympathetic nervous system, which also occurs in obesity. Coexistent insulin resistance and impaired glucose tolerance also may be present in these patients.

Renovascular hypertension may cause resistant hypertension but is less common than sleep apnea. In addition, the patient's age, obesity, plethora, and daytime sleepiness are more suggestive of sleep apnea than renovascular hypertension. Atherosclerotic renovascular hypertension usually develops in older patients, whereas fibromuscular dysplasia of the renal arteries often presents in younger patients and is more common in women.

Primary hyperaldosteronism may be present in as many as 10% of patients with resistant hypertension and should be included in the differential diagnosis. However, this condition is less likely in a patient who takes hydrochlorothiazide and has a normal potassium level.

Pheochromocytoma is a rare form of hypertension mediated by excess catecholamines. This condition causes palpitations, diaphoresis, tremor, flushing, and headaches. Diagnosis of pheochromocytoma may be difficult, and the clinical manifestations vary significantly. This patient's presentation is not fully consistent with this condition, and sleep apnea is more likely because it is more common and more likely to be associated with obesity, plethora, and daytime sleepiness.

KEY POINT

• Sleep apnea is associated with resistant hypertension and is particularly prevalent in obese patients.

Bibliography
1. **Poirier P, Giles TD, Bray GA, Hong Y, Stern JS, Pi-Sunyer FX, Eckel RH; American Heart Association; Obesity Committee of the Council on Nutrition, Physical Activity, and Metabolism.** Obesity and cardiovascular disease: pathophysiology, evaluation, and effect of weight loss: an update of the 1997 American Heart Association Scientific Statement on Obesity and Heart Disease from the Obesity Committee of the Council on Nutrition, Physical Activity, and Metabolism. Circulation. 2006;113:898-918. Epub 2005 Dec 27. [PMID: 16380542]

Item 66   Answer: A

The most appropriate next step in this patient's management is ambulatory blood pressure monitoring. White coat hypertension due to this patient's anxiety regarding a new physician and medication change is highly possible, and ambulatory blood pressure monitoring would confirm this diagnosis. In addition, overtreatment of hypertension in elderly patients is associated with increased adverse effects of medication, particularly symptoms associated with hypotension. Moreover, this patient's fatigue, weakness, and dizziness suggest that she is already overmedicated. Although current blood pressure targets for the elderly have not been clearly defined, a systolic blood pressure ≤160 mm Hg in this population has been associated with better outcomes. Ambulatory blood pressure monitoring is useful in this setting to document the level of blood pressure control.

Performing magnetic resonance angiography would be premature in this patient. Renovascular hypertension is a possible cause of resistant hypertension in the elderly, but her symptoms are consistent with overmedication. In addition, her long-standing history of stable hypertension is consistent with primary or essential hypertension. Increasing her hydrochlorothiazide dose before excluding a white coat effect could lead to increased symptoms. Lower doses of medication are indicated for many elderly patients, and 50 mg/d of hydrochlorothiazide most likely will be poorly tolerated in this patient.

Discontinuation of metoprolol may be reasonable. However, because of her elevated office blood pressure measurements, this agent should be discontinued only after documenting that her blood pressure is adequately controlled.

KEY POINT

• In selected patients, ambulatory blood pressure monitoring can exclude white coat hypertension.

Bibliography
1. **Fisher M, Blackwell J, Saseen J.** Clinical inquiries. What is the best way to identify patients with white-coat hypertension? J Fam Pract. 2005;54:549-50, 552. [PMID: 15939009]

Item 67   Answer: C

Poorly controlled diabetes mellitus or hypertension, proteinuria, and cigarette smoking are all risk factors for chronic kidney disease progression. However, treatment of hypertension is the cornerstone in preserving renal function in patients with diabetic nephropathy. Reduction in blood pressure has been shown to influence progression of renal disease and the development of cardiovascular disease in patients with diabetes. The goal of treatment of blood pressure in patients with both type 1 and type 2 diabetes mellitus is to maintain a blood pressure ≤130/80 mm Hg in the absence of significant proteinuria and ≤125/75 mm Hg if accompanied by a urine protein concentration >1 g/24 h. Angiotensin-converting enzyme inhibitors or angiotensin receptor blockers constitute first-line treatment of hypertension, even in patients with advanced diabetic nephropathy.

The beneficial effect of strict metabolic control of diabetes on the progression of advanced renal disease is less established than is strict control of blood pressure. Nevertheless, metabolic control should be improved in this setting in order to minimize the risk for metabolic, microvascular, and macrovascular complications of diabetes. Proteinuria is a well-recognized risk factor for the progression of renal disease, including diabetic nephropathy. Cigarette smoking has been shown to have significant detrimental effects on the kidney and may cause increased proteinuria and an accelerated decline in renal function. Nevertheless, uncontrolled hypertension is the major factor contributing to progressive renal failure.

• Reduction in blood pressure slows the progression of renal disease and the development of cardiovascular disease in patients with diabetes mellitus.

Bibliography

1. Barnett A. Prevention of loss of renal function over time in patients with diabetic nephropathy. Am J Med. 2006;119:S40-7. [PMID: 16563947]

Item 68   Answer: D

Therapy with a thiazide diuretic is indicated for this patient. This patient has type 2 diabetes mellitus, coronary artery disease, possible early diabetic nephropathy, and inadequate blood pressure control. His current regimen of a β-blocker and angiotensin-converting enzyme inhibitor is appropriate for cardiovascular disease and target organ protection. The addition of a thiazide diuretic is likely to improve blood pressure control, which is indicated to prevent further progression of target organ damage.

The addition of an angiotensin receptor blocker or potassium-sparing diuretic may provide renal protection and additional blood pressure control but would likely further exacerbate his hyperkalemia. Therapy with α-blockers has not been shown to have particular advantages compared with use of the other agents listed and may not lower blood pressure sufficiently.

• Diuretics potentiate the blood pressure–lowering effects of angiotensin-converting enzyme inhibitors and β-blockers.

Bibliography

1. Einhorn PT, Davis BR, Massie BM, Cushman WC, Piller LB, Simpson LM, Levy D, Nwachuku CE, Black HR; ALLHAT Collaborative Research Group. The Antihypertensive and Lipid Lowering Treatment to Prevent Heart Attack Trial (ALLHAT) Heart Failure Validation Study: diagnosis and prognosis. Am Heart J. 2007;153:42-53. [PMID: 17174636]

Item 69   Answer: D

Hypertension is an independent risk factor for peripheral artery disease, and current guidelines support aggressive blood pressure management. For the general population, a blood pressure target of <140/90 mm Hg is associated with a decrease in cardiovascular complications, and a target pressure of <130/80 mm Hg is indicated for patients with diabetes mellitus (such as this patient) or renal failure.

• The target blood pressure for patients with diabetes mellitus or renal failure is <130/80 mm Hg.

Bibliography

1. Chobanian AV, Bakris GL, Black HR, Cushman WC, Green LA, Izzo JL Jr, et al. The Seventh Report of the Joint National Committee on Prevention, Detection, Evaluation, and Treatment of High Blood Pressure: the JNC 7 report. JAMA. 2003;289:2560-72. [PMID: 12748199]

Item 70   Answer: B

The addition of hydrochlorothiazide to this patient's medication regimen is the most appropriate next step. Patients with concomitant diabetes mellitus and hypertension typically require multidrug therapy to achieve target blood pressure goal (<130/80 mm Hg in this patient). Because this patient also has mild chronic kidney disease (calculated creatinine clearance, 69 mL/min) with microalbuminuria, ischemic heart disease, and congestive heart failure, blood pressure control is imperative. Adding a diuretic to a multidrug antihypertensive regimen may help to achieve a patient's blood pressure goal, and a regimen is not considered ineffective until a diuretic has been included.

Hydrochlorothiazide is administered once daily and is inexpensive and effective. Black patients usually respond less predictably well to angiotensin-converting enzyme (ACE) inhibitors, but the addition of a diuretic can help to equalize the effectiveness of these agents to that of white patients. Multiple trials have shown that β-blockers and ACE inhibitors are indicated in this setting. These agents prevent the progression of diabetic nephropathy, improve survival in heart failure, and provide secondary prevention of the acute coronary syndrome. Routine questioning of the patient about compliance is indicated, because compliance with therapy is a significant problem in hypertension management.

Clonidine has more side effects than similar agents and is not vasculo- or renoprotective; therefore, it is not indicated until all first-line agents have been tried. Hydralazine combined with nitrates is used as an alternative to ACE inhibitors or angiotensin-receptor blockers in patients intolerant to both, and can be added to standard heart failure therapy in black patients with heart failure. Hydralazine and nitrates have not been shown to have the same cardioprotective properties as ACE inhibitors. Patients with diabetes typically require three to four antihypertensive drugs, and this patient's medication regimen should not raise suspicion for a secondary cause of hypertension, such as pheochromocytoma. Moreover, this patient has no additional signs or symptoms suggestive of pheochromocytoma. Measurement of 24-hour urine catecholamines is therefore not indicated. Reevaluation in 2 to 3 months is not appropriate because blood pressure control in this setting is imperative to prevent morbidity and mortality.

• Multidrug antihypertensive therapy is often needed to achieve optimal blood pressure control in patients with diabetes mellitus.

• An ineffective multidrug antihypertensive regimen should be considered a failure only if it includes a diuretic.

Bibliography
1. Chobanian AV, Bakris GL, Black HR, Cushman WC, Green LA, Izzo JL Jr, Jones DW, Materson BJ, Oparil S, Wright JT Jr, Roccella EJ; National Heart, Lung, and Blood Institute Joint National Committee on Prevention, Detection, Evaluation, and Treatment of High Blood Pressure; National High Blood Pressure Education Program Coordinating Committee. The Seventh Report of the Joint National Committee on Prevention, Detection, Evaluation, and Treatment of High Blood Pressure: the JNC 7 report. JAMA. 2003;289:2560-72. Epub 2003 May 14. Erratum in: JAMA. 2003;290:197. [PMID: 12748199]

Item 71　　Answer: B

The most appropriate treatment for this patient is labetalol therapy. This agent has been used extensively in pregnancy because of its combined α-and β-blocking properties. Methyldopa also has been used extensively in pregnancy and is one of the only agents in which long-term follow-up of infants exposed in utero has proved to be safe.

Diuretic agents may interfere with the normal physiologic volume expansion associated with pregnancy. Therefore, initiation of diuretic therapy during pregnancy usually is not recommended in the absence of renal insufficiency. However, if needed, patients with hypertension treated with chronic diuretic therapy before conception may continue treatment with these agents at lower doses. Angiotensin-converting enzyme inhibitors and angiotensin receptor blockers are contraindicated in pregnancy because of adverse effects on fetal renal function, particularly after second- and third- trimester exposure. There is no clear association between these drugs and teratogenic effects after first-trimester exposure. However, avoidance of these drugs is indicated during all trimesters of pregnancy because of the risk for negative fetal outcomes.

KEY POINT

• Labetalol or methyldopa is the preferred treatment for chronic hypertension in pregnant patients.

Bibliography
1. Podymow T, August P, Umans JG. Antihypertensive therapy in pregnancy. Semin Nephrol. 2004;24:616-25. [PMID: 15529297]

Item 72　　Answer: B

This patient most likely has a dissecting aortic aneurysm associated with a hypertensive crisis that requires immediate treatment with intravenous antihypertensive agents. Clues to the diagnosis include hypertension, back pain, and a diastolic murmur (suggesting involvement of the aortic valve). Most hypertensive crises result from inadequately treated blood pressure or noncompliance with medications. Patients with hypertensive crisis and end-organ damage should be treated in the intensive care unit with parenteral antihypertensive agents. Patients are placed on a cardiac monitor and serial noninvasive blood pressure measurements or continuous measurements with an indwelling arterial catheter are taken. The goal of therapy is not to decrease the blood pressure to "normal" levels but to prevent further end-organ damage. It is dangerous to lower the blood pressure quickly and excessively, particularly in elderly hypovolemic patients and in patients with chronic hypertension. Precipitous decreases predispose the patient to cerebral, cardiac, and renal ischemia. A progressive reduction in the blood pressure should be undertaken. Decreasing the mean arterial pressure (MAP) by 20% to 25% or decreasing the diastolic blood pressure to <120 mm Hg is recommended. This level has been suggested by studies of autoregulation of the cerebral blood flow when MAP was safely reduced by 20% to 25% in normotensive and hypertensive patients. Other authorities advocate decreasing the MAP to 110 to 115 mm Hg within the first hour with a return to normal or baseline blood pressure over the next 24 hours. The diagnosis of dissecting aortic aneurysm is made by either CT scan of the chest, bedside echocardiogram, or aortic angiogram.

This patient does not have evidence of an acute myocardial infarction or unstable angina, and there is no need for thrombolytic therapy or heparin. Even if acute coronary syndrome was present, the use of thrombolytic therapy or heparin is contraindicated by the elevated blood pressure and possibility of aortic dissection. Oral antihypertensive agents are not adequate treatment to prevent further end-organ damage and are not indicated.

KEY POINT

• Patients with hypertensive crisis and end-organ damage should be treated in the intensive care unit with parenteral antihypertensive agents.

Bibliography
1. Ince H, Nienaber CA. Diagnosis and management of patients with aortic dissection. Heart. 2007;93:266-70.[PMID: 17228080]

Item 73　　Answer: C

Ramipril therapy is indicated for this patient. His long-standing uncontrolled hypertension, black race, bland urine sediment with non-nephrotic-range proteinuria, and ultrasonographic findings of small kidneys are consistent with hypertensive nephrosclerosis. Treatment of this condition relies on strict blood pressure control to slow the rate of progressive renal failure.

In the African American Study of Kidney Disease and Hypertension (AASK) trial, patients treated with the angiotensin-converting enzyme inhibitor ramipril were significantly less likely to develop the secondary outcomes of a reduced glomerular filtration rate, development of renal failure, or death compared with those treated with metoprolol or amlodipine. Terazosin, an α-blocker, is not an effective agent when used as monotherapy. Other studies also have demonstrated the beneficial effects of medications that block the renin–angiotensin system and of slowing progression of kidney disease. Therefore, these agents are recommended for first-line therapy for patients with both diabetic and nondiabetic kidney disease.

KEY POINT

• Angiotensin-converting enzyme inhibitors or angiotensin receptor blockers are the agents of choice for the treatment of hypertension in chronic kidney disease.

Bibliography

1. Chobanian AV, Bakris GL, Black HR, Cushman WC, Green LA, Izzo JL Jr, et al. Seventh report of the Joint National Committee on Prevention, Detection, Evaluation, and Treatment of High Blood Pressure. Hypertension. 2003;42:1206-52. [PMID: 14656957]

Item 74   Answer: C

This patient's young age and refractory hypertension warrant consideration of a secondary cause of hypertension. The classic triad of symptoms—headaches, palpitations, and diaphoresis—is suggestive of pheochromocytoma. These tumors are present in less than 1% of hypertensive patients, are derived from chromaffin cells, and elaborate norepinephrine, epinephrine, and dopamine. Tumors originating in the adrenal glands are referred to as pheochromocytomas, whereas those originating along the sympathetic paraganglia are referred to as paragangliomas. Hypertension is present in more than 90% of patients with pheochromocytoma: more than 50% of these patients have sustained elevations in blood pressure; 30% to 40% have episodic elevations, and up to 10% have no hypertension. Lability of blood pressure is due to episodic catecholamine release, volume depletion, and adrenergic receptor desensitization due to chronic stimulation. Other symptoms include anxiety, tremor, and pallor. Chronic complications of excess catecholamine release include cardiac arrhythmias, both dilated and hypertrophic cardiomyopathy, and accelerated atherosclerosis related to hypertension. Propranolol for this patient's migraine headaches worsened his symptoms because of the unopposed α-tone resulting from β-blockade.

Serum potassium levels are usually decreased in patients with primary aldosteronism and Cushing's syndrome; furthermore, these conditions are not associated with headaches, palpitations, and diaphoresis. Carcinoid syndrome is the term applied to symptoms mediated by humoral factors released by some carcinoid tumors. Episodic flushing is most characteristic of the carcinoid syndrome; it begins suddenly and lasts up to 30 minutes. Severe flushes are accompanied by a fall in blood pressure and rise in heart rate. The patient does not have flushing or hypotension, making carcinoid syndrome an unlikely diagnosis.

KEY POINT

• The classic symptoms for pheochromocytoma consist of hypertension, headaches, palpitations, and diaphoresis.

Bibliography

1. Lenders JW, Eisenhofer G, Mannelli M, Pacak K. Phaeochromocytoma. Lancet. 2005;366:665-75. [PMID: 16112304]

Item 75   Answer: D

Patients with pheochromocytoma should be treated with α-blockade therapy (e.g., phenoxybenzamine) for at least 2 weeks before surgery. Phenoxybenzamine provides complete α-blockade, and dosages of this agent should be titrated to achieve blood pressure control.

Calcium-channel blockers do not provide α-blockade and therefore are not indicated. Because unopposed α-tone can exacerbate hypertension in this setting, β-blockade is not indicated for pheochromocytoma unless adequate therapy with an α-blocker has already been administered. Before surgery, patients with pheochromocytoma should be euvolemic or slightly volume expanded. High sympathetic tone and pressure natriuresis associated with pheochromocytoma may cause volume depletion, which may result in secondary stimulation of the renin–angiotensin system and worsening hypertension. Diuretics are contraindicated because these agents may exacerbate this situation.

KEY POINT

• Patients with pheochromocytoma should receive an α-blocker before surgery.

Bibliography

1. Manger WM, Gifford RW. Pheochromocytoma. J Clin Hypertens (Greenwich). 2002;4:62-72. [PMID: 11821644]

Item 76   Answer: C

Renovascular hypertension is an increasingly common cause of uncontrolled hypertension. This condition should be suspected in elderly patients with evidence of diffuse atherosclerosis; a history of cigarette smoking; and chronic kidney disease characterized by modest elevations in creatinine levels, non-nephrotic-range proteinuria, and a bland urine sediment. Increased renal echogenicity on ultrasonography is a nonspecific finding of diffuse renal disease. Another important clue is the discrepancy in kidney size as detected by ultrasonography; the smaller kidney is the result of reduced renal blood flow and suggests the presence of renovascular hypertension. Hyperreninemia secondary to renal ischemia often causes recurrent episodes of pulmonary edema, as seen in this patient. Evaluation in this setting warrants imaging of the renal arteries.

Hypertension caused by sleep apnea syndrome characteristically occurs in obese men who snore and experience daytime somnolence and carbon dioxide retention. Sleep apnea syndrome would not explain this patient's difference in kidney size or chronic kidney disease. Cushing's syndrome is recognized by cushingoid (moon-shaped) facies, central obesity, striae, proximal myopathy, and easy bruising. Hypokalemia is common. In the absence of any of these clinical features, Cushing's syndrome is unlikely. Patients with hyperthyroidism are likely to experience mainly systolic hypertension, heat intolerance, palpitations, tachycardia, and weight loss. Systolic and diastolic hypertension resistant to multiple drug therapy in the absence of other signs of hyperthyroidism is unlikely.

KEY POINT

- Individuals with uncontrolled hypertension and recurrent episodes of flash pulmonary edema should be screened for renovascular disease.

Bibliography

1. **Garovic VD, Textor SC.** Renovascular hypertension and ischemic nephropathy. Circulation. 2005;112:1362-74. [PMID: 16129817]

Item 77 Answer: A

The most appropriate next step in this patient's management is therapy with a short-acting angiotensin-converting enzyme (ACE) inhibitor, such as captopril. This patient has scleroderma renal crisis with new-onset hypertension, increased creatinine concentration, decreased platelets, and anemia with lower-extremity edema. Close monitoring and aggressive titration of a short-acting ACE inhibitor are indicated to rapidly decrease her blood pressure to the low-normal range.

Scleroderma renal crisis is associated with an increase in renin levels. Therefore, treatment with an ACE inhibitor is more appropriate than diuretic therapy or calcium-channel blockers. Intravenous labetalol is not a first-line agent for treating scleroderma renal crisis. In addition, labetalol may worsen this patient's symptoms of Raynaud's phenomenon and is therefore not the most appropriate choice in this clinical scenario. However, this agent may be used if additional blood pressure control is needed.

KEY POINT

- Short-acting angiotensin-converting enzyme inhibitors are the drugs of choice in the treatment of scleroderma renal crisis.

Bibliography

1. **Rhew EY, Barr WG.** Scleroderma renal crisis: new insights and developments. Curr Rheumatol Rep. 2004;6:129-36. [PMID: 15016343]

Chapter 5
Hematology

Hematology contains self-assessment items that correspond to the following chapters in the *Internal Medicine Essentials for Clerkship Students 2* textbook:

Anemia
Bleeding Disorders
Sickle Cell Anemia
Thrombocytopenia
Thrombophilia
Common Leukemias
Multiple Myeloma

Hematology contains self assessment items that correspond to the following Training Problems in the *Core Medicine Clerkship Guide*:

Anemia

Chapter 5

Hematology

Questions

Item 1

A 50-year-old man is evaluated in the office for the recent onset of pruritus while showering. He has previously been in excellent health, eats a normal diet, is an occasional smoker, and does not take any medications.

On physical examination, he has a ruddy face and a palpable spleen tip. Results of fecal occult blood testing are negative. The arterial oxygen saturation is 99% on room air.

Laboratory studies show a hematocrit of 61.0% compared with a value of 44.5% documented 5 years ago, leukocyte count of 11,100/μL, mean corpuscular volume of 79 fL, and platelet count of 650,000/μL. Serum chemistry studies are normal except for a reduced ferritin concentration.

Which of the following is the most likely diagnosis?

(A) Myelodysplastic syndrome
(B) Polycythemia vera
(C) Relative erythrocytosis
(D) Secondary erythrocytosis related to smoking

Item 2

A 34-year-old woman is evaluated in the office for a 1-day history of fever, chills, and cough. She has a past history of iron deficiency anemia attributed to menorrhagia for which she has been treated effectively with ferrous gluconate daily for 1 year.

On physical examination, temperature is 38.6 °C (101.5 °F). Crackles and egophony are heard in the right posterior chest.

Laboratory studies:

Hemoglobin	11.3 g/dL
Mean corpuscular hemoglobin	27.6 pg
Mean corpuscular hemoglobin concentration	33.2 g/dL
Mean corpuscular volume	83 fL
Leukocyte count	11,000/μL (80% neutrophils, 7% band forms, 10% lymphocytes, 3% monocytes)
Platelet count	440,000/μL
Ferritin	126 ng/mL
Iron	25 μg/dL
Total iron-binding capacity	277 μg/dL

Which of the following is most likely causing this patient's anemia?

(A) Anemia of inflammation (anemia of chronic disease)
(B) Combined iron deficiency anemia and anemia of inflammation
(C) Iron deficiency anemia
(D) Sideroblastic anemia

Item 3

A 64-year-old man is evaluated in the emergency department for severe fatigue that has worsened over the past 3 months and recurrent epistaxis that has occurred over the past week. He has not had fever, a recent illness, or any risk factors for HIV infection. He has not taken any over-the-counter medications or used alcohol. His family history is significant for two siblings who died of cancer. On physical examination, petechiae are noted on the buccal mucosa and lower extremities. There is no lymphadenopathy, hepatomegaly, or splenomegaly.

Laboratory studies:

Hematocrit	23%
Leukocyte count	1200/μL
Platelet count	15,000/μL
Reticulocyte count	1000/μL (normal, 25,000–75,000/μL)
Activated partial thromboplastin time	Normal
Prothrombin time	Normal
Aspartate aminotransferase	Normal
Alanine aminotransferase	Normal

No significant red blood cell abnormalities are noted on a peripheral blood smear. Chest radiograph is unremarkable. A bone marrow biopsy specimen is shown (*see Figure 13 in Color Plates*).

Which of the following is the most likely diagnosis?

(A) Acute myeloid leukemia
(B) Aplastic anemia
(C) Chronic hepatitis B infection
(D) Myelophthisic (marrow-invasive) anemia

Item 4

An 18-year-old woman is evaluated in the office for a 3-week history of headache and exercise intolerance. She lives in Michigan and has not traveled outside the United States. The remainder of the medical history is noncontributory.

On physical examination, the patient is pale. Heart rate is 100/min, and respiration rate is 14/min. There is no evidence of jugular venous distention or an S_3, and the lungs are clear. The spleen tip is palpable on abdominal examination.

Laboratory studies indicate a hemoglobin of 5.5 g/dL and an absolute reticulocyte count of 605,000/µL (normal, 25,000–75,000/µL). The peripheral blood smear is shown (*see Figure 14 in Color Plates*).

Which of the following is the most likely diagnosis?

(A) Aplastic anemia
(B) Autoimmune hemolytic anemia
(C) Bleeding
(D) Malaria
(E) Thrombotic thrombocytopenic purpura

Item 5

A 78-year-old woman is evaluated in the office for increasing forgetfulness that has been slowly progressive over the past 7 months. She is able to live independently and has not had difficulty performing the usual activities of daily living. She has no other medical problems and takes no medications. The remainder of the medical history and physical examination are noncontributory.

Laboratory studies:

Hemoglobin	7.8 g/dL
Leukocyte count	3800/µL
Mean corpuscular volume	110 fL
Platelet count	127,000/µL
Lactate dehydrogenase	565 U/L
Direct bilirubin	0.3 mg/dL
Total bilirubin	4.8 mg/dL
Vitamin B_{12}	325 pg/mL
Folate	12 ng/mL
Homocysteine	20 µmol/L
Methylmalonic acid	400 nmol/L

Which of the following is the most likely diagnosis?

(A) Autoimmune hemolytic anemia
(B) Folate deficiency
(C) Myelodysplasia
(D) Vitamin B_{12} deficiency

Item 6

A 27-year-old woman is evaluated in the emergency department for severe left-sided abdominal pain resulting from a bad fall that occurred during a neighborhood football game. The patient indicates that she has been anemic in the past.

On physical examination, the patient is lying on her right side. Heart rate is 98/min, respiration rate is 12/min, and blood pressure is 140/88 mm Hg. The abdomen is flat with nor-mal bowel sounds. There is no guarding or rebound. The spleen tip is palpable.

The complete blood count is normal except for a hemoglobin concentration of 10.5 g/dL and a mean corpuscular hemoglobin concentration of 39 g/dL. Results of a direct antiglobulin test (direct Coombs' test) are negative. The peripheral blood smear is shown (*see Figure 15 in Color Plates*).

Which of the following is the most likely diagnosis?

(A) Hereditary spherocytosis
(B) Hypersplenism
(C) Iron deficiency anemia
(D) β-Thalassemia trait (thalassemia minor)

Item 7

A 22-year-old woman is evaluated in the office for extreme fatigue and exercise intolerance developing over 7 months. The medical history is noncontributory.

On physical examination, there is conjunctival pallor and tachycardia. The remainder of the examination is normal. Her hemoglobin is 5 g/dL. The peripheral blood smear is shown (*see Figure 16 in Color Plates*).

Which of the following is the most likely diagnosis?

(A) Autoimmune hemolytic anemia
(B) Iron deficiency anemia
(C) Thrombotic thrombocytopenic purpura
(D) Vitamin B_{12} deficiency

Item 8

A 20-year-old woman is evaluated in the office for excessive fatigue of several years' duration. The remainder of the medical history and physical examination are noncontributory. She has a family history of anemia.

Laboratory studies include a hemoglobin of 10 g/dL, a mean corpuscular volume of 60 fL, and a red blood cell count of 5.5 million cells/µL. The leukocyte and platelet counts and results of hemoglobin electrophoresis are normal. The peripheral blood smear is shown (*see Figure 17 in Color Plates*).

Which of the following is the most likely diagnosis?

(A) Autoimmune hemolytic anemia
(B) Iron deficiency anemia
(C) Sickle cell anemia
(D) α-Thalassemia trait

Item 9

A 51-year-old woman is evaluated during a routine office visit. She states that she has been fatigued for the past 6 months and has decreased exercise tolerance. She is perimenopausal and has had two menstrual periods in the past 6 months. Physical examination, including rectal examination and a single stool sample for occult blood, is normal.

Laboratory studies:

Hematocrit	30.8%
Mean corpuscular volume	76 fL
Platelet count	370,000/µL
Ferritin	11 ng/mL
Blood glucose	97 mg/dL
Iron	30 µg/dL
Total iron-binding capacity	480 µg/dL
Serum creatinine	0.9 mg/dL
Blood urea nitrogen	20 mg/dL
Thyroid-stimulating hormone	2.5 µU/mL

Results from a peripheral blood smear are pending.

Which of the following is the most appropriate next management step?

(A) Colonoscopy
(B) CT scan of the abdomen and pelvis
(C) MRI of the abdomen and pelvis
(D) Thyroxine replacement

Item 10

A 62-year-old man is evaluated during a routine office examination. His history is significant for rheumatoid arthritis that he has elected to treat only with nonsteroidal anti-inflammatory drugs. He has no fatigue or other symptoms, and the remainder of the history is noncontributory.

On physical examination, symmetrical swelling and effusions are noted, consistent with rheumatoid arthritis, in the metacarpophalangeal and proximal interphalangeal joints bilaterally.

Laboratory studies:

Hemoglobin	10.1 g/dL
Leukocyte count	6200/µL
Mean corpuscular volume	90 fL
Platelet count	234,000/µL
Reticulocyte count	6000/µL (normal, 25,000–75,000/µL)
Ferritin	250 ng/mL
Iron	37 µg/dL
Total iron-binding capacity	175 µg/dL

The peripheral blood smear is normal.

Which of the following is the most appropriate next step in management?

(A) Erythropoietin
(B) Oral ferrous sulfate
(C) Packed red blood cell transfusion
(D) No treatment is necessary

Item 11

A 27-year-old woman with a 2-year history of systemic lupus erythematosus is evaluated in the office for new-onset fatigue and shortness of breath of 10 days' duration. Her medications are hydroxychloroquine and ibuprofen. The medical history is otherwise noncontributory.

On physical examination, the heart rate is 109/min, respiration rate is 14/min, and blood pressure is 130/80 mm Hg. Other than pale conjunctivae and pallor, the physical examination is normal.

Laboratory studies indicate a hemoglobin of 5.2 g/dL, compared with a normal value 3 months ago, and an absolute reticulocyte count of 300,000/µL (normal, 25,000–75,000/µL). The peripheral blood smear shows polychromatic red blood cells and microspherocytes.

Which of the following is the most appropriate initial treatment for this patient?

(A) Corticosteroid therapy
(B) Erythropoietin
(C) Oral ferrous sulfate
(D) Plasmapheresis

Item 12

A 64-year-old man is evaluated in the office for worsening dyspnea and a gradual decrease in exercise tolerance over the past 2 months associated with his chronic obstructive pulmonary disease. He had an acute coronary syndrome 2 years ago, and his medications are daily aspirin, bronchodilators, inhaled corticosteroids, atenolol, and a statin. A routine screening colonoscopy was normal 1 year ago.

On physical examination, heart rate is 90/min, respiration rate is 20/min, and blood pressure is 130/90 mm Hg. Laboratory studies include a hemoglobin concentration of 9.6 g/dL and mean corpuscular volume of 78 fL. Stool is positive for occult blood. Iron deficiency anemia is diagnosed. Upper endoscopy reveals chronic gastritis, and the daily aspirin is stopped.

Which of the following is the most appropriate treatment for this patient's anemia?

(A) Blood transfusion
(B) Erythropoietin
(C) Intravenous iron
(D) Oral iron

Item 13

A 61-year-old man is evaluated in the office for fatigue and diminished exercise tolerance of 2 months' duration. His medical history includes hypercholesterolemia for which he takes pravastatin. He had a 30-pack-year history of cigarette smoking before quitting 5 years ago.

On physical examination, heart rate is 90/min, and blood pressure is 140/80 mm Hg. There is no abdominal tenderness, splenomegaly, or lymphadenopathy.

Laboratory studies:

Hemoglobin	8.6 g/dL
Leukocyte count	2100/µL
Platelet count	99,000/µL
Mean corpuscular volume	96 fL
Reticulocyte count	0.5% of erythrocytes

The peripheral blood smear shows dysplastic neutrophils. On bone marrow aspirate smear, dysplastic changes in myeloid and erythroid precursors are noted, with no increase in myeloblasts and no karyotypic abnormalities.

Which of the following is the most likely diagnosis?

(A) Acute myeloid leukemia
(B) Folate deficiency
(C) Lead toxicity
(D) Myelodysplastic syndrome

Item 14

A 34-year-old woman is evaluated in the office for vaginal bleeding, easy bruisability, and gingival bleeding of 2 weeks' duration. She also has a tender right thigh, which she believes began swelling after she bumped it on a table 2 days ago. She is 3 months' postpartum following the birth of a normal infant by cesarean delivery. The prothrombin time and activated partial thromboplastin time were normal prior to childbirth, and the cesarean delivery was not complicated by excessive bleeding. Her medical history and physical examination are otherwise noncontributory.

Laboratory studies:

Hemoglobin	10.8 g/dL
Leukocyte count	4500/µL
Platelet count	350,000/µL
Prothrombin time	12 s
Activated partial thrombo- plastin time	53 s
Urinalysis	3+ red blood cells; no leukocytes or cellular casts

Which of the following tests would be most likely to confirm this patient's diagnosis?

(A) Bleeding time
(B) Fibrin D-dimer measurement
(C) Fibrinogen and fibrin degradation products
(D) Inhibitor screen and factor VIII level

Item 15

A 30-year-old woman is evaluated in the office for heavy menstrual bleeding. She has a history of easy bruising, gingival bleeding when she brushes her teeth, and nose bleeds. She required a blood transfusion after the birth of her only child. She has never had surgery. Her mother also had heavy menstrual bleeding. The patient is otherwise healthy and takes no medications, including aspirin.

On physical examination, vital signs are normal. She has bruising on her shins and forearms. Pelvic examination is normal.

Laboratory studies:

Hemoglobin	11 g/dL
Leukocyte count	4300/µL
Platelet count	250,000/µL
Bleeding time	14 min (normal <10 min)
Prothrombin time	11 s
Activated partial thrombo- plastin time (aPTT)	40 s

The aPTT normalizes when mixed 1:1 with normal plasma.

Which of the following is the most likely diagnosis?

(A) Hemophilia A
(B) Hemophilia B
(C) Factor VIII inhibitor
(D) von Willebrand's disease

Item 16

A 28-year-old woman is evaluated in the emergency department for chest pain and shortness of breath of 6 hours' duration. Her history is significant for hemoglobin SS.

On physical examination, the temperature is 39 °C (102.2 °F). She is tachypneic and has decreased breath sounds with dullness to percussion at the right lung base. Arterial oxygen saturation is 85% on room air. A chest radiograph confirms the presence of a right lower lobe pulmonary infiltrate. The hemoglobin is 7.2 g/dL, and the leukocyte count is 12,500/µL. Initial electrocardiogram and cardiac enzyme values are normal.

Which of the following is the most likely diagnosis?

(A) Acute chest syndrome
(B) Acute myocardial infarction
(C) Chronic pulmonary hypertension
(D) Musculoskeletal chest pain

Item 17

A 32-year-old black man with sickle cell anemia is hospitalized for a 2-day history of acute pain in his back, chest, and extremities, along with nausea and vomiting. The pain has not responded to oral hydromorphone therapy. He has been hospitalized twice in the past year for similar symptoms.

On physical examination, the patient appears ill and uncomfortable. Temperature is 38.7 °C (101.7 °F), heart rate is 104/min, respiration rate is 20/min, blood pressure is 130/80 mm Hg, and oxygen saturation is 94% with the patient breathing room air. Wheezes are heard on auscultation of the lungs. The abdomen is nontender. Laboratory studies on admission: hemoglobin, 8 g/dL; leukocyte count, 18,000/µL; platelet count, 550,000/µL; and creatinine, 1.0 mg/dL. A urine albumin–creatinine ratio was 3 mg/g 4 months ago. Chest radiograph shows an infiltrate in the right upper lobe.

Treatment is started with intravenous normal saline, patient-controlled morphine, ceftriaxone, azithromycin, and an inhaled β-agonist. A red blood cell transfusion is also begun. Over the next 3 days, the patient's symptoms resolve.

Which of the following is the most appropriate long-term management of this patient's sickle cell anemia?

(A) Captopril
(B) Hydroxyurea
(C) Penicillin
(D) Recombinant erythropoietin

Item 18

A 46-year-old woman with a 10-year history of primary progressive multiple sclerosis is admitted to the hospital for surgical debridement and wound management of a sacral pressure ulcer. The patient is bed bound and is cared for at home by her husband. Her medications are sertraline, baclofen, and oxybutynin. The remainder of the medical history is noncontributory.

On physical examination, she is thin, is in no distress, and has normal vital signs. There are contraction deformities of the lower extremities, and a 6- × 8-cm sacral ulcer that extends to the fascia with minimal purulent exudates and no evidence of cellulitis.

Laboratory studies include a hematocrit of 34%, leukocyte count of 15,000/μL with 80% neutrophils, and a platelet count of 425,000/μL. All other laboratory studies are normal. Subcutaneous prophylactic unfractionated heparin is administered. Six days after initiation of heparin, her platelet count decreases to 210,000/μL, and on the ninth day after therapy, the platelet count has decreased to 95,000/μL. The peripheral blood smear shows decreased platelets but is otherwise normal. There is no evidence of bleeding from venous puncture sites or the wound.

Which of the following is the most likely diagnosis?

(A) Disseminated intravascular coagulation
(B) Hemolytic uremic syndrome
(C) Heparin-induced thrombocytopenia
(D) Pseudothrombocytopenia
(E) Thrombotic thrombocytopenic purpura

Item 19

A 26-year-old woman is evaluated in the office for easy bruising of 1 to 2 weeks' duration. She has had heavy menstrual bleeding since menarche. The patient is otherwise healthy, and her only medication is two aspirin tablets two or three times weekly for muscle aches associated with strenuous exercise. There is no family history of bleeding disorders.

On physical examination, vital signs are normal. There are multiple petechiae and four to five ecchymoses on her trunk and extremities. Cardiac and pulmonary examinations are normal. The spleen and liver are not palpable.

Laboratory studies:

Hemoglobin	12 g/dL
Leukocyte count	5600/μL with a normal differential
Platelet count	12,000/μL
Serum chemistry studies	Normal

A peripheral blood smear shows decreased platelets.

Which of the following is the most likely diagnosis?

(A) Aplastic anemia
(B) Aspirin-induced platelet defect
(C) Immune thrombocytopenic purpura
(D) Thrombotic thrombocytopenic purpura
(E) von Willebrand's disease

Item 20

A 27-year-old woman in the 30th week of pregnancy is evaluated during a routine office visit. The patient's pregnancy has been uneventful, with no bothersome symptoms or bleeding. The medical history and physical examination are noncontributory.

Laboratory studies include a hemoglobin of 13.8 g/dL, leukocyte count of 4600/μL, and platelet count of 90,000/μL. Platelet count values were 190,000/μL at week 12 and 177,000/μL at week 33. Serum chemistry test results, including liver chemistry tests, are normal. Recent ultrasonography showed normal fetal development.

Which of the following is the most likely diagnosis?

(A) Gestational thrombocytopenia
(B) HELLP syndrome
(C) Hemolytic uremic syndrome
(D) Thrombotic thrombocytopenic purpura

Item 21

A 70-year-old woman is evaluated in the office for a 4-month history of easy bruisability. Her medical history is otherwise noncontributory. She specifically denies blood loss.

Physical examination, including vital signs and testing for fecal occult blood, is normal. The complete blood count indicates a hemoglobin of 10.5 g/dL, leukocyte count of 4500/μL, and platelet count of 35,000/μL. Evidence of normochromic anemia and thrombocytopenia is noted on the peripheral blood smear.

Which of the following is the most appropriate next step in management?

(A) Begin prednisone
(B) Begin anti-Rh(D) immunoglobulin
(C) Perform bone marrow aspiration and biopsy
(D) Perform splenectomy

Item 22

A 30-year-old woman is evaluated in the emergency department for a 2-week history of fatigue, malaise, low-grade fever, and intermittent epistaxis. Her husband states that she has been forgetful and occasionally confused during this period. The remainder of the medical history is noncontributory. On physical examination, there are bruises over the upper and lower extremities and palatal petechiae.

Laboratory studies:

Hemoglobin	7.2 g/dL
Leukocyte count	9600/μL
Platelet count	12,000/μL
Lactate dehydrogenase	1700 U/L

The peripheral blood smear is shown (*see Figure 18 in Color Plates*).

Which of the following is the most likely diagnosis?

(A) Immune thrombocytopenic purpura
(B) Rocky Mountain spotted fever
(C) Systemic lupus erythematosus
(D) Thrombotic thrombocytopenia purpura

Item 23

A 22-year-old woman is evaluated in the office for contraceptive therapy. The patient is sexually active in a monogamous relationship. Her 55-year-old mother had pulmonary emboli 3 weeks postpartum after her only pregnancy and was recently diagnosed with proximal deep venous thrombosis of the right lower extremity. Results of her mother's laboratory evaluation for an underlying thrombophilic disorder included an antithrombin deficiency based on both functional and immunologic assays of 45% and 47% of normal, respectively. Results of the mother's genetic analysis were negative for factor V Leiden and prothrombin G20210A mutations, and plasma levels of protein C and protein S were normal. The remainder of the patient's medical and family history is noncontributory.

The physical examination, including vital signs, is normal. Laboratory studies indicate a functional antithrombin level of 50% of normal (reference range, 80% to 120% of normal); a repeated test is 48% of normal.

Which of the following contraceptive methods is contraindicated in this patient?

(A) Barrier contraceptive devices
(B) Estrogen oral contraceptive
(C) Intrauterine device
(D) Progestin (only) oral contraceptive

Item 24

A 28-year-old woman of Chinese descent is evaluated in the office for a diagnosis of right lower-extremity deep venous thrombosis during the 30th week of her first pregnancy. She took oral contraceptives for several years. Her medical and family history is otherwise noncontributory.

On physical examination, the patient is pregnant. There is painful swelling of the right leg from the ankle to the knee. The remainder of the examination is normal.

Laboratory studies, including complete blood count, prothrombin time, and activated partial thromboplastin time, are normal. Heparin and warfarin are begun.

Which of the following is the most appropriate next diagnostic test?

(A) Factor V Leiden and prothrombin G20210A mutational analysis
(B) Lupus anticoagulant and cardiolipin antibody measurement
(C) Protein C, protein S, and antithrombin measurement
(D) No further testing

Item 25

A 35-year-old woman is evaluated in the office for a 3-week history of a sense of abdominal fullness and fatigue. The remainder of the medical history is noncontributory.

On physical examination, vital signs are normal. Abdominal examination reveals a palpable spleen tip 4 cm below the left costal margin. Laboratory studies indicate a hematocrit of 42%, leukocyte count of 22,500/μL, and platelet count of 530,000/μL. A bone marrow aspirate specimen shows >60% Philadelphia chromosome (Ph)–positive cells by fluorescence in situ hybridization, and karyotypic analysis reveals no additional chromosomal abnormalities. No fibrosis or increase in blasts is noted on the bone marrow specimen.

Which of the following is the most appropriate management?

(A) Allogeneic stem cell transplantation
(B) Hydroxyurea
(C) Imatinib mesylate
(D) Interferon and low-dose cytarabine
(E) Observation

Item 26

A 45-year-old woman is evaluated in the office for a 3-week history of fatigue. The remainder of the medical history is noncontributory.

On physical examination, vital signs are normal. Abdominal examination reveals a palpable spleen tip 6 cm below the left costal margin. Laboratory studies indicate a hematocrit of 44%, leukocyte count of 28,500/μL, and platelet count of 490,000/μL. The peripheral blood smear shows increased numbers of granulocytic cells in all phases of development. The bone marrow aspirate specimen shows >65% Philadelphia chromosome (Ph)–positive cells by fluorescence in situ hybridization.

Which of the following is the most likely diagnosis?

(A) Acute myeloid leukemia
(B) Chronic lymphoid leukemia
(C) Chronic myeloid leukemia
(D) Transformed chronic myeloid leukemia

Item 27

A 56-year-old man is admitted to the hospital for excessive fatigue, fever, and nose bleeds. He was diagnosed with myelodysplastic syndrome (refractory anemia with excess blasts) 5 months ago for which he received intermittent packed red blood cell transfusions and weekly erythropoietin injections. He has not required platelet transfusions and has had no infections. His medical history is otherwise unremarkable.

On physical examination, temperature is 38.0 °C (100.4 °F), heart rate is 100/min, and blood pressure is 120/80 mm Hg. Numerous ecchymoses and petechiae are visible, particularly on the extremities. There is no abdominal tenderness, splenomegaly, or lymphadenopathy.

Laboratory studies indicate a hemoglobin of 6 g/dL, leukocyte count of 1200/μL, and a platelet count of 7000/μL. The peripheral blood smear shows 40% immature myeloid blasts and an absence of platelets.

Which of the following is the most likely diagnosis?

(A) Acute leukemia
(B) Anemia of inflammatory disease
(C) Bone marrow invasion by solid tumor
(D) Thrombotic thrombocytopenic purpura

Item 28

A 64-year-old man is evaluated in the emergency department for a 3-day history of progressive, severe fatigue, dyspnea, forgetfulness, an inability to concentrate, and excessive thirst. He has also had lower back pain for the past 3 months.

On physical examination, the patient is confused. The heart rate is 120/min, respiration rate 14/min, and the blood pressure is 110/75 mm Hg. The oral mucosa is dry, and the spine is tender to light percussion.

Laboratory studies:

Hematocrit	27%
Leukocyte count	13,500/μL with a left shift
Platelet count	160,000/μL
Calcium	13.5 mg/dL
Creatinine	3.5 mg/dL

A radiograph of the lumbar spine shows osteopenia and compression fractures at T10 and L1. A bone marrow aspirate smear is shown (*see Figure 19 in Color Plates*).

Which of the following is the most likely diagnosis?

(A) Acute myeloid leukemia
(B) Chronic lymphocytic leukemia
(C) Megaloblastic anemia
(D) Metastatic small-cell carcinoma of the lung
(E) Multiple myeloma

Item 29

A 74-year-old woman is evaluated for follow-up of a high total protein measurement found during a recent routine evaluation. She has hypertension for which she takes ramipril. Her medical history is otherwise noncontributory.

On physical examination, heart rate is 80/min, and blood pressure is 140/80 mm Hg. There is no bone tenderness, splenomegaly, or lymphadenopathy.

Laboratory studies:

Hemoglobin	13.5 g/dL
Leukocyte count	7200/μL
Platelet count	247,000/μL
Total protein	8.0 g/dL
Creatinine	Normal
Calcium	Normal

Serum protein electrophoresis reveals a 1.2-g/dL monoclonal protein spike, further identified as IgG-κ by immunofixation. Bone marrow aspirate smear shows 7% plasmacytosis. No lytic lesions are detected on bone survey.

Which of the following is the most appropriate next step in the management of this patient?

(A) Bisphosphonates
(B) Positron emission tomography
(C) Repeated serum protein electrophoresis in 3 to 6 months
(D) Thalidomide and dexamethasone

Chapter 5

Hematology

Answers and Critiques

Item 1   **Answer: B**

This patient's presenting symptom of pruritus while showering and the elevated hematocrit value are typical of polycythemia vera. Major diagnostic criteria for this disease include an elevated red blood cell mass, normal arterial oxygen saturation, and the presence of splenomegaly. It is currently difficult to obtain a red blood cell mass study in many places in the United States; therefore, the diagnosis of polycythemia vera is frequently established by identifying an elevated hematocrit value in the absence of secondary causes of erythrocytosis. The presence of a low serum ferritin concentration in this patient reflects the increased use of endogenous iron stores as a consequence of increased bone marrow erythroid activity rather than iron deficiency caused by blood loss or decreased dietary iron consumption. A major cause of morbidity in patients with polycythemia vera is thrombosis, which can be alleviated by reducing the hematocrit to <45% with phlebotomy or by administering hydroxyurea. Patients with polycythemia vera may also have a mildly increased leukocyte or platelet count.

Myelodysplastic syndrome is a definitional diagnosis requiring cytopenia of at least one lineage. The differential diagnosis of cytopenia of any single lineage is broad (especially in patients with anemia), but the finding of cytopenias of more than one lineage increases the probability of a diagnosis of myelodysplastic syndrome. This patient does not have cytopenia and therefore does not have myelodysplasia.

Relative erythrocytosis is not associated with a true increase in red blood cell mass. The hematocrit or hemoglobin concentration in patients with relative erythrocytosis appears to be increased because of a reduction in plasma volume. This finding may occur as a result of dysentery, heat exhaustion, profound perspiration, capillary leak syndrome, vomiting, and diuretic use and rarely may be idiopathic. Patients with relative erythrocytosis do not have pruritus or increased platelet and leukocyte counts.

Secondary erythrocytosis is a true increase in red blood cell mass that is often mediated by erythropoietin. In rare circumstances, however, a mutation in the erythropoietin receptor may cause secondary erythrocytosis. Erythropoietin-mediated secondary erythrocytosis may be either congenital or acquired. Examples of congenital secondary erythrocytosis include high-oxygen-affinity hemoglobinopathy (autosomal dominant), familial 2,3-diphosphoglycerate deficiency (auto-

somal recessive), benign familial erythrocytosis (autosomal dominant), or autosomal recessive familial erythrocytosis. Examples of acquired secondary erythrocytosis include either central hypoxia (chronic obstructive pulmonary disease, intracardiac shunts, smoking) or peripheral hypoxia (renal vascular disease). Acquired secondary erythrocytosis may also result from pathologic production of erythropoietin by tumors (hepatoma, hypernephroma, cerebellar hemangioblastoma). The normal arterial oxygen saturation rules out secondary erythrocytosis due to smoking in this patient.

KEY POINT

- Major diagnostic criteria of polycythemia vera include an elevated red blood cell mass, a normal arterial oxygen saturation, and the presence of splenomegaly.

Bibliography

1. **Tefferi A**. Polycythemia vera: a comprehensive review and clinical recommendations. Mayo Clin Proc. 2003;78:174-94. [PMID: 12583529]

Item 2   **Answer: A**

Anemia of inflammation is most likely causing this patient's anemia. The patient has signs and symptoms of pneumonia. During infection, iron levels decrease, reflecting sequestration of iron in body storage pools (due to increased levels of hepcidin) and binding of iron by bacterial lactoferrin (which bacteria use to support their growth). Inflammatory cytokine levels also increase during infection, which profoundly affects transferrin and ferritin expression and results in low total iron-binding capacity, low transferrin levels (200–360 mg/mL), and high ferritin levels. Therefore, expected laboratory study findings during periods of inflammation include low or low-normal iron levels and total iron-binding capacity and normal or high ferritin levels, which this patient has.

This patient's ratio of iron to total iron-binding capacity is 0.09, which suggests iron deficiency anemia. However, 20% of patients with anemia of inflammation have iron/total iron-binding capacity ratios less than 0.10. Therefore, this patient's low iron/total iron-binding capacity ratio does not necessarily support a diagnosis of iron deficiency anemia, which generally also is associated with high-normal to high transferrin levels and total iron-binding capacity. In iron deficiency anemia, decreased ferritin levels reflect reduced storage pools of iron; conversely, in anemia of inflammation, inflammatory cytokines may increase ferritin levels by as much as threefold.

Therefore, combined iron deficiency anemia and anemia of inflammation often is associated with low-normal ferritin levels, whereas this patient has high-normal ferritin levels.

This patient has a low-normal mean corpuscular hemoglobin level, low-normal mean corpuscular volume, and mid-normal mean corpuscular hemoglobin concentration. Hypochromic and/or microcytic erythrocytes are present in both iron deficiency anemia and anemia of inflammation. Sideroblastic anemia may potentially cause hypochromic anemia but also is often associated with a high iron/total iron-binding capacity ratio and high or high-normal ferritin levels, which reflect the abnormal accumulation of iron in sideroblasts.

KEY POINT

• In anemia of inflammation, expected laboratory findings include low or low-normal iron levels and total iron-binding capacity and normal or high ferritin levels.

Bibliography
1. **Weiss G, Goodnough LT**. Anemia of chronic disease. N Engl J Med. 2005;352:1011-23. [PMID: 15758012]

Item 3   Answer: B

This patient has pancytopenia and hypocellular bone marrow consistent with a diagnosis of aplastic anemia. Fifty per cent of patients with aplastic anemia have no obvious cause, such as exposure to toxins, drug administration, or viral infection, to account for the development of the disease. Immunosuppressive therapy with antithymocyte globulin and cyclosporine has been shown to be effective in reducing transfusion requirements in more than 70% of patients with aplastic anemia and would be the preferred therapy for this patient.

Although patients with acute myeloid leukemia commonly present with pancytopenia, their bone marrow is typically hypercellular rather than hypocellular. Invasion of bone marrow by any solid tumor or hematologic malignancy may result in pancytopenia. A peripheral blood smear may show teardrop cells, nucleated red blood cells, and immature cells consistent with marrow-invasive tumor or leukemia, lymphoma, or chronic inflammatory disease, findings that this patient does not have. Chronic viral diseases, granulomatous diseases (tuberculosis), or, rarely, bacterial infections may cause pancytopenia with a cellular marrow or may evolve into true aplastic anemia. However, clinical evidence of hepatitis with elevated liver chemistry test results (aspartate aminotransferase, alanine aminotransferase) that would support a diagnosis of hepatitis B is absent in this patient.

KEY POINT

• Pancytopenia and hypocellular bone marrow are consistent with a diagnosis of aplastic anemia.

Bibliography
1. **Young NS, Calado RT, Scheinberg P.** Current concepts in the pathophysiology and treatment of aplastic anemia. Blood. 2006;108:2509-19. Epub 2006 Jun 15. [PMID: 16778145]

Item 4   Answer: B

This patient most likely has autoimmune hemolytic anemia characterized by markedly accelerated destruction of erythrocytes after release from marrow accompanied by an elevated reticulocyte count. The most common type of autoimmune hemolytic anemia is warm-antibody mediated. In this condition, IgG antibodies bind to Rh-type antigens on the erythrocyte surface at 37 °C and facilitate Fc-receptor-mediated erythrocyte destruction by splenic macrophages. Patients have microspherocytes on their peripheral blood smear, as does this patient, in addition to an increased reticulocyte count. Warm antibodies are diagnosed by the direct antiglobulin test (direct Coombs' test); however, 5% to 10% of patients with warm-antibody autoimmune hemolytic anemia have a normal Coombs' test.

This patient's elevated reticulocyte count is not compatible with aplastic anemia. Bleeding can mimic hemolysis in that the hemoglobin concentration can fall rapidly and, in an iron-replete patient, the reticulocyte count is elevated. In patients with severe anemia, as in this patient, the bleeding is clinically apparent with obvious external loss of blood. Internal bleeding with resorption of hematomas is less common and sometimes occult and may cause confusion with hemolytic anemia, but the presence of microspherocytes confirms the diagnosis of autoimmune hemolytic anemia. Thrombotic thrombocytopenic purpura usually presents with neurologic symptoms of varying and variable severity, and there is always severe fragmentation anemia and thrombocytopenia; none of these signs are present in this patient. Malaria is characterized by fever, splenomegaly, and hemolysis in a patient with an appropriate travel history. Finding intraerythrocytic parasites on a peripheral blood smear is diagnostic. The lack of fever, travel history, and intraerythrocytic parasites on the blood smear excludes this diagnosis in this patient.

KEY POINT

• Autoimmune hemolytic anemia is characterized by anemia, an elevated reticulocyte count, and microspherocytes on the peripheral blood smear.

Bibliography
1. **Bain BJ.** Diagnosis from the blood smear. N Engl J Med. 2005;353:498-507. [PMID: 16079373]

Item 5   Answer: D

This patient has vitamin B_{12} deficiency, which leads to macrocytosis. Severe vitamin B_{12} deficiency can also cause ineffective hematopoiesis characterized by a relative pancytopenia. Patients with this deficiency have hemolysis typified by elevated lactate dehydrogenase and unconjugated (indirect) bilirubin levels. Low vitamin B_{12} levels are associated with neuropsychiatric findings, including increased forgetfulness. Supplemental vitamin B_{12} does not always reverse these neurologic findings, although replacement of this vitamin can prevent further deterioration of mental status. The serum vitamin B_{12} concentration is not a good measurement of tissue cobalamin levels.

Patients with a vitamin B_{12} deficiency have elevated serum methylmalonic acid and homocysteine concentrations. Conversely, patients with a folate deficiency have an elevated homocysteine concentration only. Although myelodysplasia can cause macrocytosis, it does not cause the other abnormalities found in this patient. Autoimmune hemolytic anemia is not associated with abnormalities of either homocysteine or methylmalonic acid. Neither myelodysplasia nor autoimmune hemolytic anemia is associated with memory disturbance.

KEY POINTS

- The serum vitamin B_{12} level is not a good measurement of tissue cobalamin levels.

- Patients with a vitamin B_{12} deficiency have elevated serum methylmalonic acid and homocysteine concentrations.

- Patients with a folate deficiency have an elevated homocysteine concentration only.

Bibliography
1. Cravens DD, Nashelsky J, Oh RC. Clinical inquiries. How do we evaluate a marginally low B12 level? J Fam Pract. 2007;56:62-3. [PMID: 17217902]

Item 6   Answer: A

This patient's peripheral blood smear shows evidence of hereditary spherocytosis, a disorder of the skeletal membrane proteins in the red blood cell. The most appropriate next diagnostic step is to review the peripheral blood smear of her family members. This patient's hematologic findings are characterized by spherocytic red blood cells, which are found in patients with warm-antibody autoimmune hemolytic anemia (AIHA) and hereditary spherocytosis. However, patients with hereditary spherocytosis typically have predominantly spherocytic red blood cells on the peripheral blood smear, whereas patients with warm-antibody AIHA may also have some normal-shaped cells. Hereditary spherocytosis is distinguished by a mild, Coombs'-negative hemolytic anemia, and an elevated mean corpuscular hemoglobin concentration that occurs because spherocytes contain more hemoglobin per unit of volume than normal red blood cells,. In addition, spherocytes from any cause have increased osmotic fragility and are more prone to hemolysis when placed in a hypotonic solution. This phenomenon is analogous to a "full" water balloon that is more prone to rupture than a partially deflated balloon when additional water is added.

Splenomegaly of any cause can induce hemolysis; hypersplenism may also decrease the number of leukocytes, platelets, or any combination of cell lines. Hemolysis due to hypersplenism is usually modest and somewhat proportional to the size of the spleen. Hypersplenism per se produces no morphologic changes in red blood cells, but the peripheral

blood smear may show changes related to the underlying cause (e.g., target cells with liver disease). Hypersplenism does not cause spherocytosis, making this diagnosis unlikely in this patient. The peripheral blood smear in patients with iron deficiency anemia is characterized by hypochromia, microcytosis, and increased red blood cells of various sizes and shapes. The patient's peripheral blood smear does not show any of these changes, effectively ruling out iron deficiency anemia. β-Thalassemia trait (thalassemia minor) is characterized by mild microcytic anemia due to reduced expression of the β-globin gene and occurs in persons of African, Mediterranean, Middle Eastern, and Southeast Asian ancestry. The presence of spherocytes and absence of target cells make β-thalassemia trait unlikely in this patient.

KEY POINT

- Patients with hereditary spherocytosis have predominantly spherocytic red blood cells on the peripheral blood smear and an elevated mean corpuscular hemoglobin concentration.

Bibliography
1. Bolton-Maggs PH, Stevens RF, Dodd NJ, Lamont G, Tittensor P, King MJ, et al. Guidelines for the diagnosis and management of hereditary spherocytosis. Br J Haematol. 2004;126:455-74. [PMID: 15287938]

Item 7   Answer: B

This patient has iron deficiency anemia. The peripheral blood smear of patients with iron deficiency anemia shows microcytic hypochromic red blood cells, abnormalities in the size (anisocytosis) and shape (poikilocytosis) of red blood cells, and, occasionally, red blood cells of bizarre shapes, such as cigar-shaped cells. These abnormalities can lead to an increase in the reported red cell distribution width.

Thrombotic thrombocytopenic purpura is a disease characterized by microangiopathic hemolytic anemia. Patients with microangiopathic hemolytic anemia have both fragmented and nucleated red blood cells on the peripheral blood smear and low platelet counts, whereas those with iron deficiency anemia have anisocytosis, microcytosis, thrombocytosis, and no nucleated red blood cells. Autoimmune hemolytic anemia is manifested by spherocytes on the peripheral blood smear, which are not present in this patient. Patients deficient in vitamin B_{12} have macrocytic red blood cells and hypersegmented neutrophils, a hematologic finding not present in this patient.

KEY POINT

- Hematologic findings in patients with iron deficiency anemia consist of microcytic hypochromic red blood cells, abnormalities in the size and shape of red blood cells, and occasional bizarre-shaped red blood cells.

Bibliography
1. Killip S, Bennett JM, Chambers MD. Iron deficiency anemia. Am Fam Physician. 2007;75:671-8. [PMID: 17375513]

Item 8   Answer: D

This patient has the α-thalassemia trait, which is characterized by a two-gene defect ([α,–]/[α,—]). Chromosome 16 normally contains two copies of an α gene. The α-thalassemias occur when there are defects in transcription or translation of any of the four α-globin genes. A two-gene defect leads to mild microcytic anemia with prominent target cells, as shown in this patient's peripheral blood smear; the hemoglobin electrophoretic pattern is normal in these patients. Additionally, patients with thalassemia typically have preserved or increased red blood cell counts compared with patients with iron deficiency, who have a reduced red blood cell count.

Iron deficiency anemia is characterized by findings of varying severity with hypochromia, microcytosis, an increased red blood cell distribution width, and a decreased red blood cell count. This anemia is common in women of childbearing age and is usually due to menstrual or gastrointestinal blood loss. Autoimmune hemolytic anemia is associated with an elevated reticulocyte count and microspherocytes. Target cells are not found in patients with autoimmune hemolytic anemia. Sickle cell anemia is usually associated with some manifestation of the disease during childhood, including acute pain episodes. The average hemoglobin level is 7 to 8 g/dL, and the anemia is normochromic normocytic with a high reticulocyte count because of chronic hemolysis. A microcytic anemia is not characteristic of sickle cell anemia unless there is a co-existing thalassemia.

KEY POINT

- Patients who have α-thalassemia trait have mild microcytic anemia with prominent target cells on peripheral blood smear.

Bibliography
1. **Weatherall DJ, Provan AB**. Red cells I: inherited anaemias. Lancet. 2000;355:1169-75. [PMID: 10791394]

Item 9   Answer: A

This patient has iron deficiency anemia and is symptomatic and older than 50 years. Colon cancer must therefore be considered, and colonoscopy is indicated. In iron deficiency anemia, the peripheral blood smear shows microcytic, hypochromic erythrocytes with marked anisopoikilocytosis. Thrombocytosis is common. The serum iron concentration, a poor reflection of iron stores, is usually low; the total iron-binding capacity (TIBC) is high and the ferritin level is low. Because ferritin levels can increase in inflammatory states, serum ferritin may be normal or elevated in iron deficiency but a finding <12 ng/mL is very specific for iron deficiency. A serum ferritin level of 12–20 ng/mL suggests iron deficiency or markedly depleted iron stores, possibly associated with another cause of anemia, such as inflammation. A serum ferritin concentration >20 ng/mL does not exclude iron deficiency in patients with inflammation or liver disease. The serum transferrin saturation [(serum iron/TIBC) × 100] is frequently low in the anemia of inflammation as well as in iron

deficiency. This patient's low hematocrit, microcytosis, low serum iron, and elevated TIBC support a diagnosis of iron deficiency anemia.

CT scans or MRI of the abdomen cannot diagnose colonic mucosal abnormalities associated with adenomas or early cancer and are not used in the initial evaluation of iron deficiency anemia. Virtual colonoscopy, using CT scans or MRI with three-dimensional reconstruction, may be a possible screening test in the future. A positive virtual colonoscopy requires a follow-up standard colonoscopy and biopsy of all abnormal lesions and is not an appropriate diagnostic modality in patients with iron deficiency anemia in whom the pretest probability of an abnormality is high. Hypothyroidism has been linked to iron deficiency anemia; however, this patient's thyroid-stimulating hormone level is normal, ruling out hypothyroidism. Thyroxine replacement is therefore not indicated.

KEY POINT

- In a patient with iron deficiency anemia who is older than 50 years, colon cancer must be considered and colonoscopy is therefore indicated.

Bibliography
1. **Smith RA, Cokkinides V, Eyre HJ; American Cancer Society.** American Cancer Society guidelines for the early detection of cancer, 2003. CA Cancer J Clin. 2003;53:27-43. [PMID: 12568442]

Item 10   Answer: D

This patient has asymptomatic anemia of inflammation (also called anemia of chronic disease) and does not require therapy. Anemia of inflammation is caused by increased interleukin-6 levels, which result in increased hepcidin levels. Hepcidin decreases iron absorption from the gut and decreases iron release from macrophages. Anemia of inflammation is characterized by a low or normal serum iron concentration, reduced total iron-binding capacity, and a serum ferritin concentration that is either normal or increased; a low serum ferritin concentration is most consistent with iron deficiency anemia. Anemia of inflammation usually results in a hemoglobin concentration of 8 to 10 g/dL.

Red blood cell transfusion is seldom required in patients with anemia of inflammation and, when used, is always reserved for those with symptomatic anemia regardless of its cause. Iron, supplemental erythropoietin, or any specific treatment is not required in a patient with asymptomatic anemia of inflammation and a hemoglobin concentration ≥10 g/dL. The treatment of choice is to manage the condition responsible for the chronic inflammation, in this case, the patient's rheumatoid arthritis.

KEY POINT

- Anemia of inflammation is characterized by a low or normal serum iron concentration, reduced serum total iron-binding capacity, and a serum ferritin concentration that is either normal or increased.

Bibliography

1. **Andrews NC**. Anemia of inflammation: the cytokine-hepcidin link. J Clin Invest. 2004;113:1251-3. [PMID: 15124013]

Item 11   Answer: A

This patient has warm-antibody autoimmune hemolytic anemia (AIHA); the first step in treatment is corticosteroid therapy. Polychromasia in patients with AIHA usually results from reticulocytosis. Reticulocytes contain nucleic acids that stain blue. Warm-antibody AIHA occurs when IgG antibodies bind to red blood cell antigens (usually of the Rh-type) at body temperature. These cells are eventually cleared by splenic macrophages. Spherocytes are detected in patients with warm-antibody AIHA because of membrane removal by macrophages in the spleen. Although warm-antibody AIHA is initially treated with corticosteroid therapy, intravenous immune globulin and splenectomy are also treatment options. However, intravenous immune globulin has not been shown to be as effective as corticosteroid therapy in these patients.

Red blood cells are microcytic in patients with iron deficiency, and reticulocytosis is decreased in the absence of iron. Therefore, iron and erythropoietin are not useful in the treatment of this patient. Plasmapheresis is used in the treatment of thrombotic thrombocytopenic purpura, which is a microangiopathic hemolytic anemia characterized by the presence of schistocytes.

KEY POINT

- The initial treatment in patients with warm-antibody autoimmune hemolytic anemia is corticosteroid therapy.

Bibliography

1. **Gehrs BC, Friedberg RC**. Autoimmune hemolytic anemia. Am J Hematol. 2002;69:258-71. [PMID: 11921020]

Item 12   Answer: D

This patient has iron deficiency anemia, most likely resulting from chronic gastric bleeding. He requires iron replacement therapy in addition to careful monitoring and follow-up. The response to oral iron is fast, with a response in this patient likely to occur in less than 1 week. There is no evidence of malabsorption; therefore, intravenous iron is not indicated.

This patient's chronic dyspnea is due to poor lung function and not a lack of oxygen-carrying capacity. There is little evidence that increasing the circulating red blood cell mass at his current hemoglobin concentration will improve tissue oxygenation in a patient with pulmonary disease. In the intensive-care setting, a liberal transfusion strategy to a target hemoglobin concentration of 10 to 12 g/dL in euvolemic patients was associated with a higher overall mortality rate when compared with a restrictive transfusion strategy to a target hemoglobin level of 7 to 9 g/dL. This adverse effect of the higher hemoglobin concentration may occur because the higher hematocrit increases viscosity and, consequently, impairs capillary blood flow. The patient's cardiac history is not a reason to institute blood transfusion. If he were having an acute ischemic event, some studies suggest transfusion is desirable to increase the hematocrit concentration to >30%, but even this approach has been questioned recently.

This patient's signs, symptoms, and laboratory findings are not suggestive of renal disease, which may cause a low erythropoietin level or a bone marrow disorder that would require administration of supraphysiologic levels of erythropoietin. Moreover, erythropoietin therapy would be ineffective in this patient until iron has become available for red blood cell production.

KEY POINT

- Patients with iron deficiency anemia require oral iron replacement therapy.

Bibliography

1. **Killip S, Bennett JM, Chambers MD**. Iron deficiency anemia. Am Fam Physician. 2007;75:671-8. [PMID: 17375513]

Item 13   Answer: D

This patient has myelodysplastic syndrome, which is a definitional diagnosis requiring cytopenia of at least one cell lineage. Anemia is the most common laboratory finding in myelodysplastic syndrome (54% of patients have a hemoglobin concentration of <10 g/dL). Myelodysplastic syndrome was first identified as a clinical entity separate from acute myeloid leukemia based on the findings that the former has a more indolent natural history and is a clonal neoplastic condition related to acute myeloid leukemia. The differential diagnosis of cytopenia of any single lineage is broad (especially in patients with anemia), but the finding of cytopenias of more than one lineage increases the probability of a diagnosis of myelodysplastic syndrome. Review of the peripheral blood smear or bone marrow aspirate may identify evidence of dysplasia (e.g., bilobed neutrophils) that may further support the diagnosis. In this patient, subcutaneous erythropoietin therapy may improve anemia and reduce transfusion requirements.

Lead toxicity is associated with a microcytic anemia with sideroblasts in the bone marrow and is usually, but not invariably, found in children. This patient has a normocytic anemia and lacks bone marrow sideroblasts. In addition, dysplastic neutrophils, as seen in this patient's peripheral blood smear, are not found in patients with lead toxicity. In patients with acute myeloid leukemia (AML), quantitative abnormalities on the complete blood count require direct examination of the peripheral blood smear. Direct examination will typically reveal abnormal populations of cells (e.g., blasts); some blasts may contain Auer rods. Acute myeloid leukemia is associated with >20% blasts in the bone marrow by the World Health Organization (WHO) classification, and this finding is absent in this patient. Folate deficiency is associated with a macrocytic anemia with megaloblastic bone marrow abnormalities and most commonly occurs in patients with chronic alcoholism.

KEY POINT

- Myelodysplastic syndrome is a definitional diagnosis requiring cytopenia of at least one lineage.

Bibliography

1. Steensma DP, Bennett JM. The myelodysplastic syndromes: diagnosis and treatment. Mayo Clin Proc. 2006;81:104-30. [PMID: 16438486]

Item 14   Answer: D

The test most likely to establish the diagnosis is an inhibitor screen and factor VIII level. This patient has developed an acquired, rather than an inherited, coagulopathy because all of her coagulation studies were normal before childbirth 3 months earlier, and she tolerated a surgical procedure without difficulty. Her current constellation of symptoms and laboratory abnormalities is consistent with the development of a factor VIII inhibitor. These inhibitors characteristically develop in association with certain malignancies, particularly lymphomas; in patients with autoimmune disorders; and in the postpartum setting. Diagnosis of the presence of an inhibitor occurs by first performing a mixing study, or inhibitor screen, in which the patient's plasma and normal plasma are mixed in a 1:1 ratio, and the abnormal test is repeated. If the coagulation abnormality results from a factor deficiency, the test result using the mixed plasmas will normalize. However, if an inhibitor is present, the added factor from the control plasma will also be neutralized, and the abnormal study will not be corrected. Therefore, if this patient has developed a factor VIII inhibitor, the mixing study will not correct the abnormality, and a confirmatory measurement of factor VIII activity should then be performed. If the factor VIII activity level is low, additional studies to measure the inhibitor titer would be indicated.

The bleeding time is a relatively nonspecific test, and platelet dysfunction would not result in a new prolongation of the activated partial thromboplastin time. The fibrinogen concentration is often low, and fibrin degradation products and fibrin D-dimer levels are often elevated in patients with disseminated intravascular coagulation, but this disorder would be unlikely in an otherwise healthy patient. Moreover, the prothrombin time is generally prolonged preferentially in patients with disseminated intravascular coagulation, whereas the activated partial thromboplastin time remains normal or is only mildly increased in such patients.

KEY POINTS

- Bleeding symptoms and hematologic abnormalities in patients with autoimmune disorders, malignancy, or in the postpartum setting may be due to an acquired factor VIII inhibitor.

- Diagnosis of the presence of an inhibitor occurs by first performing a mixing study, or inhibitor screen, in which the patient's

plasma and normal plasma are mixed in a 1:1 ratio, and the abnormal test is repeated.

Bibliography

1. Acharya SS, DiMichele DM. Management of factor VIII inhibitors. Best Pract Res Clin Haematol. 2006;19:51-66. [PMID: 16377541]

Item 15   Answer: D

The patient has von Willebrand's disease (vWD), which is characterized by primary hemostatic dysfunction and is associated with factor VIII deficiency. vWD is one of the most common disorders of primary hemostasis, occurring in 1:100 to 1:400 people and should be suspected if the activated partial thromboplastin time (aPTT), bleeding time or Platelet Function Analyzer (PFA-100®) test is prolonged. vWD is caused by deficiency or dysfunction of von Willebrand factor (vWF), which mediates the adhesion of platelets to sites of vascular damage. vWD is inherited as an autosomal disorder, and a family history and the patient's personal history usually reveal manifestations of a primary platelet dysfunction such as mucosal bleeding, epistaxis, gingival bleeding, menorrhagia, or purpura. Since vWF stabilizes factor VIII in the circulation, diminished levels of vWF can be associated with diminished activity of factor VIII and prolongation of the aPTT. In patients with vWD, the aPTT will correct when mixed with normal plasma. It is common for vWD to go undiagnosed for many years.

Hemophilia A and B are X-linked recessive disorders (occurring almost exclusively in men) and are characterized by joint and deep muscle bleeding rather than mucosal bleeding. Hemophilia A is characterized by deficiency of factor VIII and hemophilia B by deficiency of factor IX; however, both disorders are associated with a prolonged aPTT and both correct with mixing studies. A factor VIII inhibitor is unlikely because a mixing study would not normalize the aPTT in the presence of an inhibitor. In these cases, the inhibitor inactivates the factor VIII in the normal plasma, and the prolonged aPTT persists.

KEY POINTS

- von Willebrand's disease should be suspected if the activated partial thromboplastin time, bleeding time, or Platelet Function Analyzer (PFA-100®) test is prolonged.

- von Willebrand's disease is inherited as an autosomal disorder; clinical manifestations correspond to a primary platelet disorder characterized by mucosal bleeding, epistaxis, gingival bleeding, menorrhagia, or purpura.

Bibliography

1. Pruthi RK. A practical approach to genetic testing for von Willebrand disease. Mayo Clin Proc. 2006;8:679-91. [PMID: 16706266]

Item 16   Answer: A

Acute chest syndrome (ACS) is characterized by fever, chest pain, shortness of breath, hypoxia, and a radiographically detected pulmonary infiltrate in a patient with a sickling disorder. This syndrome may be caused by infection, in situ thrombosis, atelectasis, fat embolism, or any combination of these events. ACS is a leading cause of death in patients with a sickling disorder. Red blood cell transfusion, by simple transfusion to a target hemoglobin level of 10 g/dL or by exchange transfusion, is necessary in patients with ACS to decrease blood viscosity and increase oxygen delivery. In addition, exchange transfusion may decrease the number of inflammatory cells and mediators of inflammation to improve the course of this disease.

Acute chest pain, especially in an older adult patient, may suggest myocardial infarction, but this diagnosis cannot explain the appearance of a localized pulmonary infiltrate. The musculoskeletal involvement in patients with sickle cell disease includes bone infarcts, avascular necrosis, leg ulcers, and osteomyelitis. Musculoskeletal chest pain cannot explain this patient's hypoxemia or pulmonary infiltrate. Pulmonary hypertension is a known complication of long-standing sickle cell disease and is associated with an increased risk of death in patients with this disease. However, pulmonary hypertension tends to develop insidiously, and patients present with progressive dyspnea on exertion, syncope or lightheadedness, and signs of right-sided heart failure. This patient's acute presentation of fever, a pulmonary infiltrate, and hypoxemia is not compatible with chronic pulmonary hypertension.

KEY POINT

- Acute chest syndrome is characterized by fever, chest pain, shortness of breath, hypoxia, and a pulmonary infiltrate in a patient with a sickling disorder.

Bibliography

1. Stuart MJ, Setty BN. Acute chest syndrome of sickle cell disease: new light on an old problem. Curr Opin Hematol. 2001;8:111-22. [PMID: 11224686]

Item 17   Answer: B

This patient has the acute chest syndrome, the most common form of pulmonary disease in patients with sickle cell anemia and a major cause of morbidity and mortality, and will likely benefit from long-term hydroxyurea therapy. Therapy with hydroxyurea reduces the number of acute pain episodes in patients with sickle cell anemia by 50% and decreases the frequency of the acute chest syndrome by 40%. Nine-year follow-up data from a 2-year, multicenter, double-blind, randomized, placebo-controlled trial showed that hydroxyurea use was associated with a 40% reduction in mortality in such patients. Daily oral hydroxyurea therapy is indicated for patients who have three or more acute painful episodes yearly that require in-patient parenteral opioid therapy. The diagnosis of the acute chest syndrome is established by identify-

ing an infiltrate on chest radiograph that involves at least one lung segment and that is not thought to be due to atelectasis. Associated findings include one or more of the following: chest pain; temperature >38.5 °C (101.3 °F); tachypnea, wheezing, cough, or the appearance of increased work of breathing (such as retractions); and hypoxemia relative to baseline oxygen saturation values. Common causative organisms are *Chlamydophila* (*Chlamydia*) and *Mycoplasma*, but respiratory syncytial virus, *Staphylococcus aureus*, and *Streptococcus pneumoniae* have been identified in some patients.

Patients with sickle cell anemia are at risk for proteinuria and chronic renal failure. Angiotensin-converting enzyme inhibitors such as captopril may help to prevent renal disease in patients who show signs of developing kidney dysfunction. However, this patient has a normal creatinine level and normal levels of microalbumin; therefore, angiotensin-converting enzyme inhibitor therapy is not indicated at this time. In children up to the age of 5 years, prophylactic penicillin (or a macrolide in patients with a penicillin allergy) decreases the risk of infections known to trigger the acute chest syndrome but is not useful in older patients. Recombinant erythropoietin is used in patients with sickle cell disease primarily to manage anemia due to underproduction of erythropoietin in patients who develop chronic renal failure.

KEY POINT

- In patients with sickle cell anemia, hydroxyurea therapy reduces the number of acute pain episodes by 50% and decreases the frequency of the acute chest syndrome by 40%.

Bibliography

1. Steinberg MH, Barton F, Castro O, Pegelow CH, Ballas SK, Kutlar A, et al. Effect of hydroxyurea on mortality and morbidity in adult sickle cell anemia: risks and benefits up to 9 years of treatment. JAMA. 2003;289:1645-51. Erratum in: JAMA. 2003;290:756. [PMID: 12672732]

Item 18   Answer: C

The rapidly decreasing platelet count occurring 6 days after initiation of heparin suggests that this patient's thrombocytopenia was most likely heparin induced; heparin therapy must stopped, and alternative anticoagulation with a direct thrombin inhibitor should be instituted immediately. Absolute thrombocytopenia had not yet developed in this patient by post-therapy day 6, but the presence of absolute thrombocytopenia is not always necessary for a diagnosis of heparin-induced thrombocytopenia (HIT). Although estimates of the risk for thrombosis after discontinuation of heparin vary, current recommendations suggest that all patients with HIT, even those without thrombosis, should receive alternative anticoagulation; therefore, simply discontinuing heparin and observing this patient is not sufficient. Currently available alternative anticoagulants for patients with HIT in the United States include the direct thrombin inhibitors argatroban and lepirudin. The former is approved for treatment of HIT in patients with or without thrombosis, the latter for the treatment of HIT in those with thrombosis.

Thrombotic thrombocytopenic purpura is characterized by thrombocytopenia, fever, microangiopathic hemolytic anemia, acute neurologic symptoms, and renal disease. Hemolytic uremic syndrome is characterized by thrombocytopenia, microangiopathic hemolytic anemia, and renal disease. The patient does not meet the clinical criteria for either of these disorders. Disseminated intravascular coagulation is a coagulopathy characterized by an elevated prothrombin time and activated partial thromboplastin time, low fibrinogen levels, and thrombocytopenia. The patient has no clinical signs of a coagulopathy, including an open wound that is not actively bleeding. Pseudothrombocytopenia is caused by in vitro clumping of platelets due to EDTA-dependent agglutinins, which may lead to falsely decreased platelet counts. Pseudothrombocytopenia is excluded by examination of a peripheral blood smear and also may be excluded by obtaining a platelet count in a citrate solution (which prevents platelet clumping).

KEY POINTS

- A rapidly falling platelet count occurring within days of heparin administration is indicative of heparin-induced thrombocytopenia (HIT).

- In patients with HIT, heparin therapy must stopped and alternative anticoagulation with a direct thrombin inhibitor instituted immediately.

Bibliography
1. **Menajovsky LB.** Heparin-induced thrombocytopenia: clinical manifestations and management strategies. Am J Med. 2005;118:21S-30S. [PMID: 16125511]

Item 19   Answer: C

This patient most likely has immune thrombocytopenic purpura (ITP). There is no gold standard for diagnosing ITP, and it is therefore a diagnosis of exclusion. Severe thrombocytopenia in a patient with a normal hemoglobin level and a normal leukocyte count and differential is consistent with ITP, and the diagnosis is further suggested in patients whose only symptoms are related to bleeding in the absence of fever, headache, or other constitutional manifestations. The physical examination is unremarkable except for signs of bleeding, including petechiae and ecchymoses.

Patients with aplastic anemia have anemia and leukopenia as well as a reduced platelet count, whereas this patient's only hematologic abnormality is thrombocytopenia. A mild qualitative platelet defect develops in all patients who use aspirin therapy but generally is not sufficiently severe to cause bleeding symptoms in the absence of additional defects in hemostasis. Patients with thrombotic thrombocytopenic purpura may have bleeding and severe thrombocytopenia, but this condition is almost always associated with microangiopathic hemolytic anemia, schistocytes on the peripheral blood smear,

and an elevated lactate dehydrogenase level. Patients with this multisystem condition may have fever, fluctuating neurologic symptoms and deficits, and renal disease. In von Willebrand's disease, inherited defects in the production or metabolism of von Willebrand factor lead to a qualitative platelet defect and bleeding manifestations. Characteristically, patients have prolonged partial thromboplastin and bleeding times and a normal platelet count. In addition, the platelet count is invariably normal in patients with this condition who also take aspirin.

KEY POINT

- Immune thrombocytopenic purpura is a likely diagnosis in patients who are healthy except for bleeding-related findings accompanied by severe thrombocytopenia and a normal hemoglobin level and leukocyte count.

Bibliography
1. **Cines DB, Blanchette VS.** Immune thrombocytopenic purpura. N Engl J Med. 2002;346:995-1008. [PMID: 11919310]

Item 20   Answer: A

This patient with mild, asymptomatic thrombocytopenia in the 30th week of an uncomplicated pregnancy and previously normal platelet counts has incidental thrombocytopenia of pregnancy (gestational thrombocytopenia). She requires close follow-up monitoring of the platelet count but should be reassured that the cause of her thrombocytopenia appears to be benign.

There are many possible causes of thrombocytopenia that occurs in the third trimester of pregnancy, including thrombocytopenia associated with hypertensive disorders or the HELLP syndrome (**h**emolysis with a microangiopathic blood smear, **e**levated **l**iver enzymes, **l**ow **p**latelets), hemolytic uremic syndrome, thrombotic thrombocytopenic purpura, and idiopathic thrombocytopenic purpura. However, incidental thrombocytopenia of pregnancy is the most common cause of thrombocytopenia in this setting. This disorder is not associated with either poor pregnancy outcomes or fetal morbidity. However, a decrease in the platelet count to below approximately 70,000/µL would be cause for heightened concern.

In this patient, HELLP syndrome is unlikely because of the normal hemoglobin level and normal liver chemistry tests. Hemolytic uremic syndrome and thrombotic thrombocytopenic purpura are both unlikely in the absence of anemia. Idiopathic thrombocytopenia is a possibility, but patients usually present with platelet counts <90,000/µL; therefore, careful follow-up of the patient's platelet count is essential.

KEY POINT

- Incidental thrombocytopenia of pregnancy (gestational thrombocytopenia) is the most common cause of thrombocytopenia during pregnancy.

Bibliography
1. **McCrae KR.** Thrombocytopenia in pregnancy: differential diagnosis, pathogenesis, and management. Blood Rev. 2003;17:7-14. [PMID: 12490206]

Item 21   Answer: C

This patient requires a bone marrow examination. She has thrombocytopenia with mild anemia and therefore does not have true isolated thrombocytopenia. Although immune thrombocytopenic purpura (ITP) is often believed to be a disorder that primarily affects young women, recent population-based studies have demonstrated that the age-specific incidence of ITP may actually be highest in the elderly. Therefore, ITP is a reasonable preliminary diagnosis in this patient. However, because of the presence of another hematologic abnormality (anemia), bone marrow aspiration and biopsy should be performed now. Anemia may be present in patients with ITP as the result of bleeding, but in an elderly patient with no history of bleeding and a normal fecal occult blood test, consideration of an alternative diagnosis is reasonable.

The use of other therapies, such as intravenous anti-Rh(D) immunoglobulin or intravenous immunoglobulin G, may be considered in patients with ITP who fail to respond to prednisone, but these agents should not be used until the diagnosis of ITP is more strongly established. Splenectomy is not indicated in this patient until a diagnosis of ITP is confirmed and she fails to respond to first-line therapy with prednisone. Moreover, even in patients with classic ITP who ultimately become refractory to therapy, most experts recommend bone marrow examination before splenectomy.

KEY POINTS

- Patients with immune thrombocytopenic purpura have isolated thrombocytopenia; anemia may be present as the result of bleeding.

- The incidence of immune thrombocytopenic purpura may actually be highest in the elderly.

Bibliography

1. **Chong BH, Ho SJ.** Autoimmune thrombocytopenia. J Thromb Haemost. 2005;3:1763-72. [PMID: 16102043]

Item 22   Answer: D

This patient has at least four of the five manifestations that comprise the pentad of thrombotic thrombocytopenic purpura (TTP), including fever, neurologic abnormalities, thrombocytopenia, and microangiopathic hemolytic anemia (anemia, schistocytes, and elevated lactate dehydrogenase concentration); the fifth manifestation of TTP is renal insufficiency. The treatment of choice for TTP is plasma exchange, which should be initiated as urgently as possible.

The systemic manifestations of systemic lupus erythematosus (SLE) can mimic all clinical features of TTP, but distinguishing features include the presence of a rash and autoimmune hemolysis in patients with SLE. This patient has no other manifestations of SLE, making this diagnosis less likely. Rocky Mountain spotted fever is an acute illness progressing over a few days that is characterized by multiple-organ failure with confusion or coma. Purpura and hypotension, which may be

fulminant, are also characteristic. However, the high fever with chills and extensive purpura characteristic of Rocky Mountain spotted fever are not characteristic of TTP. Immune thrombocytopenic purpura (ITP) is a diagnosis of exclusion. ITP is not associated with anemia, fever, neurologic abnormalities, or renal dysfunction and is therefore not a tenable diagnosis for this patient.

KEY POINT

- Thrombotic thrombocytopenic purpura (TTP) is characterized by fever, neurologic abnormalities, thrombocytopenia, microangiopathic hemolytic anemia, and renal insufficiency.

Bibliography

1. **Moake JL.** Thrombotic microangiopathies. N Engl J Med. 2002;347:589-600. [PMID: 12192020]

Item 23   Answer: B

The use of estrogen-containing oral contraceptives is associated with approximately a fourfold increased relative risk for venous thromboembolism in women of childbearing age without hereditary thrombophilia. This risk is increased to 35-fold in women who are heterozygous for the factor V Leiden mutation and is probably greater in those with a hereditary antithrombin deficiency. This patient has a heterozygous type I antithrombin deficiency (plasma antithrombin levels as determined by immunologic and functional assay are reduced to approximately 50% of normal). Oral contraceptives that contain only a progestational agent appear to confer little, if any, increased risk for venous thrombosis and are the best alternative for this patient. Barrier contraceptives and intrauterine devices confer no increased risk of thrombosis in this patient and are not contraindicated.

KEY POINT

- Estrogen oral contraceptives increase the risk of venous thromboembolism in women with thrombophilia.

Bibliography

1. **Gomes MP, Deitcher SR.** Risk of venous thromboembolic disease associated with hormonal contraceptives and hormone replacement therapy: a clinical review. Arch Intern Med. 2004;164:1965-76. [PMID: 15477430]

Item 24   Answer: D

This patient requires no further diagnostic tests at this time. Although pregnancy increases the risk for venous thromboembolism, testing for the presence of a hereditary thrombophilic disorder or markers of the antiphospholipid antibody syndrome (i.e., lupus anticoagulant and cardiolipin antibody concentration) does not alter the initial management or the duration of anticoagulant therapy in such patients. The factor V Leiden and prothrombin G20210A mutations are the most common mutations predisposing to venous thrombosis in white populations; they are, however, rarely found in native Asian and black populations. Although this patient does not have a family history of venous thrombosis, there is a small chance that she has an antithrombin, protein C, or protein S deficiency; however, pregnancy reduces the levels of protein C and S and their plasma levels are also depressed by oral anticoagulants. If follow-up testing is deemed appropriate, it will need to be postponed until after discontinuation of warfarin and completion of the pregnancy.

KEY POINTS

- Factor V Leiden and prothrombin G20210A mutations are the most common mutations predisposing to venous thrombosis in white populations, but are rare in Asian and black populations.

- Levels of protein C and protein S are reduced during pregnancy and while taking oral anticoagulants, making testing for deficiency unreliable during these times.

Bibliography
1. Lim W, Eikelboom JW, Ginsberg JS. Inherited thrombophilia and pregnancy associated venous thromboembolism. BMJ. 2007;334:1318-21. [PMID: 17585161]

Item 25   Answer: C

This patient has Philadelphia chromosome (Ph)–positive chronic myeloid leukemia (CML) with no evidence of disease acceleration or blast crisis. Imatinib mesylate is an oral drug that specifically targets and inhibits *BCR-ABL* tyrosine kinase activity and leads to suppression of the CML clone. In a large trial, imatinib mesylate was compared with interferon and low-dose cytarabine, the existing standard therapy for patients with newly diagnosed CML. Complete hematologic remission was achieved in 95% of patients treated with imatinib mesylate compared with 56% of those treated with interferon and low-dose cytarabine. In addition, imatinib mesylate was better tolerated than interferon and low-dose cytarabine. Complete cytogenetic remission rates (i.e., an absence of Ph-positive cells on karyotypic analysis) were also better in patients who received imatinib mesylate compared with interferon and cytarabine (85% vs. 22%).

Given her relatively young age, this patient should be considered for high-dose chemotherapy and allogeneic stem cell transplantation if she does not respond to imatinib mesylate or becomes refractory to treatment. Hydroxyurea may be helpful in controlling this patient's blood counts but results in significantly inferior remission rates compared with imatinib therapy. Observation alone is associated with poorer patient outcomes compared with therapy with imatinib mesylate.

KEY POINT

- Imatinib mesylate treatment for chronic myeloid leukemia is associated with complete hematologic remission in 95% of patients.

Bibliography
1. Schiffer CA. BCR-ABL tyrosine kinase inhibitors for chronic myelogenous leukemia. N Engl J Med. 2007;357:258-65. [PMID: 17634461]

Item 26   Answer: C

This patient has Philadelphia chromosome (Ph)–positive chronic myeloid leukemia. Chronic myeloid leukemia is a clonal proliferation of mature granulocytes associated with a (9;22)(q34;q11) translocation (Philadelphia chromosome). Patients usually present in chronic phase and may do well for years. Chronic myeloid leukemia is recognized by an elevated leukocyte count and increased numbers of granulocytic cells in all phases of development on the peripheral blood smear. Very immature cells or blasts represent 1% to 5% of the granulocytes, with increasing numbers of promyelocytes, myelocytes, and metamyelocytes. The diagnosis is confirmed by cytogenetic study of the bone marrow aspirate showing a t(9;22) chromosomal abnormality (Philadelphia chromosome) or the presence of the novel *BCR-ABL* gene produced by the translocation. The *BCR-ABL* gene is detected and quantitated by polymerase chain reaction. Chronic myeloid leukemia may transform into acute leukemia (myeloid in two thirds of patients, lymphoid in one third). The transformation may be recognized as an accelerated phase or as a blast crisis; evidence of transformed chronic myeloid leukemia is not found on this patient's peripheral blood smear or bone marrow aspirate specimens.

Chronic lymphoid leukemia is the most common leukemia encountered in adults. Patients may be asymptomatic or have nonspecific complaints of fever, night sweats, weight loss, fatigue, or malaise. Patients with splenomegaly may have early satiety or left upper quadrant abdominal pain. Lymphadenopathy, which is often painless, may be present. The key to diagnosis is the recognition of an increased leukocyte count and increased numbers of mature lymphocytes and "smudge" cells (lymphocytes that appear flattened or distorted) on the peripheral blood smear. The diagnosis of chronic lymphoid leukemia is confirmed by an absolute increase in mature lymphocytes (>5000/µL). Immunophenotyping by flow cytometry is necessary and will show a mature B cell lymphocyte phenotype with expression of CD19 and CD20 along with expression of a T lymphocyte antigen, CD5. Acute myeloid leukemia is a malignant clonal proliferation of myeloid cells that do not fully mature. The diagnosis is suggested by an elevated leukocyte count, anemia, thrombocytopenia, and blasts on the peripheral blood smear. The diagnosis is confirmed by bone marrow aspiration and biopsy showing >20% blasts. Typical myeloblasts demonstrate antigens found on immature cells, such as CD34 (stem cell marker), and HLA-DR, as well as antigens that are more specific for granulocytic maturation, such as CD33 and CD13.

KEY POINT

- Chronic myeloid leukemia is recognized by an elevated leukocyte count and increased numbers of granulocytic cells in all phases of development on the peripheral blood smear.

Bibliography
1. Hehlmann R, Hochhaus A, Baccarani M; European LeukemiaNet. Chronic myeloid leukaemia. Lancet. 2007;370:342-50. [PMID: 17662883]

Item 27   Answer: A

This patient with underlying myelodysplastic syndrome now has signs and symptoms suggestive of disease transformation to acute myeloid leukemia, including severe pancytopenia and circulating myeloid blasts. He requires induction chemotherapy containing cytarabine and an anthracycline. A bone marrow aspiration and biopsy can confirm the diagnosis and provide additional cytogenetic information. Many patients with refractory anemia with an excessive number of blasts will undergo transformation to acute leukemia during their lifetime.

Patients with thrombotic thrombocytopenic purpura can present with severe hemolytic anemia and thrombocytopenia; however, red blood cell fragmentation is not identified on the peripheral blood smear, and the myeloid blasts and chronic course of the patient's illness do not suggest the presence of thrombotic thrombocytopenic purpura.

Anemia of inflammatory disease (sometimes called anemia of chronic disease) is a commonly employed term for the nonspecific anemia associated with infectious, inflammatory, and neoplastic disorders. Anemia of inflammatory disease was once thought to be characterized by distinct abnormalities of iron metabolism, i.e., low serum iron and transferrin concentrations, reduced transferrin saturation, normal or elevated serum ferritin level, and normal or increased bone marrow iron stores. It is now recognized that this type of anemia is common in patients with other chronic disorders, can be present without the distinctive abnormalities in iron metabolism, and that the iron abnormalities are a secondary phenomenon and not responsible for the anemia. The anemia of inflammatory disease, however, is not associated with thrombocytopenia or the appearance of blast cells.

Tumor invasion of the bone marrow produces anemia with a low reticulocyte count and extramedullary hematopoiesis. Extramedullary hematopoiesis is signaled by the presence of nucleated red blood cell and myelocytes in the peripheral blood. These features are absent in this patient, making bone marrow invasion by tumor unlikely.

KEY POINT

• Signs suggestive of disease transformation from myelodysplastic syndrome to acute myeloid leukemia include severe pancytopenia and circulating myeloid blasts on the peripheral blood smear.

Bibliography
1. Steensma DP, Bennett JM. The myelodysplastic syndromes: diagnosis and treatment. Mayo Clin Proc. 2006;81:104-30. [PMID: 16438486]

Item 28   Answer: E

This patient has hypercalcemia, bone pain, and anemia, a characteristic presentation for multiple myeloma. The bone marrow aspirate reveals clusters of large plasma cells supporting this diagnosis. These cells can be easily distinguished from megaloblastic red blood cell precursors by their dispersed nuclear chromatin pattern and perinuclear halo. Red blood cell precursors on the bone marrow aspirate do not reveal any evidence of megaloblastic changes that would be present in megaloblastic anemia. Similarly, there is no hypersegmentation of the neutrophil precursors that is associated with megaloblastic anemia. Hypercalcemia with renal failure can occasionally occur in patients with chronic lymphocytic leukemia. However, this patient's relatively low leukocyte count and the morphologic findings of the bone marrow aspirate rule out this diagnosis.

Small-cell carcinoma of the lung can cause bone metastases with compression fractures and bone marrow failure due to malignant infiltration, but this neoplasm rarely causes hypercalcemia and does not result in infiltration of the bone marrow with plasma cells. Hypercalcemia caused by acute myeloid leukemia (AML) is rare. In addition, more severe bone marrow failure and a reduced platelet count would be likely in patients with AML. Although bone pain is common in patients with AML, compression fractures of the vertebrae are not. Finally, the bone marrow aspirate morphologic findings rule out AML because the smear does not depict diffuse infiltration with leukemic blasts.

KEY POINT

• Hypercalcemia, bone pain, anemia, and clusters of large plasma cells on bone marrow aspirate are diagnostic of multiple myeloma.

Bibliography
1. Kyle RA, Rajkumar SV. Multiple myeloma. N Engl J Med. 2004;351:1860-73. Erratum in: N Engl J Med. 2005;352:1163. [PMID: 15509819]

Item 29   Answer: C

This patient is best managed with a repeated serum protein electrophoresis in 3 to 6 months. She has a monoclonal gammopathy of unknown significance (MGUS), as characterized by the presence of serum monoclonal γ-globulin in the absence of clinical features of multiple myeloma, a relatively low paraprotein level (<3.5 g/dL), and <10% plasmacytosis in the bone marrow. The incidence of MGUS increases with age and may affect 5% of individuals >80 years of age. No anti–plasma cell treatment (i.e., thalidomide and dexamethasone) should be initiated for this patient. A routine follow-up examination to identify any signs and symptoms of progression to multiple myeloma and periodic measurement of monoclonal protein concentration are sufficient. The risk for progression to plasma cell malignancy appears to correlate with the initial paraprotein level, with the lowest risk in patients with a paraprotein concentration of ≤0.9 g/dL and the highest in those with a concentration of ≥3 g/dL.

This patient does not require further disease staging, and positron emission tomography is not the preferred staging technique for multiple myeloma. Bisphosphonate therapy is not indicated in the absence of bone disease.

KEY POINT

• Monoclonal gammopathy of unknown significance (MGUS) is characterized by the presence of serum monoclonal γ-globulin without the clinical features of multiple myeloma, a paraprotein level <3.5 g/dL, and <10% plasmacytosis in the bone marrow.

Bibliography

1. **Blade J.** Clinical practice. Monoclonal gammopathy of undetermined significance. N Engl J Med. 2006;355:2765-70. [PMID: 17192542]

Chapter 6

Infectious Disease Medicine

Infectious Disease Medicine contains self-assessment items that correspond to the following chapters in the *Internal Medicine Essentials for Clerkship Students 2* textbook:

Approach to Fever
Sepsis Syndrome
Common Upper Respiratory Problems
Urinary Tract Infection
Sexually Transmitted Diseases
Human Immunodeficiency Virus Infection
Nosocomial Infection
Tuberculosis
Community-Acquired Pneumonia
Infective Endocarditis
Osteomyelitis

Infectious Disease Medicine contains self assessment items that correspond to the following Training Problems in the *Core Medicine Clerkship Guide*:

Dysuria
Fever
Upper Respiratory Complaints
HIV Infection
Nosocomial Infections
Pneumonia

Chapter 6

Infectious Disease Medicine

Questions

Item 1

A 36-year-old man is evaluated in the office because of frothy, watery stools that are found to be positive for *Giardia lamblia* antigen. This is his third episode of giardiasis in the past 10 months. Previous episodes were treated with metronidazole, following which symptoms resolved and *G. lamblia* antigen was no longer found in stool specimens. The patient has also had two episodes of bronchitis and three episodes of sinusitis over the past 2 years. He is HIV negative and is a lifelong nonsmoker.

Metronidazole is prescribed.

Which of the following diagnostic studies should be done at this time?

(A) Bone marrow biopsy
(B) Colonoscopy with biopsies
(C) Measurement of cytoplasmic antineutrophil cytoplasmic antibody (c-ANCA)
(D) Measurement of serum IgG levels
(E) Upper endoscopy with duodenal aspirates for pathogens

Item 2

A 25-year-old woman is evaluated in the office for a 3-day history of a malodorous vaginal discharge. She does not have itching or irritation. She has been sexually active with the same partner for 6 months and uses condoms. Her medical history is unremarkable.

On physical examination, external genitalia are normal. Pelvic examination reveals a homogeneous, white, malodorous vaginal discharge that does not adhere to the vaginal walls. There is no vaginal erythema. Bimanual examination shows no cervical motion tenderness. Microscopic appearance of a stained wet prep of the vaginal material is shown (*see Figure 20 in Color Plates*).

Which of the following is the most likely diagnosis?

(A) Bacterial vaginosis
(B) *Candida* vaginitis
(C) Physiologic discharge
(D) *Trichomonas* vaginitis

Item 3

A 25-year-old woman is evaluated in the office because of a white, 'cottage cheese–like" vaginal discharge. She has no dysuria or hematuria and no history of sexually transmitted diseases. The patient has been sexually active with a single male partner for more than 3 years. Her only medication is an oral contraceptive. She and her partner do not use condoms.

Pelvic examination discloses a moderately thick, white vaginal discharge. The cervix is normal, and no ulcers are seen. The pH of the vaginal secretions is <4.5. A wet prep shows no motile organisms, and cervical specimens are sent for ligase chain reaction testing for both gonorrhea and chlamydial infection. A stained specimen of the vaginal material is shown (*see Figure 21 in Color Plates*).

Which of the following is the most likely diagnosis?

(A) Bacterial vaginosis
(B) *Candida* vaginitis
(C) *Chlamydia* cervicitis
(D) Gonorrhea
(E) Trichomoniasis

Item 4

A 45-year-old man is evaluated in the office for fever of 1 week's duration. Ten days ago, he was seen for upper respiratory tract congestion, cough, right maxillary pain, purulent nasal drainage, and generalized malaise for the previous 2 weeks. He was diagnosed with acute sinusitis and given a 14-day course of cephalexin. He noted improvement in all symptoms within 3 days. On day 4 of treatment, he felt warm and took his temperature; it was 38.5 °C (101.3 ° F). Fever has persisted daily for the past 7 days. His original symptoms have completely resolved, and he reports feeling well otherwise. He has no prior medical problems, has never been hospitalized, and takes no medications other than the cephalexin. He reports no allergies.

On physical examination, temperature is 38.3 °C (101.1 °F), blood pressure is 130/70 mm Hg, and heart rate is 88/min. The throat is normal without postnasal drip, erythema, or exudate. There is no sinus tenderness to palpation. Tympanic membranes are without evidence of inflammation or effusion. There is no lymphadenopathy. Lungs and cardiac examination are normal. There is no hepatic or splenic enlargement. Skin is normal.

Urinalysis and complete blood count are normal.

Which of the following is the most likely cause of his fever?

(A) Antibiotic-resistant sinusitis
(B) Drug fever
(C) Factitious fever
(D) Lymphoma
(E) Viral infection

Item 5

A 72-year-old woman who lives in a nursing home is brought to the emergency department because of a 2-day decline in alertness. She is normally ambulatory and communicative but requires assistance completing her activities of daily living. She has a history of Alzheimer's dementia and hypertension, and her medications are donepezil and atenolol.

On physical examination, the temperature is 35.0 °C (95.0 °F), blood pressure is 90/60 mm Hg, heart rate is 110/min, and respiration rate is 18/min. She is easily aroused but not communicative, and her skin is cool and mottled. Oxygen saturation is 90% with the patient breathing oxygen, 2 L/min, by nasal cannula. The mucous membranes are dry and crusted. Cardiac examination reveals tachycardia. The lungs are clear. The abdomen is soft, and there is suprapubic tenderness.

Laboratory studies: hemoglobin, 11.5 g/dL; leukocyte count, 15,000/µL (60% neutrophils, 15% band forms, 25% lymphocytes); serum creatinine, 1.6 mg/dL (baseline creatinine, 0.9 mg/dL). Urinalysis reveals 100 leukocytes/hpf; dipstick is positive for leukocyte esterase and nitrite.

Which of the following diagnoses is most consistent with this patient's presentation?

(A) Sepsis
(B) Septic shock
(C) Severe sepsis
(D) Systemic inflammatory response syndrome

Item 6

A 71-year-old woman is brought to the emergency department from a nursing home because of confusion, fever, and flank pain. On physical examination, temperature is 38.5 °C (101.3 °F), blood pressure is 82/48 mm Hg, heart rate is 123/min, and respiration rate is 27/min. Examination shows dry mucous membranes, costovertebral angle tenderness, poor skin turgor, and no edema. Leukocyte count is 15,600/µL; urinalysis shows 50–100 leukocytes and many bacteria/hpf. The patient has an anion-gap metabolic acidosis and high lactic acid levels. Antibiotic therapy is started.

Which of the following is most likely to improve survival for this patient?

(A) Aggressive fluid resuscitation
(B) 25% albumin infusion
(C) Hemodynamic monitoring with a pulmonary artery catheter
(D) Maintaining hemoglobin above 12 g/dL
(E) Maintaining P_{CO_2} below 50 mm Hg

Item 7

A 45-year-old man with rheumatoid arthritis calls the office because his teenage daughter has just been diagnosed with influenza. His current medications are prednisone and methotrexate. He has not received an influenza vaccination.

Which of the following is the most appropriate management for this patient?

(A) Intramuscular trivalent inactivated influenza vaccine
(B) Intranasal trivalent live-attenuated, cold-adapted influenza vaccine
(C) Oseltamivir
(D) Oseltamivir and intramuscular trivalent inactivated influenza vaccine

Item 8

A 45-year-old man with asthma is evaluated in the office because of malaise, myalgias, coryza, and a cough. Both influenza A and B are occurring in the community, and the patient has not been immunized against influenza. He takes an inhaled bronchodilator and inhaled corticosteroids. The patient has never traveled outside the United States.

On physical examination, he appears ill. Temperature is 38.3 °C (101 °F), blood pressure is 130/78 mm Hg, heart rate is 95/min, and respiration rate is 24/min. Expiratory wheezing is present.

A chest radiograph is normal.

Which of the following antiviral agents is most appropriate for this patient?

(A) Amantadine
(B) Oseltamivir
(C) Rimantadine
(D) Zanamivir

Item 9

A 24-year-old man requests antibiotics during an office evaluation for symptoms he has attributed to a sinus infection. He reports sinus congestion and clear nasal drainage that have persisted for 1 month after he developed a cold; he has no fever, sinus pain, purulent nasal drainage, sneezing, or nasal itching. Since the onset of his symptoms, he has been using a nasal decongestant spray twice daily with only short-term symptomatic relief, but he states that antibiotics have been effective in the past for treating his sinus infections. His history includes allergic rhinitis, but his primary allergens are not in season.

Nasal examination shows congested nasal mucosa with a profuse watery discharge. The nasal septum appears normal, the turbinates are pale, and there are no polyps. The remainder of the physical examination is normal.

Which of the following is the most likely diagnosis?

(A) Allergic rhinitis
(B) Bacterial sinusitis
(C) Nonallergic rhinitis
(D) Rhinitis medicamentosa
(E) Viral upper respiratory tract infection

Item 10

A 37-year-old woman is evaluated in the office for a 2-week history of sinus congestion. She initially thought she had a cold and felt better after taking an over-the-counter combination of oral pseudoephedrine and diphenhydramine; however, her symptoms returned, and she began having low-grade fevers and increased nasal secretions. She has no drug allergies.

On physical examination, the temperature is 37.4 °C (99.4 °F). There is right maxillary tenderness, erythematous turbinates, and yellowish-green nasal secretions.

Which of the following is the most appropriate management for this patient?

(A) Oral amoxicillin
(B) Oral amoxicillin–clavulanate
(C) Oral antihistamine
(D) Sinus CT scan
(E) Sinus radiograph

Item 11

A 30-year-old woman is evaluated in the office for a 2-day history of cough, nasal congestion, rhinorrhea, and constant frontal headache. She is otherwise healthy and takes no medications. She has no known drug allergies.

On physical examination, temperature is 37.9 °C (100.2 °F), heart rate is 68/min, and blood pressure is 120/70 mm Hg. She appears uncomfortable. The forehead is tender to palpation. The posterior pharynx is slightly erythematous with a visible white postnasal drip. The nasal mucosa is erythematous and congested, but there is no purulent discharge. The tympanic membranes are normal.

Which of the following is the most appropriate initial management for this patient?

(A) Amoxicillin
(B) Frontal and maxillary sinus radiography
(C) Sinus puncture and aspiration
(D) Symptomatic treatment

Item 12

A 27-year-old woman is evaluated in the office because of a 1-day history of dysuria, left flank pain, and fever. She does not have nausea or vomiting. The patient is sexually active. She had one episode of cystitis 3 months ago that was treated successfully with trimethoprim–sulfamethoxazole. Urine cultures were not obtained at that time.

On physical examination, the patient appears uncomfortable but not acutely ill. Temperature is 38.5 °C (101.3 °F), heart rate is 100/min, respiration rate is 18/min, and blood pressure is 120/78 mm Hg. There is pain on percussion of the left flank.

The leukocyte count is 20,000/µL with 80% segmented neutrophils and 5% band forms. Urinalysis shows 100 leukocytes/hpf and a positive test for leukocyte esterase. Pregnancy test is negative.

Which of the following is the most appropriate empiric therapy for this patient?

(A) Intravenous levofloxacin
(B) Intravenous trimethoprim–sulfamethoxazole
(C) Oral amoxicillin–clavulanate
(D) Oral levofloxacin
(E) Oral trimethoprim–sulfamethoxazole

Item 13

A 28-year-old woman is evaluated in the office for dysuria of 2 days' duration. She is healthy, sexually active, takes no medications and has no drug allergies.

On physical examination, vital signs are normal. There is mild suprapubic tenderness. A urine dipstick test is positive for leukocyte esterase and nitrite, and a urine pregnancy test is negative.

Which of the following is the most appropriate management for this patient?

(A) Amoxicillin for 7 days
(B) Cephalexin for 7 days
(C) Ciprofloxacin for 3 days
(D) Trimethoprim–sulfamethoxazole for 3 days
(E) Urine culture

Item 14

A 35-year-old man is evaluated in the office because of a 2-day history of painful sores on his penis without fever, headache, dysuria, or photophobia. He has never had similar lesions. The patient reports a new sexual partner for the past 6 months but does not know if his partner has a history of any sexually transmitted diseases.

On physical examination, vital signs are normal. There is no rash or evidence of meningismus. Nontender right inguinal lymphadenopathy is noted. Examination of the genitals is shown (*see Figure 22 in Color Plates*).

Which of the following is the most likely diagnosis?

(A) Group B streptococcal infection
(B) Herpes simplex virus infection
(C) Herpes zoster
(D) Syphilis

Item 15

A 23-year-old woman is evaluated in the office because of a 1-day history of genital pain, dysuria, and fever. She has never had similar symptoms and has not had photophobia, nausea, vomiting, or urinary retention. The patient has had only one sexual partner in her life, and he does not have genital lesions. They last had intercourse 5 days ago.

General physical examination is normal except for a temperature of 38.1 °C (100.6 °F). There is no nuchal rigidity. Findings on the vulva include red, eroded mucosa. The inguinal lymph nodes are moderately tender and enlarged bilaterally.

Which of the following antiviral agents is most appropriate at this time?

(A) Intravenous acyclovir
(B) Oral valacyclovir
(C) Topical acyclovir
(D) Topical penciclovir

Item 16

A 50-year-old man is evaluated in the office for a diffuse rash. One week ago, a nonpruritic red rash developed on his chest and back and was accompanied by malaise and a low-grade fever. He does not have headache, cough, abdominal pain, or dysuria. He has been otherwise healthy and takes no medications. He recently returned from a 2-week trip to Europe where he had multiple episodes of unprotected sex with men.

On physical examination, temperature is 37.3 °C (99.2 °F), blood pressure is 135/80 mm Hg, and heart rate is 82/min. The oropharynx is normal. There is generalized lymphadenopathy and a rash on his trunk, arms, and legs, with lesions on his palms, as shown (*see Figure 23 in Color Plates*). A serologic test for HIV is ordered.

Which of the following tests is most likely to establish the diagnosis?

(A) Herpes simplex virus IgG test
(B) Heterophile antibody test
(C) Polymerase chain reaction for *Chlamydia trachomatis*
(D) Potassium hydroxide stain of skin scrapings
(E) Rapid plasma reagin test

Item 17

A 28-year-old man with long-standing HIV infection is evaluated in the office for a 1-week history of dysphagia and mild odynophagia and a 2.3-kg (5-lb) weight loss. He has not had fever or hematemesis. History is significant for oropharyngeal candidiasis and *Pneumocystis jiroveci* (formerly *Pneumocystis carinii*) pneumonia. The patient is noncompliant about taking his highly active antiretroviral therapy (HAART).

Physical examination is normal except for oral thrush. His most recent CD4 cell count was 68/μL.

He is counseled regarding the importance of adhering to his HAART regimen.

Which of the following is the most appropriate next step in managing this patient's dysphagia and odynophagia?

(A) Barium swallow
(B) CT scan of the chest
(C) Fluconazole
(D) Omeprazole
(E) Upper endoscopy

Item 18

A 28-year-old man is evaluated at a community health center for a 10-day history of sore throat, headache, fever, anorexia, and muscle aches. Two days ago, a rash became apparent on his trunk and abdomen. He had been previously healthy and has not had any contacts with ill persons; he has had multiple male and female sex partners and infrequently uses condoms. He has been tested for HIV infection several times, most recently 8 months ago; all tests were negative.

On physical examination, his temperature is 38.6 °C (101.4 °F). He has several small ulcers on his tongue and buccal mucosa and cervical and supraclavicular lymphadenopathy. A faint maculopapular rash is present on his trunk and abdomen.

A rapid plasma reagin test is ordered.

Which of the following diagnostic studies should also be done at this time?

(A) CD4 cell count
(B) Epstein-Barr virus IgM
(C) HIV viral load
(D) Skin biopsy

Item 19

A 35-year-old man is diagnosed with HIV infection after he sought testing because of sexual exposure to another man approximately 5 years ago who he subsequently learned was HIV-infected. The patient is asymptomatic. Medical history is unremarkable, and he takes no medications.

On physical examination, he appears healthy. Vital signs and general examination are normal. The liver and spleen are not enlarged. CD4 cell count is 184/μL, and HIV RNA viral load is 13,043 copies/mL.

Which of the following is the most appropriate management at this time?

(A) Begin treatment with zidovudine
(B) Begin treatment with zidovudine, didanosine, and nelfinavir
(C) Delay treatment until the HIV RNA viral load is >100,000 copies/mL
(D) Delay treatment until the patient becomes symptomatic

Item 20

A 24-year-old man is evaluated in the office because of a lesion on his right arm that he first noticed 2 weeks ago. The patient has a 4-year history of HIV infection, most likely acquired after having sex with another man. He has been asymptomatic until now and has never received antiretroviral therapy. Currently, the CD4 cell count is 402/μL, and HIV RNA viral load is 14,355 copies/mL.

On physical examination, the patient appears well. Vital signs are normal. The skin lesion is shown (*see Figure 24 in Color Plates*). Examination of the skin and mucous membranes is otherwise normal. There is no lymphadenopathy or peripheral edema. Abdominal examination, including rectal examination, is normal.

Which of the following is the most likely diagnosis?

(A) Cherry angioma
(B) Dermatofibroma
(C) Hypersensitivity vasculitis
(D) Kaposi's sarcoma

Item 21

A 44-year-old man with HIV infection is hospitalized because of a 1-week history of progressive left lower extremity weakness and inability to walk. For the past 2 months, he has also had rapid weight loss, night sweats, and low-grade fever. Although HIV infection was diagnosed 2 years ago, the patient never returned for follow-up evaluation and treatment. His CD4 cell count at the time of diagnosis was 88/µL.

On physical examination on admission, he appears cachectic and chronically ill. Temperature is 38.1 °C (100.6 °F). Significant findings include thrush, splenomegaly, bilateral lower extremity weakness, and hyperreflexia.

MRIs of the brain are shown.

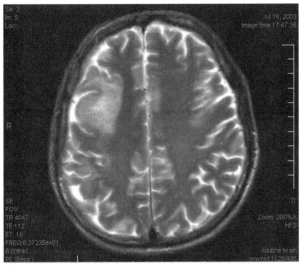

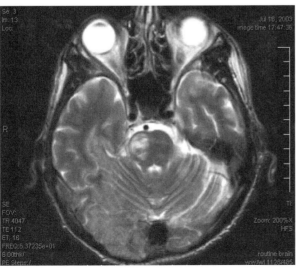

Lumbar puncture is performed; cerebrospinal fluid examination shows the following:

Opening pressure	Normal
Leukocyte count	21/µL with 98% lymphocytes and 2% neutrophils
Erythrocyte count	1/µL
Protein	85 mg/dL
Glucose	55 mg/dL
India ink stain	Negative
Cryptococcal antigen	Negative

Polymerase chain reaction is positive for polyomavirus JC and negative for Epstein–Barr virus.

Which of the following is the most likely diagnosis?

(A) Cerebral lymphoma
(B) Cerebral toxoplasmosis
(C) Cryptococcal meningitis
(D) Progressive multifocal leukoencephalopathy

Item 22

An excessive number of central line catheter-related bloodstream infections are occurring in an intensive care unit. The infections develop within 1 week of catheter placement.

A physician is observed placing a central venous catheter. She washes her hands with alcohol gel, selects the subclavian site for insertion, and cleanses the site with povidone-iodine. The patient is covered in a single, large sterile drape, and the physician wears a mask, sterile gown, and gloves.

Which of the observed practices is most likely to have contributed to the increased rate of bloodstream infections?

(A) Cleansing the insertion site with povidone-iodine
(B) Hand washing with alcohol gel
(C) Protective garb (mask, gown, gloves)
(D) Single draping of the patient
(E) Subclavian site for catheter insertion

Item 23

A 52-year-old man underwent right hip replacement surgery 2 days ago. Today he develops watery diarrhea with bowel movements every 1 to 2 hours. A stool assay is positive for *Clostridium difficile* toxin, and appropriate treatment is begun. The patient is in a two-bed hospital room.

Which of the following should be done to prevent the spread of *C. difficile* to the roommate and to other persons in the hospital?

(A) Bathe the patient with antiseptic soap
(B) Place the patient in contact isolation
(C) Place the patient in droplet isolation
(D) Place the patient in respiratory isolation

Item 24

A 39-year-old migrant worker from Central America comes to the emergency department because of a 2-month history of cough, occasional fever, night sweats, a 4.5-kg (10-lb) weight loss, and one episode of hemoptysis. The patient does not smoke or use alcohol or illicit drugs. Family members and friends are well, and he is unaware of exposure to anyone with tuberculosis. He has never received bacille Calmette–Guérin vaccine. The patient is in a monogamous sexual relationship and has never been tested for HIV.

Which of the following precautions is needed before evaluating this patient?

(A) Airborne isolation of the patient
(B) A mask for the patient
(C) Droplet precautions
(D) No special precautions are required

Item 25

An unusually high number of urinary tract infections are occurring in residents in a long-term-care facility. Many residents are infirm and incontinent and have indwelling urinary catheters in place.

Which of the following will most likely decrease the frequency of urinary tract infections in these residents?

(A) Acidification of the urine
(B) Administration of prophylactic antibiotics
(C) Changing of the indwelling catheters weekly
(D) Removal of the indwelling catheters whenever possible
(E) Washing the collecting bags with hydrogen peroxide

Item 26

A 25-year-old man is admitted to the intensive care unit after sustaining a closed head injury and a pneumothorax in a motor vehicle accident. He scores 5/15 on the Glasgow Coma Scale. A ventriculostomy tube and chest tube are placed, and intubation and mechanical ventilation are required to reduce elevated intracranial pressure.

Which of the following may reduce the risk of ventilator-associated pneumonia in this patient?

(A) Avoiding subglottic suctioning
(B) Changing the ventilator tubing every 3 days
(C) Keeping the patient at a 45-degree angle
(D) H_2-receptor antagonists
(E) Prophylactic intravenous antibiotics

Item 27

A 76-year-old woman is transferred to the intensive care unit after developing respiratory failure 48 hours after being admitted to the hospital for community-acquired pneumonia. She was hospitalized 2 weeks ago for urosepsis treated with ciprofloxacin for 10 days. At the time of the second admission, she had right lower and right middle lobar pulmonary consolidation but appeared clinically stable. Ceftriaxone therapy and heparin prophylaxis were started, but the following day her condition deteriorated, with worsening dyspnea, progressive hypox-

emia, and persistent fever, with oxygen saturation ranging from 80% to 85% with the patient breathing 100% oxygen.

On transfer to the intensive care unit, she is in severe respiratory distress, her heart rate is 124/min, and her respiration rate is 40/min, using the accessory muscles of respiration. She has rhonchi in all lung fields, and cardiac examination reveals no murmurs or gallops.

Chest radiograph shows diffuse bilateral pulmonary infiltrates.

Which of the following is the most appropriate next step in managing this patient?

(A) Bronchoscopy
(B) Change to vancomycin, cefepime, and ciprofloxacin
(C) CT scan of the chest
(D) Doppler ultrasonography of the legs

Item 28

A 40-year-old male high school teacher is evaluated because of a reactive tuberculin skin test of 12 mm of induration done as part of a pre-employment physical examination. The patient has always been in good health and takes no medications. At the end of the last school term, he relocated to a different state and will begin teaching at a new school. He has an occasional dry cough but is otherwise asymptomatic and has no known contact with persons with tuberculosis. His last annual tuberculin skin test induced 10 mm of induration. Physical examination is normal.

Which of the following is the most appropriate management at this time?

(A) Begin isoniazid
(B) Collect sputum for acid-fast stain and culture
(C) Obtain a chest radiograph
(D) No intervention is necessary

Item 29

A 44-year-old woman is evaluated in the office because of a 3-week history of cough and fever. Six months ago, when she was working as a hospital nurse, her annual tuberculin skin test result was positive for the first time at 15 mm of induration. She was advised to take isoniazid prophylaxis but declined because of concerns about her age and the risk of hepatotoxicity. Subsequently, she decided to seek employment in a non–health care setting.

On physical examination, temperature is 38.3 °C (101 °F); other vital signs are normal. Crackles are heard over the left posterior chest. A chest radiograph confirms a density in the posterior left upper lobe.

Which of the following is the most appropriate management at this time?

(A) Begin empiric therapy with intravenous ceftriaxone and azithromycin
(B) Begin empiric therapy with isoniazid
(C) Begin empiric therapy with isoniazid, pyrazinamide, ethambutol, and rifampin
(D) Obtain sputum for acid-fast stain and culture
(E) Repeat the tuberculin skin test

Item 30

A 48-year-old man is evaluated in the office because of fever, night sweats, dyspnea and fatigue with exertion, and anorexia of 4 weeks' duration. He has a 5-year history of rheumatoid arthritis. His initial therapeutic regimen was prednisone, methotrexate, and hydroxychloroquine. Six months ago, infusion therapy with infliximab was added.

On physical examination today, temperature is 38.2 °C (100.8 °F), heart rate is 90/min, respiration rate is 18/min, and blood pressure is 100/60 mm Hg. Pulmonary examination reveals diffuse crackles bilaterally. On abdominal examination, there is evidence of hepatosplenomegaly. Musculoskeletal examination reveals no signs of arthritis. The remainder of the examination is unremarkable.

Laboratory studies:

Hemoglobin	8.7 g/dL
Leukocyte count	11,500/μL
Platelet count	98,000/μL
Erythrocyte sedimentation rate	90 mm/h

Chest radiograph shows a pattern of diffuse, fine patchy densities.

Which of the following is the most appropriate next step in this patient's management?

(A) Add clarithromycin
(B) Discontinue methotrexate; add azathioprine
(C) Increase prednisone dose
(D) Place in respiratory isolation; evaluate for tuberculosis

Item 31

A 32-year-old man is evaluated in the office because of a 2-month history of fever, night sweats, weight loss, and cough. Ten months ago, he was incarcerated because of drug possession charges related to injection drug use. At that time, a tuberculin skin test and serologic studies for HIV were negative. A follow-up HIV test 6 weeks later was also negative. Since release from jail, he has been drug-free, lives alone, and is employed as a nighttime office janitor.

On physical examination, he has an occasional cough and appears chronically ill. Temperature is 38 °C (100.4 °F); other vital signs are normal. Fine crackles are auscultated over the right posterior thorax.

A chest radiograph shows a right upper lobe infiltrate with a small cavity. A stained sputum specimen is positive for acid-fast organisms; sputum culture results are pending.

Which of the following is the most appropriate initial therapy for this patient?

(A) Isoniazid alone for 9 months
(B) Isoniazid, pyrazinamide, and ethambutol
(C) Isoniazid, pyrazinamide, and ethionamide
(D) Isoniazid, rifampin, pyrazinamide, and ethambutol
(E) No therapy until cultures confirm *Mycobacterium tuberculosis*

Item 32

A 62-year-old female social worker is screened for tuberculosis with a tuberculin skin test during a pre-employment physical examination. Forty-eight hours later she has 16 mm of induration at the site of the injection. She has never had a reactive tuberculin skin test and has no known exposure to tuberculosis. History reveals no risk factors for tuberculosis. She has no other medical problems and takes no medications; physical examination and review of systems are normal.

Results of blood tests, including HIV and aminotransferase levels, are normal, as are results of chest radiography.

Which of the following is the most appropriate management for this patient?

(A) Bacille Calmette-Guérin vaccination
(B) Isoniazid for 9 months
(C) Isoniazid, rifampin, pyrazinamide, and ethambutol for 9 months
(D) Retesting in 3 weeks
(E) Observation

Item 33

A 25-year-old man has a pre-employment physical examination before beginning a medical residency program at an urban teaching hospital. He is from India, where he completed his medical training. He is in good health and takes no medications.

Physical examination is normal. A tuberculin skin test induces 22 mm of induration. The patient subsequently remembers having received bacille Calmette–Guérin vaccine as a child and has a scar on his right shoulder compatible with such a vaccination. A follow-up chest radiograph is normal.

Which of the following is most appropriate at this time?

(A) Obtain an induced sputum sample for *Mycobacterium tuberculosis*
(B) Repeat the chest radiograph in 6 months
(C) Treat with isoniazid for 9 months
(D) Treat with isoniazid, pyrazinamide, and ethambutol for 1 month

Item 34

A 39-year-old woman is evaluated in the office for a malar rash, arthralgias, and serositis. Complete blood count and renal and liver chemistry studies are normal. Assays for antinuclear antibodies, anti–double-stranded DNA antibodies, and anti-Smith antibodies are positive. Serologic studies for HIV are negative.

Chest radiograph is normal. Tuberculin skin testing reveals 8 mm of induration.

Before initiating prednisone, which of the following is the most appropriate next step in this patient's management?

(A) Isoniazid for 9 months
(B) Isoniazid, pyrazinamide, rifampin, and ethambutol for 12 months
(C) Rifampin and pyrazinamide for 2 months
(D) No antituberculous therapy

Item 35

A 68-year-old woman with polymyositis is evaluated in the office because of increased difficulty swallowing and a 2-week history of low-grade fever, intermittent cough, and sputum production.

On physical examination, temperature is 37.9 °C (100.2 °F), and crackles are heard at the base of the right lung posteriorly. The leukocyte count is 9700/μL with 85% neutrophils, 12% lymphocytes, 2% monocytes, and 1% eosinophils.

A chest radiograph shows patchy pulmonary infiltrates in the right lower lobe. Sputum Gram stain shows many neutrophils, a few squamous epithelial cells, and several morphologic types of both gram-negative rods and gram-positive cocci. Results of sputum culture are pending.

Which of the following is the most appropriate management at this time?

(A) Bronchoscopy
(B) Clindamycin
(C) Metronidazole
(D) Penicillin

Item 36

A 73-year-old man is evaluated in the office because of a 1-day history of increasing cough, dyspnea, fever, and chills. He has chronic obstructive pulmonary disease and type 2 diabetes mellitus complicated by mild azotemia. The patient has a 60-pack-year smoking history and continues to smoke. Current medications are inhaled ipratropium bromide, inhaled salmeterol, lisinopril, hydrochlorothiazide, low-dose aspirin, and glyburide.

On physical examination, he is in mild respiratory distress. Temperature is 38 °C (100.4 °F), heart rate is 100/min, respiration rate is 20/min, and blood pressure is 135/85 mm Hg. Oxygen saturation is 86% with the patient breathing room air. Chest examination discloses decreased breath sounds bilaterally, scattered rhonchi, and a few crackles at the left base posteriorly.

The leukocyte count is 9700/μL with 72% neutrophils, 10% band forms, and 18% lymphocytes. Blood urea nitrogen is 40 mg/dL, and serum creatinine is 2.4 mg/dL. A chest radiograph shows a patchy infiltrate at the left lung base. The patient is hospitalized on a general medicine ward.

Which of the following is the most appropriate intravenous antibiotic therapy at this time?

(A) Ampicillin–sulbactam
(B) Ceftriaxone and azithromycin
(C) High-dose penicillin
(D) Ticarcillin and tobramycin
(E) Trimethoprim–sulfamethoxazole

Item 37

A 72-year-old male smoker with chronic obstructive pulmonary disease was hospitalized 2 days ago because of patchy left lower lobe pneumonia accompanied by fever, cough, and dyspnea. His initial leukocyte count was 14,300/μL. Intravenous levofloxacin and supplemental oxygen, 2 L/min by nasal prongs, were started on admission.

On hospital day 3, the patient has been afebrile for the past 18 hours. He has good oral intake, his cough has decreased, and he is no longer dyspneic. Oxygen saturation is 92% with the patient breathing room air, and his leukocyte count is now 9600/μL. A repeat chest radiograph shows no change in the size of the left lower lobe infiltrate.

Which of the following is most appropriate at this time?

(A) Addition of intravenous ceftriaxone
(B) Change to oral levofloxacin
(C) CT scan of the chest
(D) Fiberoptic bronchoscopy

Item 38

A 35-year-old woman is evaluated in the office because of a 3-day history of fever, productive cough, and wheezing. Her 2-year old son recently had a cough and fever to 38.9 °C (102 °F) that subsequently resolved. The patient has mild asthma that has not required treatment. She has a 10-pack-year smoking history but stopped smoking 3 years ago.

On physical examination, she coughs frequently and has mildly audible wheezing. Temperature is 38.2 °C (100.8 °F), heart rate is 100/min, respiration rate is 16/min, blood pressure is 115/75 mm Hg, and oxygen saturation is 98% with the patient breathing room air. Examination of the chest shows bronchial breath sounds and a few crackles in the lateral right lower chest near the mid-axillary line.

The leukocyte count is 11,900/μL with 80% neutrophils, 2% band forms, 14% lymphocytes, and 4% monocytes. A chest radiograph shows right middle lobe consolidation. Sputum culture is obtained.

In addition to starting inhaled bronchodilators, which of the following is most appropriate at this time?

(A) Await results of sputum culture
(B) Azithromycin
(C) Ciprofloxacin
(D) Gentamicin
(E) Trimethoprim–sulfamethoxazole

Item 39

A 67-year-old-man is evaluated in the emergency department for a productive cough, headache, fever, and shortness of breath for 2 weeks. The patient was seen in the office 1 week ago because of flu-like symptoms and diarrhea. He is a current smoker and has a history of coronary artery disease and diabetes mellitus; his medications are aspirin, pravastatin, metoprolol, and glyburide. He has been working part time at a pet store since he moved from Arizona 1 year ago.

On physical examination, temperature is 39.8 °C (103.7 °F), blood pressure is 124/60 mm Hg, heart rate is 72/min and regular, and respiration rate is 24/min. Auscultation of the chest discloses crackles, diminished breath sounds, and egophony at the left lung base.

Laboratory results:

Hemoglobin	10.8 g/dL
Leukocyte count	12,000/μL (3% segmented neutrophils and 7% band forms)
Blood urea nitrogen	28 mg/dL
Creatinine	0.9 mg/dL
Sodium	129 meq/L
Alanine aminotransferase	68 U/L
Aspartate aminotransferase	54 U/L

Sputum examination shows only a large number of neutrophils. A chest radiograph shows a left lower lobe pulmonary infiltrate.

Which of the following is the most appropriate therapy for this patient?

(A) Azithromycin and cefuroxime
(B) Doxycycline
(C) Fluconazole
(D) Piperacillin–tazobactam and ciprofloxacin

Item 40

A 62-year-old man comes to the emergency department because of a 2-day history of fever, cough, and yellow-green sputum production. The patient had severe pneumonia at age 40 years, following which he developed a daily cough and whitish-yellow sputum production; a diagnosis of bronchiectasis was made. He typically receives one or two courses of antibiotics each year when his sputum increases in volume and becomes darker. He is a lifelong nonsmoker.

On physical examination, temperature is 38.7 °C (101.6 °F). Coarse breath sounds are heard at the posterior base of the right lung. Scattered crackles and rhonchi are also auscultated. The leukocyte count is 13,500/μL. A chest radiograph shows a patchy right lower lobe infiltrate. A chest film obtained 2 years ago showed nonspecific increased markings at the base of the right lung but was otherwise unremarkable.

In choosing an antimicrobial regimen for this patient, coverage should be included for which of the following organisms?

(A) *Mycobacterium tuberculosis*
(B) *Nocardia brasiliensis*
(C) *Pseudomonas aeruginosa*
(D) Respiratory syncytial virus

Item 41

A 36-year-old woman is evaluated in the emergency department for fever and dyspnea. She reports a 4-week history of recurrent fevers. She has had intermittent night sweats and decreased appetite. She admits to injection heroin use; her last use was 3 days ago.

On physical examination, temperature is 39.6 °C (103.2 °F), heart rate is 70/min and irregular, blood pressure is 100/52 mm Hg, and oxygen saturation is 91% with the patient breathing room air. Jugular venous pressure is 12 cm H_2O. She has bibasilar crackles. Cardiac examination shows a soft S_1 with a muffled S_2. An S_3 and S_4 are not present. A grade 2/6 diastolic murmur is heard that is loudest at the second left intercostal space. The electrocardiogram is shown. An echocardiogram is obtained.

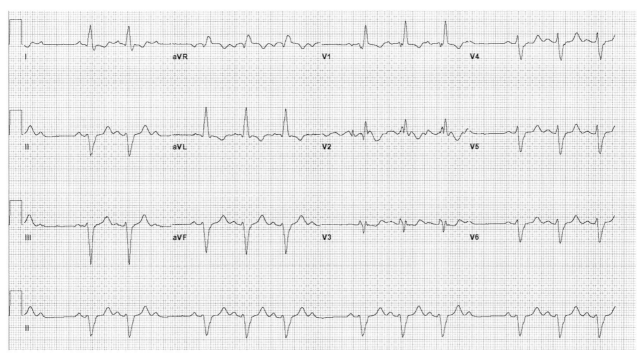

Item 41

Which of the following findings on echocardiography will best explain this patient's findings?

(A) Aortic valve perforation and paravalvular abscess
(B) Aortic valve thrombosis
(C) Mitral valve perforation
(D) Pulmonic valve perforation
(E) Tricuspid valve vegetations and perforation

Item 42

A 65-year-old man is scheduled to undergo dental extraction. The patient has a history of hyperlipidemia, hypertension, type 2 diabetes mellitus, and chronic stable angina. He had an episode of exercise-associated chest pain 6 weeks ago and was found to have three-vessel coronary artery disease and underwent coronary artery bypass graft surgery. He has no known allergies.

Which of the following is the most appropriate antibiotic prophylaxis for this patient before his dental procedure?

(A) Amoxicillin, 2 g orally, 1 hour before the procedure
(B) Ampicillin, 2 g intravenously, 30 minutes before the procedure
(C) Clindamycin, 600 mg orally, 1 hour before the procedure
(D) Vancomycin, 1 g intravenously, 30 minutes before the procedure
(E) No antibiotic prophylaxis

Item 43

A 34-year-old asymptomatic woman is seen in the office for a routine annual physical examination. She has no significant medical history. She is on no medications and has no medication allergies.

The cardiac examination reveals a normal S_1 and a split S_2 that widens with respiration. A grade 2/6 midsystolic murmur is heard in the fourth left intercostal space. The rest of her physical examination is unremarkable.

An echocardiogram demonstrates normal left and right ventricular size and function. Valvular anatomy and motion are normal. There is mild tricuspid and mitral regurgitation. The patient is scheduled for dental procedures in the next 2 weeks.

Which of the following is the most appropriate recommendation regarding antibiotic prophylaxis for this patient prior to her dental procedure?

(A) Amoxicillin orally 1 hour before the procedure
(B) Amoxicillin orally 4 times daily for 7 days
(C) Ampicillin intravenously 30 minutes before the procedure
(D) Antibiotic prophylaxis is not needed

Item 44

A 40-year-old male injection drug user is hospitalized because of a 1-week history of fever and arthralgias. The patient has a long history of alcohol abuse and has been admitted to the hospital on two previous occasions with alcohol withdrawal symptoms.

On physical examination, temperature is 38.7 °C (101.7 °F), heart rate is 110/min and regular, and blood pressure is 130/74 mm Hg. His fingernails are shown (*see Figure 25 in Color Plates*).

Which of the following must be included in the differential diagnosis of this patient's fever?

(A) Cirrhosis
(B) Congenital heart disease
(C) Infective endocarditis
(D) Thrombotic thrombocytopenic purpura

Item 45

A 14-year-old girl with sickle cell disease is brought to the emergency department because of a typical vaso-occlusive crisis. Although intravenous fluids, supplemental oxygen, and narcotic analgesics are administered, the crisis does not abate, and she is hospitalized.

On physical examination, her temperature is 39.1 °C (102.4 °F), heart rate is 130/min, respiration rate is 20/min, and blood pressure is 110/60 mm Hg. She has diffuse bone and abdominal pain that is most severe in the area of her right hip. A radiograph of the right hip reveals evidence of bony destruction in the femur at the level of the metaphysis. Two sets of blood cultures are obtained, and the patient is sent for urgent CT-guided bone biopsy for cultures and histopathologic studies.

While waiting culture results, empiric antimicrobial therapy should cover which of the following organisms?

(A) *Aspergillus, Proteus,* and *Vibrio*
(B) *Clostridium, Nocardia,* and *Listeria*
(C) *Neisseria, Pseudomonas,* and *Escherichia*
(D) *Staphylococcus, Streptococcus,* and *Salmonella*

Item 46

A 60-year-old man with type 2 diabetes mellitus has a chronic ulcer over the sole of his right foot directly under the first metatarsal that has been draining purulent material for several weeks. He does not have fever or other associated symptoms.

On physical examination, he is afebrile. There is a draining sinus tract on the sole of his right foot. Placement of a steel probe through the sinus tract goes directly to bone. Cultures of the pus from the tract grow *Escherichia coli* and *Enterococcus faecalis*.

Which of the following is the most appropriate management at this time?

(A) Amputation of the right foot
(B) Begin intravenous ampicillin–sulbactam
(C) Begin intravenous vancomycin and piperacillin–tazobactam
(D) Begin oral amoxicillin–clavulanate
(E) Bone biopsy

Item 47

A 72-year-old woman has a laceration of her left ankle sutured in the emergency department. One week later, she returns to the emergency department because of pain and discharge from the suture site.

On physical examination, she is afebrile. The left ankle shows purulent drainage from the previous suture site and dehiscence of the wound over the lateral malleolus. There is no evidence of exposed bone.

Which of the following studies will be most sensitive and specific for diagnosing osteomyelitis in this patient?

(A) Gallium scan
(B) Indium-labeled leukocyte scan
(C) MRI scan
(D) Plain radiograph
(E) Triple-phase bone scan

Item 48

Four months ago, a 23-year-old man sustained open fractures of his distal left tibia and fibula in a motor cycle accident and underwent surgical repair with placement of titanium plates. He now returns with increasing pain, swelling, and redness in the area of the fractures.

On physical examination, the area above the left ankle is swollen and tender, with erythema extending 2 cm from the surgical margin. A small amount of purulent discharge is apparent from a sinus tract at the distal end of the surgical wound, and Gram stain of the material reveals gram-positive cocci. A radiograph of the leg reveals bone resorption around several of the screws holding the titanium plates.

Which of the following is the best management option for this patient?

(A) Intravenous cefazolin for 4 to 6 weeks
(B) Intravenous vancomycin for 4 to 6 weeks
(C) Intravenous vancomycin for 4 to 6 weeks plus hyperbaric oxygen therapy
(D) Surgical removal of the orthopedic implant with intravenous antibiotics for 4 to 6 weeks

Chapter 6
Infectious Disease Medicine
Answers and Critiques

Item 1   Answer: D

Common variable immunodeficiency (also called acquired hypogammaglobulinemia) should be suspected in a patient with recurrent gastrointestinal infections (especially giardiasis) and respiratory infections. The diagnosis is established by the presence of decreased serum IgG levels. Patients may also develop malabsorption secondary to villous atrophy that does not respond to a gluten-free diet.

Patients with common variable immunodeficiency may also develop small bowel bacterial overgrowth; however, upper endoscopy with duodenal aspirates would not identify a specific diagnosis for the underlying condition. Although patients with common variable immunodeficiency are at risk for autoimmune or neoplastic diseases, there is no indication for bone marrow biopsy in this patient at this time. Wegener's granulomatosis, which is diagnosed by a positive cytoplasmic antineutrophil cytoplasmic antibody (c-ANCA) assay, may be associated with recurrent respiratory infections. However, patients with Wegener's granulomatosis rarely develop gastrointestinal complications, and there is no association with recurrent episodes of giardiasis. Unless other gastrointestinal disorders are present, patients with common variable immunodeficiency will have normal colonoscopic examinations. In addition, disorders that are diagnosed by colonoscopy (e.g., inflammatory bowel disease, microscopic colitis, colonic neoplasia) would not be associated with a prodrome of recurrent giardiasis.

KEY POINT

- Common variable immunodeficiency should be suspected in a patient with recurrent gastrointestinal infections (especially giardiasis) and respiratory infections.

Bibliography
1. Bonilla FA, Bernstein IL, Khan DA, Ballas ZK, Chinen J, Frank MM, et al. Practice parameter for the diagnosis and management of primary immunodeficiency. Ann Allergy Asthma Immunol. 2005;94:S1-63. [PMID: 15945566]

Item 2   Answer: A

Symptoms of bacterial vaginosis include increased malodorous discharge without irritation or pain. On physical examination, clinical criteria for bacterial vaginosis include a homogeneous, white discharge that smoothly coats the vaginal walls, absence of vaginal erythema, presence of clue cells (as seen in the figure), vaginal pH >4.5, and vaginal discharge that develops a fishy odor either before or after the addition of 10% potassium hydroxide to the slide preparation. Clue cells are squamous epithelial cells so densely covered with bacteria that their edges are obscured. Symptomatic patients who have at least three of these criteria should be treated with metronidazole or clindamycin, either orally or vaginally.

Patients with candidal vaginitis are likely to have a "cottage cheese–like" vaginal discharge, moderate to significant vaginal irritation, inflammation, and lack of odor on physical examination. Patients with *Trichomonas vaginalis* infection often note a discharge that is typically yellow–green and pruritic. On physical examination, the discharge may be "frothy." Physiologic discharge is not usually malodorous and would not likely change as suddenly as this patient's history suggests.

KEY POINT

- Clinical criteria for bacterial vaginosis include homogeneous, white discharge, absence of vaginal erythema, presence of clue cells, vaginal pH >4.5, and vaginal discharge with a fishy odor.

Bibliography
1. Eckert LO. Clinical practice. Acute vulvovaginitis. N Engl J Med. 2006;355:1244-52. Erratum in: N Engl J Med. 2006;355:2797. [PMID: 16990387]

Item 3   Answer: B

This patient has *Candida* vaginitis. The three most likely diagnoses in a patient with a vaginal discharge are a candidal infection, trichomoniasis, and bacterial vaginosis. A thick, milky vaginal discharge is characteristic of *Candida*, and a malodorous discharge with a high pH is characteristic of either trichomoniasis or bacterial vaginosis. The diagnosis is determined by the appearance of the stained specimens. The figure shows the pseudohyphae and budding yeast indicative of candidal vaginitis, and this infection can be treated with either intravaginal clotrimazole cream or a single oral dose of fluconazole.

The normal appearance of the cervix indicates that a chlamydial infection or gonorrhea is unlikely, since these infections cause cervicitis and not vaginitis. Furthermore, the absence of gram-negative cocci within neutrophils on stained specimens is inconsistent with gonorrhea.

- A thick, milky vaginal discharge is characteristic of *Candida* vaginitis, and a malodorous discharge with a high pH is characteristic of either trichomoniasis or bacterial vaginosis.

- Stained specimens of vaginal discharge from patients with candidal vaginitis show pseudohyphae and budding yeast.

Bibliography

1. **Sobel JD.** Vulvovaginal candidosis. Lancet. 2007;369:1961-71. [PMID: 17560449]

Item 4   Answer: B

This patient most likely has a drug fever. Antibiotics can cause or prolong fever, creating confusion for the clinician. A common cause of drug fever is the β-lactam antibiotics. This patient was treated for an obvious sinusitis and responded well to treatment. He is otherwise asymptomatic and feels well despite having a documented fever; importantly, his physical examination is normal. Eosinophilia and rash accompany drug fever in only 25% of cases; their absence does not rule out drug fever. The diagnosis of drug fever is made by stopping the suspected drug; in certain cases the patient may be rechallenged with the drug to document the source of fever. In most patients, the fever will abate within 72 hours after stopping the drug. Do not substitute the suspected drug with a drug from the same class because fever is likely to persist or recur. In this patient, the appropriate management is to stop the cephalexin. Because the recommended treatment for sinusitis is 5 to 14 days of antibiotics and he is on day 10 without evidence of sinusitis, this can be done without substituting another antibiotic. He should be observed as an outpatient for defervescence or the development of new signs or symptoms suggesting an alternative diagnosis.

Antimicrobial resistance is always possible, but the patient's symptoms quickly responded to the antibiotic with complete resolution of symptoms, eliminating this diagnosis. Whereas the patient may have acquired a new viral infection, he has no associated symptoms or findings of infection other than fever, making this unlikely. Factitious fever, although rare, does occur. Patients with factitious fever often have a serious underlying psychiatric disease. They tend to be demanding, manipulative, and may seek care at multiple hospitals. Their social histories are sketchy, and it is frequently difficult to pin down exact dates of their many past medical diagnoses and procedures. Many have worked in health care settings or have a spouse working in a health care field. Such patients can cause fever in a variety of ways, but most take substances surreptitiously, inject substances to which they are allergic, or hide warm devices to raise their temperature in the office or hospital. This patient does not match the typical psychological profile of someone with factitious fever. Lymphoma is always a consideration in a patient with a troublesome fever, but the lack of other symptoms (such as night sweats, anorexia, weight loss, or pruritus) and absence of lymphadenopathy or hepatosplenomegaly lowers the probability of this diagnosis.

- Drug fever should be suspected in patients in whom a new drug, particularly an antibiotic, was recently started and who have fever without other obvious signs of infection or inflammation.

- Eosinophilia and rash accompany drug fever in only 25% of cases; their absence does not rule out drug fever.

Bibliography

1. **Johnson DH, Cunha BA**. Drug fever. Infect Dis Clin North Am. 1996;10:85-91. [PMID: 8698996]

Item 5   Answer: C

This patient has severe sepsis. In 1992, the American College of Chest Physicians and the Society of Critical Care Medicine developed standard definitions for the various components of the sepsis syndrome, which are as follows:

1. Systemic inflammatory response syndrome (SIRS) is defined as the presence of two or more of the following (in the absence of a known cause): temperature >38.0 °C (100.4 °F) or <36.0 °C (96.8 °F); heart rate >90/min; respiration rate >20/min or $P\text{CO}_2$ <32 mm Hg; leukocyte count >12,000/μL or <4000/μL, or >10% band forms.

2. Sepsis is defined as SIRS in response to a confirmed infectious process.

3. Severe sepsis is defined as sepsis with organ dysfunction, hypoperfusion, or hypotension.

4. Septic shock is defined as sepsis-induced hypotension or hypoperfusion abnormalities despite adequate fluid resuscitation.

This patient meets the criteria for SIRS, has an identifiable source of infection (the urinary tract), and has evidence of end-organ damage and hypoperfusion (altered mental status; cool, mottled skin; and an elevated serum creatinine level). She also has evidence of hypotension and therefore meets the criteria for severe sepsis. Proper identification of the severity of infection in this setting allows for early resuscitation, evaluation of the intensity of necessary care, and prevention of morbidity and mortality.

SIRS represents a significant alteration to homeostasis but is not specific to sepsis. Noninfectious SIRS may exist in numerous conditions, including trauma, pancreatitis, and severe burns. Sepsis is SIRS with an identified infectious source but without evidence of end-organ damage or hypoperfusion, which this patient has. A diagnosis of septic shock cannot be established until fluid resuscitation has been administered and the response to this therapy has been evaluated.

- Sepsis is defined as the systemic inflammatory response syndrome in response to documented or suspected infection without evidence of end-organ damage or hypoperfusion.

- Severe sepsis is defined as sepsis with organ dysfunction, hypoperfusion, or hypotension.

- Septic shock is defined as sepsis-induced hypotension or hypoperfusion abnormalities despite adequate fluid resuscitation.

Bibliography

1. **Russell JA.** Management of sepsis. N Engl J Med. 2006;355:1699-713. Erratum in: N Engl J Med. 2006;355:2267. [PMID: 17050894]

Item 6   Answer: A

Aggressive fluid resuscitation with resolution of lactic acidosis within 6 hours would have a beneficial effect on this patient's survival. The patient has severe sepsis presumptively from pyelonephritis. The timing of resuscitation matters to survival. In a landmark study, early goal-directed therapy that included interventions delivered within the first 6 hours to maintain a central venous oxygen saturation of >70% and to effect resolution of lactic acidosis resulted in higher survival rates than more delayed resuscitation attempts. Over the first 72 hours, patients in the control arm of the study received the same quantity of fluid for resuscitation but had a significantly higher likelihood of dying by hospital discharge or at 60 days than those who received interventions within the first 6 hours.

Crystalloid is given much more frequently than colloid, and there are no data to support routinely using colloid in lieu of crystalloid, especially in patients who are as obviously volume depleted as this patient. Blood transfusions may be part of the resuscitation effort for anemic patients in shock, but the need to achieve hemoglobin levels above 12 g/dL is not supported by evidence. In stable patients in the intensive care unit who are not in shock, a transfusion threshold of 7 g/dL of hemoglobin is an acceptable conservative approach, but this does not apply to the treatment of patients with severe sepsis. There are no data to support that maintaining a lower PCO_2 or using a pulmonary artery catheter would help to increase survival in this patient.

KEY POINT

- Aggressive fluid resuscitation with resolution of lactic acidosis within 6 hours has a beneficial effect on survival in patients with severe sepsis.

Bibliography

1. **Rhodes A, Bennett ED.** Early goal-directed therapy: an evidence-based review. Crit Care Med. 2004;32:S448-50. [PMID: 15542954]

Item 7   Answer: D

This patient should be treated with oseltamivir and intramuscular trivalent inactivated influenza vaccine. Influenza virus is a common community-acquired infection that may cause fatal pneumonitis and secondary bacterial pneumonia in immunosuppressed patients. Prophylactic therapy with zanamivir or oseltamivir may prevent spread of infection to close contacts within the family setting. The Centers for Dis-

ease Control and Prevention recently advised against the use of amantadine and rimantadine because of a high rate of influenza virus resistance. Administration of antiviral therapy does not affect the immune response to inactivated influenza vaccine. Vaccination should be performed now, because oseltamivir provides short-term (2 weeks) prophylaxis against influenza.

Intranasal trivalent live-attenuated vaccine is contraindicated in immunosuppressed patients.

KEY POINTS

- Postexposure prophylaxis with zanamivir or oseltamivir and trivalent inactivated influenza vaccine may benefit immunosuppressed patients exposed to influenza virus.

- Intranasal trivalent live-attenuated influenza vaccine is contraindicated in immunosuppressed patients.

Bibliography

1. Antiviral drugs prophylaxis and treatment of influenza. Med Lett Drugs Ther. 2006;48:87-8. [PMID: 17051136]

Item 8   Answer: B

This patient should be treated with oseltamivir. The presumptive diagnosis of influenza in this patient is based on the history, clinical findings, and influenza activity in the community. Differentiating between influenza A and B is not possible without performing a diagnostic study. However, both viruses are circulating in the community, and an antiviral agent that is effective against both pathogens is required. Oseltamivir and zanamivir are neuraminidase inhibitors, which are a class of antiviral agents licensed for treatment of influenza A and B. Meta-analyses and some individual trials of zanamivir and oseltamivir show approximately 40% to 50% reductions in lower respiratory tract complications and associated antibiotic use following administration of these antiviral agents. However, only oseltamivir is appropriate for this patient because zanamivir, an inhaled anti-viral agent, is associated with bronchospasm in 5% to 10% of patients with asthma.

Amantadine and rimantadine should not be used because they are only active against influenza A. On January 14, 2006, the Centers for Disease Control and Prevention (CDC) reported that >90% of circulating influenza A virus isolates were resistant to amantadine and rimantadine. Furthermore, the CDC issued a health alert advising against the use of amantadine or rimantadine for prophylaxis or treatment of influenza. This recommendation was restated for the 2006–2007 influenza season and is likely to remain in effect beyond 2007.

KEY POINTS

- The neuraminidase inhibitors oseltamivir and zanamivir are both active against influenza A and B.

- Because zanamivir may induce bronchospasm, it is contraindicated in patients with asthma.

Bibliography
1. **Moscona A.** Neuraminidase inhibitors for influenza. N Engl J Med. 2005;353:1363-73. [PMID: 16192481]

Item 9   Answer: D

Persistent rhinitis symptoms in the setting of nasal decongestant spray overuse suggest rhinitis medicamentosa. Repeated use of nasal decongestants causes a decreased sensitivity to their vasoconstrictor effect and a rebound phenomenon with increased nasal congestion and discharge. Management involves immediately withdrawing the vasoconstrictor and initiating treatment with a nasal corticosteroid spray.

Allergic rhinitis is unlikely in this patient given his lack of allergy symptoms, such as sneezing and nasal itching, and because the symptoms are occurring when the patient's allergens are not in season. The absence of purulent drainage, fever, and sinus pain and the presence of pale turbinates argue against a diagnosis of bacterial sinusitis. Although nonallergic or vasomotor rhinitis can possibly be a complication of allergic rhinitis, environmental changes, such as air pollution, temperature or humidity changes, or nonspecific irritants, such as spicy foods, strong odors, perfume, exhaust fumes, cigarette smoke, and solvents, usually precipitate vasomotor symptoms. Most viral upper respiratory tract infections resolve within 1 week; long-term symptoms usually indicate a secondary bacterial infection.

KEY POINT

• Persistent rhinitis symptoms in the setting of chronic use of nasal decongestant sprays suggest rhinitis medicamentosa.

Bibliography
1. **Lockey RF.** Rhinitis medicamentosa and the stuffy nose. J Allergy Clin Immunol. 2006;118:1017-8. Epub 2006 Jul 24. [PMID: 17088123]

Item 10   Answer: A

The patient meets the criteria for acute bacterial rhinosinusitis: duration of symptoms >1 week and worsening symptoms after initial improvement, maxillary tenderness, purulent drainage, and poor response to decongestants. Generally, antibiotics should be reserved for patients who meet these criteria or for those with severe symptoms of rhinosinusitis (high fever, periorbital swelling, and severe facial pain) of any duration. Antibiotics targeting *Streptococcus pneumoniae* and *Haemophilus influenzae* reduce symptom duration. A 3- to 10-day course of a narrow-spectrum antibiotic, such as amoxicillin, trimethoprim–sulfamethoxazole, or doxycycline, is the preferred initial treatment.

Broad-spectrum antibiotics (amoxicillin–clavulanate) are no more effective than narrow-spectrum antibiotics in treating acute sinusitis. However, broad-spectrum antibiotics are more expensive, more likely to cause adverse reactions, and potentially more likely to increase antibiotic resistance. Although

oral antihistamines may be effective in patients with chronic sinusitis related to allergic rhinitis, there is insufficient evidence for recommending their use in patients with acute bacterial rhinosinusitis. Sinus radiographs and sinus CT scans are not recommended for acute, uncomplicated sinusitis. CT is more sensitive than plain radiography, but neither test can distinguish bacterial from viral infection.

KEY POINTS

• The criteria for acute bacterial rhinosinusitis are duration of symptoms >1 week and worsening symptoms after initial improvement, maxillary tenderness, purulent drainage, and poor response to decongestants.

• A 3- to 10-day course of a narrow-spectrum antibiotic, such as amoxicillin, trimethoprim–sulfamethoxazole, or doxycycline, is the preferred initial treatment for acute bacterial rhinosinusitis.

Bibliography
1. **Ah-See KW, Evans AS.** Sinusitis and its management. BMJ. 2007;334:358-61. [PMID: 17303885]

Item 11   Answer: D

Most cases of sporadic acute rhinosinusitis are caused by viral infection, and related symptoms usually improve with symptomatic treatment only. Various inexpensive, nontoxic interventions, including drinking additional fluids, saltwater gargle, throat lozenges, and saline nasal spray, may alleviate symptoms of upper respiratory tract infection. Heated vapor inhalation has been shown to improve nasal patency and decrease nasal resistance. Subjective and objective measures of nasal symptoms have been shown to improve with a single dose of an oral or topical nasal decongestant, whereas rhinorrhea, sneezing, and symptom scores have been shown to improve with first-generation antihistamines.

It is unlikely that this patient has bacterial sinusitis. Patients with only one of the three following clinical criteria have a less than 25% probability of having bacterial sinusitis: upper respiratory tract infection lasting more than 7 days, facial pain, and purulent nasal discharge. However, antibiotic therapy may be warranted in patients with at least two of these clinical criteria or in patients who have had symptoms for longer than 7 to 10 days and in whom symptomatic therapy is ineffective. Imaging studies are not indicated for uncomplicated acute rhinosinusitis. Sinus radiography is not cost effective compared with symptomatic treatment or use of clinical criteria to guide antibiotic therapy.

Sinus infection may spread locally, resulting in osteitis of the sinus bones or orbital cellulitis, or spread to the central nervous system, resulting in meningitis, brain abscess, or infection of the intracranial venous sinuses. Therefore, patients with ophthalmic or neurologic symptoms or signs may require diagnostic imaging studies. Sinus puncture and aspiration with culture is the gold standard for the diagnosis of acute bacterial sinusitis in the research setting. However, sinus puncture is painful and requires expertise and therefore should be considered only if a precise diagnosis is needed to determine optimal therapy, such as in immunocompromised patients.

KEY POINT

• Viral infection causes most cases of sporadic acute rhinosinusitis, and related symptoms usually improve with only symptomatic treatment.

Bibliography
1. Poole MD, Portugal LG. Treatment of rhinosinusitis in the outpatient setting. Am J Med. 2005;118:45S-50S. [PMID: 15993677]

Item 12   Answer: D

This patient has pyelonephritis, is not pregnant, and can be treated with oral levofloxacin. The most important first step in treating pyelonephritis is to determine the route of therapy. In general, oral therapy is used for a highly compliant patient who can eat and drink, and the parenteral route is used for a patient who is nauseated or vomiting. A parenteral regimen can be changed to oral therapy once the patient has been stabilized and can tolerate oral drugs. Oral therapy is suitable for the patient described here, and levofloxacin for 7 to 14 days is the most appropriate of the regimens listed. Levofloxacin is classified as pregnancy category C (no adequate and well-controlled studies in pregnant women). Until recently, a 14-day course of levofloxacin was the standard of care. There is good evidence, however, that a 7-day course is sufficient for patients with uncomplicated acute pyelonephritis. The following classes of alternative antimicrobial agents may be considered for empiric therapy for this disorder: third-generation or extended-spectrum cephalosporins, extended-spectrum penicillins or aminoglycosides, monobactams, and carbapenems.

Because of increasing bacterial resistance to trimethoprim–sulfamethoxazole, this drug should not be used for empiric treatment of acute pyelonephritis. Although oral β-lactams such as amoxicillin–clavulanate are sometimes effective, published studies to date show that they are inferior to levofloxacin.

KEY POINT

• Oral levofloxacin is indicated for empiric treatment of a highly compliant, nonpregnant patient with acute pyelonephritis who can eat and drink.

Bibliography
1. Ramakrishnan K, Scheid DC. Diagnosis and management of acute pyelonephritis in adults. Am Fam Physician. 2005;71:933-42. Erratum in: Am Fam Physician. 2005;72:2182. [PMID: 15768623]

Item 13   Answer: D

A 3-day course of trimethoprim–sulfamethoxazole (TMP-SMZ) is the appropriate treatment for this patient with an uncomplicated urinary tract infection. A urine pregnancy test is indicated in this sexually active patient before antibiotic treatment is started. Urine cultures are seldom needed. Urine dipstick testing has superseded microscopy and urine culture because the dipstick method is cheaper, faster, and more con-

venient. Cultures are warranted to identify unusual or resistant organisms in women whose symptoms either do not respond to therapy or recur within 2 to 4 weeks after therapy.

Standard management of an acute, uncomplicated urinary tract infection in an otherwise healthy, nonpregnant woman requires only a 3-day course of a first-line antimicrobial agent such as TMP-SMZ. This should be sufficient to eradicate the infection and corroborate the diagnosis by alleviating the symptoms. Because of the increasing incidence of bacterial resistance to fluoroquinolones, use of fluoroquinolone-sparing regimens is encouraged; however, this approach may result in lower cure rates and therefore should not be used in patients with severe symptoms.

Ciprofloxacin is appropriate for patients with unrelieved dysuria and bacteriuria after treatment with TMP-SMZ or for patients who live in geographic locations where resistance to TMP-SMZ exceeds 15%. Longer courses of antibiotic therapy (7 to 10 days) are not more effective in eradicating infection or preventing recurrence and are associated with a higher rate of adverse effects (30% versus 18%).

Amoxicillin is less effective than TMP-SMZ and fluoroquinolones but is the drug of choice for culture-proven *Enterococcus* infection and may be useful during pregnancy for susceptible organisms when TMP-SMZ and fluoroquinolones are contraindicated. First-generation cephalosporins (for example, cephalexin) are more expensive and less effective than TMP-SMZ or fluoroquinolones. First-generation cephalosporins may be an option during pregnancy, although resistance to these agents is common.

KEY POINTS

• A 3-day course of trimethoprim–sulfamethoxazole is recommended initial therapy for acute uncomplicated urinary tract infection in a young, healthy, nonpregnant woman.

• Urine dipstick testing has superseded microscopy and urine culture in the diagnosis of cystitis because the dipstick method is cheaper, faster, and more convenient.

Bibliography
1. Warren JW, Abrutyn E, Hebel JR, Johnson JR, Schaeffer AJ, Stamm WE. Guidelines for antimicrobial treatment of uncomplicated acute bacterial cystitis and acute pyelonephritis in women. Infectious Diseases Society of America (IDSA). Clin Infect Dis. 1999;29:745-58. [PMID: 10589881]
2. Fihn SD. Clinical practice. Acute uncomplicated urinary tract infection in women. N Engl J Med. 2003;349:259-66. [PMID: 12867610]

Item 14   Answer: B

The diagnosis is genital herpes simplex virus infection. Primary genital herpes appears as vesicles progressing to pustules and then to ulcers or erosions. At the time of presentation, only ulcers or erosions may be present. Tender inguinal lymphadenopathy usually develops after the genital lesions develop and lasts after the genital lesions resolve. Extra-genital herpes may be seen on the buttocks, thighs, anus, rectum, fingers (whitlow), or conjunctiva. The first episodes may be severe or so mild as to be unrecognized.

Herpes zoster lesions would be more extensive and would involve other areas in a dermatomal distribution. Lesions in patients with syphilis are not painful and tend to be larger. Group B streptococcal infection is manifested as a diffuse cellulitis or abscess formation rather than as vesicular, pustular, or erosive lesions.

KEY POINT

- Primary genital herpes appears as vesicles progressing to pustules and then to ulcers or erosions.

Bibliography

1. **Sen P, Barton SE.** Genital herpes and its management. BMJ. 2007;334:1048-52. [PMID: 17510153]

Item 15   Answer: B

This patient has primary genital herpes without systemic complications such as meningitis or urinary retention and should be treated with oral valacyclovir. Genital herpes lesions typically begin as vesicles that ulcerate and are quite painful. Depending upon when the patient is examined, vesicles may not be present. Look for abnormalities in the genital area, such as cracks, fissures, red areas, abraded areas, and ulcers. The incubation period for genital herpes simplex virus is 3 to 5 days, and transmission of the virus usually results from asymptomatic shedding of viral organisms, as most likely occurred in her male partner. Treatment of initial episodes decreases the duration and severity of symptoms. Of the drugs listed, only oral valacyclovir is appropriate for therapy. An ester of acyclovir, valacyclovir is converted to acyclovir in the liver. Oral valacyclovir is better absorbed and produces higher drug levels than oral acyclovir.

Systemic, not topical, therapy should be used for all patients with first episodes of genital herpes because topical therapy is ineffective in the management of either primary or recurrent genital herpes. Despite a lack of controlled trials, intravenous acyclovir is used for patients who have complications from primary infection, such as meningitis or urinary retention. Penciclovir is not licensed for either topical or oral administration in the management of genital herpes and is only minimally effective in the treatment of herpes simplex labialis infection (cold sores, fever blisters).

KEY POINT

- Oral valacyclovir is the most appropriate antiviral agent for a patient with genital herpes simplex virus infection without systemic complications.

Bibliography

1. **Sen P, Barton SE.** Genital herpes and its management. BMJ. 2007;334:1048-52. [PMID: 17510153]

Item 16   Answer: E

The patient most likely has secondary syphilis characterized by a generalized rash, low-grade fever, and generalized lymphadenopathy in the context of recent high-risk sexual behavior. The rash of secondary syphilis may be diffuse and include the palms and soles or may be patchy. The lesions may be macular, papular, maculopapular, papulosquamous, or papulopustular; vesicular lesions are rare. A rapid plasma reagin test for syphilis is an appropriate initial screening test, but given its lack of specificity, a positive test should be confirmed with a specific treponemal antibody test. In addition to secondary syphilis, this patient must be evaluated for acute retroviral syndrome (primary HIV infection). This diagnosis should be considered if a febrile illness occurs within several weeks of a potential exposure. There is not a clinically reliable "cluster" of signs and symptoms that is sensitive and specific for the diagnosis of acute retroviral syndrome, but the most consistently reported findings include fever (97%), fatigue (90%), lymphadenopathy (50% to 77%), pharyngitis (73%), transient rash (40% to 70%), and headache (30% to 60%).

Chlamydia infection is a common sexually transmitted disease that is associated with urethritis, but systemic symptoms and rash do not occur. Herpes simplex virus is a common cause of genital ulcers, erosions, and vesicular lesions. Herpes simplex virus IgG positivity simply implies a past exposure, but not necessarily recent or active disease, and would not be helpful in assessing this patient's (nonvesicular) rash and constitutional symptoms. Mononucleosis is a viral syndrome caused by infection with the Epstein-Barr virus and is typically associated with sore throat, fever, posterior cervical lymphadenopathy, and often splenomegaly. A rash is uncommon, although a generalized exanthem characterized by bright red macules and papules that may become confluent is frequently present if the patient received ampicillin or amoxicillin. This patient did not receive antibiotics, and his high-risk sexual behavior makes secondary syphilis a more likely diagnosis; therefore, the heterophile antibody test (Monospot test) is not needed. Tinea corporis, a dermatophyte infection, occurs on the trunk or extremities and characteristically consists of circular or oval, scaling, erythematous lesions that spread outward with central clearing. It may be diagnosed by scraping the skin and examination with a potassium hydroxide stain, which demonstrates hyphal elements. Importantly, superficial dermatophyte infections are not associated with systemic symptoms, making this diagnosis unlikely.

KEY POINT

- Secondary syphilis and acute retroviral syndrome should always be considered in a sexually active patient with a rash, fever, and generalized lymphadenopathy.

Bibliography

1. **Golden MR, Marra CM, Holmes KK.** Update on syphilis: resurgence of an old problem. JAMA. 2003;290:1510-4. [PMID: 13129993]

Item 17   Answer: C

This patient should be started on fluconazole. He is at risk for development of opportunistic infections because of his low CD4 cell count (<100/µL). Candidiasis is the most common esophageal disorder in patients with HIV infection. Approximately two-thirds of patients with *Candida* esophagitis have concomitant thrush. Because of the strong association between oral and esophageal candidiasis, patients with symptomatic thrush should receive a brief course of systemic antifungal therapy with fluconazole. If his symptoms do not improve in several days, upper endoscopy is indicated for diagnosis. Upper endoscopy would also have been indicated initially if his dysphagia had been so severe that he was unable to swallow.

Gastroesophageal reflux disease is relatively uncommon in patients with HIV infection and would present with heartburn rather than with dysphagia and odynophagia. Since this patient is unlikely to have gastroesophageal reflux disease, omeprazole is not indicated. Although a barium swallow may demonstrate some esophageal abnormalities, it is often nondiagnostic in a patient with esophagitis. A CT scan of the chest may show thickening of the esophagus in patients with severe esophagitis but is not indicated for the initial evaluation of esophageal complaints.

KEY POINT

• Patients with HIV infection and odynophagia associated with oral thrush should receive an empiric trial of fluconazole.

Bibliography
1. **Pappas PG, Rex JH, Sobel JD, Filler SG, Dismukes WE, Walsh TJ, et al.** Guidelines for treatment of candidiasis. Clin Infect Dis. 2004;38:161-89. [PMID: 14699449]

Item 18   Answer: C

This patient's prolonged febrile syndrome in the setting of HIV risk factors should raise concerns for recent infection with HIV. The most appropriate test for diagnosing acute HIV is the measurement of HIV viral load. Three to six weeks after developing HIV infection, most patients have a cluster of mononucleosis-like symptoms corresponding with the initial burst of HIV replication and dissemination. The measurement of HIV viral load is the most sensitive test for HIV infection during the acute symptomatic phase. Tests for HIV-specific antigens, such as p24, can also detect the presence of virus in the acute setting. Antibodies to HIV do not commonly occur until about 6 weeks after infection, and therefore may be negative during the acute symptomatic phase. In addition to the acute retroviral syndrome, this patient must be evaluated for secondary syphilis, using the rapid plasma regain test. Secondary syphilis and acute retroviral syndrome should always be considered in a sexually active patient with a rash, fever, and generalized lymphadenopathy.

Patients with acute HIV infection usually have nonspecific symptoms such as fever, pharyngitis, lymphadenopathy, rash,

and/or headache, often persisting for several weeks. Mucocutaneous ulceration is present less often. The CD4 cell count may be profoundly depressed in patients with acute HIV infection, but the CD4 cell count is insensitive in the diagnosis of acute infection. Although acute HIV infection can mimic the signs and symptoms of mononucleosis, testing for Epstein-Barr virus is less an immediate concern in this patient who has multiple risk factors for HIV infection. The histopathology of the rash in acute HIV infection is nonspecific and is not useful in diagnosis; therefore, a skin biopsy is not indicated.

KEY POINTS

• The presentation of acute HIV infection can be nonspecific and obtaining a history of risk factors is essential.

• Antibodies to HIV are not detectable until about 6 weeks after infection; the measurement of HIV viral load is the most sensitive test for infection during the acute stage.

Bibliography
1. **Kahn JO, Walker BD.** Acute human immunodeficiency virus type 1 infection. N Engl J Med. 1998;339:33-9. [PMID: 9647878]

Item 19   Answer: B

This patient should begin treatment with zidovudine, didanosine, and nelfinavir. The HIV RNA viral load and especially the CD4 cell count are the best available predictors of disease progression and AIDS-related death. The most recent treatment guidelines by the Clinical Practices Panel convened by the U.S. Department of Health and Human Services recommend initiating treatment for patients with HIV-related constitutional symptoms, those with a major AIDS-related opportunistic infection, and those with CD4 cell counts <200/µL. The CD4 cell count is a more important prognostic determinant than the HIV RNA viral load, although older age and viral load values >100,000 copies/mL are also significant predictors of progression to AIDS. Although this patient is asymptomatic, his CD4 cell count is <200/µL. He is therefore at risk for AIDS-related complications, and antiretroviral therapy is indicated now.

Because of the low CD4 cell count, therapy should not be delayed until symptoms appear or the viral load exceeds 100,000 copies/mL. Drug regimens containing three or more agents are more effective and provide a survival advantage compared with one- or two-drug regimens among patients with advanced disease; therefore, zidovudine monotherapy is not appropriate.

KEY POINTS

• Antiretroviral therapy should be initiated for a treatment-naïve patient with HIV infection and a CD4 cell count <200/µL, even if the patient is asymptomatic.

• Drug regimens containing three or more agents are more effective and provide a survival advantage compared with one- or two-drug regimens among patients with advanced disease.

Bibliography

1. **Phillips AN, Gazzard BG, Clumeck N, Losso MH, Lundgren JD.** When should antiretroviral therapy for HIV be started? BMJ. 2007;334:76-8. [PMID: 17218713]

Item 20   Answer: D

This patient most likely has Kaposi's sarcoma. Kaposi's lesions commonly involve the face, trunk, and lower extremities and range from erythematous or violaceous macules to larger nodules and plaques that may ulcerate. Early skin lesions may present as palpable nodules before skin discoloration occurs, and faint, light-brown lesions are often indistinguishable from other skin abnormalities. A yellow "halo" around nodular lesions is associated with rapidly progressive disease. Kaposi's sarcoma is caused by human herpesvirus 8. It occurs in men who have sex with men and can develop even before suppression of the CD4 cell count. Kaposi's sarcoma frequently regresses and sometimes resolves completely when highly active antiretroviral therapy (HAART) is successful.

Dermatofibromas appear as discrete, flesh-colored, button-like nodules or papules, which range from 3–10 mm in diameter. They are common and benign, are often present for long periods of time, and characteristically umbilicate when lateral pressure is applied to the lesion. Cherry angiomas are common, asymptomatic bright-red to violaceous vascular papules. The lesions begin to appear at the age of 30 years and increase in number as the patient ages. They are principally located on the trunk. The sudden appearance of a new lesion on the arm of a young man is not compatible with a cherry angioma. Hypersensitivity vasculitis typically presents as "palpable purpura" on the lower extremities. These lesions are bright red, well-demarcated papules and macules with a central dot of hemorrhage. Numerous lesions appear at the same time and can be discrete or confluent. An isolated lesion on the arm is not compatible with hypersensitivity vasculitis.

KEY POINTS

- Kaposi's sarcoma lesions commonly involve the face, trunk, and lower extremities and range from erythematous or violaceous macules to larger nodules and plaques that may ulcerate.

- In patients with HIV infection and Kaposi's sarcoma, the sarcoma frequently regresses and sometimes resolves completely after successful treatment with highly active antiretroviral therapy.

Bibliography

1. **Cattelan AM, Calabrò ML, De Rossi A, Aversa SM, Barbierato M, Trevenzoli M, et al.** Long-term clinical outcome of AIDS-related Kaposi's sarcoma during highly active antiretroviral therapy. Int J Oncol. 2005;27:779-85. [PMID: 16077928]

Item 21   Answer: D

The most likely diagnosis is progressive multifocal leukoencephalopathy (PML). PML is an opportunistic infection caused by polyomavirus JC, leading to demyelination of the central nervous system that causes gradually progressive neurologic deficits. Radiographically, there is no mass effect, in contrast to primary central nervous system lymphoma and toxoplasmosis in which mass effect may occur. The lesions are generally bilateral, asymmetric, nonenhancing, and periventricular or subcortical in distribution. This patient has late-stage HIV infection based on a CD4 cell count that was <100/µL 2 years ago without treatment and the presence of thrush, which typically indicates a risk for AIDS-related opportunistic infections. He also has focal neurologic signs and an MRI that shows multiple white matter lesions without mass effect involving the right lateral frontal, right frontoparietal, and left frontal lobes; right pons; bilateral brachium pontis; and right cerebellum. In addition, a polymerase chain reaction is positive for polyomavirus JC. These findings are diagnostic of PML. While the gold standard for diagnosis of PML is brain biopsy, the patient's lesions are quite deep and relatively inaccessible. Given the preponderance of evidence supporting a diagnosis of PML, biopsy can be deferred. Approximately 50% of patients with AIDS and PML will survive the PML if highly active antiretroviral therapy is administered, presumably because of the effects of immune reconstitution in arresting the disease process. Unfortunately, neurologic deficits typically persist in survivors proportionate to the disease severity at the time of presentation.

In patients with HIV infection and CD4 cell counts <200/µL, localized or focal encephalitis is the most common presentation of toxoplasmosis and is the most common central nervous system mass lesion. However, the positive polymerase chain reaction for polyomavirus JC is strong evidence for PML and excludes toxoplasmosis. Central nervous system lymphoma occurs in approximately 2% to 12% of HIV-infected individuals. It develops when the CD4 cell counts are <200/µL and often <50/µL and, unlike in immunocompetent hosts, is strongly associated with Epstein–Barr virus infection. In patients with AIDS, lymphoma was second only to toxoplasmosis as the most common central nervous system mass lesion. The negative polymerase chain reaction for Epstein–Barr virus and the diffuse nature of the MRI abnormality exclude central nervous system lymphoma. Cryptococcal meningitis is a subacute central nervous system infection associated with a cerebrospinal fluid pleocytosis of 40-400 cells/µL with lymphocyte predominance and slightly low glucose levels. India ink stain of the cerebrospinal fluid has limited sensitivity, but the cerebrospinal fluid is positive for cryptococcal polysaccharide antigen in 90% of patients. The patient's negative cryptococcal antigen makes this diagnosis unlikely.

- Progressive multifocal leukoencephalopathy is an opportunistic infection caused by polyomavirus JC, leading to demyelination of the central nervous system causing progressive neurologic deficits.

- Approximately 50% of patients with AIDS and progressive multifocal leukoencephalopathy will survive the latter disease if highly active antiretroviral therapy is administered.

Bibliography

1. Benson CA, Kaplan JE, Masur H, Pau A, Holmes KK; CDC; National Institutes of Health; Infectious Diseases Society of America. Treating opportunistic infections among HIV-exposed and infected children: recommendations from CDC, the National Institutes of Health, and the Infectious Diseases Society of America.MMWR Recomm Rep. 2004;53(RR-15):1-112. Erratum in: MMWR Morb Mortal Wkly Rep. 2005;54:311. [PMID: 15841069]

Item 22   Answer: A

In the insertion procedure described here, chlorhexidine would have been more effective than povidone-iodine for cleansing the patient's skin. Chlorhexidine is a superior skin cleanser and has residual activity for at least 30 minutes after it is applied. A meta-analysis showed that use of chlorhexidine reduced catheter-associated colonization and bloodstream infections by 50% when compared with use of povidone-iodine.

Hand washing before any procedure is critical. Either washing with soap and water for at least 15 seconds or using alcohol-based gels is appropriate. Use of a subclavian site is also appropriate. A subclavian site is associated with a lower risk of colonization and infection than other intravascular sites. In addition, a subclavian site is easier to keep dressed. Single draping the patient and use of protective garb are also correct because maximal barrier precautions (large sterile drape to cover the patient and sterile gown, gloves, and mask for the operator) reduce intravascular line infections 3- to 6-fold.

- Chlorhexidine is superior to povidone-iodine for cleaning a catheter insertion site.

Bibliography

1. O'Grady NP, Alexander M, Dellinger EP, Gerberding JL, Heard SO, Maki DG, et al. Guidelines for the prevention of intravascular catheter-related infections. Centers for Disease Control and Prevention. MMWR Recomm Rep. 2002;51:1-29. [PMID: 12233868]

Item 23   Answer: B

In-hospital epidemics of *Clostridium difficile* colitis frequently occur, and the efficacy of contact isolation techniques in limiting the spread of infection has been well documented. Gowns, gloves, and careful hand washing are the main preventive measures, but care in moving apparatus of all kinds from room to room is also important, since *C. difficile* spores can easily be found on the surface of almost any item. Alcohol rubs are not effective for killing *C. difficile* spores.

Bathing the patient with antiseptic soap is ineffective because even if the organisms could be removed from the patient's skin, they would be replenished with the next bowel movement. Also, organisms on bed clothing and other items in the room are probably more likely to contaminate the hands and clothes of hospital staff and possibly the roommate. Respiratory isolation will be ineffective because the organisms are not spread by the respiratory route. Droplet isolation is not required because droplet spread is not a factor in the transmission of *C. difficile*.

- Contact isolation is most effective for reducing spread of *Clostridium difficile* in hospitals.

Bibliography

1. Guerrant RL, Van Gilder T, Steiner TS, Thielman NM, Slutsker L, Tauxe RV, et al. Practice guidelines for the management of infectious diarrhea. Clin Infect Dis. 2001;32:331-51. [PMID: 11170940]

Item 24   Answer: A

This patient's symptoms are highly suggestive of tuberculosis. He must be placed in airborne isolation to protect health care workers and other patients. In addition, health care workers must wear approved respirators with increased filtration capacity, such as an N95 mask or a powered-air purifying respirator (PAPR). Most mycobacterial infections are transmitted from person to person by airborne particles. Preventing these particles from contacting nonimmune hosts interrupts transmission. Droplet precautions are not sufficient protection to prevent the spread of tuberculosis. The patient should wear a surgical mask when being transported.

- Prevention of nosocomial mycobacterial infections requires airborne isolation of the patient and personal respirators for health care workers.

Bibliography

1. Guidelines for prevention of nosocomial pneumonia. Centers for Disease Control and Prevention. MMWR Recomm Rep. 1997;46:1-79. [PMID: 9036304]

Item 25   Answer: D

Ninety percent of urinary tract infections are related to indwelling catheters, and removing the catheters whenever possible is critical for preventing infections. The risk of colonization and infection increases the longer the catheters are in place. Physicians need to weigh the risk of infection against the difficulties associated with the care of incontinent patients. In patients who require an indwelling catheter, suprapubic catheters and intermittent catheterization can be used. Men can also use condom catheters.

There is no role for administering prophylactic antibiotics, acidifying the urine, or using any type of disinfecting wash, as none of these interventions has been shown to prevent urinary tract infections. No studies have shown that routinely changing the catheters decreases the risk of infection.

KEY POINT

• Ninety percent of urinary tract infections are associated with indwelling urinary catheters.

Bibliography

1. **Nicolle LE.** Urinary tract infection in geriatric and institutionalized patients. Curr Opin Urol. 2002;12:51-5. [PMID: 11753134]

Item 26   Answer: C

Proper positioning of the patient can reduce the risk of ventilator-associated pneumonia. This patient is at high risk for ventilator-associated (nosocomial) pneumonia because of chest trauma, a Glasgow Coma Scale score of <9, and the need for mechanical ventilation. To prevent nosocomial pneumonia, the Centers for Disease Control and Prevention recommend interventions to decrease aspiration, such as raising the head of the bed to a 45-degree angle, maintaining gastric acidity, maximizing nutrition, preventing colonization or cross-contamination by the hands of heath care workers, and manipulating respiratory-tract equipment in a sterile fashion and disinfecting the equipment appropriately. Maintaining patients in a semi-recumbent position has been shown to decrease ventilator-associated pneumonia by 34% compared with patients kept supine.

H_2-receptor antagonists are a risk factor for development of ventilator-associated pneumonia because these agents reduce gastric acidity. There are no data to confirm that use of prophylactic intravenous antibiotics prevents pneumonia, and antibiotics may increase the risk of colonization with resistant organisms. Changing tubing every 3 days is not necessary. Several clinical trials have shown that changing circuit tubing only every 2 weeks in adult patients does not increase the risk of infection. Use of endotracheal tubes that do not allow suctioning of subglottic secretions increases, rather than decreases, the risk of pneumonia in patients who are intubated for long periods of time.

KEY POINT

• Keeping mechanically ventilated patients at a 45-degree angle helps prevent development of ventilator-associated pneumonia.

Bibliography

1. Guidelines for prevention of nosocomial pneumonia. Centers for Disease Control and Prevention. MMWR Recomm Rep. 1997;46:1-79. [PMID: 9036304]

Item 27   Answer: B

This patient most likely has a nosocomial (health care-acquired) pneumonia that has failed to respond to initial antibiotic therapy and requires broader antibiotic coverage. The history of a prior hospital admission within 90 days places the patient at risk for resistant organisms, and antibiotic coverage should reflect this. She needs coverage for methicillin-resistant *Staphylococcus aureus* (MRSA) as well as for *Pseudomonas* species.

Bronchoscopy with protected specimen sampling has not been shown to improve outcomes and is not recommended. A CT scan of chest is unlikely to provide further information about this patient's pneumonia and will not guide the proper selection of antibiotics. The risk of deep venous thrombosis increases once a patient is intubated for respiratory failure, but this does not occur for a few days, and the clinical picture is that of a respiratory infection with sepsis. Prophylaxis with heparin has been initiated, reducing the likelihood of deep venous thrombosis; therefore, a Doppler study of the lower extremities is not indicated at this time.

KEY POINT

• Patients with nosocomial (health care-acquired) pneumonia require initial coverage for resistant organisms including methicillin-resistant *Staphylococcus aureus* and *Pseudomonas* species.

Bibliography

1. Guidelines for the management of adults with hospital-acquired, ventilator-associated, and healthcare-associated pneumonia. Am J Respir Crit Care Med. 2005;171:388-416. [PMID: 15699079]

Item 28   Answer: D

This low-risk, asymptomatic person has a nondiagnostic tuberculin skin test reaction for latent or active tuberculosis. Three cut-points have been defined for a positive tuberculin reaction: >5 mm, >10 mm, and >15 mm of induration. The cut-off threshold of >15 mm is used for all low-risk persons, such as the person in this case. Since his tuberculin skin test is not diagnostic for either active or latent tuberculosis, neither additional diagnostic studies nor therapy is indicated at this time.

The cut-off threshold of >5 mm is for persons at highest risk of developing active tuberculosis (e.g., HIV-infected patients, immunosuppressed patients, persons with close contact with anyone with active tuberculosis, or those with a chest radiograph consistent with prior tuberculosis). The cut-off threshold of >10 mm is used for persons who have immigrated to the United States from high-risk countries within the past 5 years, injection drug users, prisoners, health care workers, and patients with silicosis, diabetes mellitus, chronic renal failure, leukemia and lymphoma, carcinoma of the head and neck or lung, recent significant weight loss, and a history of gastrectomy or jejunoileal bypass. Healthy adolescents who are exposed to adults in high-risk categories should also be screened using this >10-mm cut-off.

Current recommendations do not support the use of tuberculin skin testing as a screening test in otherwise healthy persons with no personal or occupational exposure to tuberculosis because a large number of healthy adults need to be screened to prevent a single case of active tuberculosis, and the possibility of harm caused by extensive preventive treatment exceeds the benefit of the few cases of tuberculosis prevented.

KEY POINT

- The tuberculin skin test cut-off threshold of >15 mm is used for all low-risk persons.

Bibliography

1. **Sharma U, Morris C, Safranek S.** What is the recommended approach to asymptomatic patients who develop a reactive PPD? J Fam Pract. 2006;55:163-5; [PMID: 16451786]

Item 29   Answer: D

This patient requires a sputum stain and culture for acid-fast bacilli. Reactivation tuberculosis often closely follows conversion of a tuberculin skin test, and 50% of the lifetime risk of tuberculosis occurs within 2 years of conversion. Treatment of latent tuberculosis is indicated for anyone with known conversion, regardless of age, since the risk of tuberculosis exceeds the risk of the medication. However, in patients with more chronic, stable disease, such as the patient described here, therapy can wait until the diagnosis is confirmed.

In certain situations, empiric treatment for suspected *Mycobacterium tuberculosis* infection should precede establishing the diagnosis, particularly when treatment delay may be associated with increased morbidity or mortality, such as significant cavitary disease with pulmonary compromise or tuberculous meningitis. In these critical situations, initiating therapy with four antituberculous drugs shortly after obtaining necessary sputum samples for culture and staining is reasonable. Treatment with isoniazid alone is indicated for latent tuberculosis, not active disease. Single-drug therapy with isoniazid would have been ideal for this patient at the time that her skin test converted to positive. Repeating the tuberculin skin test will not provide useful information regarding diagnosis or treatment and should not be done.

Empiric therapy with intravenous ceftriaxone and azithromycin is used for patients with suspected community-acquired pneumonia. However, this patient's recent tuberculin skin test conversion, upper lobe pulmonary infiltrate, and relatively chronic symptoms are more suggestive of reactivation tuberculosis than of community-acquired pneumonia.

KEY POINTS

- Treatment of latent tuberculosis is indicated for any person with a known tuberculin skin test conversion, regardless of the person's age.

- Reactivation tuberculosis often closely follows conversion of a tuberculin skin test, and 50% of the lifetime risk of tuberculosis occurs within 2 years of conversion.

Bibliography

1. **Yew WW, Leung CC.** Update in tuberculosis 2006. Am J Respir Crit Care Med. 2007;175:541-6. [PMID: 17341648]

Item 30   Answer: D

The most appropriate management for this patient is hospitalization for respiratory isolation and evaluation for tuberculosis. He is immunosuppressed and has symptoms and signs of an indolent infection. He also demonstrates significant constitutional symptoms that should raise suspicion for a systemic infection. Most patients using anti–tumor necrosis factor-α agents (e.g., infliximab) who develop reactivation tuberculosis have extrapulmonic disease. His presentation with new pulmonary infiltrates is consistent with reactivation pulmonary tuberculosis; his anemia and thrombocytopenia suggest the possibility of bone marrow involvement, and his hepatosplenomegaly suggests gastrointestinal involvement.

Because this patient has fever, dyspnea, and diffuse pulmonary infiltrates, clinical suspicion for methotrexate pneumonitis also should be raised. However, this is not the most likely diagnosis because it does not explain all of the patient's signs and symptoms. Discontinuing methotrexate is therefore not indicated.

Pending results of this patient's microbiologic studies, a diagnosis of community-acquired pneumonia may be pursued, and empiric antibiotic therapy would be appropriate in this setting. However, clarithromycin alone is not recommended for patients admitted to the hospital with community-acquired pneumonia, particularly those who are immunosuppressed. The reason for this patient's recent decline is most likely infection, not a flare of rheumatoid arthritis. Therefore, an increase in his prednisone dose is not indicated and may be deleterious.

KEY POINT

- Anti–tumor necrosis factor-α therapy increases the risk for reactivation tuberculosis.

Bibliography

1. **Mutlu GM, Mutlu EA, Bellmeyer A, Rubinstein I.** Pulmonary adverse events of anti-tumor necrosis factor-alpha antibody therapy. Am J Med. 2006;119:639-46. [PMID: 16887405]

Item 31   Answer: D

The initial treatment of this patient with active tuberculosis must include four antituberculous drugs. The American Thoracic Society, U.S. Centers for Disease Control and Prevention, and the Infectious Diseases Society of America have published recommendations for the management of tuberculosis. The guidelines recommend one of the following drug combinations: 1) isoniazid, rifampin, and pyrazinamide; 2) isoniazid, rifampin, pyrazinamide, and ethambutol; or 3) isoniazid, rifampin, pyrazinamide, and streptomycin. The guidelines also recommend that if the probability of resistance to isoniazid is greater than 4%, a fourth drug must be included to decrease the possibility of selecting for further drug-resistant mycobacteria. When susceptibility tests become available and the organism is shown to be susceptible to isoniazid, rifampin, and pyrazinamide, the fourth drug can eventually be stopped. As of 1997, 84% of the U.S. population met the threshold of greater than 4% resistance to isoniazid. Consequently, unless there is compelling evidence to the contrary, most patients with newly diagnosed tuberculosis in the United States are treated, at least initially, with four-drug therapy. This patient is most likely to have acquired his infection in prison. Because the likelihood of isoniazid resistance is extremely high in the prison population, initial treatment with a four-drug regimen is the best option. Therapy cannot be delayed until a definitive diagnosis of tuberculosis is made because this might take weeks and the infection could worsen or spread to other persons in the interim.

KEY POINT

• When initiating antituberculous therapy, a four-drug regimen is initially used.

Bibliography
1. American Thoracic Society; CDC; Infectious Diseases Society of America. Treatment of tuberculosis. MMWR Recomm Rep. 2003;52(RR-11):1-77. [PMID: 12836625]

Item 32   Answer: B

This patient meets the clinical criteria for latent tuberculosis infection and should receive treatment with isoniazid for 9 months to prevent reactivation tuberculosis. She has a >15-mm induration on tuberculin skin testing, which identifies her as high risk (5% to 10%) for the development of reactivation tuberculosis. Because the patient has no signs or symptoms of active tuberculosis or HIV infection and has normal results on chest radiography, she has latent infection, and treatment with isoniazid for 9 months is the appropriate therapy. In U.S. Public Health Service trials, patients taking 80% of their medication over a 10-month period had an 88% reduction of reactivation tuberculosis in the first year and a 68% reduction over the next 10 years.

Although the incidence of isoniazid-related hepatotoxicity is slightly increased in older patients, age is not a limitation to treatment of latent tuberculosis. The U.S. Centers for Disease Control and Prevention, the American Thoracic Society, and the Infectious Diseases Society of America have guidelines that call for treatment for all high-risk persons with latent tuberculosis unless prior treatment can be documented or such treatment is medically contraindicated.

Bacille Calmette-Guérin (BCG) vaccination has no role in the prevention or treatment of tuberculosis in the United States. BCG vaccine efficacy for the prevention of tuberculosis has varied among different controlled trials conducted with different populations around the world. Recent data suggest an approximately 50% protection when BCG is used in Native Americans, which is inferior to the protection provided by

isoniazid therapy. Retesting may be useful in patients with negative skin tests, especially in high-risk persons or those with either distant or recent (<12 weeks prior) exposure to active disease, but would provide no additional information in this patient. Four-drug antituberculous treatment with isoniazid, rifampin, pyrazinamide, and ethambutol is not indicated in the absence of active disease. Observation alone is insufficient protection for this patient who is at risk for reactivation tuberculosis.

KEY POINT

• In patients at high risk for developing active tuberculosis, treatment may reduce the risk of active disease up to 90%.

Bibliography
1. **American Thoracic Society; Centers for Disease Control and Prevention; Infectious Diseases Society of America.** American Thoracic Society/Centers for Disease Control and Prevention/Infectious Diseases Society of America: controlling tuberculosis in the United States. Am J Respir Crit Care Med. 2005;172:1169-227. [PMID: 16249321]

Item 33   Answer: C

This patient requires treatment for latent tuberculosis with a 9-month course of isoniazid despite his previous inoculation with bacille Calmette–Guérin (BCG) vaccine. Prior vaccination with BCG does not change the interpretation of the tuberculin skin test in most adults. Persons who received BCG vaccine usually have a negative tuberculin skin test (as defined by standard criteria) unless they are infected with *Mycobacterium tuberculosis* or are given a second tuberculin skin test shortly after the first. Occasional persons who have received BCG vaccine may have positive skin test results without having latent tuberculosis. However, no currently available test or prediction rule can distinguish true-positive from false-positive skin test reactivity. Because a 22-mm test reaction is most likely related to infection rather than to BCG vaccine, this patient should receive a 9-month course of isoniazid.

Observing him for 6 months and then repeating the chest radiograph jeopardizes his health as well as the health of his patients. His normal physical examination and chest radiograph help rule out active tuberculosis, and patients with a normal chest radiograph do not require sputum examination. Alternative treatments for latent tuberculosis include rifampin and pyrazinamide for 2 months or rifampin alone for 4 months. Treatment with isoniazid, pyrazinamide, and ethambutol for 1 month is not an acceptable alternative regimen.

Although not listed as an option, blood tests for tuberculosis based on interferon-γ production after exposure to *M. tuberculosis* are available and have a sensitivity and specificity comparable to tuberculin skin testing. However, these tests have not been as widely used as the tuberculin skin test and are not yet part of algorithms used for prevention and treatment of health care workers with a positive tuberculin skin test.

KEY POINTS

- Prior vaccination with bacille Calmette–Guérin (BCG) does not change the interpretation of the tuberculin skin test in most adults.

- The recommended treatment for latent tuberculosis is isoniazid for 9 months.

Bibliography

1. **Rowland K, Guthmann R, Jamieson B, Malloy D.** Clinical inquiries. How should we manage a patient with a positive PPD and prior BCG vaccination? J Fam Pract. 2006;55:718-20. [PMID: 16882448]

Item 34   Answer: A

Isoniazid therapy for 9 months is recommended for this patient. Immunosuppressed patients have an increased risk for developing primary or reactivation tuberculosis. Prednisone may cause false-negative tuberculin skin test results. Therefore, tuberculin skin testing in immunosuppressed patients is recommended before initiation of prednisone therapy. The American Thoracic Society recommends that patients who use prednisone, ≥15 mg/d, or any other immunosuppressive agent and who have ≥5 mm of induration on tuberculin skin testing begin prophylactic therapy with isoniazid, 300 mg/d, for 9 months.

Concomitant administration of rifampin and pyrazinamide is associated with substantial hepatic toxicity and is not indicated for patients with latent tuberculosis unless the benefits of this treatment outweigh the risks or other regimens cannot be used. Since this patient has no evidence of active tuberculosis, four-drug treatment for 1 year is not needed. Compared with isoniazid, rifampin for 4 months may be associated with better compliance and fewer side effects and therefore may be used as alternative therapy for latent tuberculosis.

KEY POINT

- Prophylactic isoniazid therapy is beneficial in patients who use prednisone, ≥15 mg/d, or any other immunosuppressive agent and who have ≥5 mm of induration on tuberculin skin testing.

Bibliography

1. Targeted tuberculin testing and treatment of latent tuberculosis infection. Am J Respir Crit Care Med. 2000;161:S221-47. [PMID: 10764341]

Item 35   Answer: B

This patient should be started on clindamycin. The presence of underlying polymyositis and difficulty swallowing place this patient at risk for aspiration and the development of aspiration pneumonia. Other risk factors for aspiration pneumonia include episodes of depressed consciousness (e.g., patients with alcoholism) or mechanical factors that increase the likelihood of secretions entering the tracheobronchial tree (e.g., patients with esophageal obstruction). Although aspiration of acidic gastric contents can result in a chemical pneumonitis, aspiration of oral secretions typically results in an anaerobic pneumonia caused by anaerobic organisms that are normally present in the mouth. A sputum Gram stain often shows both gram-positive and gram-negative organisms of different morphologic types, as was found in this patient. The typical location of aspiration pneumonia depends upon the patient's position at the time of aspiration. Based on gravitational flow of airway secretions, the pneumonia is preferentially localized in the dependent regions of the lung at the time of aspiration. In an upright patient, the lower lobes are usually affected, more so on the right than on the left. In a supine patient, common sites of aspiration pneumonia are the posterior segment of the right upper lobe and the superior segment of the right lower lobe.

Although options for antibiotic coverage of anaerobic aspiration pneumonia have generally included either penicillin or clindamycin, controlled studies have shown that antibiotic failure rates have been higher for penicillin than for clindamycin. Metronidazole does not adequately cover microaerophilic and aerobic streptococci from the mouth, which are contributing organisms in many patients with aspiration pneumonia. Bronchoscopy is not indicated because it is unable to confirm anaerobic infection, since anaerobic organisms from the mouth will contaminate the specimens obtained.

KEY POINTS

- Risk factors for aspiration pneumonia include difficulty swallowing, episodes of depressed consciousness, and mechanical factors such as esophageal obstruction.

- Clindamycin provides effective treatment for anaerobic aspiration pneumonia.

Bibliography

1. **Niederman MS.** Recent advances in community-acquired pneumonia: inpatient and outpatient. Chest. 2007;131:1205-15. [PMID: 17426229]

Item 36   Answer: B

This patient should be started on ceftriaxone and azithromycin. Recommendations for initial empiric antibiotic therapy for a patient with community-acquired pneumonia are based upon specific factors that determine a particular subset into which the patient can be categorized. These factors include the place of treatment (outpatient, inpatient, or intensive care unit), the presence or absence of underlying cardiopulmonary diseases, and the presence or absence of other modifying factors that may increase the risk that a particular organism, especially *Pseudomonas aeruginosa*, is causing the infection. This patient has an underlying cardiopulmonary disease and is hospitalized. The recommended empiric antibiotic therapy for a hospitalized patient with community-acquired pneumonia who is not in an intensive care unit is 1) an intravenous β-lactam plus an intravenous or oral macrolide or doxycycline or 2) monotherapy with an intravenous fluoroquinolone. The recommended treatment for a patient in the intensive care unit is an intravenous β-lactam (ceftriaxone or cefotaxime) plus either an intravenous macrolide (azithromycin) or an intravenous fluoroquinolone. If the patient is at risk for *P. aeruginosa* infection, an antipseudomonal β-lactam should be used.

The most appropriate treatment for this patient is the combination of ceftriaxone and azithromycin. The other regimens do not cover the atypical pathogens that commonly cause community-acquired pneumonia, including *Mycoplasma pneumoniae*, *Chlamydophila pneumoniae* (formerly *Chlamydia pneumoniae*), and *Legionella pneumophila*.

KEY POINTS

- The recommended empiric therapy for a patient with community-acquired pneumonia who is hospitalized on a general medical floor is either monotherapy with an intravenous fluoroquinolone or combination therapy with an intravenous β-lactam plus either an intravenous or oral macrolide or doxycycline.

- The recommended empiric therapy for a patient with community-acquired pneumonia who is hospitalized in an intensive care unit is an intravenous β-lactam plus either an intravenous macrolide or an intravenous fluoroquinolone.

Bibliography
1. **Niederman MS.** Recent advances in community-acquired pneumonia: inpatient and outpatient. Chest. 2007;131:1205-15. [PMID: 17426229]

Item 37 Answer: B

This patient with community-acquired pneumonia has been responding well to therapy, as indicated by resolution of his fever, cough, and dyspnea by day 3 of hospitalization, and can be changed to oral antibiotics. Specific criteria for changing from intravenous to oral antibiotics include improvement in fever, cough, and dyspnea and a decrease in the leukocyte count. In addition, the patient must have a functioning gastrointestinal tract and be able to take oral medication. This patient meets all criteria, and intravenous levofloxacin should therefore be changed to the oral agent. In most patients, oral therapy can usually be instituted within 3 days.

The unchanged chest radiograph findings are not of concern because the patient is improving by all other clinical measures. Only about two thirds of patients demonstrate chest radiographic clearing of pneumonia by the fourth week of therapy. In addition, radiographic clearing is generally slower in patients who are older than 50 years of age, have multilobar involvement, or have an underlying chronic disease or alcoholism.

Neither a CT scan nor bronchoscopy is indicated because the patient is responding to therapy. However, one or both of these procedures may be required in someone who is not responding adequately to treatment. Since this patient is doing well on levofloxacin, there is no reason to switch to or add another antibiotic.

- Hospitalized patients with community-acquired pneumonia can usually be changed from an intravenous to an oral antibiotic regimen when fever, cough, and dyspnea have resolved; oral intake is satisfactory; and the leukocyte count is returning towards normal.

Bibliography
1. **Niederman MS.** Recent advances in community-acquired pneumonia: inpatient and outpatient. Chest. 2007;131:1205-15. [PMID: 17426229]

Item 38 Answer: B

This patient has community-acquired pneumonia in association with mild lung disease and can be treated with azithromycin. The most likely pathogens include the common causes of community-acquired pneumonia, particularly *Streptococcus pneumoniae*, and atypical organisms, especially *Mycoplasma pneumoniae*, *Chlamydophila pneumoniae* (formerly *Chlamydia pneumoniae*), and *Legionella pneumophila* (especially in patients with more severe illness). This patient's mild asthma does not put her at risk for community-acquired pneumonia due to unusual pathogens. The current recommendation for management of outpatients who have uncomplicated community-acquired pneumonia without other risk factors is empiric antibiotic therapy to cover both *S. pneumoniae* and atypical pathogens. The primary choices are an advanced-generation macrolide (such as azithromycin or clarithromycin), a ketolide (telithromycin), or doxycycline. Azithromycin is therefore the most appropriate of the antibiotics listed.

Because sputum Gram stain and culture are neither sensitive nor specific, initial therapy for uncomplicated community-acquired pneumonia is empiric and is based upon the coverage of usual pathogens rather than the results of either study. The role of culture in the management of acute pneumonia is somewhat controversial. Most clinicians do not obtain cultures for patients with uncomplicated community-acquired pneumonia. However, cultures are often helpful for patients who fail to respond to therapy or for tracking pathogens and resistance patterns in selected geographic areas. Trimethoprim–sulfamethoxazole provides limited coverage for *S. pneumoniae* and almost no coverage for atypical organisms. Ciprofloxacin is effective against atypical pathogens but has limited activity against *S. pneumoniae*. Gentamicin is generally not recommended for treatment of outpatient pneumonia because it must be administered either intravenously or intramuscularly, provides minimal coverage for *S. pneumoniae*, and has no activity against atypical organisms.

KEY POINTS

- Options for treatment of community-acquired pneumonia in an outpatient without additional risk factors include an advanced-generation macrolide or a ketolide or doxycycline.

- **Treatment of an outpatient with community-acquired pneumonia should be started without waiting for results of Gram stain and culture.**

Bibliography

1. **Niederman MS.** Recent advances in community-acquired pneumonia: inpatient and outpatient. Chest. 2007;131:1205-15. [PMID: 17426229]

Item 39   Answer: A

Azithromycin and cefuroxime is the appropriate treatment for this patient who has community-acquired pneumonia, with *Legionella pneumophila* as the probable pathogen. Azithromycin monotherapy is used in patients without cardiopulmonary disease or modifying factors. Otherwise, it is combined with a β-lactam agent. Macrolide monotherapy is associated with breakthrough bacteremia in patients with underlying medical conditions who are infected with either macrolide-resistant or macrolide-sensitive organisms. Breakthrough bacteremia is more common in patients with resistant organisms. However, when it occurs in patients infected with macrolide-sensitive organisms, these patients are more often older than 65 years, have underlying heart disease, or are residents of a nursing home. An alternative therapy is monotherapy with an antipneumococcal fluoroquinolone (levofloxacin, gatifloxacin, moxifloxacin), which will also cover *Legionella* sp.

Community-acquired pneumonia caused by *Legionella pneumophila* should be considered in all patients with the appropriate risk factors and presenting symptoms. The most common risk factors include cigarette smoking, advanced age, and predisposing underlying conditions, such as chronic lung disease, immunodeficiency, malignancy, end-stage renal disease, and diabetes mellitus. The signs and symptoms of *Legionella* disease are nonspecific and range in severity from mild illness to fatal multilobar pneumonia. High fever is a hallmark of legionellosis, and relative bradycardia may be present. Extrapulmonary manifestations include headache, lethargy, and confusion as well as diarrhea, nausea, vomiting, and abdominal pain. Hyponatremia and elevated liver enzymes are reported in approximately 50% of patients. Hypophosphatemia, azotemia, and an elevated creatine kinase level may also be found.

Doxycycline may be less effective than macrolides or fluoroquinolones for the treatment of legionellosis. It is the agent of choice for psittacosis, which is an occupational disease of zoo and pet shop employees and is caused by the intracellular bacterium *Chlamydophila* (formerly *Chlamydia*) *psittaci*. However, gastrointestinal manifestations are very uncommon, and the leukocyte count is usually normal to mildly decreased.

Fluconazole is indicated for treatment of coccidioidomycosis, which is endemic in Arizona. The dimorphic fungus *Coccidioides immitis* usually causes a self-limited pneumonia in which chest radiography exhibits a patchy pneumonitis. Patients with impaired cell-mediated immunity (such as those with AIDS), pregnant women, and certain ethnic groups (African-Americans and Filipinos) may develop severe pneumonia and disseminated disease.

The combination of piperacillin–tazobactam and ciprofloxacin is appropriate to treat *Pseudomonas aeruginosa* infection; however, this patient lacks risk factors for infection with this pathogen, such as bronchiectasis, corticosteroid therapy or recent administration of broad-spectrum antibiotics, or malnutrition.

KEY POINTS

- *Legionella* pneumonia is likely in a patient with extrapulmonary manifestations and hyponatremia, azotemia, and elevated liver enzymes or creatine kinase.
- Empiric therapy for patients with underlying medical conditions and community-acquired pneumonia should include a macrolide and a β-lactam agent; alternatively, a fluoroquinolone alone may be used.

Bibliography

1. **Mandell LA, Bartlett JG, Dowell SF, et al.** Update of practice guidelines for the management of community-acquired pneumonia in immunocompetent adults. Clin Infect Dis. 2003;37:1405-33. PMID: 14614663.

Item 40   Answer: C

This patient should receive antibiotic coverage for *Pseudomonas* infection. His diagnosis of bronchiectasis is based on the development of chronic cough and sputum production following a severe episode of pneumonia 22 years ago and the chest radiographic findings from 2 years ago. Although bronchiectatic airways may be colonized by more common respiratory pathogens, such as *Streptococcus pneumoniae* and *Haemophilus influenzae*, additional pathogens often become prominent in patients with long-standing disease, especially patients who have received multiple courses of antibiotics. Pathogens of particular concern include *Staphylococcus aureus* and *Pseudomonas aeruginosa*. Because he has bronchiectasis, this patient is at significant risk for community-acquired pneumonia due to *Pseudomonas*, with which his airways may be chronically colonized. The antibiotic regimen selected to treat his pneumonia should therefore include coverage for this organism.

This patient has no particular diagnostic clues to suggest infection with *Mycobacterium tuberculosis*. In addition, the acute onset of his current illness is more suggestive of a nontuberculous bacterial infection. Respiratory syncytial virus (RSV) probably does play a role in adult pulmonary infections, although it is rarely the life-threatening infection that may occur in children with severe heart or lung disease. However, findings due to RSV infection tend to be less local than the findings in this patient. RSV infection in adults is difficult to diagnose and is almost impossible to treat. Although inhaled ribavirin is used to treat RSV infection in children, ribavirin is seldom given to adult patients other than those who are already hospitalized with a diagnosis of severe RSV infection. *Nocardia* pulmonary infections are uncommon and occur most often in immunosuppressed patients who are usually receiving high-dose systemic corticosteroids. Patients have fever and minimal pulmonary signs and symptoms and tend to have localized "coin lesions" on chest radiographs that may already have metastasized to other body sites (especially the brain). In addition, *Nocardia asteroides* is much more likely to cause pulmonary infections than is *Nocardia brasiliensis*.

KEY POINT

• Bronchiectasis is a risk factor for the development of *Pseudomonas aeruginosa* community-acquired pneumonia.

Bibliography

1. **Barker AF.** Bronchiectasis. N Engl J Med. 2002;346:1383-93. [PMID: 11986413]

Item 41   Answer: A

This patient had severe aortic valve endocarditis and will have echocardiographic evidence of valve perforation and paravalvular extension. On cardiac examination, the soft S_1 is due to premature closure of the mitral valve secondary to the rapid rise in left ventricular pressure resulting from regurgitant blood flow through the incompetent aortic valve. The damaged aortic valve fails to close properly and is associated with a muffled S_2. A grade 2/6 diastolic murmur that is heard loudest at the second left intercostal space is typical of aortic regurgitation. There is probable extension of the infection producing a paravalvular abscess, as clued by the conduction abnormalities seen on the electrocardiogram (right bundle branch block, left anterior fascicular block, and Mobitz type II second-degree atrioventricular block). The aortic valve and its adjacent ring are the most susceptible of all the valves to abscess formation and the associated cardiac conduction complications because this anatomic site overlies the intraventricular septum that contains the ventricular conduction system. This patient meets several criteria for surgery, including presentation in congestive heart failure, severe valvular regurgitation with destruction, and evidence of paravalvular extension.

None of the other valve conditions are capable of producing the precise combination of a soft or absent S_1 and a diastolic murmur at the base of the heart and cardiac conduction abnormalities. Aortic valve thrombosis would produce a basal systolic and diastolic murmur, and mitral and tricuspid valve perforation would produce a holosystolic murmur at the cardiac apex. The murmur of acute pulmonary regurgitation may be indistinguishable from aortic regurgitation, but it does not significantly alter the S_1 and S_2 and is not associated with cardiac conduction abnormalities.

KEY POINT

• The aortic valve and its adjacent ring are the most susceptible of all the valves to abscess formation and subsequent cardiac conduction complications.

Bibliography

1. **Beynon RP, Bahl VK, Prendergast BD.** Infective endocarditis. BMJ. 2006;333:334-9. [PMID: 16902214]

Item 42   Answer: E

Patients with low-risk cardiac conditions, including previous coronary artery bypass graft surgery, have no greater risk of developing infective endocarditis compared with the general population. Therefore, these patients do not need antibiotic prophylaxis before undergoing a procedure likely to result in transient bacteremia. Other low-risk cardiac conditions that do not require antibiotic prophylaxis include isolated secundum atrial septal defect; surgical repair of atrial septal defect, ventricular septal defect, or patent ductus arteriosus; mitral valve prolapse without valvular regurgitation; physiologic, functional, or innocent heart murmurs; previous Kawasaki's disease or rheumatic fever without valvular dysfunction; and cardiac pacemakers as well as implanted defibrillators.

Antibiotic prophylaxis is indicated for patients with moderate-risk and high-risk cardiac conditions. High-risk conditions include prosthetic cardiac valves, such as bioprosthetic and homograft valves; previous bacterial endocarditis; complex cyanotic congenital heart diseases, such as single-ventricle states, transposition of the great arteries, tetralogy of Fallot; and surgically constructed systemic pulmonary shunts or conduits. Moderate-risk conditions include most congenital cardiac malformations other than high- and low-risk conditions; acquired valve dysfunction, such as rheumatic heart disease; hypertrophic cardiomyopathy; mitral valve prolapse with regurgitation and/or thickened leaflets; and intracardiac defects repaired within the preceding 6 months.

Transient bacteremia is likely to result from dental, respiratory, gastrointestinal, and genitourinary procedures. High-risk dental procedures include dental extractions; periodontal procedures, such as surgery, scaling and root planing, probing, and routine maintenance; dental implant placement; endodontic (root canal) instrumentation; and prophylactic cleaning of teeth or implants during which bleeding is anticipated. Other high-risk procedures include tonsillectomy and/or adenoidectomy, surgery that involves respiratory mucosa, bronchoscopy with a rigid bronchoscope, sclerotherapy for esophageal varices, esophageal stricture dilation, endoscopic retrograde cholangiopancreatography in patients with biliary obstruction, biliary tract surgery, surgery that involves intestinal mucosa, prostate gland surgery, cystoscopy, and urethral dilation.

Patients with moderate- and high-risk cardiac conditions who undergo high-risk dental procedures associated with viridans streptococcal bacteremia and who have no history of penicillin allergy should receive amoxicillin, 2 g orally, 1 hour before the procedure. Patients unable to take oral medications should receive ampicillin, 2 g intramuscularly or intravenously, 30 minutes before the procedure. Clindamycin or azithromycin is indicated for patients with a penicillin allergy. Vancomycin is indicated for moderate-risk patients with a penicillin allergy undergoing high-risk genitourinary or gastrointestinal procedures that are associated with enterococcal bacteremia.

KEY POINT

• Patients with low-risk cardiac conditions, including coronary artery bypass graft surgery, have no greater risk for infective endocarditis than the general population and therefore do not require antibiotic prophylaxis before medical or dental procedures.

Bibliography

1. **Morris AM**. Coming clean with antibiotic prophylaxis for infective endocarditis. Arch Intern Med. 2007;167:330-2; discussion 333-4. [PMID: 17325293]

Item 43   Answer: D

This is a healthy person without cardiovascular symptoms. Her cardiac examination is benign, with a physiologically split S$_2$ and a mild midsystolic murmur. Physiologic (trivial or mild) valvular regurgitation identified by echocardiography does not pose a risk of endocarditis, and antibiotic prophylaxis is not needed.

Echocardiography was not indicated but was ordered in this case. Transthoracic echocardiography is indicated when a systolic murmur grade ≥3/6 or any diastolic murmur is heard on examination or if a new murmur is diagnosed in the interval since a previous normal physical examination. However, with widespread use of echocardiography, valvular abnormalities that are not clinically relevant are becoming increasingly diagnosed. Such abnormalities include physiologic regurgitation (mild or less in severity) of the mitral, tricuspid, and pulmonic valves. Aortic regurgitation is not "physiologic" and is most commonly associated with aortic sclerosis.

Cardiac findings and abnormalities classified as low risk in the American College of Cardiology/American Heart Association guidelines do not warrant antibiotic prophylaxis prior to dental procedures. Low-risk lesions include benign (innocent) cardiac flow murmurs, prior coronary artery bypass graft surgery, presence of a pacemaker or an implantable cardioverter-defibrillator, secundum atrial septal defects, and mitral valve prolapse without mitral regurgitation. With the exception of secundum atrial septal defects, all other congenital heart disease is classified as moderate or high risk.

Moderate-risk lesions include bicuspid aortic valves, any acquired valvular heart disease, hypertrophic cardiomyopathy, and mitral valve prolapse with greater than mild mitral regurgitation. High-risk lesions include patients with prosthetic heart valves, a history of endocarditis, and complex con-

genital heart disease. The dental procedures that warrant prophylaxis include teeth cleaning and any procedure in which bleeding is anticipated, such as extractions, periodontal procedures, implants, root canals, and the initial placement of orthodontic bands. Prophylaxis is not indicated for local anesthetic injections, restorative dentistry (fillings), or any procedure in which bleeding is not expected.

Patients with cardiac lesions that carry a moderate or higher risk of developing endocarditis should receive antibiotic prophylaxis. The current guideline for patients without allergy to penicillin or cephalosporins is amoxicillin, 2 g orally, 1 hour before each procedure. For moderate-risk patients undergoing more invasive procedures that are prone to causing bacteremia (e.g., genitourinary and gastrointestinal procedures), ampicillin, 2 g, is given intravenously 30 minutes before each procedure. For high-risk patients undergoing these procedures (such as those with prosthetic heart valves, a history of endocarditis, or complex congenital heart disease), gentamicin, 1.5 mg/kg, is added to ampicillin. A 7-day course of amoxicillin is not a prescribed protocol for antibiotic prophylaxis prior to dental procedures.

KEY POINT

• Physiologic (trivial or mild) valvular regurgitation does not require antibiotic prophylaxis.

Bibliography

1. **Morris AM**. Coming clean with antibiotic prophylaxis for infective endocarditis. Arch Intern Med. 2007;167:330-2; discussion 333-4. [PMID: 17325293]

Item 44   Answer: C

The figure shows multiple splinter hemorrhages beneath the fingernails. Infective endocarditis is a known cause of these physical findings (mean frequency of occurrence in proven infective endocarditis 23%, reported range 3% to 39%), which should alert the clinician to include infective endocarditis in the differential diagnosis of fever, particularly in an injection drug user. Since trauma secondary to manual labor is also associated with splinter hemorrhages, care must be taken to interpret this physical examination finding in the proper context.

Congenital heart disease, particularly cyanotic heart disease, is associated with clubbing of the fingers but not splinter hemorrhages. Thrombotic thrombocytopenic purpura is associated with petechiae and purpura caused by thrombocytopenia, and jaundice caused by hemolysis may be present but not splinter hemorrhages. Cirrhosis is associated with Terry's nails, which are white proximal nail beds. Greater than 80% of the proximal nail is white and the remaining distal nail is pink; cirrhosis is not associated with splinter hemorrhages.

KEY POINT

• Infective endocarditis is a cause of splinter hemorrhages, and their presence should alert the clinician to include infective endocarditis in the differential diagnosis of fever.

Bibliography
1. Fanning WL, Aronson M. Osler node, Janeway lesions, and splinter hemorrhages. Arch Dermatol. 1977;113:648-9. [PMID: 856054]

Item 45   Answer: D

This patient with sickle cell disease most likely has osteomyelitis of her right femur. Potential causative organisms are staphylococci (including methicillin-resistant *Staphylococcus aureus*), streptococci, and *Salmonella* species. The preferred antimicrobial regimen for this patient is vancomycin plus ceftriaxone in order to cover all possible pathogens. The other options are not common causes of osteomyelitis in either normal persons or patients with sickle cell disease.

KEY POINT

- In a patient with sickle cell disease and osteomyelitis, potential causative organisms are staphylococci, streptococci, and *Salmonella* species.

Bibliography
1. Chambers JB, Forsythe DA, Bertrand SL, Iwinski HJ, Steflik DE. Retrospective review of osteoarticular infections in a pediatric sickle cell age group. J Pediatr Orthop. 2000;20:682-5. [PMID: 11008753]

Item 46   Answer: E

This patient needs a bone biopsy to guide antimicrobial therapy. In patients with suspected osteomyelitis of the foot, such as this patient with diabetes mellitus and a contiguous ulcer, palpation of the bone with a steel probe through the ulcer is often performed. This test has a positive predictive value of 89% and negative predictive value of 56% for the diagnosis of osteomyelitis. Since the diagnosis has been established in this patient, it is important to identify the causative organism to guide appropriate antimicrobial therapy. Although cultures of the drainage fluid are positive in this patient, such cultures may grow organisms that are not necessarily present in the underlying infected bone. In one study, sinus tract cultures were compared with cultures of operative specimens from 40 patients with chronic osteomyelitis. Only 44% of the sinus tract cultures contained the operative pathogen. However, isolation of *Staphylococcus aureus* from sinus tracts does correlate with the presence of *S. aureus* in the operative specimen Therefore, bone biopsy with appropriate cultures and histopathologic examination should optimally be done for definitive identification of the causative organism before beginning antimicrobial therapy. This patient requires additional studies and a trial of antimicrobial therapy before amputation is considered.

KEY POINT

- In patients with a contiguous foot ulcer and possible osteomyelitis, bone biopsy with cultures and histopathologic examination should be performed before initiating antimicrobial therapy.

Bibliography
1. Edmonds ME, Foster AV. Diabetic foot ulcers. BMJ. 2006;332:407-10. [PMID: 16484268]

Item 47   Answer: C

This patient should be evaluated with an MRI scan. All patients with pain contiguous to a bone and drainage from a fistulous sinus tract should be evaluated for osteomyelitis. MRI is an invaluable study for detecting osteomyelitis (with a sensitivity of 95% and a specificity of 88%). MRI is better able to distinguish soft-tissue infection from osteomyelitis, is more sensitive than plain radiographs, and allows better identification of optimal areas for needle aspiration or biopsy. MRI and CT scans are considered the imaging procedures of choice in the diagnosis of patients with suspected osteomyelitis.

When the presence of hardware precludes use of MRI or creates imaging artifacts with CT, nuclear imaging studies (e.g., bone scan, gallium scan, or indium-labeled leukocyte scan) may be helpful and provide reasonable sensitivity and specificity. Bone scans, however, may be difficult or impossible to interpret in patients with contiguous-focus osteomyelitis because adjacent inflammation, infection, or postoperative changes may result in false-positive results. Plain radiographs may be normal early in the disease. Soft- tissue swelling and subperiosteal elevation are the earliest abnormalities, and they may not be seen for several weeks; 30% to 50% of the bone must be destroyed before lytic lesions appear, and they typically do not appear for 2 to 6 weeks after onset of the illness.

KEY POINT

- MRI and CT scans are the imaging procedures of choice in the diagnosis of patients with suspected osteomyelitis.

Bibliography
1. Kapoor A, Page S, Lavalley M, Gale DR, Felson DT. Magnetic resonance imaging for diagnosing foot osteomyelitis: a meta-analysis. Arch Intern Med. 2007;167:125-32. [PMID: 17242312]

Item 48   Answer: D

This patient probably has osteomyelitis, and the orthopedic implant should be removed and intravenous antibiotic therapy started. Patients who have periprosthetic pain after surgery are more likely to have a periprosthetic infection than patients who are pain-free after surgery. Plain radiographs may not show signs of infection early in the disease. Soft tissue swelling (as seen in this patient) and subperiosteal elevation are the earliest abnormalities, which may not occur for several weeks. In addition, 30% to 50% of the bone must be destroyed before lytic lesions are apparent on radiographs, and such lesions typically do not appear until 2 to 6 weeks after onset of the infection. Surgical débridement is often warranted for the successful eradication of infection caused by orthopedic implant–associated osteomyelitis. Failure to remove the infected orthopedic implant allows the microorganisms to form a biofilm and therefore escape the effects of host defenses and antimicrobial agents. Surgical intervention is also important for the débridement of necrotic soft tissue and resection of necrotic or dead bone.

Antibiotic therapy without removal of the infected hardware will likely result in a relapse of the infection. Furthermore, sinus tract cultures are often contaminated with skin flora and correlate poorly with deep wound cultures. Ideally, deep wound cultures are obtained at the time of surgery before antibiotics are started. Orthopedic implant–associated osteomyelitis has high rates of infection with methicillin-resistant *Staphylococcus aureus* and *Staphylococcus epidermidis*, either of which would be resistant to cefazolin. Vancomycin may be an appropriate antibiotic in this setting but should be used in conjunction with surgical débridement and be guided by operative cultures. Hyperbaric oxygen therapy does not have a role in the treatment of acute osteomyelitis.

KEY POINT

• Surgical débridement and removal of the infected implant are often warranted for the successful eradication of infection due to orthopedic implant–associated osteomyelitis.

Bibliography

1. **Trampuz A, Zimmerli W.** Diagnosis and treatment of infections associated with fracture-fixation devices. Injury. 2006;37:S59-66. [PMID: 16651073]

Chapter 7

Nephrology

Nephrology contains self-assessment items that correspond to the following chapters in the *Internal Medicine Essentials for Clerkship Students 2* textbook:

Acute Renal Failure
Chronic Kidney Disease
Acid-Base Disorders
Fluid and Electrolyte Disorders
Calcium and Phosphorus Metabolism

Nephrology contains self assessment items that correspond to the following Training Problems in the *Core Medicine Clerkship Guide*:

Fluid, Electrolyte, and Acid-Base Disorders
Acute Renal Failure and Chronic Renal Disease

Chapter 7

Nephrology

Questions

Item 1

A 69-year-old man is evaluated during a routine physical examination. He has a history of hypertension, hyperlipidemia, osteoarthritis of the knees, and a 40-pack-year smoking history. Medications are hydrochlorothiazide, atenolol, simvastatin, and acetaminophen as needed. Physical examination is unchanged from 1 year ago.

Laboratory studies:

Blood urea nitrogen	12 mg/dL
Creatinine	1.1 mg/dL
Sodium	138 meq/L
Potassium	4.2 meq/L
Bicarbonate	25 meq/L
Urinalysis	pH 5.0, specific gravity 1.015, 2+ blood, 5–10 intact erythrocytes/hpf without casts

Repeated urinalysis 14 days later is unchanged. Spiral CT scan of the abdomen is normal.

Which of the following is the most appropriate next step in the management of this patient's hematuria?

(A) Ciprofloxacin
(B) Cystoscopy
(C) Renal biopsy
(D) Repeat urinalysis in 6 months

Item 2

A 60-year-old man with a 10-year history of hypertension is hospitalized for headache and uncontrolled blood pressure. The patient has a 58-pack-year smoking history. Medications are metoprolol and hydrochlorothiazide.

Physical examination on admission reveals a blood pressure of 180/120 mm Hg, heart rate of 100/min, respiration rate of 12/min, and decreased pedal pulses. Laboratory studies show a potassium level of 4.2 meq/L and a creatinine level of 1.5 mg/dL.

Over the next week, the blood pressure gradually normalizes after enalapril and amlodipine are added. On follow-up examination, his blood pressure is 132/76 mm Hg and heart rate is 60/min without orthostatic changes.

Laboratory studies 1 week after admission:

Blood urea nitrogen	45 mg/dL
Creatinine	3.5 mg/dL
Sodium	140 meq/L
Potassium	5.1 meq/L
Chloride	105 meq/L
Bicarbonate	20 meq/L
Urinalysis	Trace protein; several hyaline casts/hpf

Which of the following is the most appropriate next step in this patient's treatment?

(A) Discontinue amlodipine
(B) Discontinue enalapril
(C) Switch amlodipine to verapamil
(D) Switch enalapril to losartan

Item 3

A 56-year-old man is hospitalized for substernal chest pain. He has a history of peripheral arterial disease, hypertension, hyperlipidemia, and type 2 diabetes mellitus. His medications include hydrochlorothiazide, pravastatin, enalapril, aspirin, and glyburide.

On physical examination, blood pressure is 156/90 mm Hg and pulse rate is 88/min. There is an S_4 gallop, bilateral carotid artery bruits, and diminished lower extremity pulses.

Cardiac enzymes are normal; serum creatinine level is 1.4 mg/dL (confirmed as baseline creatinine level). Because of persistent pain and ST-T–wave changes on electrocardiography, he undergoes cardiac catheterization, which shows nonobstructive coronary artery disease. Metoprolol and sublingual nitroglycerin are added to his medical program. He is discharged 2 days later, at which time his serum creatinine level is 1.5 mg/dL.

He is evaluated in follow-up 2 weeks later. He has been free of chest pain. His blood pressure is 164/94 mm Hg and heart rate is 60/min; there are no orthostatic changes. Physical examination reveals a rash (*see Figure 26 in Color Plates*). The serum creatinine level is 3.4 mg/dL and blood urea nitrogen is 34 mg/dL. Urinalysis shows 1+ protein, specific gravity 1.010, and no formed elements.

Which of the following is the most likely cause of this patient's acute renal failure?

(A) Atheroembolic disease
(B) Contrast nephropathy
(C) Diabetic nephropathy
(D) Hypertensive nephrosclerosis
(E) Volume depletion

Item 4

A 62-year-old man with chronic kidney disease, long-standing type 2 diabetes mellitus, and hypertension is hospitalized for a 2-week history of progressive lower extremity edema and dyspnea on exertion. Two weeks ago, he came to the emergency department for left shoulder pain and began therapy with ibuprofen; his other medications are low-dose aspirin, simvastatin, glipizide, and atenolol.

On admission, his creatinine level is 3.5 mg/dL; 2 months ago, it was 1.6 mg/dL. A urinalysis yields 120 mL of blood-tinged urine; his total urine output on the first day of admission is 800 mL.

On physical examination, he is afebrile, heart rate is 54/min, respiration rate is 18/min, and blood pressure is 110/46 mm Hg. Funduscopic examination shows proliferative changes and microaneurysms. The jugular venous pressure is 10 cm H_2O. On cardiac examination, an S_4 gallop is present. Pulmonary examination reveals bibasilar crackles. There is bilateral lower extremity edema.

Urinalysis shows a specific gravity of 1.010, trace leukocyte esterase, 1+ protein, and trace blood. On microscopic examination there are numerous leukocyte casts/hpf. Urine sodium is 20 meq/L.

Renal ultrasonography shows that both kidneys are 11.6 cm in length. There is no hydronephrosis, perinephric fluid collection, or nephrolithiasis.

Which of the following is the most appropriate next step in this patient's management?

(A) Discontinue ibuprofen
(B) Initiate ciprofloxacin
(C) Initiate dialysis
(D) Perform renal biopsy

Item 5

An 83-year-old male nursing-home resident with a history of dementia is evaluated in the emergency department for abdominal pain. According to the nursing-home staff, he had become increasingly agitated over the past day.

On physical examination, temperature is 36.7 °C (98 °F), heart rate is 96/min, and blood pressure is 150/92 mm Hg. The patient appears frail and confused and is clutching his abdomen and writhing in pain. He is unable to answer questions. Skin turgor is normal. Pulmonary examination reveals crackles at both lung bases. There is suprapubic tenderness. The prostate is smooth and enlarged.

Laboratory studies:

Blood urea nitrogen	63 mg/dL
Creatinine	3.6 mg/dL
Sodium	137 meq/L
Potassium	6.2 meq/L
Chloride	107 meq/L
Bicarbonate	18 meq/L
Urinalysis	Specific gravity 1.014, trace protein, 0 leukocytes/hpf, 0 erythrocytes/hpf

Which of the following is most likely to establish a diagnosis?

(A) Blood urea nitrogen–creatinine ratio
(B) Measurement of fractional excretion of sodium
(C) Placement of a urinary bladder catheter
(D) Response to intravenous normal saline

Item 6

A 58-year-old man is brought to the emergency department after he was unable to arise from a chair because of muscle pain and weakness, which he has had for 2 to 3 weeks. He began taking simvastatin 1 month ago for treatment of hypercholesterolemia. He takes no other medications and does not use illicit drugs.

On physical examination, temperature is 37.3 °C (99.2 °F), heart rate is 105/min, and blood pressure is 178/98 mm Hg. Funduscopic examination shows no retinal hemorrhages or papilledema. Cardiac examination reveals a grade 2/6 systolic ejection murmur. There is bilateral lower-extremity proximal muscle weakness.

Laboratory studies:

Blood urea nitrogen	38 mg/dL
Creatinine	2.6 mg/dL (1.0 mg/dL 4 months ago)
Sodium	132 meq/L
Potassium	5.6 meq/L
Bicarbonate	18 meq/L
Calcium	8.8 mg/dL
Phosphorus	8.0 mg/dL
Urinalysis	pH 5.5, specific gravity 1.015, 4+ blood, trace protein, occasional hyaline casts/hpf, no erythrocytes or erythrocyte casts

Renal ultrasonography shows normal-sized kidneys and no hydronephrosis.

Which of the following is the most likely cause of this patient's renal failure?

(A) Acute glomerulonephritis
(B) Acute interstitial nephritis
(C) Acute rhabdomyolysis
(D) Hypertensive nephrosclerosis

Item 7

A 43-year-old woman with advanced cirrhosis secondary to hepatitis C is hospitalized for tense ascites and leg edema. She undergoes therapeutic paracentesis with removal of 4 L of ascitic fluid and begins treatment with intravenous furosemide. Her usual dose of spironolactone is continued.

Over the next 3 days, she has a net diuresis of 3 kg (6.6 lb) during which the creatinine level increases from a baseline level of 0.8 mg/dL to 1.6 mg/dL. Her urine output decreases to 480 mL/24 h.

On physical examination, blood pressure is 96/40 mm Hg. There is scleral icterus. Pulmonary examination reveals decreased breath sounds at the lung bases. She has modest ascites and no edema.

Laboratory studies:

Blood urea nitrogen	20 mg/dL
Creatinine	1.6 mg/dL
Sodium	117 meq/L
Potassium	3.6 meq/L
Chloride	80 meq/L
Bicarbonate	28 meq/L
Urinalysis	Several granular and epithelial casts/hpf
Urine sodium	12 meq/L

In addition to discontinuing spironolactone and furosemide, which of the following is the most appropriate next step in this patient's management?

(A) Intravenous normal (0.9%) saline
(B) Octreotide and midodrine
(C) Placement of a transjugular intrahepatic portosystemic shunt
(D) Repeated large-volume paracentesis

Item 8

A 64-year-old man with a 10-day history of fever and cough is hospitalized for lethargy and confusion. His wife reports decreased oral intake for the past 7 days. In the emergency department, he develops worsening hypotension, hypoxemia, and increased respiratory distress, and intubation and mechanical ventilation are required.

On physical examination, temperature is 40.2 °C (104.3 °F), heart rate is 120/min, and blood pressure is 70/48 mm Hg. Cardiac examination reveals tachycardia. On pulmonary examination, there are decreased breath sounds at both lung bases. The remainder of the examination is normal. Bladder catheterization produces 350 mL of dark urine.

Laboratory studies:

Hematocrit	44% (normal peripheral blood smear)
Leukocyte count	19,700/μL
Platelet count	285,000/μL
Blood urea nitrogen	69 mg/dL
Creatinine	5 mg/dL
Urine creatinine	25 mg/dL
Urine sodium	70 meq/L

A photomicrograph of the urine sediment is shown (*see Figure 27 in Color Plates*). Chest radiograph shows an endotracheal tube in place and bilateral lower-lobe pulmonary infiltrates.

Which of the following is the most likely diagnosis?

(A) Acute tubular necrosis
(B) Acute interstitial nephritis
(C) Prerenal acute renal failure
(D) Thrombotic thrombocytopenic purpura

Item 9

A 50-year-old woman is hospitalized for lower-extremity edema and accelerated hypertension. She has a 3-year history of diet-controlled type 2 diabetes mellitus and hypertension treated with enalapril.

On physical examination, she is afebrile, heart rate is 60/min, respiration rate is 25/min, and blood pressure is 198/106 mm Hg. There is no jugular venous distention. Cardiopulmonary examination is normal. There is pitting edema in the bilateral lower extremities.

Laboratory studies:

Blood urea nitrogen	21 mg/dL
Creatinine	1.7 mg/dL
Albumin	3.2 g/dL
Urinalysis	pH 5.0, specific gravity 1.015, 1+ blood, 4+ protein
Urine protein/ creatinine ratio	3.5 mg/mg

A photomicrograph of the urine sediment is shown (*see Figure 28 in Color Plates*). Renal ultrasonography reveals small bilateral 1-cm simple cysts, normal-sized kidneys, and no hydronephrosis.

Which of the following is the most likely diagnosis?

(A) Acute glomerulonephritis
(B) Acute interstitial nephritis
(C) Acute tubular necrosis
(D) Prerenal azotemia

Item 10

A 60-year-old man is evaluated in the office for a 1-month history of progressive bilateral lower extremity edema; during this time, he has also had increasing blood pressure readings as measured on his home monitor. He has no cardiac, respiratory, genitourinary, or musculoskeletal complaints. The patient has a 25-year history of type 2 diabetes mellitus and hypertension; his current medications include hydrochlorothiazide, metoprolol, lisinopril, glyburide, metformin, pravastatin, and aspirin. He has been taking these medications for 7 years without any recent changes in dosage. He takes no over-the-counter medications or herbal or nutritional supplements.

On physical examination, blood pressure is 155/100 mm Hg (120/75 mm Hg 2 months ago) and heart rate is 60/min. BMI is 24. He has no evidence of diabetic retinopathy or neuropathy. Cardiac and pulmonary examinations are normal.

He has pitting edema of his feet and ankles and periorbital edema.

Laboratory studies:

Hemoglobin A$_{1c}$	6.5%
Creatinine	1.9 mg/dL
Albumin	2.0 g/dL
LDL cholesterol	205 mg/dL
Urinalysis	Proteinuria and lipiduria
Urine protein/ creatinine ratio	6.3 mg/mg

Laboratory results 3 months ago were all normal, including screening for microalbuminuria.

Which of the following is the most accurate description of this patient's renal disease?

(A) Acute tubulointerstitial nephritis
(B) Diabetic nephropathy
(C) Hypertensive nephrosclerosis
(D) Primary glomerular disease

Item 11

A 19-year-old woman is evaluated for sudden-onset periorbital and pretibial edema. Three weeks ago, she was diagnosed with pharyngitis that has since resolved without treatment.

On physical examination, blood pressure is 150/100 mm Hg. Cardiac examination reveals a normal S$_1$ and S$_2$ with a soft S$_3$. The lungs are clear and the abdominal examination is normal. There is periorbital and bilateral pitting pretibial edema. There are no rashes.

Laboratory studies:

Blood urea nitrogen	30 mg/dL
Creatinine	1.5 mg/dL
Albumin	3.8 g/dL
Complement (C3)	15 mg/dL
Complement (C4)	48 mg/dL
Urinalysis	1+ protein; several erythrocytes, dysmorphic erythrocytes, and erythrocyte casts/hpf

Which of the following is the most likely diagnosis?

(A) Antineutrophil cytoplasmic antibody–associated small-vessel vasculitis
(B) Goodpasture's syndrome
(C) IgA glomerulonephritis
(D) Postinfectious glomerulonephritis
(E) Systemic lupus erythematosus nephritis

Item 12

An 18-year-old man is evaluated in the emergency department for hemoptysis. He felt well until 4 weeks ago, when he developed an upper respiratory tract infection with cough, sinus pressure, and rhinorrhea, but no pharyngitis.

On physical examination, heart rate is 90/min and blood pressure is 170/100 mm Hg. The conjunctivae are pale. Car-

diac examination reveals a grade 2/6 systolic murmur along the left sternal border. There is no jugular venous distention or extra heart sounds. Diffuse crackles are present in both lung bases. The abdomen is soft and nontender with no masses. There is 1+ edema in the lower extremities.

Laboratory studies:

Hemoglobin	8.5 g/dL
Leukocyte count	10,500/µL
Platelet count	250,000/µL
Blood urea nitrogen	70 mg/dL
Creatinine	4.3 mg/dL
Complement (C3)	140 mg/dL
Complement (C4)	35 mg/dL
Antinuclear antibodies	Negative
Urinalysis	15–20 dysmorphic erythrocytes and 1 erythrocyte cast/hpf

Chest radiograph reveals bilateral fluffy pulmonary infiltrates.

Which of the following is the most likely diagnosis?

(A) Goodpasture's syndrome
(B) Henoch-Schönlein purpura
(C) Postinfectious glomerulonephritis
(D) Systemic lupus erythematosus

Item 13

A previously healthy 19-year-old man had a 2-day history of increasing watery diarrhea, nausea, mild abdominal pain, and fever. On the second day, his stools became bloody. Ciprofloxacin was prescribed, and the diarrhea abated after several days.

Nine days after the diarrhea ended, the patient develops decreased urine output, darkening of his urine, dyspnea on exertion, and swelling of his legs and feet. On physical examination, temperature is 37.5 °C (99.5 °F), heart rate is 118/min, respiration rate is 22/min, and blood pressure is 184/102 mm Hg. Prominent bibasilar crackles are auscultated. Cardiac rhythm is regular, and an S$_3$ is heard. Abdominal examination is normal. There is 2+ pitting edema of the lower legs and feet. Neurologic examination is normal.

Laboratory studies:

Hemoglobin	7.9 g/dL
Leukocyte count	33,500/µL
Platelet count	90,000/µL
Blood urea nitrogen	88 mg/dL
Creatinine	7.2 mg/dL
Urinalysis	2+ blood, 15–20 leukocytes and 25–50 erythrocytes/hpf; protein 550 mg/dL

A peripheral blood smear shows many fragmented erythrocytes (schistocytes) and platelet clumping. A chest radiograph shows pulmonary congestion and small bilateral pleural effusions. Plain radiographs of the abdomen and renal ultrasonography are normal.

Which of the following pathogens is most likely causing this patient's diarrheal disease?

(A) *Campylobacter jejuni*
(B) *Escherichia coli* O157:H7
(C) Norovirus
(D) *Salmonella enteritidis*
(E) *Staphylococcus aureus*

Item 14

A 66-year-old woman is evaluated in the office for fatigue, decreased exercise tolerance of 1 month's duration, and new-onset dyspnea on exertion. Over-the-counter ibuprofen was unsuccessful in relieving the symptoms of fatigue, and she discontinued its use after 3 days. She has a history of hypertension and was diagnosed with diet-controlled type 2 diabetes mellitus 2 years ago. Medications are low-dose aspirin, lisinopril, and hydrochlorothiazide.

On physical examination, heart rate is 74/min, respiration rate is 14/min, and blood pressure is 148/86 mm Hg. The conjunctivae are pale. Cardiac examination reveals a grade 2/6 systolic ejection murmur. There is bilateral lower-extremity edema.

Laboratory studies:

Hemoglobin	7.2 g/dL
Leukocyte count	7100/μL
Blood urea nitrogen	64 mg/dL
Creatinine	5.2 mg/dL
Sodium	133 meq/L
Potassium	4.1 meq/L
Chloride	110 meq/L
Bicarbonate	20 meq/L
Glucose	142 mg/dL
Albumin	4.0 g/dL
Calcium	11.0 mg/dL
Phosphorus	5.4 mg/dL
Urinalysis	pH 5.0, specific gravity 1.015, no blood, 1+ protein, 0–1 leukocytes/hpf
Urine protein–creatinine ratio	2.5 mg/mg

Which of the following is the most likely cause of this patient's renal failure?

(A) Acute interstitial nephritis
(B) Chronic interstitial nephritis
(C) Diabetic nephropathy
(D) Myeloma kidney

Item 15

A 21-year-old woman is evaluated in the office for facial and lower-extremity edema of 1 week's duration. For the past 3 weeks, she has had fatigue. She has no history of diabetes mellitus, cigarette smoking, or illicit drug use.

On physical examination, blood pressure is 90/55 mm Hg. Cardiac and pulmonary examinations are normal. The abdomen is soft and without masses. There is periorbital edema and 2+ lower-extremity edema.

Laboratory studies:

Creatinine	0.7 mg/dL
Total cholesterol	325 mg/dL
Albumin	2.9 g/dL
Complement (C3 and C4)	Normal
Urinalysis	Specific gravity 1.026, 3+ protein
24-Hour urine protein excretion	15 g/24 h

A photomicrograph of the urine sediment under polarized light microscopy is shown (*see Figure 29 in Color Plates*).

Which of the following is the most likely diagnosis?

(A) Focal segmental glomerulosclerosis
(B) Membranoproliferative glomerulonephritis
(C) Membranous nephropathy
(D) Minimal change glomerulopathy
(E) Systemic lupus erythematosus nephritis

Item 16

A 51-year-old man with a history of chronic lymphocytic leukemia with transformation to prolymphocytic leukemia is hospitalized for chemotherapy. Before initiation of chemotherapy, he receives allopurinol and normal saline at a rate of 250 mL/h. One day later, his creatinine level is 2.3 mg/dL (baseline creatinine is 0.8 mg/dL), and his urine output over the past 12 hours is 200 mL despite continued saline hydration.

On physical examination, he is afebrile, heart rate is 98/min, respiration rate is 16/min, and blood pressure is 134/78 mm Hg. There is lymphadenopathy involving the cervical and submental chains and supraclavicular areas bilaterally, as well as bulky axillary and inguinal lymphadenopathy. Cardiac and pulmonary examinations are normal. The spleen is palpable approximately 3 to 4 cm below the left costal margin, and there is no hepatomegaly. There is no edema, cyanosis, or clubbing of the extremities.

Laboratory studies:

Leukocyte count	72,000/μL
Blood urea nitrogen	63 mg/dL
Uric acid	19 mg/dL
Creatinine	2.3 mg/dL
Potassium	5.5 meq/L
Bicarbonate	17 meq/L
Calcium	7.5 mg/dL
Phosphorus	11 mg/dL
Urinalysis	pH 5, numerous finely granular casts/hpf, no protein

Which of the following is the most likely diagnosis?

(A) Acute interstitial nephritis
(B) Prerenal azotemia
(C) Renal vein thrombosis
(D) Tumor lysis syndrome

Item 17

A 74-year-old man is evaluated in the office for a 5-month history of sinusitis and intermittent otitis media. He also has lost 4.1 kg (9 lb) and has occasional monoarthritis migrating from joint to joint. He has not had a fever.

On physical examination, he is afebrile. Cardiac examination reveals a grade 2/6 early systolic murmur at the left sternal border. Pulmonary examination demonstrates occasional rhonchi. There is crusting in his right naris and an opaque right tympanic membrane. He has mild bilateral maxillary sinus tenderness. The abdomen is soft and nontender with no masses. There is 1+ peripheral edema.

Laboratory studies:

Hemoglobin	11.5 g/dL
Leukocyte count	10,800/μL
Blood urea nitrogen	28 mg/dL
Creatinine	1.6 mg/dL
Albumin	3.8 g/dL
Complement (C3)	100 mg/dL
Complement (C4)	32 mg/dL
Urinalysis	18 dysmorphic erythrocytes and 1 erythrocyte cast/hpf

Chest radiograph shows several nodules in the right upper pulmonary lobe and a hazy density in the left lower pulmonary lobe.

Which of the following is the most likely diagnosis?

(A) Goodpasture's syndrome
(B) Polyarteritis nodosa
(C) Systemic lupus erythematosus
(D) Wegener's granulomatosis

Item 18

A 54-year-old woman is evaluated in the office for a creatinine level of 1.3 mg/dL; 18 months ago, this value was 0.9 mg/dL. She has a 5-year history of type 2 diabetes mellitus, hyperlipidemia, and hypertension that is well controlled with lisinopril, hydrochlorothiazide, and atenolol. She also takes low-dose aspirin, glipizide and simvastatin. Laboratory studies show a normal hemoglobin level and metabolic panel.

Which of the following diagnostic studies is most appropriate for this patient?

(A) Measurement of hemoglobin A_{1c}
(B) Measurement of urine microalbumin
(C) Renal ultrasonography
(D) Serum protein electrophoresis

Item 19

A 55-year-old man with chronic kidney disease presumed secondary to diabetic nephropathy is evaluated in the office prior to a planned débridement of his left great toe for a chronic nonhealing diabetic ulcer. His creatinine level is 2.4 mg/dL. Medications are lisinopril, atenolol, furosemide, and glyburide. In addition, he is currently taking a 14-day course of amoxicillin–clavulanate.

On physical examination, heart rate is 72/min and blood pressure is 148/68 mm Hg. Cardiac examination reveals a normal S_1 and S_2 and a grade 2/6 systolic murmur radiating to the left axilla. Pulmonary examination is normal. There is a 7-mm ulcer extending across the left great toe with purulent drainage.

Which of the following is recommended to determine the stage of this patient's chronic kidney disease?

(A) 24-Hour urine for creatinine clearance
(B) ^{125}I-iothalamate radionuclide scanning
(C) Mathematical formula for estimation of the glomerular filtration rate
(D) Renal ultrasonography

Item 20

A 68-year-old man is brought to the emergency department after an intentional toxic ingestion.

On physical examination, temperature is 36.7 °C (98 °F), heart rate is 79/min, respiration rate is 32/min, and blood pressure is 156/80 mm Hg. He is lethargic and weak, in moderate respiratory distress, and oriented only to place and person. Cardiovascular and pulmonary examinations are normal.

Laboratory studies:

Sodium	141 meq/L
Potassium	3.9 meq/L
Chloride	103 meq/L
Bicarbonate	11 meq/L
Arterial blood gas studies (on room air):	
pH	7.49
P_{CO_2}	15 mm Hg
P_{O_2}	67 mm Hg

Which of the following best characterizes the patient's acid–base disorder?

(A) Mixed anion gap metabolic acidosis and respiratory acidosis
(B) Mixed anion gap metabolic acidosis and respiratory alkalosis
(C) Mixed metabolic alkalosis and respiratory alkalosis
(D) Mixed non–anion gap metabolic acidosis and respiratory alkalosis

Item 21

A 64-year-old man is admitted to the intensive care unit with pneumonia and septic shock. Over the past 4 days, he has had increasing shortness of breath and fever. His only medical problem prior to hospitalization was hypertension. Surgical history is significant for a cholecystectomy. Medications are amlodipine and hydrochlorothiazide.

On physical examination, temperature is 38.8 °C (98.8 °F), heart rate is 110/min, respiration rate is 22/min, and blood pressure is 85/50 mm Hg. Other than tachycardia, cardiac examination is normal. On pulmonary examination, there are crackles over the entire right lung field.

Laboratory studies on admission:

Sodium	136 meq/L
Potassium	4.8 meq/L
Chloride	100 meq/L
Bicarbonate	10 meq/L

Arterial blood gas studies (on room air):

pH	6.94
P_{CO_2}	48 mm Hg
P_{O_2}	51 mm Hg

Which of the following acid–base conditions is most likely present in this patient?

(A) Anion gap metabolic acidosis

(B) Mixed anion gap metabolic acidosis and respiratory acidosis

(C) Mixed anion gap metabolic acidosis and respiratory alkalosis

(D) Mixed non–anion gap metabolic acidosis and respiratory acidosis

(E) Mixed non–anion gap metabolic acidosis and respiratory alkalosis

Item 22

A 44-year-old woman with cirrhosis secondary to autoimmune hepatitis is hospitalized for a progressively worsening 2-day history of fever and abdominal pain. She is currently on the orthotopic liver transplantation waiting list and has been clinically stable for the past month. Medications are spironolactone, furosemide, and oral lactulose.

On physical examination, temperature is 38.2 °C (100.8 °F), heart rate is 72/min, respiration rate is 24/min, and blood pressure is 74/55 mm Hg. Cardiac and pulmonary examinations are normal. The abdomen is distended with diffuse tenderness.

Laboratory studies:

Blood urea nitrogen	20 mg/dL
Creatinine	1.3 mg/dL
Sodium	132 meq/L
Potassium	5.1 meq/L
Chloride	98 meq/L
Bicarbonate	12 meq/L

Arterial blood gas studies (on room air):

pH	7.25
P_{CO_2}	26 mm Hg
P_{O_2}	78 mm Hg

Which of the following is the most likely acid–base disorder?

(A) Anion gap metabolic acidosis

(B) Mixed anion gap metabolic acidosis and respiratory acidosis

(C) Mixed anion gap metabolic acidosis and respiratory alkalosis

(D) Mixed non–anion gap metabolic acidosis and respiratory acidosis

(E) Non–anion gap metabolic acidosis

Item 23

A 56-year old man with a history of alcoholism is found lying on the street with impaired consciousness. On arrival at the emergency department, he is unresponsive and is intubated.

On physical examination, temperature is 36.1 °C (97 °F), heart rate is 70/min, and blood pressure is 126/80 mm Hg. Funduscopic examination shows no papilledema. Cardiac, pulmonary, and abdominal examinations are normal.

Laboratory studies:

Glucose	86 mg/dL
Blood urea nitrogen	45 mg/dL
Creatinine	2.8 mg/dL
Sodium	138 meq/L
Potassium	5.4 meq/L
Chloride	94 meq/L
Bicarbonate	14 meq/L

Arterial blood gas studies:

pH	7.28
P_{CO_2}	29 mm Hg
P_{O_2}	60 mm Hg
Plasma osmolality	316 mosm/kg H_2O
Urinalysis	Calcium oxalate crystals

Which of the following is the most likely diagnosis?

(A) Alcoholic ketoacidosis

(B) Diabetic ketoacidosis

(C) Ethylene glycol poisoning

(D) Lactic acidosis

Item 24

A 68-year-old woman is admitted to a rehabilitation hospital 1 week after a total hip arthroplasty. Her postoperative course has been uncomplicated. She has hypertension, type 2 diabetes mellitus, and closed-angle glaucoma. Current medications are warfarin, enalapril, atenolol, acetazolamide, pioglitazone, and glipizide.

On physical examination, temperature is 37.3 °C (99.1 °F), heart rate is 66/min, respiration rate is 22/min, and blood pressure is 146/80 mm Hg. BMI is 35.1. The remainder of the examination is normal except for a well-healing surgical wound over her hip.

Laboratory studies:

Blood urea nitrogen	13 mg/dL
Creatinine	0.8 mg/dL
Sodium	141 meq/L
Potassium	4.2 meq/L
Chloride	117 meq/L
Bicarbonate	14 meq/L

Arterial blood gas studies (on room air):

pH	7.29
P_{CO_2}	30 mm Hg
P_{O_2}	70 mm Hg

Which of the following best describes this patient's acid–base disturbance?

(A) Mixed non–anion gap metabolic acidosis and respiratory acidosis
(B) Mixed anion gap metabolic acidosis and respiratory alkalosis
(C) Non–anion gap metabolic acidosis
(D) Respiratory acidosis

Item 25

A 66-year-old man with type 2 diabetes mellitus and hypertension is evaluated in emergency department for an 8-day history of severe diarrhea, abdominal pain, and decreased food intake. His intake of liquids has been adequate. He believes that he became sick after babysitting for his grandson, who had similar symptoms.

On physical examination, temperature is 37.1 °C (98.8 °F), heart rate is 66/min with no orthostatic changes, and respiration rate is 26/min. The remainder of the physical examination is normal.

Laboratory studies:

Sodium	136 meq/L
Potassium	3.9 meq/L
Chloride	114 meq/L
Bicarbonate	13 meq/L
Arterial blood gas studies (on room air):	
pH	7.26
P_{CO_2}	27 mm Hg
P_{O_2}	90 mm Hg

Which of the following most accurately describes this patient's acid–base disorder?

(A) Anion gap and non–anion gap metabolic acidosis
(B) Mixed non–anion gap metabolic acidosis and respiratory acidosis
(C) Mixed non–anion gap metabolic acidosis and respiratory alkalosis
(D) Non–anion gap metabolic acidosis

Item 26

A 44-year-old man diagnosed with cryptogenic cirrhosis 2 years ago is hospitalized for a fractured left hip sustained after a car accident. He is asymptomatic except for pain in his hip. He has felt well recently and is currently on the liver transplantation waiting list. He has a 25-pack-year smoking history and does not drink alcoholic beverages or use illicit drugs. Medications are spironolactone, lactulose, propranolol, and furosemide.

On physical examination, temperature is 36 °C (96.8 °F), heart rate is 72/min, respiration rate is 18/min, and blood pressure is 98/55 mm Hg. He is cachectic and has scleral icterus and palmar erythema. Mentation is normal, and no asterixis is noted. Cardiac examination reveals no murmurs or rubs, and his lungs are clear. The abdomen is distended but nontender. There is peripheral edema.

Laboratory studies:

Sodium	134 meq/L
Potassium	3.3 meq/L
Chloride	107 meq/L
Bicarbonate	18 meq/L
Arterial blood gas studies (on room air):	
pH	7.48
P_{CO_2}	25 mm Hg
P_{O_2}	92 mm Hg

Which of the following is best describes this patient's acid–base disorder?

(A) Metabolic alkalosis
(B) Mixed anion gap metabolic acidosis and respiratory alkalosis
(C) Mixed metabolic alkalosis and respiratory acidosis
(D) Non–anion gap metabolic acidosis
(E) Respiratory alkalosis

Item 27

A 19-year-old man is brought to the emergency department by his friend because of altered mental status. His friend reports that the patient was fine 12 hours ago. Medical history is noncontributory, and he takes no medications. He does not drink alcoholic beverages or use illicit drugs.

On physical examination, he is comatose. Heart rate is 110/min, respiration rate is 28/min, and blood pressure is 90/60 mm Hg. Cardiac and pulmonary examinations are normal. Oxygen saturation is 96% by pulse oximetry with the patient breathing room air. Neurologic examination is normal.

Laboratory studies:

Glucose	114 mg/dL
Blood urea nitrogen	14 mg/dL
Electrolytes:	
Sodium	142 meq/L
Potassium	3.6 meq/L
Chloride	112 meq/L
Bicarbonate	14 meq/L
Arterial blood gas studies (patient breathing room air):	
pH	7.42
P_{CO_2}	20 mm Hg
P_{O_2}	94 mm Hg
Serum osmolality	290 mosm/kg H_2O
Urinalysis	3+ ketones, no glucose

Which of the following is the most likely cause of this patient's acid–base disorder?

(A) Alcoholic ketoacidosis
(B) Diabetic ketoacidosis
(C) Ethylene glycol toxicity
(D) Methanol toxiciTY
(E) Salicylate toxicity

Item 28

A 34-year-old woman is evaluated in the office for polyuria and polydipsia. She has no other medical problems, and she is taking no medications. Her physical examination is normal.

Fasting glucose is 100 mg/dL, and there is no glucose on urinalysis. Serum sodium is 140 meq/L; other electrolytes are likewise normal. Her measured urine output is 7 to 8 L/24 h.

A water deprivation test is performed. During the test, the serum sodium increases to 148 meq/L, the urine osmolality remains <300 mosm/kg H$_2$O, and the plasma osmolality increases to 299 mosm/kg H$_2$O. Despite no oral intake during the test, her urine output remains on average 275 mL/h. At this time, 0.3 µg of desmopressin is administered subcutaneously. One hour later, the urine osmolality increases to 600 mosm/kg H$_2$O, and the urine output decreases to less than 100 mL/h.

Which of the following is the most likely diagnosis?

(A) Central diabetes insipidus
(B) Nephrogenic diabetes insipidus
(C) Normal, no evidence of pathology
(D) Primary polydipsia

Item 29

A 55-year-old man with coronary artery disease is evaluated in the office 2 weeks after having had a myocardial infarction. On hospital discharge, his medications were aspirin, sustained-release metoprolol, isosorbide mononitrate, lisinopril, furosemide, and atorvastatin. Echocardiogram at that time showed inferior and posterior wall akinesis and a left ventricular ejection fraction of 40%.

On examination today, heart rate is 60/min and blood pressure is 130/70 mm Hg. Jugular venous pressure is normal and the lungs are clear. Cardiac rhythm is regular, with normal S$_1$ and S$_2$ and no murmurs or extra heart sounds. Laboratory results from yesterday are potassium 5.7 meq/L, serum creatinine 1.0 mg/dL, and LDL cholesterol 65 mg/dL.

Which of the following medications should be stopped in this patient?

(A) Atorvastatin
(B) Aspirin
(C) Furosemide
(D) Lisinopril
(E) Metoprolol

Item 30

A 73-year-old woman is brought to the emergency department after falling at home. Her family states that she has been very confused and disoriented over the past 2 days and that she began therapy with a new medication 4 days ago. She has type 2 diabetes mellitus, hypertension, and glaucoma. A bag containing the patient's medications includes glyburide, metformin, hydrochlorothiazide, acetazolamide, and enalapril.

On physical examination, temperature is 37 °C (98.6 °F), heart rate is 68/min, respiration rate is 12/min, and blood pressure is 115/65 mm Hg. She is confused and unable to

answer questions appropriately. Cardiac examination is normal. The lungs are clear. There is no edema.

Laboratory studies:

Blood urea nitrogen	17 mg/dL
Creatinine	1.1 mg/dL
Sodium	107 meq/L
Potassium	2.9 meq/L
Chloride	76 meq/L
Bicarbonate	24 meq/L

Therapy with which of the following drugs was most likely recently started in this patient?

(A) Acetazolamide
(B) Enalapril
(C) Glyburide
(D) Hydrochlorothiazide
(E) Metformin

Item 31

A 61-year-old woman is hospitalized for a 5-day history of nausea and vomiting and decreased oral intake and a 2-day history of postural lightheadedness. Her creatinine level is 7 mg/dL (creatinine level 1 month ago was 1 mg/dL). She has a history of hypertension and type 2 diabetes mellitus. Medications are aspirin, glipizide, enalapril, and chlorthalidone.

On physical examination, heart rate is 98/min and blood pressure is 85/60 mm Hg. Skin turgor is decreased. Cardiac and pulmonary examinations are normal. There is no peripheral edema. On neurologic examination, she is alert and oriented and there are no focal neurologic signs.

Laboratory studies:

Blood urea nitrogen	85 mg/dL
Creatinine	8 mg/dL
Sodium	120 meq/L
Potassium	3.7 meq/L
Chloride	86 meq/L
Bicarbonate	26 meq/L
Urinalysis	Several hyaline casts/hpf
Urine sodium	4 meq/L

Which of the following is the next best step in this patient's management?

(A) Dialysis
(B) Fluid restriction
(C) Intravenous normal (0.9%) saline
(D) Intravenous 3% sodium chloride

Item 32

A 23-year-old man with HIV infection is evaluated in the office during a follow-up examination. He was hospitalized 1 week ago with *Pneumocystis jiroveci* (formerly *Pneumocystis carinii*) pneumonia, which is being treated with trimethoprim–sulfamethoxazole and prednisone. During his hospitalization, he was diagnosed with hyponatremia. He feels well, and his condition has significantly improved since his discharge 3 days ago.

On physical examination, temperature is 36.6 °C (97.8 °F), heart rate is 84/min, respiration rate is 12/min, and blood pressure is 110/60 mm Hg without orthostatic changes. He appears thin and in no apparent distress. Cardiac examination is normal. The lungs are clear. There is no peripheral edema. Neurologic examination, including mental status, is normal.

Laboratory studies:

Glucose	122 mg/dL
Blood urea nitrogen	12 mg/dL
Creatinine	0.7 mg/dL
Sodium	111 meq/L
Potassium	3.6 meq/L
Chloride	96 meq/L
Bicarbonate	22 meq/L
Serum osmolality	246 mosm/kg H_2O
Urine sodium	117 meq/L
Urine osmolality	453 mosm/kg H_2O

Which of the following is the most likely cause of this patient's hyponatremia?

(A) Adrenal insufficiency
(B) Pseudohyponatremia
(C) Psychogenic polydipsia
(D) Syndrome of inappropriate antidiuretic hormone secretion
(E) Volume depletion

Item 33

A 66-year-old woman is evaluated in the emergency department for malaise and confusion of 8 days' duration. She has a 40-pack-year smoking history. She takes hydrochlorothiazide for hypertension. Physical examination reveals distant breath sounds. Chest radiograph shows a 1.5-cm mass in the proximal upper lobe of the left lung and infiltrates distal to the mass. A bone scan indicates no evidence of focal or metastatic disease.

Laboratory studies:

Calcium	15.8 mg/dL
Phosphorus	3.0 mg/dL
Chloride	97 meq/L
Intact parathyroid hormone	<1.0 pg/mL

Serum protein electrophoresis shows polyclonal gammopathy.

Which of the following is the most likely cause of the patient's hypercalcemia?

(A) Humoral hypercalcemia of malignancy
(B) Multiple myeloma
(C) Parathyroid adenoma
(D) Parathyroid hyperplasia
(E) Thiazide-induced hypercalcemia

Item 34

A 34-year-old man is evaluated in the emergency department for progressive nausea and poor appetite for the past 3 months and a decreased ability to concentrate. The patient has a history of hypertension, sarcoidosis, and nephrolithiasis. Sarcoidosis was diagnosed 5 years ago as a result of lymph node biopsy during an evaluation for fever, generalized lymphadenopathy, and elevated aminotransferase levels. He was treated with corticosteroids with good response; after 6 months the corticosteroids were discontinued. He has not taken corticosteroids for 2 years. A small calcium oxalate kidney stone passed spontaneously 6 months ago. At that time, he was found to have hypercalciuria but not hypercalcemia; he elected not to undergo further evaluation. His only medication at this time is metoprolol.

On physical examination, temperature is 37.7 °C (99.9 °F), blood pressure is 130/80 mm Hg, and heart rate is 68/min. Lymphadenopathy is present in the supraclavicular, epitrochlear, and axillary areas. There is mild hepatosplenomegaly.

Laboratory studies:

Sodium	145 meq/L
Potassium	4.9 meq/L
Chloride	103 meq/L
Bicarbonate	31 meq/L
Serum creatinine	1.2 mg/dL
Blood urea nitrogen	34 mg/dL
Calcium	12.6 mg/dL
Phosphorus	5.1 mg/dL
Parathyroid hormone	3 pg/mL
1,25-Dihydroxyvitamin D_3	168 pg/mL

Which of the following is the most likely cause of this patient's hypercalcemia?

(A) Metastatic bone disease
(B) Primary hyperparathyroidism
(C) Secondary hyperparathyroidism
(D) Vitamin D toxicity

Item 35

A 48-year-old woman is evaluated in the office for a serum calcium concentration of 11.6 mg/dL discovered on routine screening. There is no history or evidence of renal stones, bone fracture, cognitive impairment, or fatigue. The intact parathyroid hormone level is elevated at 115 pg/mL. The serum creatinine is 0.9 mg/dL. Phosphorus is 2.4 mg/dL. The 24-hour urine calcium excretion is 270 mg (normal for women, <250 mg).

Which of the following is the most likely diagnosis?

(A) Benign familial hypocalciuric hypercalcemia
(B) Humoral hypercalcemia of malignancy
(C) Metastatic bone disease
(D) Multiple myeloma
(E) Primary hyperparathyroidism

Item 36

A 70-year-old woman with hypertension and chronic kidney disease is evaluated in the office during a follow-up visit. On physical examination, heart rate is 80/min and blood pressure is 140/80 mm Hg. BMI is 21. Cardiac examination reveals a regular rhythm with no murmurs. The lungs are clear. Bowel sounds are normal. There is 1+ pedal edema.

Laboratory studies:

Blood urea nitrogen	30 mg/dL
Creatinine	2.5 mg/dL
Sodium	140 meq/L
Potassium	5 meq/L
Chloride	105 meq/L
Bicarbonate	20 meq/L
Phosphorus	7 mg/dL
Calcium	9 mg/dL
Albumin	3.5 g/dL

Which of the following is the most likely cause of this patient's hyperphosphatemia?

(A) Decreased glomerular filtration rate
(B) High phosphorus intake
(C) Hypocalcemia
(D) Primary hyperparathyroidism
(E) Vitamin D deficiency

Item 37

A 48-year-old man is evaluated in the office for 3 months of weakness and fatigue. He has a history of hypertension and gout. Medications are hydrochlorothiazide and colchicine. Social history is significant for having lost his job 2 years ago, after which he has been drinking 2 six-packs of beer every day. He has never had an episode of delirium tremens.

Physical examination reveals a disheveled man in no acute distress. The blood pressure is 135/80 mm Hg, and heart rate is 78/min. Chvostek's sign is positive on the right. The liver is palpated 3 cm below the right costal margin and is tender to palpation. No spider angiomata or palmar erythema is noted.

Laboratory studies:

Sodium	133 meq/L
Potassium	3.4 meq/L
Creatinine	1.2 mg/dL
Alkaline phosphatase	55 U/L
Albumin	3.6 g/dL
Calcium	7.2 mg/dL
Phosphorus	5.3 mg/dL

Measurement of which of the following is the most appropriate first test in the evaluation of this patient's hypocalcemia?

(A) 25-Hydroxyvitamin D
(B) Magnesium
(C) Parathyroid hormone
(D) Phosphate

Chapter 7

Nephrology
Answers and Critiques

Item 1   Answer: B

Cystoscopy is the most appropriate next step in the management of this patient's hematuria. Hematuria is a common finding that occurs in 1% to 3% of all patients and in as many as 10% of all men. One of the most important initial steps in the evaluation of microscopic hematuria is microscopic analysis of urine sediment to assess erythrocyte morphology to distinguish between glomerular and nonglomerular hematuria of the urinary tract. Monomorphic or intact erythrocytes characterize nonglomerular hematuria, whereas dysmorphic erythrocytes are associated with glomerular hematuria. In men >50 years of age with persistent hematuria, genitourinary tract malignancy must be excluded by cystoscopy, especially in the setting of associated risk factors such as cigarette smoking, analgesic abuse, benzene exposure, or a history of voiding abnormalities.

Repeated urinalysis is not indicated, and the associated risk factors for genitourinary tract malignancy mandate further evaluation. Urinary tract infection is commonly associated with pyuria and bacteriuria but not persistent hematuria. Moreover, a treatment course with antibiotics may delay diagnosis of urinary tract malignancy. Renal biopsy is the procedure of choice for patients with glomerular disease but has a low yield in identifying the cause of hematuria in the absence of demonstrable glomerular bleeding, proteinuria, or renal insufficiency.

KEY POINT

• Patients >50 years of age with persistent hematuria should be evaluated for genitourinary tract malignancy.

Bibliography
1. **Cohen RA, Brown RS**. Clinical practice. Microscopic hematuria. N Engl J Med. 2003;348:2330-8. [PMID: 12788998]

Item 2   Answer: B

This patient most likely has angiotensin-converting enzyme (ACE) inhibitor–induced prerenal acute renal failure. Therefore, the most appropriate initial step in this patient's management is discontinuing enalapril. Generally, an increase in the creatinine level up to 30% is acceptable after initiation of ACE inhibitors or angiotensin receptor blockers. A recent study demonstrated that continued ACE inhibitor therapy is associated with sustained renoprotective benefit in patients with stage III and IV chronic kidney disease. However, this patient demonstrated a >100% increase in the creatinine level, which should raise suspicion for bilateral renal artery stenosis or advanced intrarenal small-vessel disease. ACE inhibitors are contraindicated in this circumstance. This patient likely has atherosclerotic bilateral renal artery stenosis, given his diminished pulses in the lower extremities and long smoking history.

The glomerular filtration rate (GFR) in patients with bilateral renal artery stenosis is maintained to a great extent by an angiotensin II–induced vasoconstriction at the efferent arterioles. Both ACE inhibitors and angiotensin receptor blockers (ARBs) cause loss of efferent arteriolar vasoconstriction with a resultant decrease in the glomerular capillary pressure and GFR. Therefore, switching from an ACE inhibitor to an ARB will not improve the patient's renal function. The addition of the calcium channel blocker amlodipine was not responsible for the patient's acute renal failure. Stopping this drug or switching to another calcium channel blocker will not improve the patient's renal function.

KEY POINT

• An increase in the creatinine level ≤30% is acceptable after initiation of angiotensin-converting enzyme inhibitors or angiotensin receptor blockers.

Bibliography
1. **Garovic VD, Textor SC**. Renovascular hypertension and ischemic nephropathy. Circulation. 2005;112:1362-74. [PMID: 16129817]

Item 3   Answer: A

This patient has atheroembolic acute renal failure. Atheroembolic disease is caused by the showering of cholesterol crystals when atheromatous plaques are disrupted by arterial catheters. The renal failure usually becomes apparent between 1 and 4 weeks after the procedure. A fine reticular rash (livedo reticularis) is characteristic of this process, and its presences helps to establish the diagnosis. Patients with atheroembolic acute renal failure may have eosinophiluria. There is no treatment, and renal function does not usually return.

Although this patient has diabetes mellitus and chronic kidney disease and is at risk for developing contrast nephropathy, this diagnosis is unlikely because he has had no significant change in his serum creatinine level 48 hours after receiving contrast media. Physical examination findings, blood urea nitrogen to creatinine ratio, and urine specific gravity are not consistent with a prerenal state, making volume depletion an unlikely diagnosis. The rate of decline in glomerular filtration rate is too rapid for either diabetic nephropathy or hypertensive nephrosclerosis. Finally, contrast nephropathy, prerenal azotemia, diabetic nephropathy, or hypertensive nephrosclerosis cannot account for the patient's rash.

KEY POINTS

• Atheroembolic acute renal failure is caused by the showering of cholesterol crystals when atheromatous plaques are disrupted by arterial catheters.

• A fine reticular rash, livedo reticularis, is characteristic of atheroembolic acute renal failure and helps to establish the diagnosis.

Bibliography
1. **Dursun B, Edelstein CL.** Acute renal failure. Am J Kidney Dis. 2005; 45:614-8. [PMID: 15754287]

Item 4   Answer: A

The most important next step in this patient's management is to discontinue ibuprofen and closely monitor renal function. This patient demonstrates many features consistent with acute on chronic kidney disease following exposure to nonsteroidal anti-inflammatory drugs (NSAIDs). Intrarenal prostaglandin secretion is increased in patients with chronic kidney disease and maintains afferent arteriolar vasodilation. Prostaglandin secretion also may increase in patients with hypercalcemia, heart failure, cirrhosis, and true volume depletion. Inhibition of prostaglandin synthesis with an NSAID in these settings can lead to reversible renal vasoconstriction, decreased glomerular capillary pressure, and acute renal failure. The low urine sodium is consistent with this process. Additionally, the presence of leukocyte casts in the urine suggests concurrent tubulointerstitial nephritis.

Pyelonephritis, which would warrant empiric antibiotic therapy, is unlikely in the absence of fever and bacteriuria. Renal biopsy and dialysis would be helpful only if the renal failure persists despite discontinuation of ibuprofen or if fluid overload, acidosis, or hyperkalemia that cannot be managed medically develops.

KEY POINT

• Nonsteroidal anti-inflammatory drugs can cause acute interstitial nephritis as well as prerenal acute renal failure as a result of changes in local glomerular hemodynamics.

Bibliography
1. **Huerta C, Castellsague J, Varas-Lorenzo C, Garcia Rodriguez LA.** Nonsteroidal anti-inflammatory drugs and risk of ARF in the general population. Am J Kidney Dis. 2005;45:531-9. [PMID: 15754275]

Item 5   Answer: C

Placement of a urinary bladder catheter is most likely to establish a diagnosis in this patient. Urinary tract obstruction is common in elderly men, and evaluation for obstruction is indicated for all patients with acute renal failure. However, this patient's limited ability to give a reliable history complicates the establishment of a diagnosis.

Acute urinary retention commonly causes abdominal pain and always should be suspected in patients with this symptom and an increasing creatinine level. Placement of a urinary bladder catheter is essential in the management of acute urinary retention, and drainage of a large amount of urine with concurrent relief of symptoms would support this diagnosis. The presence of hydronephrosis on renal ultrasonography also would help to establish a definitive diagnosis, but this finding may not be present acutely.

Suspicion for prerenal failure would warrant a fluid challenge with normal saline. However, this patient's elevated blood pressure does not support this diagnosis. The blood urea nitrogen–creatinine ratio can support a diagnosis of prerenal azotemia but is not sufficiently specific to be diagnostically useful in this patient. The fractional excretion of sodium in obstructive nephropathy varies from <1% in the early phases to >2% once tubular injury has developed. Therefore, this finding will not help to establish a diagnosis of obstruction. The fractional excretion of sodium is most diagnostically useful in acute oliguric renal failure, after obstruction has been excluded.

KEY POINT

• Acute renal failure caused by urinary tract obstruction should be suspected in elderly men with abdominal pain or suprapubic fullness.

Bibliography
1. **Curtis LA, Dolan TS, Cespedes RD.** Acute urinary retention and urinary incontinence. Emerg Med Clin North Am. 2001;19:591-619. [PMID: 11554277]

Item 6   Answer: C

Statins increasingly have been recognized as a cause of acute rhabdomyolysis presenting with muscle weakness, kidney failure, and an increase in creatine kinase levels (not measured in this patient). Classically in rhabdomyolysis, release of myoglobin from skeletal muscle causes a false-positive result for blood on dipstick urinalysis, but microscopic analysis of the urine sediment shows no intact erythrocytes or erythrocyte casts, as in this case.

Patients with acute glomerulonephritis may have an associated myositis similar to that in patients with vasculitic syndromes and autoimmune disorders. However, this patient's urine sediment does not show dysmorphic erythrocytes and erythrocyte casts, which makes this diagnosis unlikely. Hypertensive nephrosclerosis is characterized by hypertension and non-nephrotic proteinuria with a bland urine sediment and slowly progressive loss of kidney function, which is not consistent with this patient's clinical presentation. Acute interstitial nephritis presents with the classic triad of fever, rash, and arthralgias. This condition typically is associated with a medication exposure, and urinalysis reveals sterile pyuria and occasionally eosinophiluria rather than hematuria. Neither hypertensive nephrosclerosis nor acute interstitial nephritis can explain the patient's muscle symptoms or metabolic abnormalities.

KEY POINT

• Rhabdomyolysis-associated acute renal failure presents with dipstick-positive hematuria but no intact erythrocytes on microscopic analysis of the urine sediment.

Bibliography

1. Sauret JM, Marinides G, Wang GK. Rhabdomyolysis. Am Fam Physician. 2002;65:907-12. [PMID: 11898964]

Item 7   Answer: A

The most appropriate next step in this patient's management is infusion of normal saline over the next 24 hours. The differential diagnosis of renal failure in this patient includes prerenal azotemia, hepatorenal syndrome, ischemic tubular injury, and sepsis-induced acute renal failure. The first step in differentiating among these conditions is expansion of the plasma volume with either isotonic saline or colloid in order to exclude a prerenal cause. Evaluation for an infectious process, particularly spontaneous bacterial peritonitis, also is indicated.

Use of octreotide and midodrine or placement of a transjugular intrahepatic portosystemic shunt (TIPS) is premature because the diagnosis of hepatorenal syndrome has not yet been established. However, evidence suggesting that combination therapy with octreotide and midodrine is effective in improving renal function and perhaps survival in patients with hepatorenal syndrome is growing. TIPS may provide short-term improvement in renal function in patients with hepatorenal syndrome but should be used only as a last resort because of the associated increased risk for encephalopathy. Absolute contraindications to TIPS include heart failure, systemic infection, and severe pulmonary hypertension. Repeated large-volume paracentesis may increase the risk for further ischemic renal injury in this patient. However, a diagnostic paracentesis to evaluate the presence of spontaneous bacterial peritonitis would be warranted.

KEY POINT

• The first step in differentiating among causes of acute renal failure in patients with cirrhosis is expansion of the plasma volume with isotonic saline to exclude a prerenal cause.

Bibliography

1. Wu CC, Yeung LK, Tsai WS, Tseng CF, Chu P, Huang TY, Lin YF, Lu KC. Incidence and factors predictive of acute renal failure in patients with advanced liver cirrhosis. Clin Nephrol. 2006;65:28-33. [PMID: 16429839]

Item 8   Answer: A

This patient's urine sediment findings and clinical presentation support a diagnosis of acute tubular necrosis (ATN). In this patient, ATN was precipitated by sepsis syndrome and associated hypotension and hypoxemia. Aside from prerenal acute renal failure, ATN is the most common cause of acute renal failure in the hospital setting. The urine findings of muddy brown casts, tubular epithelial cell casts, high urine sodium concentration (>20 meq/L) in an oliguric patient, and a fractional excretion of sodium (FENa) >1% are characteristic of ATN.

Prerenal acute renal failure also occurs in the setting of volume depletion, cirrhosis (including hepatorenal syndrome), heart failure, sepsis, or impaired renal autoregulation. However, prerenal azotemia is associated with a blood urea nitrogen/creatinine ratio >15, sodium retention as evidenced by urine sodium <10 meq/L, FENa <1%, and bland urine sediment. Acute interstitial nephritis is characterized by pyuria, leukocyte casts, and urine eosinophils; often there is a history of drug use (especially methicillin or nonsteroidal anti-inflammatory drugs but almost any drug can be causative) and rash. Thrombotic thrombocytopenic purpura is classically associated with the pentad of fever, renal failure, thrombocytopenia, microangiopathic hemolytic anemia, and neurologic findings. More frequently, only three findings of the pentad are present. This patient does not have thrombocytopenia or microangiopathic hemolytic anemia, which excludes this diagnosis.

KEY POINT

• Acute tubular necrosis is associated with muddy brown casts and tubular epithelial cell casts in the urine sediment, and in an oliguric patient, high urine sodium and a fractional excretion of sodium (FENa) >1%.

Bibliography

1. Gill N, Nally JV Jr, Fatica RA. Renal failure secondary to acute tubular necrosis: epidemiology, diagnosis, and management. Chest. 2005;128:2847-63. [PMID: 16236963]

Item 9   Answer: A

This patient has acute glomerulonephritis characterized by hypertension, edema, and findings of proteinuria and glomerular hematuria and erythrocyte casts on microscopic examination of a urine sample. Serologic studies to assess the underlying cause of glomerular disease, such as assays for antineutrophil cytoplasmic antibodies in patients with small-vessel vasculitis, antinuclear antibodies in patients with lupus nephritis, and hepatitis C antibodies in those with cryoglobulinemia, may help to narrow the differential diagnosis. However, these studies should not preclude a renal biopsy to determine the diagnosis, indicate the cause, predict the natural history and prognosis of the injury, and, most importantly, direct treatment.

The absence of leukocytes and leukocyte casts in the urine excludes the diagnosis of acute interstitial nephritis. Prerenal azotemia is unlikely in the absence of any evidence for volume depletion, heart failure, or cirrhosis. Acute tubular necrosis is unlikely in the absence of any predisposing event such as a new medication, hypotension, or sepsis. Furthermore, the urinalysis in patients with acute tubular necrosis is either bland early in the course or associated with muddy brown casts.

KEY POINTS

- Acute glomerulonephritis is characterized by hypertension, edema, and findings of proteinuria and glomerular hematuria on urinalysis.

- Renal biopsy is indicated for patients with acute glomerulonephritis of unknown cause.

Bibliography
1. Chadban SJ, Atkins RC. Glomerulonephritis. Lancet. 2005;365:1797-806. [PMID: 15910953]

Item 10   Answer: D

The patient has a primary glomerular disease manifesting as nephrotic syndrome (proteinuria greater than 3.5 g/d, hyperlipidemia, hypoalbuminemia, and edema) and should be referred urgently to a nephrologist for evaluation and management. The patient's urine protein/creatinine ratio of 6.3 mg/mg corresponds to 6.3 g/d urine protein excretion. Although diabetes mellitus is the most common cause of nephrotic syndrome and renal failure in adults in the United States, diabetic nephropathy is unlikely in this patient. The natural history of diabetic nephropathy usually follows a predictable clinical course first manifested by microalbuminuria (often referred to as "incipient" nephropathy), then proteinuria, and ultimately loss of renal function. This patient did not have microalbuminuria only 3 months ago. Furthermore, diabetic retinopathy precedes diabetic nephropathy in most patients with diabetes mellitus, and the absence of diabetic retinopathy also argues against diabetic nephropathy as the cause of the nephrotic syndrome in this patient.

Acute tubulointerstitial nephritis can also cause nephrotic syndrome, particularly in patients with nonsteroidal anti-inflammatory drug (NSAID)–induced minimal change disease. A drug history is important for ruling out tubulointerstitial nephritis, which can be caused by almost any drug. A physical examination clue to tubulointerstitial nephritis is a skin rash in some patients. Other typical findings on urinalysis include pyuria, leukocyte casts, and eosinophils. This patient has not had any recent new medications and no urinalysis findings commonly associated with acute tubulointerstitial dis-

ease, making this diagnosis unlikely. Hypertensive nephrosclerosis is usually not associated with significant proteinuria, and the patient has no evidence of hypertensive retinopathy or left-ventricular hypertrophy, which makes this diagnosis unlikely.

KEY POINTS

- Nephrotic syndrome is characterized by urine protein excretion of more than 3.5 g/day, hyperlipidemia, hypoalbuminemia, and edema.

- The natural history of diabetic nephropathy usually follows a predictable clinical course first manifested by microalbuminuria, then proteinuria, and ultimately loss of renal function.

Bibliography
1. KDOQI Clinical Practice Guidelines and Clinical Practice Recommendations for Diabetes and Chronic Kidney Disease. Am J Kidney Dis. 2007;49:S12-S154. [PMID: 17276798]

Item 11   Answer: D

Postinfectious glomerulonephritis is the most likely diagnosis in a young woman who develops glomerular disease 3 weeks after the onset of an untreated pharyngitis. In addition, the complement study results (low C3 levels and normal C4 levels) strongly suggest this diagnosis.

IgA glomerulonephritis, Goodpasture's syndrome, and antineutrophil cytoplasmic antibody–associated small-vessel vasculitis are not associated with low complement levels. IgA glomerulonephritis develops at the same time as pharyngitis, not 3 weeks later. Goodpasture's syndrome, a renal-pulmonary syndrome, typically develops in young patients. However, this patient's lack of respiratory symptoms and normal lung examination do not raise suspicion for pulmonary bleeding. Systemic lupus erythematosus (SLE) nephritis is unlikely in a patient who suddenly develops glomerulonephritis without any other previous symptoms typically associated with SLE. Similarly, this condition is associated with significantly decreased C3 and C4 levels.

KEY POINT

- Postinfectious glomerulonephritis may present 3 weeks after onset of the inciting infection and is associated with low C3 levels and normal C4 levels.

Bibliography
1. Hahn RG, Knox LM, Forman TA. Evaluation of poststreptococcal illness. Am Fam Physician. 2005;71:1949-54. [PMID: 15926411]

Item 12   Answer: A

This patient most likely has Goodpasture's syndrome in which circulating anti–glomerular basement membrane (anti-GBM) antibodies cause rapidly progressive glomerulonephritis and alveolar injury (renal-pulmonary vasculitis syndrome). The combination of glomerulonephritis and alveolar hemorrhage with anti-GBM antibodies is known as Goodpasture's syndrome. Seventy per cent of patients with Goodpasture's syndrome have hemoptysis. Pulmonary hemorrhage is more common in smokers and may be precipitated by infection or volume overload. Glomerular damage is indicated by the presence of dysmorphic erythrocytes and erythrocyte casts in the urine. The most useful diagnostic study for this condition is an assay for anti-GBM antibodies, which have been found to react with the noncollagenous portion of the α3 chain of type IV collagen in affected patients.

Classically, symptoms of upper respiratory tract infection (e.g., fever, sore throat) precede the development of postinfectious glomerulonephritis by 1 to 3 weeks. Other streptococcal infections (e.g., skin infections) can also precipitate postinfectious glomerulonephritis. It typically presents as an acute glomerulonephritis, manifesting as a systemic illness, including edema, hypertension, hematuria, and renal failure. Originally described as poststreptococcal glomerulonephritis, postinfectious glomerulonephritis can occur after infections by organisms other than streptococci, such as staphylococci or meningococci. Complement levels (C3 and C4) are usually low, and the presence of anti-DNAase B antibodies documents streptococcal infection with high sensitivity. Antistreptolysin O titers also can be followed to document streptococcal infection and resolution. Postinfectious glomerular disease may be associated with a renal-pulmonary vasculitis syndrome that is marked by pulmonary edema, but this condition is unlikely in the absence of low C3 levels. In addition, this patient has no history of pharyngitis or cellulitis to suggest that he has postinfectious glomerulonephritis and no evidence of heart failure.

This patient's condition seems limited to the lungs and kidneys and an antinuclear antibody assay is negative, which are not consistent with a diagnosis of systemic lupus erythematosus with lupus nephritis. If systemic lupus erythematosus were a diagnostic consideration, positive findings on assays for antinuclear antibodies, anti–double-stranded DNA antibodies, or anti-Sm antibodies would support the diagnosis.

Henoch-Schönlein purpura is a nongranulomatous small-vessel vasculitis typically involving the kidneys, skin, and gastrointestinal tract. Patients often present with abdominal pain, occasionally bloody diarrhea, and palpable purpura (leukocytoclastic vasculitis) involving the lower extremities. Henoch-Schönlein purpura is categorized as a dermal-renal vasculitis syndrome, not a renal-pulmonary vasculitis syndrome as seen in this patient.

KEY POINTS

• Goodpasture's syndrome is associated with circulating anti–glomerular basement membrane (anti-GBM) antibodies that cause rapidly progressive glomerulonephritis and alveolar injury (renal-pulmonary vasculitis syndrome).

• An anti–glomerular basement membrane antibody assay is indicated to diagnose Goodpasture's syndrome.

Bibliography
1. **Hudson BG, Tryggvason K, Sundaramoorthy M, Neilson EG**. Alport's syndrome, Goodpasture's syndrome, and type IV collagen. N Engl J Med. 2003;348:2543-56. [PMID: 12815141]

Item 13   Answer: B

The patient has a typical presentation of diarrhea associated with the hemolytic uremic syndrome (HUS) caused by Shiga toxin–producing *Escherichia coli*, of which *E. coli* O157:H7 is the most common pathogen. As many as 8% of patients with *E. coli* O157:H7 infection subsequently develop HUS. A high proportion of patients with HUS have permanent renal impairment, and the syndrome is associated with significant mortality. Although controversial, administration of antibiotics during the acute phase of a diarrheal illness may be associated with the development of HUS. HUS is closely related to thrombotic thrombocytopenic purpura (TTP), and the clinical syndromes of each may overlap. Both are associated with inherited low levels or inhibitors of von Willebrand factor–cleaving protease, which results in high levels of platelet-associated von Willebrand factor during attacks. Shiga toxin from *E. coli* O157:H7 or other sources may lead to antibodies directed against this protease

Campylobacter jejuni infection is unlikely because this organism is not a known cause of hemolysis or renal disease. Similarly, infection with *Salmonella enteritidis* is unlikely to induce HUS. Although the noroviruses are a common cause of diarrhea, they do not cause HUS. *Staphylococcus aureus* enterotoxin causes a self-limited acute gastroenteritis rather than the progressive findings noted in this patient.

KEY POINT

• Shiga toxin–producing *Escherichia coli* is associated with development of the hemolytic uremic syndrome.

Bibliography
1. **Razzaq S.** Hemolytic uremic syndrome: an emerging health risk. Am Fam Physician. 2006;74:991-6. [PMID: 17002034]

Item 14   Answer: D

Myeloma kidney is most likely causing this patient's renal failure. Abnormalities in renal function are common in multiple myeloma, and nearly 50% of patients with this condition have an elevated creatinine level at the time of diagnosis. Myeloma kidney is characterized by an intratubular obstruction with light-chain casts that results in renal failure. Classically, hypercalcemia, severe anemia, and a low anion gap (in this patient, the anion gap is 3) due to an increase in unmeasured cations such as calcium and immunoglobulins in the setting of kidney disease should raise suspicion for myeloma-related kidney disease. In addition, myeloma kidney is associated with a discrepancy in proteinuria detection between the dipstick urinalysis and timed urine collection in which dipstick urinalysis reveals only albumin and not light chains. However, the addition of sulfosalicylic acid to the urine specimen precipitates all proteins, including light chains. Urine protein electrophoresis also confirms the presence and type of light chains excreted in the urine.

Chronic tubulointerstitial disease secondary to analgesic use is unlikely in a patient with no history of chronic analgesic use. Acute interstitial nephritis due to nonsteroidal anti-inflammatory drug use has developed in patients with minimal exposure to these agents. However, this condition is uncommon in the absence of rash, sterile pyuria, or peripheral eosinophilia. Diabetic nephropathy is the most common cause of chronic kidney disease but is unlikely to cause a discrepancy concerning the presence of proteinuria between the urinalysis and the timed urine collection. Diabetes mellitus also would not cause this patient's anemia, low anion gap, or hypercalcemia.

KEY POINT

• Myeloma-related kidney disorders should be suspected in patients with anemia, a low anion gap, and renal failure.

Bibliography
1. **Rajkumar SV, Kyle RA.** Multiple myeloma: diagnosis and treatment. Mayo Clin Proc. 2005;80:1371-82. [PMID: 16212152]

Item 15   Answer: D

This patient most likely has minimal change glomerulopathy. Minimal change disease is the most common cause of the nephrotic syndrome in children and young adults. A low albumin level in the presence of proteinuria is consistent with this condition. Minimal change disease associated with the nephrotic syndrome presents with edema, hypoalbuminemia, hypercholesterolemia, urine protein excretion >3.5 g/24 h, and numerous oval fat bodies seen on urinalysis, which is another hallmark of a proteinuric state. The figure shows urine sediment with fatty casts under polarized light microscopy. The fat droplets have a characteristic "Maltese cross" appearance under polarized light.

Membranous nephropathy and focal segmental glomerulosclerosis, which may also cause the nephrotic syndrome, should be included in the differential diagnosis. This patient's symptoms are consistent with membranous nephropathy, but this condition typically presents in older individuals and develops less rapidly. Similarly, the development of focal segmental glomerulosclerosis is less rapid compared with this patient's disease course. Membranoproliferative glomerulonephritis is associated with a low complement (C3) level, whereas both the C3 and C4 levels are low in systemic lupus erythematosus. In addition, membranoproliferative glomerulonephritis and systemic lupus erythematosus are unlikely in the absence of hematuria.

KEY POINTS

• Minimal change disease is the most common cause of the nephrotic syndrome in children and young adults.

• The presence of oval fat bodies on urinalysis is a hallmark for proteinuria.

Bibliography
1. **Saha TC, Singh H**. Minimal change disease: a review. South Med J. 2006;99:1264-70. [PMID: 17195422]

Item 16   Answer: D

This patient has tumor lysis syndrome. Tumor lysis syndrome occurs as a function of the rapid breakdown of malignant cells, resulting in dramatic and potentially dangerous increases in serum uric acid, potassium, and phosphorus concentrations. This condition may complicate chemotherapy in patients with a high tumor burden but occasionally develops spontaneously. Despite appropriate hydration, this patient developed oliguric acute renal failure associated with marked hyperuricemia and hyperphosphatemia. Failure of medical therapy to adequately control the metabolic abnormalities of tumor lysis syndrome warrants initiation of dialysis, particularly in patients with acute renal failure. Prevention of this condition includes aggressive hydration, as well as allopurinol therapy, which typically is initiated at least 2 days before starting chemotherapy. Recently, a recombinant urate oxidase, rasburicase, has become available for the treatment of hyperuricemia. This agent is more effective in preventing renal failure in patients with severe hyperuricemia rather than in reversing established renal failure.

Acute interstitial nephritis is characterized by pyuria, leukocyte casts, and occasionally urine eosinophils and rash. Nephrotic-range proteinuria can develop in patients with minimal change disease induced by nonsteroidal anti-inflammatory drugs or other medications. The acute onset of renal failure over 24 hours, diminished urine output, metabolic disturbances, and urinalysis findings in this patient are not consistent with acute interstitial nephritis. Prerenal azotemia occurs in the setting of volume depletion, cirrhosis (including hepatorenal syndrome), heart failure, sepsis, or impaired renal autoregulation. These conditions are not present in this patient, making prerenal azotemia an unlikely diagnosis. Renal vein thrombosis is characterized by hematuria and nephrotic-range proteinuria; associated conditions include membranous nephropathy, clotting disorders, malignancy, trauma, and external compression. The absence of protein in the urine and the patient's metabolic abnormalities make this diagnosis unlikely.

KEY POINT

• Tumor lysis syndrome occurs as a function of the rapid breakdown of malignant cells, resulting in dramatic and potentially dangerous increases in serum uric acid, potassium, and phosphorus concentrations.

Bibliography
1. **Higdon ML, Higdon JA.** Treatment of oncologic emergencies. Am Fam Physician. 2006;74:1873-80. [PMID: 17168344]

Item 17   Answer: D

This patient most likely has Wegener's granulomatosis, which is a renal-pulmonary vasculitis syndrome. The diagnosis is established by positive results of a proteinase-3 antineutrophil cytoplasmic antibody (ANCA) assay. This patient's older age, sinusitis, intermittent otitis media, and crusting in his right naris are consistent with this condition. His chest radiograph findings are indicative of pulmonary disease, and the presence of dysmorphic erythrocytes on microscopic analysis of the urine, peripheral edema, and his abnormal renal function suggest glomerulonephritis.

Systemic lupus erythematosus (SLE) is capable of causing a renal-pulmonary vasculitis syndrome, but this patient's age and sex, as well as his normal complement levels, exclude this diagnosis. Furthermore, SLE does not cause upper respiratory tract disease. Like Wegener's granulomatosis, Goodpasture's syndrome is a renal-pulmonary vasculitis syndrome; it usually affects young men and does not cause upper respiratory tract disease. Polyarteritis nodosa does not cause a renal-pulmonary vasculitis syndrome and is not associated with erythrocytes or erythrocyte casts on urinalysis.

KEY POINT

- Wegener's granulomatosis is characterized by upper and lower airway disease, glomerulonephritis, and positive findings on a proteinase-3 antineutrophil cytoplasmic antibody assay.

Bibliography

1. Frankel SK, Cosgrove GP, Fischer A, Meehan RT, Brown KK. Update in the diagnosis and management of pulmonary vasculitis. Chest. 2006;129:452-65.[PMID: 16478866]

Item 18   Answer: B

Measurement of urine microalbumin is the most appropriate diagnostic study for this patient. Diabetic nephropathy is characterized by abnormal renal function and albuminuria in the setting of diabetes mellitus. Albuminuria may present as micro- or macroalbuminuria, based on the amount of albumin excreted in the urine. Microalbuminuria is characterized by a urine albumin–creatinine ratio of 30 to 300 mg/g, whereas macroalbuminuria is characterized by a urine albumin–creatinine ratio of >300 mg/g on two separate urine samples performed at least 6 months apart.

The development of microalbuminuria is believed to represent an early stage of diabetic nephropathy. Therefore, urine microalbumin measurement is recommended at least annually in all patients with diabetes. Dipstick urinalysis is a sensitive marker for macroalbuminuria, but negative results on this study do not exclude the presence of microalbuminuria and early diabetic nephropathy. Because dipstick urinalysis only detects urine albumin levels >30 to 50 mg/dL, this diagnostic study does not detect microalbuminuria.

Imaging studies such as renal ultrasonography are useful for estimating the kidney size and revealing obstructive nephropathy in patients with chronic kidney disease but not for diagnosing and assessing risk in patients with diabetic nephropathy.

Serum protein electrophoresis is effective for diagnosing myeloma-related kidney disorders in patients with chronic kidney disease of unknown cause. However, this patient has no symptoms or laboratory abnormalities associated with myeloma-related kidney disorders, such as anemia or hypercalcemia. Therefore, diabetic nephropathy is a more likely diagnosis. The hemoglobin A_{1c} level is useful for determining glycemic control, and poorly controlled diabetes is a risk factor for the development of diabetic nephropathy. However, results of hemoglobin A_{1c} measurement would not confirm the diagnosis, whereas a finding of persistent albuminuria would.

KEY POINT

- Measurement of urine microalbumin is the screening test of choice for diabetic nephropathy.

Bibliography

1. Marshall SM, Flyvbjerg A. Prevention and early detection of vascular complications of diabetes. BMJ. 2006;333:475-80. [PMID: 16946335]

Item 19   Answer: C

Practice guidelines from the National Kidney Foundation Kidney/Disease Outcomes Quality Initiative (K/DOQI) recommend the use of mathematical equations such as Cockroft–Gault or Modification of Diet in Renal Disease (MDRD) to calculate the creatinine clearance to estimate the glomerular filtration rate (GFR).

Timed urine collections are cumbersome and often inaccurate because of collection of too much or too little urine; therefore, mathematical equations are preferred to estimate the GFR. Imaging studies used to estimate the GFR, such as ^{125}I-iothalamate radionuclide scanning, are considered the gold standard for an accurate measurement of the GFR. However, these studies are costly and technically difficult to perform on all patients with chronic kidney disease and are used more commonly when precise estimations of the GFR are necessary, such as in research settings and for evaluation of potential kidney donors. Renal ultrasonography is an important tool in the assessment of kidney size and anatomy in chronic kidney disease but is not helpful in the assessment of the stage of chronic kidney disease.

KEY POINT

- Mathematical equations such as Cockroft–Gault or Modification of Diet in Renal Disease are recommended for the assessment of the glomerular filtration rate.

Bibliography

1. Stevens LA, Coresh J, Greene T, Levey AS. Assessing kidney function—measured and estimated glomerular filtration rate. N Engl J Med. 2006;354:2473-83. [PMID: 16760447]

Item 20   Answer: B

This patient has a mixed anion gap metabolic acidosis and respiratory alkalosis. The presence of an alkaline pH with a low serum bicarbonate level suggests either a respiratory alkalosis with ongoing renal compensation or a metabolic acidosis with a respiratory alkalosis. His elevated anion gap indicates the presence of a metabolic acidosis. Suspicion for a mixed disorder also should be raised in a patient whose pH is above normal in the presence of a metabolic acidosis. This presentation is not consistent with a simple metabolic acidosis with respiratory compensation because the compensation would not raise the pH above normal. To confirm the suspicion of a mixed disorder, Winter's formula can be used to estimate the expected P_{CO_2}:

Expected $P_{CO_2} = 1.5 \times [HCO_3^{-}] + 8 \pm 2 = 24.5 \pm 2$ mm Hg.

According to this formula, the expected P_{CO_2} is approximately 25 mm Hg, but the measured P_{CO_2} was 15 mm Hg, which confirms the presence of a respiratory alkalosis. The most likely cause of a mixed anion gap metabolic acidosis and respiratory alkalosis in this patient is salicylate toxicity.

Since the patient's pH is elevated, he cannot have a mixed anion gap metabolic acidosis and respiratory acidosis and because his anion gap measures 27, calculated as $[Na^+] - ([Cl^-] + [HCO_3^{-}])$, the diagnosis of mixed non–anion gap metabolic acidosis and respiratory alkalosis is incorrect. Finally, the low bicarbonate level excludes the diagnosis of mixed metabolic alkalosis and respiratory alkalosis.

KEY POINT

- In a patient with a toxic ingestion, the presence of mixed anion gap metabolic acidosis and respiratory alkalosis suggests salicylate toxicity.

Bibliography

1. **Krause DS, Wolf BA, Shaw LM**. Acute aspirin overdose: mechanisms of toxicity. Ther Drug Monit. 1992;14:441-51. [PMID: 1485363]

Item 21   Answer: B

This patient most likely has a mixed anion gap metabolic acidosis and respiratory acidosis. The pH <7.38 indicates an acidosis. The decreased bicarbonate level accompanied by an elevated anion gap is consistent with an anion gap metabolic acidosis, most likely due to septic shock–associated lactic acidosis. Winter's formula can be used to estimate the expected P_{CO_2} for the degree of acidosis:

Expected $P_{CO_2} = 1.5 \times [HCO_3^{-}] + 8 \pm 2 = 23 \pm 2$ mm Hg.

According to this formula, this patient's P_{CO_2} is significantly elevated above the expected level, which indicates the presence of relative carbon dioxide retention and respiratory acidosis. This may be due to ventilatory failure secondary to the patient's pneumonia.

KEY POINTS

- A decrease in the pH and bicarbonate level is consistent with a primary metabolic acidosis.

- In a patient with a primary metabolic acidosis, a P_{CO_2} that is higher than expected indicates a mixed metabolic and respiratory acidosis.

Bibliography

1. **Narins RG, Emmett M.** Simple and mixed acid-base disorders: a practical approach. Medicine (Baltimore). 1980;59:161-87. [PMID: 6774200]

Item 22   Answer: A

This patient most likely has an anion gap metabolic acidosis. In patients with severe liver disease, decreased clearance of lactate from the circulation can lead to lactic acidosis and may account for this patient's anion gap acidosis. The anion gap is 22, calculated as $[Na^+] - ([Cl^-] + [HCO_3^{-}])$.

Mixed anion gap metabolic acidosis and respiratory alkalosis is not correct because there is no respiratory alkalosis. The P_{CO_2} in this patient is consistent with a normal compensation for the degree of acidemia, which excludes respiratory alkalosis and respiratory acidosis. Winter's formula can be used to estimate the expected P_{CO_2}:

Expected $P_{CO_2} = 1.5 \times [HCO_3^{-}] + 8 \pm 2 = 26 \pm 2$ mm Hg.

Because the expected P_{CO_2} approximates the measured P_{CO_2}, it can be concluded that respiratory compensation is appropriate.

KEY POINTS

- The anion gap is calculated as $[Na^+] - ([Cl^-] + [HCO_3^{-}])$.

- Winter's formula can be used to estimate the expected P_{CO_2}: $1.5 \times [HCO_3^{-}] + 8 \pm 2$ mm Hg.

Bibliography

1. **Hassan H, Joh JH, Bacon BR, Bastani B**. Evaluation of serum anion gap in patients with liver cirrhosis of diverse etiologies. Mt Sinai J Med. 2004;71:281-4. [PMID: 15365595]

Item 23   Answer: C

This patient has ethylene glycol poisoning. The presence of acute renal failure associated with an increased anion gap metabolic acidosis and an increased osmolar gap is highly suggestive of ethylene glycol poisoning. The osmolar gap is the difference between calculated osmolality and measured osmolality. In this case the osmolality is calculated as:

$2 \times [Na^+] + [glucose]/18 + [BUN]/2.8 = 296$ mosm/kg H_2O.

The difference between the measured and calculated osmolality = 20 mosm/kg H_2O. The normal osmolar gap is approximately 10 mosm/kg H_2O. An elevated osmolar gap suggests the presence of an unmeasured osmole, most commonly ethanol, but can be ethylene glycol or methanol. However, only ethylene glycol is associated with renal failure and calcium oxalate crystals in the urine.

Although alcoholic and diabetic ketoacidosis and lactic acidosis can cause an anion gap metabolic acidosis, none is associated with an osmolar gap.

KEY POINT
- Ethylene glycol poisoning is associated with an anion and osmolar gap metabolic acidosis and calcium oxalate crystals in the urine.

Bibliography
1. **Megarbane B, Borron SW, Baud FJ.** Current recommendations for treatment of severe toxic alcohol poisonings. Intensive Care Med. 2005;31:189-95. [PMID: 15627163]

Item 24   Answer: C

This patient has a non–anion gap metabolic acidosis with appropriate respiratory compensation, which is most consistent with use of the carbonic anhydrase inhibitor acetazolamide. In the proximal tubule, inhibition of carbonic anhydrase impairs proximal tubular bicarbonate reabsorption, which frequently leads to a non–anion gap metabolic acidosis. This presentation is essentially the pharmacologic equivalent of a proximal (type 2) renal tubular acidosis. The appropriateness of the respiratory compensation can be checked using Winter's formula to calculate the expected P_{CO_2}:

$$\text{Expected } P_{CO_2} = 1.5 \times [HCO_3^-] + 8 \pm 2 = 29 \pm 2 \text{ mm Hg.}$$

Since the expected P_{CO_2} equals the measured P_{CO_2}, there is appropriate respiratory compensation and the acid–base disturbance is not a mixed disorder. Respiratory acidosis can be excluded because the P_{CO_2} is not elevated.

KEY POINT
- Acetazolamide may cause non–anion gap metabolic acidosis.

Bibliography
1. **Maisey DN, Brown RD.** Acetazolamide and symptomatic metabolic acidosis in mild renal failure. Br Med J (Clin Res Ed). 1981;283:1527-8. [PMID: 6799050]

Item 25   Answer: D

This patient's low pH, decreased bicarbonate level, and normal anion gap indicate the presence of non–anion gap metabolic acidosis. His adequate respiratory compensation excludes a mixed acid–base disorder. The expected respiratory compensation for metabolic acidosis can be checked by using Winter's formula:

$$\text{Expected } P_{CO_2} = 1.5 \times [HCO_3^-] + 8 \pm 2 = 27.5 \pm 2 \text{ mm Hg.}$$

Since the calculated P_{CO_2} equals the measured P_{CO_2}, the patient has normal respiratory compensation for the metabolic acidosis. The patient's anion gap is 9; he therefore cannot have a mixed anion gap and non–anion gap metabolic acidosis.

KEY POINT
- A low pH and decreased bicarbonate level indicate a metabolic acidosis.

Bibliography
1. **Narins RG, Emmett M.** Simple and mixed acid-base disorders: a practical approach. Medicine (Baltimore). 1980;59:161-87. [PMID: 6774200]

Item 26   Answer: E

The acid–base disturbance in this patient is a respiratory alkalosis, related to increased minute ventilation, which commonly develops in patients with end-stage liver disease. The liver helps to metabolize circulating steroid hormones. Elevated levels of progestins in end-stage liver disease lead to stimulation of the respiratory drive, which causes a primary respiratory alkalosis.

If the pH is not measured, this disturbance can be misdiagnosed as metabolic acidosis (low serum bicarbonate); however, the high pH excludes this diagnosis. In patients with severe liver disease, decreased clearance of lactate from the circulation can lead to lactic acidosis. However, the absence of an anion gap in this patient excludes this condition. Mixed metabolic alkalosis and respiratory acidosis is not supported by the low bicarbonate and low P_{CO_2} levels.

KEY POINT
- Respiratory alkalosis commonly develops in patients with end-stage liver disease.

Bibliography
1. **Lustik SJ, Chhibber AK, Kolano JW, Hilmi IA, Henson LC, Morris MC, et al.** The hyperventilation of cirrhosis: progesterone and estradiol effects. Hepatology. 1997;25:55-8. [PMID: 8985264]

Item 27   Answer: E

This patient most likely has salicylate toxicity. He has an anion gap metabolic acidosis and respiratory alkalosis. Metabolic acidosis is indicated by the low serum bicarbonate level and the anion gap of 16, which can be calculated according to the following formula:

$$[Na^+] - ([Cl^-] + [HCO_3^-])$$

This patient's expected P_{CO_2} is 29 ± 2 mm Hg, which can be calculated using Winter's formula:

$$\text{Expected } P_{CO_2} = 1.5 \times [HCO_3^-] + 8 \pm 2 \text{ mm Hg}$$

However, his measured P_{CO_2} of 20 mm Hg is lower than expected for the degree of metabolic acidosis present, which confirms the presence of a concurrent respiratory alkalosis. A common cause of mixed anion gap metabolic acidosis and respiratory alkalosis is salicylate toxicity, which can be confirmed by measuring the blood level of salicylate. In this case, ketonuria is likely related to increased tissue (especially fat) catabolism in the face of severe metabolic acidosis.

Alcoholic ketoacidosis, ethylene glycol toxicity, and methanol toxicity can cause anion gap metabolic acidosis but not respiratory alkalosis. In addition, alcohol poisoning is accompanied by an increased osmolal gap. The osmolal gap is obtained by calculating the difference between the calculated and measured serum osmolality. This patient's calculated serum osmolality of 295 mosm/kg H_2O can be obtained using the following formula:

$$2 \times [Na+] + [Glucose/18] + [Blood\ Urea\ Nitrogen/2.8]$$

The measured osmolality is 290 mosm/kg H_2O. Therefore, the osmolal gap is 5 mosm/kg H_2O (normal <10 mosm/kg H_2O), which excludes alcohol poisoning. Diabetic ketoacidosis usually is associated with more profound anion gap metabolic acidosis with an elevated plasma glucose level and without respiratory alkalosis.

KEY POINTS

• A common cause of mixed anion gap metabolic acidosis and respiratory alkalosis is salicylate toxicity.

• Alcohol poisoning is accompanied by an increased osmolal gap.

Bibliography
1. **Kamel KS, Halperin ML.** An improved approach to the patient with metabolic acidosis: a need for four amendments. J Nephrol. 2006;9:S76-85. [PMID: 16736445]

Item 28   Answer: A

This patient has central diabetes insipidus (DI). She presents with typical signs of DI, namely polydipsia and polyuria with excretion of large amounts of dilute urine. During the water deprivation phase of the test, the patient demonstrates impaired ability to concentrate her urine, which is consistent with either nephrogenic or central DI. Her values do not indicate a normal response to water deprivation, which would be increasing urine osmolality. She does, however, show an increase in urine osmolality after the administration of desmopressin, which is indicative of central DI. She would not have responded to the desmopressin if she had nephrogenic DI (resistance to antidiuretic hormone). Finally, primary polydipsia is unlikely, as patients with this disorder can usually partially concentrate their urine in response to water deprivation.

KEY POINT

• In the water deprivation test, impaired ability to concentrate urine is consistent with either nephrogenic or central diabetes insipidus.

Bibliography
1. **Maghnie M.** Diabetes insipidus. Horm Res. 2003;59 Suppl 1:42-54. [PMID: 12566720]

Item 29   Answer: D

This patient developed hyperkalemia as a side effect of angiotensin-converting enzyme (ACE) inhibitor therapy. The incidence of hyperkalemia is similar among patients taking ACE inhibitors or angiotensin-receptor blockers (ARBs). In patients who cannot tolerate an ACE inhibitor or an ARB, the combination of hydralazine and a nitrate should be used. This combination improves mortality compared with a placebo (although not as much as with an ACE inhibitor).

In general, discontinuation of an ACE inhibitor should be considered if the potassium level rises above 5.5 meq/L despite interventions to prevent hyperkalemia, such as discontinuation of other drugs that cause hyperkalemia, concurrent use of loop diuretics, or lowering the dose of the ACE inhibitor. Another side effect of ACE inhibitor therapy that occurs rarely is renal insufficiency, although renal insufficiency alone should not preclude treatment with ACE inhibitors. Although the risk of worsening renal function with ACE inhibitor therapy increases with the degree of baseline renal dysfunction, patients with the greatest degree of renal insufficiency generally derive the greatest long-term renoprotective effect from ACE inhibitor therapy. Some experts have proposed continuation of ACE inhibitor therapy if creatinine level increases are ≤30% above baseline and stabilize within 2 to 3 weeks. If the creatinine level remains elevated more than 30% above baseline after 4 weeks of ACE inhibitor therapy, dose reduction and/or further evaluation for other causes of renal insufficiency (such as nonsteroidal anti-inflammatory drug use or renal artery stenosis) may be indicated.

Nonselective β-adrenergic blockers interfere with potassium uptake by the cells. This causes a <0.5-meq/L increase in serum potassium levels in normal subjects and is even less when β_1-selective blockers such as atenolol or metoprolol are used. True hyperkalemia is rare in the absence of hypoaldosteronism or renal failure. Aspirin and other nonsteroidal drugs can cause hyperkalemia by inducing a hyporenin hypoaldosteronemic state via their inhibition of prostaglandin synthesis; however, these agents do not typically cause hyperkalemia by themselves in the setting of normal renal function and the euvolemic state, as in this patient. Atorvastatin does not cause hyperkalemia. Furosemide, by enhancing potassium excretion, can cause hypokalemia, not hyperkalemia.

KEY POINTS

• Hyperkalemia is a side effect of angiotensin-converting enzyme (ACE) inhibitor therapy.

• A hydralazine/nitrate combination should be considered in patients with heart failure who develop hyperkalemia while taking an ACE inhibitor or an angiotensin-receptor blocker.

Bibliography
1. **Palmer BF.** Managing hyperkalemia caused by inhibitors of the renin-angiotensin-aldosterone system. N Engl J Med. 2004;351:585-92. [PMID: 15295051].

Item 30   Answer: D

Hydrochlorothiazide is a common cause of hyponatremia in the outpatient setting. It is especially common in the elderly. Thiazide diuretics work at the level of the cortical collecting duct. Therefore, these agents maintain urinary concentrating capacity but not diluting capacity, which makes them prone to cause hyponatremic encephalopathy. By inducing relative volume depletion, antidiuretic hormone secretion is stimulated, which leads to urine concentration and water retention.

Acetazolamide acts in the proximal tubule as a carbonic anhydrase IV inhibitor. Blocking this enzyme in the proximal tubule impairs bicarbonate reabsorption but not diluting capacity and is most often associated with hypokalemia and metabolic acidosis. Acetazolamide is not associated with the development of hyponatremia. Metformin and glyburide do not affect fluid and electrolyte balance. Enalapril competes with the natural substrate, angiotensin I, thereby inhibiting its conversion to angiotensin II. Decreases in plasma angiotensin II levels also reduce aldosterone secretion, with a subsequent decrease in sodium and water retention and potassium retention.

KEY POINT

• Hydrochlorothiazide can cause severe hyponatremia.

Bibliography

1. Ayus JC, Arieff AI. Chronic hyponatremic encephalopathy in postmenopausal women: association of therapies with morbidity and mortality. JAMA. 1999;281:2299-304. [PMID: 10386554]

Item 31   Answer: C

The next best step in this patient's management is bolus therapy with 1000 mL of normal saline (0.9%). This patient's history of decreased intake, vomiting, and ongoing diuretic use is consistent with extracellular fluid volume contraction. Her decreased skin turgor, tachycardia, and hypotension also support this diagnosis. The low urine sodium (<10 meq/L) is consistent with prerenal azotemia. Initial therapy should aim to correct the extracellular fluid deficit by using isotonic saline. However, overzealous hydration in the setting of oliguric acute tubular necrosis, which may be present in this patient, may cause pulmonary edema. Therefore, close monitoring of urine output and volume status is warranted.

Because this patient has hyponatremia in the setting of volume depletion, normal saline is preferred over hypertonic saline. Dialysis is indicated only if the renal function and urine output fail to improve after hydration. Fluid restriction would help to correct the hyponatremia but would not resolve the volume deficit and resultant impaired organ perfusion.

KEY POINT

• The initial treatment of prerenal azotemia complicated by hyponatremia is volume replacement with normal saline.

Bibliography

1. Schrier RW, Wang W, Poole B, Mitra A. Acute renal failure: definitions, diagnosis, pathogenesis, and therapy. J Clin Invest. 2004;114:5-14. [PMID: 15232604]

Item 32   Answer: D

This patient's laboratory findings are consistent with the syndrome of inappropriate antidiuretic hormone secretion (SIADH). This condition is characterized by hypotonic hyponatremia with a urine osmolality >100 mosm/kg H_2O in the absence of volume depletion, adrenal insufficiency, congestive heart failure, hypothyroidism, cirrhosis, and/or renal impairment. Hypotonicity is established by the abnormally low serum osmolality measurement. The urine osmolality is inappropriately elevated in relation to the serum osmolality, indicating that the patient is retaining water. SIADH is a state in which the patient abnormally retains water despite a low serum osmolality.

Volume depletion is unlikely in the absence of a low urine sodium level and a history of vomiting or diarrhea and normal vital signs. This patient's history and normal physical examination findings and low-normal potassium concentration do not suggest adrenal insufficiency.

Hyponatremia and hypo-osmolality are usually synonymous, but there are two important exceptions in which hyponatremia may not indicate hypo-osmolality. First, pseudohyponatremia can be caused by marked elevation of plasma lipids, proteins, or both. In such patients, the concentration of sodium per liter of plasma water is unchanged, but the concentration of sodium per liter of plasma is artifactually decreased because of the increased relative proportion occupied by lipids or proteins. Measured serum osmolality will not be affected by the increased lipids or proteins, but calculated osmolality ($2 \times$ serum [Na^+] + glucose/18 + BUN /2.8) will be abnormal. This is why patients with hyponatremia should have the serum osmolality measured as well as calculated. Second, high concentrations of effective solutes other than sodium can cause relative decreases in serum sodium levels despite an unchanged serum osmolality; this occurs most commonly in patients with hyperglycemia. Again, misdiagnosis can be avoided by direct measurement of serum osmolality, as was done in this case, or by correcting the serum sodium by 1.6 to 2.4 meq/L for each 100 mg/dL increase in plasma glucose concentration above 100 mg/dL. By direct measurement, this patient has hypo-osmolal hyponatremia, which excludes hyperglycemia or other causes of hyperosmolal states that cause a relative dilution of the serum sodium as well as pseudohyponatremia. In pseudohyponatremia, the patient's osmolality would be normal. Hyponatremia due to excessive water ingestion in the absence of renal disease is associated with a very low urine osmolality (<50–100 mosm/kg H_2O). Any increase of the urine osmolality >100 mosm/kg H_2O, as in this patient, signifies an impairment of water excretion and is not compatible with psychogenic polydipsia.

- The syndrome of inappropriate antidiuretic hormone secretion (SIADH) is defined as hypotonic hyponatremia with a urine osmolality >100 mosm/kg H_2O in the absence of volume depletion, adrenal insufficiency, congestive heart failure, hypothyroidism, cirrhosis, and/or renal impairment.

Bibliography

1. **Ellison DH, Berl T**. Clinical practice. The syndrome of inappropriate antidiuresis. N Engl J Med. 2007;356:2064-72. [PMID: 17507705]

Item 33   Answer: A

Hypercalcemia with a suppressed serum parathyroid hormone (PTH) level in a patient who smokes and who has a lung mass is highly likely to be due to lung cancer. The humoral mediator of hypercalcemia of malignancy in the vast majority of patients, especially in patients with lung cancer, is parathyroid hormone–related protein (PTHrP), which is secreted by the tumor into the circulation. PTHrP binds to the PTH receptor and to the PTH/PTHrP receptor where it stimulates increased bone resorption with release of calcium into the circulation.

Hydrochlorothiazide sometimes causes mild hypercalcemia but seldom raises serum calcium levels to this degree. The suppressed serum PTH rules out hyperparathyroidism, due to either a parathyroid adenoma or hyperplasia. Multiple myeloma, which can cause hypercalcemia by producing high levels of local bone marrow cytokines, is far less likely in this patient who has a polyclonal gammopathy related to the infectious process present in the lungs, not a monoclonal gammopathy related to a malignant proliferation of plasma cells.

- Most cases of hypercalcemia of malignancy are mediated by parathyroid hormone–related protein (PTHrP), which is secreted by the tumor.

Bibliography

1. **Stewart AF.** Hypercalcemia associated with cancer. N Engl J Med 2005; 352:373-9. [PMID: 15673803]

Item 34   Answer: D

The most likely cause of this patient's hypercalcemia is vitamin D toxicity. Sarcoid granulomatous tissue can produce 1-α-hydroxylase, which converts 25-hydroxyvitamin D to the active form, 1,25-dihydroxyvitamin D_3. Normally, the conversion of 25-hydroxyvitamin D to 1,25-dihydroxyvitamin D_3 occurs via renal 1-α-hydroxylase activity that is regulated by parathyroid hormone (PTH). Hypercalcemia suppresses the release of PTH and therefore the production of 1,25-dihydroxyvitamin D_3. In this patient, the lack of suppression is due to PTH-independent extrarenal production of 1,25-dihydroxyvitamin D_3 by activated macrophages in the lungs and lymph nodes, which results in excess calcium absorption from the gut leading to hypercalciuria, hypercalcemia and

hyperphosphatemia. Symptoms of hypercalcemia include anorexia, nausea, vomiting, lethargy, and even coma. The patient's kidney stone is probably the result of hypercalciuria. Polyuria with volume depletion may also occur and is suggested by this patient's elevated blood urea nitrogen to serum creatinine ratio of greater than 20.

Both primary and secondary hyperparathyroidism are associated with increased PTH levels. In this patient, PTH is suppressed by the elevated serum calcium levels, excluding these diagnoses. Hypercalcemia due to metastatic bone disease is rare; most cases of malignancy-related hypercalcemia are due to increased levels of PTH-related protein (PTHrP). In addition, metastatic bone disease would be unlikely in a young patient without a history of cancer and without bone-related symptoms such as pain.

- Sarcoid granulomatous tissue can produce 1-α-hydroxylase, which converts 25-hydroxyvitamin D to the active form, 1,25-dihydroxyvitamin D_3, resulting in hypercalciuria and hypercalcemia.

Bibliography

1. **Sharma OP.** Vitamin D, calcium, and sarcoidosis. Chest. 1996;109:535-9. [PMID: 8620732]

Item 35   Answer: E

This patient has mild, asymptomatic hypercalcemia secondary to primary hyperparathyroidism. In patients with primary hyperparathyroidism, the calcium is elevated, phosphorus is low, and intact parathyroid hormone (PTH) is inappropriately normal for the level of hypercalcemia (in 20% of patients) or elevated (in 80% of patients). Other findings include normal or elevated calcitriol and alkaline phosphatase levels and a normal or elevated urine calcium concentration. The cause of primary hyperparathyroidism in most patients is a single parathyroid adenoma. Primary hyperparathyroidism is most often seen as an incidental finding in the absence of obvious symptoms. The prevalence of symptoms depends on the intensity by which they are sought, particularly vague symptoms of being unwell. It is rare for primary hyperparathyroidism to present as acute symptomatic hypercalcemia.

Humoral hypercalcemia of malignancy is the most common cause of hypercalcemia in patients with cancer, even in those with skeletal metastases, and is the most common cause of symptomatic hypercalcemia in hospitalized patients. In patients with humoral hypercalcemia of malignancy, the serum calcium is elevated, phosphorus may be normal or low (elevated if the glomerular filtration rate is <35 mL/min), and PTH is suppressed. Other changes include a normal or low calcitriol, normal or elevated alkaline phosphatase, and increased urine calcium concentrations. Parathyroid hormone–related protein (PTHrP) is normal or elevated, but this finding is seldom needed to make a diagnosis.

The true prevalence of hypercalcemia due to metastatic bone disease is uncertain. Hypercalciuria without hypercalcemia is much more prevalent but infrequently evaluated or monitored. In patients with hypercalcemia due to metastatic bone disease, serum calcium is elevated, phosphorus may be normal or elevated, and PTH is suppressed. Other notable changes include an elevated alkaline phosphatase value, low calcitriol level, and a PTHrP that may be low, normal, or elevated.

Multiple myeloma is the most common cause of hypercalcemia in patients with increased serum calcium, elevated serum creatinine level, and anemia. In multiple myeloma, serum protein immunoelectrophoresis is abnormal, calcium and phosphorus levels are elevated, and PTH is suppressed. Alkaline phosphatase is generally normal because there is only a limited osteoblastic response to the myelomatous infiltrate in the marrow. PTHrP is normal or low.

Benign familial hypocalciuric hypercalcemia is due to a constitutive over-expression of the calcium-sensing receptor gene. Homozygotes develop fatal neonatal primary hyperparathyroidism, whereas heterozygotes have benign familial hypocalciuric hypercalcemia. In this disorder, the serum calcium level is elevated but the urine calcium concentration is low, serum phosphorus is low, and PTH is normal. The key to recognizing the disorder is a history of hypercalcemia without elevated PTH in other family members.

KEY POINT

• In primary hyperparathyroidism, the serum calcium is elevated, phosphorus is low, and parathyroid hormone (PTH) is elevated or inappropriately normal for the level of hypercalcemia.

Bibliography

1. Bilezikian JP, Silverberg SJ. Clinical practice. Asymptomatic primary hyperparathyroidism. N Engl J Med. 2004;350:1746-51. [PMID: 15103001]

Item 36   Answer: A

A decrease in the glomerular filtration rate (GFR) is the most likely cause of this patient's hyperphosphatemia. In patients with chronic kidney disease, phosphorus excretion decreases and phosphate retention occurs when the GFR declines to <60 to 80 mL/min. The increase in phosphorus levels causes a decrease in ionized calcium, and both the elevated phosphorus levels and the hypocalcemia stimulate parathyroid hormone secretion. This secondary hyperparathyroid response is a "trade-off" in which serum levels of calcium and phosphorus normalize at the expense of persistently elevated parathyroid hormone levels. As renal function worsens, deficiency of 1,25-dihydroxyvitamin D contributes to the hypocalcemia and results in further stimulation of parathyroid hormone secretion. As the GFR continues to decline, the decrease in phosphate excretion results in hyperphosphatemia.

High phosphorus intake may worsen hyperphosphatemia in patients with chronic kidney disease, but the main cause of hyperphosphatemia is a decreased GFR. Vitamin D deficiency causes hypocalcemia but not hyperphosphatemia. Primary hyperparathyroidism is characterized by hypercalcemia and hypophosphatemia.

KEY POINT

• A low glomerular filtration rate is the cause of hyperphosphatemia in chronic kidney disease.

Bibliography

1. Slatopolsky E, Brown A, Dusso A. Role of phosphorus in the pathogenesis of secondary hyperparathyroidism. Am J Kidney Dis. 2001;37:S54-7. [PMID: 11158862]

Item 37   Answer: B

Hypomagnesemia is common and clinically significant in patients with alcoholism. It is involved in the pathogenesis of alcohol withdrawal tremors, delirium, seizures, and cardiac arrhythmias. Hypomagnesemia in such patients can mimic hypoparathyroidism, including severe hypocalcemia and hyperphosphatemia. It causes both suppression of parathyroid hormone (PTH) secretion and resistance to PTH action. Therapy for hypocalcemia in this situation is seldom successful unless the magnesium level is normalized. Although serum magnesium levels correlate poorly with intracellular magnesium stores, serum magnesium determination is the only feasible clinical measurement.

Acute alcohol ingestion induces urine magnesium loss comparable with calcium loss. When patients with chronic alcoholism abstain, serum magnesium levels rise. Poor nutritional intake, malabsorption, and diuretic therapy can worsen magnesium depletion.

Measurement of PTH, vitamin D, and phosphate should be done if the magnesium level is normal in the setting of hypocalcemia.

KEY POINT

• Hypomagnesemia in a patient with alcoholism can mimic hypoparathyroidism, including severe hypocalcemia and hyperphosphatemia.

Bibliography

1. Tong GM, Rude RK. Magnesium deficiency in critical illness. J Intensive Care Med. 2005;20:3-17. [PMID: 15665255]

Chapter 8
Neurology

Neurology contains self-assessment items that correspond to the following chapters in the *Internal Medicine Essentials for Clerkship Students 2* textbook:

Approach to the Altered Mental State
Headache
Dementia
Approach to Meningitis and Encephalitis
Stroke and Transient Ischemic Attack
Peripheral Neuropathy

Neurology contains self assessment items that correspond to the following Training Problems in the *Core Medicine Clerkship Guide*:

Altered Mental Status

Chapter 8

Neurology

Questions

Item 1

A 60-year-old morbidly obese man becomes difficult to arouse 12 hours after undergoing elective right knee replacement. He has a history of osteoarthritis, hypertension, and sleep apnea. Outpatient medications are acetaminophen and hydrochlorothiazide. He also uses nocturnal bilevel positive airway pressure ventilation. His surgery was uncomplicated, and he has received regularly scheduled doses of intravenous morphine sulfate for pain.

On physical examination, temperature is 36.6 °C (97.8 °F), heart rate is 80/min, respiration rate is 10/min and shallow, and blood pressure is 130/85 mm Hg. Cardiac examination is normal and unchanged from his examination on admission. Pulmonary examination reveals distant breath sounds without wheezes or crackles. He is moderately responsive to sternal rub. Oxygen saturation is 90% by pulse oximetry with the patient breathing oxygen, 2 L/min, by nasal cannula. The pupils are equal, round, and reactive to light. Neurologic examination is normal.

Which of the following diagnostic studies is most likely to determine the cause of this patient's diminished level of consciousness?

(A) Arterial blood gas measurement
(B) CT scan of the head
(C) Finger-stick blood glucose
(D) Lumbar puncture

Item 2

A 78-year-old woman who has acute respiratory distress syndrome and was admitted to the medical intensive care unit for mechanical ventilation 2 days ago is evaluated for disorientation. Prior to hospitalization, she lived alone and functioned well independently. The patient is on a ventilator, has received small doses of lorazepam over the past 48 hours, and had initially appeared comfortable. The nurse indicates that the patient recently became disoriented and is not interacting as clearly with her family as she had before. Her mental status has fluctuated over the past 24 hours.

On physical examination, vital signs are normal except for slight tachycardia. She is calm and awake but cannot follow directions and cannot answer simple questions by nodding her head. There is no evidence of hallucinations. Neurologic examination shows no focal abnormalities, and cranial nerve examination is normal.

Laboratory studies show hemoglobin of 9.9 g/dL and a leukocyte count of 11,000/µL with a normal differential. Comprehensive metabolic panel is normal. Serum total T_4 and thyroid-stimulating hormone levels are normal.

Which of the following is the most likely cause of her current symptoms?

(A) Cerebrovascular accident
(B) Delirium
(C) Dementia
(D) Paranoid psychosis

Item 3

A 73-year-old woman who lives in a nursing home is evaluated for a 6-month history of frequent awakening during the night, although she falls asleep without difficulty. The patient is distressed because she is fatigued throughout the day. Her medical history is significant for dementia secondary to cerebrovascular disease. Her Mini–Mental State Examination score is 20/30. A diagnosis of primary insomnia is established, and the patient is asked to avoid drinking caffeinated beverages and eating before bedtime and to minimize nighttime disturbances. When nighttime awakening persists, the patient begins taking triazolam before bedtime. After a few days of treatment, the nursing-home staff note that she is even more confused.

On physical examination, she is afebrile. The heart rate is 63/min, respiration rate is 12/min, and blood pressure is 120/72 mm Hg. The neurologic examination indicates no new focal findings. She is oriented to person but not to place or time. Laboratory studies, including complete blood count, serum chemistry studies, and urinalysis, are normal.

Which of the following is the most appropriate next step in management?

(A) Decrease triazolam dose
(B) Discontinue triazolam
(C) Initiate cognitive behavioral therapy
(D) Perform CT scan of the head and blood and urine cultures
(E) Substitute diphenhydramine for triazolam

Item 4

A 32-year-old woman is evaluated in the office for chronic headaches that have increased in frequency from severe headaches occurring monthly and milder headaches occurring weekly to daily headaches. The daily headaches have been present for 1 month. The headaches have no prodrome or aura, are located mostly on the right side of the head, and are associated with nausea, rare emesis, and photophobia. Occasionally, the headaches are bad enough that she must spend the day in bed. There is no fever, chills, neck stiffness, paresthesias or weakness, or other constitutional symptoms. The patient has had migraine headaches since she was 19 years old. In the past, her severe headaches have responded well to sumatriptan and her mild headaches to acetaminophen or naproxen; however, because her headaches have become less responsive to these agents, she has been taking butalbital-aspirin-caffeine three to four times daily over the past month. The physical examination, including vital signs and neurologic evaluation, is normal.

Which of the following is the most likely diagnosis?

(A) Basilar-type migraine
(B) Cerebral artery aneurysm
(C) Chronic daily headache
(D) Tension headache

Item 5

A 55-year-old man with coronary artery disease is evaluated in the emergency department for a severe right retro-orbital throbbing headache associated with right-sided rhinorrhea and ptosis. The headaches began 2 weeks ago and recur daily at 5 AM and 5 PM. They last 20 to 40 minutes and are usually followed by complete remission. Similar headaches occurred 2 years ago and lasted for 6 weeks.

On physical examination, the patient is comfortable and has normal vital signs. General examination, including funduscopic examination, is normal. MRI of the head and cervical spine with and without contrast is normal. Lumbar puncture shows an opening cerebrospinal fluid pressure of 180 mm H_2O with no xanthochromia, erythrocytes, or pleocytosis.

Which of the following is the most likely diagnosis?

(A) Cluster headache
(B) Migraine headache
(C) Subarachnoid hemorrhage
(D) Tension headache

Item 6

A 54-year-old woman is evaluated in the office for a 4-day history of an acute headache that has been gradually worsening and is located diffusely on the left side of her head. The patient is nauseated but does not have photophobia, fever, chills, trauma, stiff neck, muscle weakness, paresthesias, or bowel or bladder problems. She awakens with the headache, which gradually worsens during the day. She experiences slight relief with acetaminophen and ibuprofen. She has a family history of migraine headache and, as a teenager and in her mid-30s, had a few migraine headaches that were more severe than her current episode and were associated with photophobia and severe fatigue. However, since those episodes, she had been headache free until now.

Her medical history includes hypertension, diabetes mellitus, breast cancer for which she underwent lumpectomy and radiation therapy 4 years ago, and osteoarthritis. Current medications are atenolol, simvastatin, metformin, tamoxifen, and aspirin.

On physical examination, the patient appears to be in distress, but vital signs are normal. The neurologic evaluation is significant for decreased vibratory and monofilament perception in both lower extremities in a stocking distribution.

Which of the following is the most appropriate management for this patient?

(A) Bone scan
(B) Lumbar puncture and cerebrospinal fluid analysis
(C) MRI of the head
(D) Sumatriptan therapy

Item 7

A 29-year-old woman is evaluated in an urgent care clinic for a headache of 10 hours' duration. The headache began gradually but quickly became debilitating. It is now a throbbing headache localized to the left side of her head and associated with nausea and vomiting. She took ibuprofen at the onset of the headache without significant relief; she now prefers to rest in a dark, quiet room. She has had similar headaches in the past, which were triggered by stress at work.

On physical examination, she is resting on her side in a darkened room holding an emesis basin. Temperature is 37 °C (98.6 °F), blood pressure is 138/90 mm Hg, and heart rate is 88/min. Physical examination, including neurologic examination, is unremarkable.

Which of the following is the most likely diagnosis?

(A) Cluster headache
(B) Intracerebral mass
(C) Migraine headache
(D) Sinus headache
(E) Tension headache

Item 8

A 44-year-old woman is evaluated in the office for headache that occurs three to four times a week. She has no accompanying nausea but does have mild sensitivity to sound, but no sensitivity to light, with the headaches. The pain is a constant pressure in the back of her head. She can function during the headaches but would prefer not to have them. She has had these headaches since her teenage years and notes that they seem to be more frequent with less sleep, increased stress, and missed meals. Headaches may last several hours but remit within 30 minutes or an hour after taking acetaminophen.

On physical examination, she is fatigued and thin. Temperature is 36.9 °C (98.4 °F), heart rate 92/min, respiration rate 18/min, and blood pressure 138/85 mm Hg. Examination, including neurologic evaluation, shows no abnormalities.

Which of the following is the most likely diagnosis?

(A) Cluster headache
(B) Migraine headache without aura
(C) Paroxysmal hemicrania
(D) Tension headache

Item 9

A 22-year-old woman is evaluated in the office for daily headaches that seemed to be initially worse in the supine position for 1 to 2 weeks, waking her from sleep, but now have been present continuously for the last month. She previously had occasional headaches with photophobia and phonophobia beginning at age 14 years. She has had intermittent blurred vision for the past month.

Physical examination is significant only for obesity (BMI 30). Funduscopic examination is shown (*see Figure 30 in Color Plates*).

Which of the following is the most appropriate next step in the management of this patient's headache?

(A) Begin therapy for migraine headaches
(B) Begin therapy for tension headaches
(C) Lumbar puncture
(D) MRI of the head

Item 10

A 72-year-old woman is brought to the office by her son for evaluation of gradually progressive forgetfulness over the past 18 months. On a recent week-long visit, she could not learn the name of the hosts' dog. She frequently re-reads the daily paper and tends to ask the same questions repeatedly. She has no significant medical history and no abnormalities of gait, posture, coordination, speech, or dexterity. Personality is preserved. She takes no medications.

On physical examination, vital signs are normal, as is attention. Her score on the Mini–Mental State Examination is 21/30, and she recalls none of three words after brief distraction. She has difficulty copying a geometric figure. Neurologic examination is otherwise normal.

Which of the following is the most likely diagnosis?

(A) Alzheimer's dementia
(B) Dementia secondary to vitamin B_{12} deficiency
(C) Dementia with Lewy bodies
(D) Frontotemporal dementia
(E) Vascular dementia

Item 11

A 78-year-old man is brought to the office by his family for evaluation of confusion and memory problems, which have been worsening over the past 3 weeks. Initially, his symptoms were evident mainly in the morning, but they now seem to occur throughout the day. He wanders from the house and sometimes does not recognize his wife. He has visual hallucinations, and, while sitting in the kitchen, believes that he is on a bus. His medical history includes type 2 diabetes mellitus with painful peripheral neuropathy, coronary artery disease, depression, and heart failure. Medications are glyburide, nortriptyline, digoxin, lorazepam, metoprolol, lisinopril, aspirin, and pravastatin. His daughter does not know how long he has been taking these medications. There is no family history of neurologic disease.

On physical examination, the patient has asterixis and findings consistent with peripheral neuropathy. Oxygen saturation is normal with the patient breathing room air. He is mildly lethargic and inattentive and is not oriented to time or place. His score on the Mini–Mental State Examination is 13/30, and he recalls two of three words after a delay. Laboratory studies, including electrolyte levels and liver chemistry and renal function studies, are normal. CT scan of the head without contrast is also normal.

Which of the following conditions is most likely causing this patient's cognitive impairment?

(A) Alzheimer's disease
(B) Dementia with Lewy bodies
(C) Depression
(D) Toxic encephalopathy
(E) Vascular dementia

Item 12

A 70-year-old woman is evaluated in the office for an episode of abrupt cognitive decline that began 2 weeks ago when she was suddenly unable to read the newspaper during breakfast. She could not find the bathroom in her own home but could carry on a conversation and recognize family members. Her condition has since improved. She has a history of hypertension and coronary artery disease and has had spells of forgetfulness over the past few years. She takes metoprolol, hydrochlorothiazide, pravastatin, and low-dose aspirin.

On physical examination, vital signs and general examination are normal. Her score on the Mini–Mental State Examination is 22/30. She is not oriented to time or place. Neurologic examination is normal except for an extensor plantar response on the left. CT scan of the head shows bilateral periventricular white matter hypodensity.

The patient returns 3 months later. She is oriented to place and has improved daily function, a score on the Mini–Mental State Examination of 24/30, and a normal neurologic examination, except for the extensor plantar response.

Which of the following is the most likely diagnosis?

(A) Alzheimer's disease
(B) Frontotemporal dementia
(C) Dementia with Lewy bodies
(D) Vascular dementia

Item 13

A 68-year-old man is brought to the office by his daughter for evaluation of memory loss. She has noticed that her father has had declining memory over the past 12 months. He has forgotten to pay utility bills, has gotten lost while driving, and has had two motor vehicle accidents during this time. He has a history of hypertension and hyperlipidemia for which he takes hydrochlorothiazide, pravastatin, and aspirin. The patient's wife died 1 year ago.

On physical examination he is cooperative and in no distress. Blood pressure is 120/70 mm Hg and heart rate is 70/min. The remainder of the examination, including a detailed neurologic examination, is normal.

Which of the following is the most appropriate next step in the evaluation of this patient's memory loss?

(A) Lumbar puncture
(B) Metabolic panel
(C) Mini-Mental State Examination
(D) MRI of the head
(E) Toxicology screen

Item 14

A 78-year-old woman is evaluated in the office for progressive impairments of memory and other aspects of intellect, which have developed insidiously over 3 years. The patient's score on the Mini–Mental State Examination is 22/30, and she recalls none of three words after a 3-minute delay. There are no other significant findings on physical examination.

Which of the following is most likely to improve this patient's symptoms?

(A) Central cholinesterase inhibitor
(B) Estrogen replacement therapy
(C) Ginkgo biloba
(D) Memantine
(E) Vitamin E

Item 15

A 45-year-old man, who lives in Minnesota, is brought to the emergency department in January because of expressive aphasia and fever. His wife reports that he had been feeling unwell for 3 days but had only nonspecific symptoms. He developed a fever the afternoon before coming to the emergency department, and aphasia occurred several hours before his arrival at the hospital. The patient has not had nausea, vomiting, or diarrhea. He has always been healthy, takes no medications, has not traveled outside the United States, and has no pets.

On physical examination, his temperature is 38.3 °C (101 °F); other vital signs are normal. Expressive aphasia is noted. The pupils are equal and reactive to light, and the fundi are normal. There is no nuchal rigidity, and no petechial lesions are seen on the skin, nail beds, or conjunctivae. Weakness of the right lower extremity is noted.

Lumbar puncture is performed; cerebrospinal fluid findings are as follows:

Leukocyte count	150/µL with 90% lymphocytes
Erythrocyte count	1500/µL
Protein	125 mg/dL
Glucose	Normal
Gram stain	Negative

Which of the following organisms is most likely causing this patient's current findings?

(A) Cytomegalovirus
(B) Echovirus
(C) Epstein–Barr virus
(D) Herpes simplex virus
(E) West Nile virus

Item 16

A 25-year-old man is evaluated in the emergency department for fever, headache, and mental status changes of 4 hours' duration. He underwent cadaveric kidney transplantation 10 months ago, and his immunosuppressive regimen includes prednisone and azathioprine. He has no allergies.

On physical examination, temperature is 38.7 °C (101.6 °F), heart rate is 115/min, respiration rate is 25/min, and blood pressure is 100/60 mm Hg. He is oriented to the year and his name but cannot recall the month, his current location, or the reason for his hospitalization. The neck is supple, and Kernig's sign is absent. Neurologic examination is normal. Leukocyte count is 20,000/µL.

CT scan of the head shows no sign of hemorrhage, hydrocephalus, mass effect, or midline shift. Lumbar puncture is performed, and cerebrospinal fluid examination shows the following.

Leukocyte count	2000/µL (60% neutrophils, 40% lymphocytes)
Erythrocyte count	20/µL
Glucose	25 mg/dL
Protein	150 mg/dL
Gram stain	Negative
Opening pressure	Normal

Results of blood, urine, and cerebrospinal fluid cultures are pending.

Which of the following is the most appropriate empiric antibiotic therapy until culture results are available?

(A) Ampicillin and ceftriaxone
(B) Ampicillin, ceftriaxone, and vancomycin
(C) Ceftriaxone and moxifloxacin
(D) Ceftriaxone and vancomycin
(E) Moxifloxacin

Item 17

A 45-year-old woman who has a 3-day history of progressive earache and fever is hospitalized after becoming unresponsive. Medical history is unremarkable; she has no allergies; and she takes no medications.

On physical examination, temperature is 40 °C (104 °F), heart rate is 120/min, respiration rate is 32/min, and blood pressure is 80/50 mm Hg. The patient is obtunded and has meningismus. The leukocyte count is 25,000/µL with 25% band forms, and the platelet count is 20,000/µL.

Lumbar puncture is performed; cerebrospinal fluid examination shows the following.

Appearance	Cloudy
Leukocyte count	2500/µL with 99% neutrophils
Glucose	20 mg/dL
Protein	230 mg/dL

A Gram stain of unspun cerebrospinal fluid is shown (*see Figure 31 in Color Plates*).

In addition to dexamethasone, which of the following empiric treatment regimens should be initiated?

(A) Ceftriaxone
(B) Penicillin
(C) Vancomycin
(D) Vancomycin and ceftriaxone

Item 18

A 78-year-old woman is brought to the emergency department after she was unable to be awakened by her husband this morning. When paramedics arrived at her home, she was intubated for airway protection.

On physical examination, her eyes are closed, but in response to a command, she appears to consistently blink her eyes appropriately. When her eyes are opened by the examiner, intermittent spontaneous downward eye movements are seen. There are no spontaneous horizontal eye movements, and her eyes do not move laterally when her head is turned to either side. Pupils are pinpoint but reactive. She has intermittent spontaneous extensor posturing of her arms and legs but does not move any of her extremities on command. Reflexes are brisk, and an extensor plantar response is present bilaterally.

Which of the following is the most likely cause of this patient's findings?

(A) Cerebral anoxia
(B) "Locked-in" syndrome
(C) Status epilepticus
(D) Thiamine deficiency

Item 19

A 42-year-old woman who is unresponsive is brought to the emergency department by her husband. He had last seen her behaving normally when he left for work 9 hours earlier. She has no significant medical history and takes no medications.

Physical examination is normal. Neurologic examination reveals deep coma with normal pupil reactivity. CT scan of the head shows a small left temporal lobe parenchymal hemorrhage with extensive subarachnoid hemorrhage but without evidence of significant brain edema.

Which of the following is the most likely diagnosis?

(A) Amyloid angiopathy
(B) Carotid artery stenosis
(C) Middle cerebral artery embolism
(D) Ruptured arteriovenous malformation

Item 20

A 22-year-old man is evaluated in the emergency department 8 hours after the sudden onset of moderate neck pain followed by vertigo, ataxia, slurred speech, and difficulty swallowing. His medical history is unremarkable, and he is not taking any medications. Physical examination shows left ptosis, anisocoria with the left pupil smaller than the right, nystagmus, left-sided dysmetria, and decreased pain and temperature sensation on the left side of the face and right side of the body.

Which of the following arteries is most likely responsible for these findings?

(A) Anterior cerebral artery
(B) Middle cerebral artery
(C) Posterior cerebral artery
(D) Vertebral artery

Item 21

A 71-year-old man is evaluated in the emergency department. The patient felt well when he went to bed at midnight but awoke at 8:00 AM with left upper-extremity weakness and numbness. He arrives at the emergency department at 9:00 AM.

The patient's medical history includes hypertension and hyperlipidemia for which he takes a thiazide diuretic and a statin. On physical examination, blood pressure is 178/92 mm Hg. Neurologic examination shows mild left-sided hemi-attention (neglect), a mild left central facial palsy, mild left upper- and lower-extremity weakness, and a mild left hemisensory deficit. Complete blood count and serum electrolytes and glucose are normal. CT scan of the head is normal.

Which of the following is the most appropriate next step in this patient's management?

(A) Lower blood pressure to 140/90 mm Hg
(B) Start aspirin
(C) Start intravenous heparin
(D) Start intravenous tissue plasminogen activator

Item 22

A 60-year-old man is evaluated in the emergency department 30 minutes after the onset of clumsiness of the right hand and slurred speech. His medical history includes hypertension, hyperlipidemia, and migraine headaches. He is otherwise healthy and has never been hospitalized or had surgery. His medications are hydrochlorothiazide, enalapril, pravastatin, and ibuprofen as needed.

On physical examination, the temperature is 37 °C (98.6 °F), blood pressure is 140/90 mm Hg, heart rate is 73/min, and oxygen saturation is 98% by pulse oximetry with the patient receiving oxygen, 2 L/min by nasal cannula. Carotid pulsations are normal without bruits. Cardiac examination shows a regular rhythm with normal heart sounds and no murmurs. Neurologic examination reveals dysarthria and subtle right-sided weakness, more prominent in the arm than the leg.

Electrocardiogram shows sinus rhythm. CT scan of the head without contrast is normal. The patient is admitted to the stroke unit.

Which of the following is the most appropriate treatment for this patient?

(A) Alteplase
(B) Aspirin
(C) Heparin
(D) Metoprolol
(E) Warfarin

Item 23

A 55-year-old woman is evaluated in the emergency department for mild weakness of the right face and arm that began about 1 hour ago; she has normal sensation, vision, and cognition. About 7 days ago, she bent over and felt a "pop" in her head, followed by a very severe headache that dissipated over the next 3 days. She has no significant medical history and is not taking any medications. She has a 35-pack-year smoking history.

On physical examination, her blood pressure is 135/82 mm Hg. Neurologic examination shows only a mild right central facial palsy and mild right arm weakness. CT scan of the head is normal.

Which of the following is the most appropriate next step in the evaluation of this patient?

(A) Carotid duplex ultrasonography
(B) Echocardiography
(C) Lumbar puncture
(D) Magnetic resonance angiography of the head

Item 24

A 62-year-old woman is evaluated in the emergency department for sudden loss of vision in the left eye. Her symptoms lasted for 25 minutes and resolved while she was in transit to the emergency department. She had a similar, less severe episode 1 week ago also involving the left eye. She has a history of hypertension and hyperlipidemia. Current medications are aspirin, a thiazide diuretic, and a statin. She has a 42-pack-year smoking history.

On physical examination, her temperature is 37 °C (98.6 °F) and blood pressure is 136/88 mm Hg. There are no carotid bruits. She has a normal cardiac rhythm with no murmurs and normal distal pulses. Neurologic evaluation is unremarkable. Complete blood count and serum electrolytes and glucose are normal. CT scan of the head shows no abnormalities. She is begun on aspirin.

Which of the following diagnostic studies will most likely suggest the correct therapeutic course?

(A) Carotid duplex ultrasonography
(B) Electroencephalography
(C) Lumbar puncture
(D) MRI of the head

Item 25

A 32-year-old woman is hospitalized because of symptoms that began as numbness and tingling in both feet and progressed over several days to include gait instability, weakness of both hands, diplopia, and dyspnea. The symptoms began 11 days after a viral illness. She has a 5-year history of diet-controlled type 2 diabetes mellitus.

On admission, the patient is unable to walk. Physical examination shows sinus tachycardia, proximal and distal weakness in her upper and lower extremities bilaterally, areflexia, and marked vibratory and position sense loss in the fingers and toes bilaterally.

Which of the following is the most likely diagnosis?

(A) Amyotrophic lateral sclerosis
(B) Diabetic lumbosacral polyradiculopathy
(C) Guillain–Barré syndrome
(D) Myasthenia gravis

Item 26

A 68-year-old man is evaluated in the office for weakness and tingling in his arms and legs that began 5 months ago with mild weakness and have progressed to more profound weakness associated with numbness and tingling in his hands and feet. The patient has a 2-year history of type 2 diabetes mellitus treated with glyburide and metformin.

On physical examination, the patient has difficulty rising from his chair without pushing off with his arms. He has moderate weakness (4/5) of hip flexion bilaterally and more severe weakness (3/5) of ankle plantar flexion and grip strength bilaterally. Deep tendon reflexes are 1+ in his upper extremities and absent in his lower extremities. Vibration sensation and position sense are diminished in his feet. Pinprick and light touch sensations are normal throughout.

Fasting plasma glucose is 104 mg/dL and hemoglobin A_{1c} has ranged from 6.3% to 7.1% over the past year.

Which of the following is the most likely diagnosis?

(A) Chronic inflammatory demyelinating polyneuropathy
(B) Diabetic peripheral neuropathy
(C) Hemispheric stroke
(D) Polymyositis

Chapter 8

Neurology

Answers and Critiques

Item 1 Answer: A

Measurement of arterial blood gases is likely to determine the cause of this patient's diminished consciousness. His history of obesity and sleep apnea and the recent general anesthesia and regular narcotic therapy make the obesity hypoventilation syndrome likely. If he has obesity hypoventilation syndrome as well as obstructive sleep apnea, he is likely to be very sensitive to the respiratory depressant effect of narcotics. Pulse oximetry is useful in monitoring oxygenation but does not adequately assess ventilation in patients receiving supplemental oxygen. Measurement of blood gases in patients who are hypoventilating shows an elevated P_{CO_2} and a decreased pH (respiratory acidosis). In narcotic-related hypoventilation, intravenous naloxone, a short-acting opioid antagonist, can quickly reverse the effects that narcotic agents have on ventilation.

Brain imaging is used in patients with a history of head trauma or evidence of focal neurologic impairment on clinical examination. Finger-stick blood glucose measurement is rapid and simple and is most likely warranted in this patient. However, without a history of diabetes mellitus or liver disease, the level of suspicion for hypo- or hyperglycemia is low. Lumbar puncture is rarely helpful in diagnosing the cause of diminished consciousness in the absence of clinical signs supporting a diagnosis of meningitis or subarachnoid hemorrhage, such as fever, nuchal rigidity, or focal neurologic signs.

KEY POINTS

- An elevated P_{CO_2} may cause diminished consciousness.

- Patients with obesity hypoventilation syndrome have respiratory acidosis; measurement of arterial blood gases in these patients shows an elevated P_{CO_2} and a decreased pH.

Bibliography
1. Caples SM, Gami AS, Somers VK. Obstructive sleep apnea. Ann Intern Med. 2005;142:187-97. [PMID: 15684207]

Item 2 Answer: B

This patient has the most common type of delirium in the intensive care unit (ICU), which is hypoactive or "quiet" delirium. Delirium is a form of acute brain dysfunction that occurs in 50% to 80% of mechanically ventilated patients in the ICU. It is associated with a 3-fold higher rate of death by 6 months, much longer stays in the ICU and hospital, higher costs, and a 10-fold higher rate of chronic cognitive deficits after ICU

survival. Delirium can be diagnosed quickly using the Confusion Assessment Method-ICU (CAM-ICU), which takes 20 to 30 seconds to perform in most patients. The four cardinal features of the diagnosis are: 1) acute onset or fluctuations in mental status over a 24-hour period, 2) inattention, 3) disorganization of thinking, and 4) an altered level of consciousness at the time of the evaluation. This patient has features 1, 2, and 3. She is having fluctuations in her mental status, cannot follow directions, and is inattentive, as evidenced by her inability to correctly answer simple questions that would require organization of thinking. Hallucinations may be a symptom of delirium, but they are not required for the diagnosis. She is not hyperactive or in "distress," and this also is not required for the diagnosis of delirium. In fact, only 5% of ICU delirium is of the pure hyperactive subtype. Although most CAM-ICU monitoring is done by nurses, physicians should be familiar with these criteria so that they can detect this form of organ dysfunction and recognize the many potential causes, such as acute respiratory distress syndrome or administration of benzodiazepines, as in this patient.

She exhibits no signs of acute focal neurologic events such as a cerebrovascular accident. Since she was functioning independently prior to hospitalization and her mental status changes occurred while in the ICU, dementia is an unlikely diagnosis. The fluctuating mental status and absence of a premorbid history of mental illness make psychosis unlikely.

KEY POINTS

- The most common form of delirium in the intensive care unit is hypoactive or "quiet" delirium.

- The cardinal features of delirium are 1) acute onset or fluctuations in mental status over a 24-hour period, 2) inattention, 3) disorganization of thinking, and 4) an altered level of consciousness at the time of the evaluation.

Bibliography
1. Ely EW, Inouye SK, Bernard GR, Gordon S, Francis J, May L, et al. Delirium in mechanically ventilated patients: validity and reliability of the confusion assessment method for the intensive care unit (CAM-ICU). JAMA. 2001;286:2703-10. [PMID: 11730446]

Item 3 Answer: B

Given the recent initiation of a benzodiazepine, the most likely cause of this patient's confusion is a reaction to triazolam, and the appropriate intervention is to discontinue this medication. Benzodiazepines are the class of psychotropic agents most frequently implicated in causing delirium and exacerbating pre-existing cognitive impairment in elderly patients.

Doses of hypnotic medications should be decreased in the elderly, but once an adverse effect such as delirium occurs, prescribing a different medication is preferable to reducing the dose of the causative agent. The patient's physical examination findings and laboratory studies were normal; therefore, it is not necessary to perform a full workup to evaluate for an infectious cause or occurrence of a new cerebrovascular accident. Diphenhydramine is used as an off-label treatment for insomnia but is also associated with delirium in the elderly and would not be an appropriate substitute medication. Cognitive behavioral therapy has established efficacy in many randomized-controlled trials in the treatment of primary insomnia. However, it is less likely to be effective in patients with significant cognitive impairment.

KEY POINT

• Benzodiazepines are one of the most frequently implicated classes of drugs causing delirium and exacerbating pre-existing cognitive impairment in elderly patients.

Bibliography
1. **Young J, Inouye SK.** Delirium in older people. BMJ. 2007;334:842-6. [PMID: 17446616]

Item 4   Answer: C

This patient has chronic daily headache, or "transformed" headache due to the daily use of butalbital-aspirin-caffeine. Migraine or tension headaches can "transform" into chronic daily headaches if analgesic use becomes too frequent. Although there are no data on how frequently analgesic preparations may be safely taken, most experts recommend taking them no more than three times per week. Nearly any analgesic, including acetaminophen, nonsteroidal anti-inflammatory drugs, butalbital-aspirin-caffeine, isometheptene-dichloralphenazone-acetaminophen, and the triptans, can lead to chronic daily headache.

Cerebral artery aneurysm is unlikely in this patient because she has a history of migraine headache and her headaches have been chronic, not acute in onset. Basilar-type migraine affects young women and is characterized by any combination of dysarthria, vertigo, diplopia, tinnitus, decreased hearing, ataxia, simultaneous bilateral paresthesias, and altered consciousness, which this patient does not have. Tension headaches last from 30 minutes to 7 days, typically have a bilateral location, have a nonpulsating pressing or tightening quality described by patients as a "band-like" constriction around their head, are mild to moderate in intensity, and do not prohibit activity. There is no aggravation of tension headache by using stairs or by doing any similar routine activity, no association with nausea or vomiting (although anorexia may occur), and no association with concomitant photophobia and phonophobia (although either may occur singularly). While the patient's history has some elements of tension

headache, the key to the diagnosis is the daily headache and daily medication use.

KEY POINT

• Migraine or tension headache can "transform" into chronic daily headaches if analgesic use becomes too frequent.

Bibliography
1. **Gladstein J.** Headache. Med Clin North Am. 2006;90:275-90. [PMID: 16448875]

Item 5   Answer: A

This patient's history is most consistent with cluster headache. Cluster headache is a painful, disabling headache that is typically unilateral and periorbital/temporal and is associated with at least one of the following features on the same side as the headache: conjunctival irritation/lacrimation, rhinorrhea/nasal congestion, eyelid edema, facial/forehead sweating, and miosis/ptosis. Agitation may also occur. Cluster headaches may recur several times daily or at the same time each day. Cluster headaches also present in a cluster period, typically a 3- to 6-week time period during which patients experience episodes of headache. Prednisone is the most appropriate treatment for cluster headache.

The symptoms meeting criteria for migraine headache include worsening of the headache with movement, limitation of activities, and the need for absence of light and sound (a dark, quiet room). An excellent mnemonic for remembering the diagnostic criteria for migraine headache is POUND: pulsatile, one-day duration, unilateral, nausea or vomiting, and disabling. The more features of POUND that are present, the more likely the diagnosis is migraine headache. In this patient, the periodicity, prominent autonomic symptoms, and predictable occurrence of the headache are more compatible with cluster headache than migraine headache. The patient does not have a headache due to subarachnoid hemorrhage, which has been ruled-out with a normal MRI scan and lumbar puncture. Tension headache can be ruled out because of the disabling characteristics of this patient's headache, its episodic nature, and the quality of the pain.

KEY POINT

• Cluster headache is a painful, disabling headache that is typically unilateral and periorbital/temporal and is associated with autonomic symptoms.

Bibliography
1. **Lipton RB, Bigal ME, Steiner TJ, Silberstein SD, Olesen J.** Classification of primary headaches. Neurology. 2004;63:427-35. [PMID: 15304572]

Item 6   Answer: C

This patient has several "red flags" (headache onset that is acute and occurring after age 50 years and a history of malignancy) that should prompt immediate neuroradiologic imaging in the form of an MRI of the head.

A lumbar puncture is not the first diagnostic test for headache; if an intracranial mass is present, lumbar puncture may precipitate fatal brainstem herniation. A bone scan is not indicated because the patient is not displaying any symptoms suggesting bone involvement at this time, and the more immediate need is to evaluate the source of her headache pain with an MRI. Although she has a history of migraine headaches, her current headache is different from the migraines she experienced in the past, and she has been headache free for over 2 decades; therefore, triptans, which are specific agents for treating migraines, are not indicated.

KEY POINT

- Headaches that are acute in onset, occur after age 50 years, and are associated with a history of malignancy are "red flags" prompting immediate neuroradiologic evaluation.

Bibliography

1. Detsky ME, McDonald DR, Baerlocher MO, Tomlinson GA, McCrory DC, Booth CM. Does this patient with headache have a migraine or need neuroimaging? JAMA. 2006;296:1274-83. [PMID: 16968852]

Item 7   Answer: C

This patient has a migraine headache. A careful review of symptoms can easily discriminate between migraine, tension, and other types of headaches. A three-item migraine screen was recently validated to assist in discriminating migraine from tension headaches in which the presence of two of the following three criteria is highly predictive of migraines: nausea, photophobia, and headache-related disability. The distinguishing symptoms of migraine headache can also be remembered, perhaps more easily, by the mnemonic "POUND": the more characteristics present, the more likely the headache is a migraine headache—pounding, one-day duration, unilateral, nausea or vomiting, and disabling.

Tension headache is the most common headache, lasting from 30 minutes to 7 days. Such headaches are typically bilateral and are generally described as a nonpulsating pressing or tightening sensation or as a "band-like" constriction around the head. The pain is mild to moderate in intensity and does not prohibit activity. Tension headaches are not aggravated by using stairs or doing any similar routine activity, and they are not associated with nausea or vomiting.

Cluster headache is more common in men than women and is usually periorbital or frontotemporal. Pain becomes very severe in minutes and can be excruciating. Accompanying autonomic symptoms include ipsilateral lacrimation, conjunctival injection, nasal congestion, miosis, rhinorrhea, ptosis, or eyelid edema. A cluster headache can sometimes be experienced several times per day, which almost never happens with migraines; cluster headaches also characteristically repeat over a course of weeks and then may not recur for months or years.

Sinus headaches are usually worse when the patient is lying down and are most characteristically associated with nasal congestion and tenderness overlying the affected sinus. A headache caused by an intracerebral mass is typically chronic and worse on awakening; generally progressive; aggravated by coughing, straining, or changing position; and usually accompanied by an abnormal neurologic examination.

KEY POINT

- The distinguishing symptoms of migraine headache can be remembered by the mnemonic "POUND": pounding; one-day duration; unilateral; nausea; and disability.

Bibliography

1. Lipton RB, Bigal ME, Steiner TJ, Silberstein SD, Olesen J. Classification of primary headaches. Neurology. 2004;63:427-35. [PMID: 15304572]

Item 8   Answer: D

This patient has tension headache, the most prevalent of all headache types. Patients with tension headache may experience a sensation of squeezing or pressure around the head or neck and may be sensitive to light or sound. These headaches may last minutes to days, are constant (not pulsatile), and are never associated with nausea. Tension headaches may occur alone or with migraine. Compared with migraine headaches, tension headaches are less likely to prevent patients from engaging in activities of daily living in a normal, expedient manner.

This patient does not describe disability or any other abnormalities with the headaches. She does not describe enough features to meet migraine criteria in that she does not have unilateral pain, pulsatile pain, pain that limits activities, or pain of moderate to severe intensity. She has no nausea with the headaches and does not have both photophobia and phonophobia to meet migraine diagnostic criteria. Although the patient does not meet the criteria for migraine, the key feature that establishes a diagnosis of tension headache is the lack of disabling pain.

Paroxysmal hemicrania is a unilateral headache of seconds to minutes in duration that, despite its brevity, can be disabling. Cluster headache is a painful, disabling headache that may be associated with autonomic symptoms such as tearing or rhinorrhea. Cluster headaches are typically unilateral and periorbital/temporal and are associated with at least one of the following features on the same side as the headache: conjunctival irritation/lacrimation, rhinorrhea/nasal congestion, eyelid edema, facial/forehead sweating, and miosis/ptosis. Agitation may also occur. Cluster headaches may recur several times daily at the same time each day. Cluster headaches also present in a cluster period, typically a 3- to 6-week time period during which patients experience episodes of headache.

- Tension headache is distinguished from migraine by the fact that patients with tension headache are not disabled and can carry out activities of daily living in a normal, expedient manner.

Bibliography

1. **Davenport R.** Diagnosing acute headache. Clin Med. 2004;4:108-12. [PMID: 15139725]

Item 9   Answer: D

This patient requires a neuroimaging procedure. She has several "red flags" suggesting an underlying serious condition as the cause of the headache. The odds of a significant abnormality on neuroimaging are increased if the patient reports rapidly increasing headache frequency, dizziness or lack of coordination, paresthesias, or awakening from sleep because of the headache. A neurologic abnormality on physical examination, such as focal weakness, sensory loss, or, as in this patient, papilledema, is an indication for neuroimaging. This patient's symptoms and signs of headache, intermittent blurred vision, and papilledema are most consistent with increased intracranial pressure, which may be due to a mass lesion or obstruction to cerebrospinal fluid flow.

A lumbar puncture is indicated to rule out infection but not until an imaging study has ruled out an intracranial mass that might result in brainstem herniation. Based upon the patient's symptoms and ophthalmological examination, migraine and tension headache are unlikely, and treatment for these conditions is not appropriate.

- A neuroimaging study is indicated for patients with headache and "red flags," including rapidly increasing headache frequency, dizziness or lack of coordination, paresthesias, awakening from sleep because of the headache, or abnormal neurologic examination.

Bibliography

1. **Detsky ME, McDonald DR, Baerlocher MO, Tomlinson GA, McCrory DC, Booth CM.** Does this patient with headache have a migraine or need neuroimaging? JAMA. 2006;296:1274-83. [PMID: 16968852]

Item 10   Answer: A

This patient has a syndrome of primary dementia (i.e., dementia with a normal neurologic examination and prominent amnesia), which are the defining characteristics of dementia of the Alzheimer type. The prominent amnesia in Alzheimer's disease is related to the vulnerability of mesial temporal lobe structures. Importantly, this patient's course has been gradual, not abrupt, and she has preservation of her personality and no hallucinations.

Although frontotemporal dementia is also a primary dementia, the early changes are alterations in personality, decision-making, initiative, and, sometimes, language. Moderately advanced frontotemporal dementia also is characterized by significant memory impairment, and, at this stage, may be clinically misdiagnosed as Alzheimer's disease. However, Alzheimer's disease is the much more common of the two disorders and, given the prominence of the memory difficulty early in the course, is the more likely diagnosis in this patient.

Dementia with Lewy bodies is characterized by fluctuating cognition, parkinsonism, and/or visual hallucinations, none of which is present in this patient. This form of dementia may have a cognitive profile similar to that in Alzheimer's disease, but this may be due to the high rate of the presence of both Alzheimer's disease and dementia with Lewy bodies. Vascular dementia is unlikely in this patient who has no vascular risk factors, stroke-like course of illness, or focal signs on neurologic examination. Occult medical disorders, such as hypothyroidism or vitamin B_{12} deficiency, account for a very small number of cases of dementia (approximately 2%). These forms of dementia usually cause attentional impairment and slowing of thought and rarely mimic the amnesic profile of Alzheimer's dementia.

- Alzheimer's disease is characterized by primary dementia with prominent amnesia.

Bibliography

1. **Blennow K, de Leon MJ, Zetterberg H.** Alzheimer's disease. Lancet. 2006;368:387-403. [PMID: 16876668]

Item 11   Answer: D

Fluctuating lethargy and inattention, hallucinations, and asterixis suggest a toxic/metabolic cause of this patient's impairment. The patient is taking several medications that might impair cognition. Nortriptyline has anticholinergic properties and is likely to cause impairment in patients with latent cholinergic deficiency (the elderly or patients with mild cognitive impairment, early dementia, or Parkinson's disease). The sedative-hypnotic lorazepam and digoxin may also contribute to cognitive impairment.

Vascular dementia, particularly that due to small-vessel cerebrovascular disease, is unlikely, given the absence of a stepwise course and absence of evidence of a cerebrovascular accident on CT scan. Depression may cause chronic cognitive impairment (pseudodementia), but not asterixis and an altered level of consciousness.

In patients with incipient Alzheimer's disease, anticholinergic delirium is produced more readily by anticholinergic medications. This diagnosis cannot be ruled out in this patient, but establishing the diagnosis would require removal of the causative agent and re-evaluation after recovery. However, asterixis, a sign of metabolic encephalopathy, would be unusual in this setting and points strongly to a metabolic encephalopathy.

Dementia with Lewy bodies is associated with fluctuation of cognitive status and visual hallucinations. It is a consideration in this patient, but is less likely because of the subacute onset, absence of parkinsonism, and presence of asterixis.

KEY POINT

• Cognitive impairment accompanied by fluctuating lethargy and inattention, hallucinations, and asterixis is likely the result of a toxic encephalopathy.

Bibliography

1. **Inouye SK.** Delirium in older persons. N Engl J Med. 2006;354:1157-65. Erratum in: N Engl J Med. 2006;354:1655. [PMID: 16540616]

Item 12   Answer: D

This patient probably has vascular dementia because of the history of vascular risk factors, abrupt onset with subsequent improvement, periventricular white matter ischemia on imaging, and a focal neurologic sign (extensor plantar response). Follow-up imaging may demonstrate a recent infarct not evident on the earlier scan that can be temporally associated with the episode of cognitive decline.

The prominent features of Alzheimer's disease are gradual short-term memory loss and a normal neurologic examination. Frontotemporal dementia is recognized by the early alterations in personality, decision making, initiative, and, sometimes, language. Dementia with Lewy bodies is characterized by fluctuating cognition, parkinsonism, and/or visual hallucinations, none of which is present in this patient.

KEY POINT

• Vascular dementia is suggested by a history of vascular risk factors, abrupt onset with subsequent improvement, periventricular white matter ischemia on imaging, and focal neurologic findings.

Bibliography

1. **Nelson NW.** Differential diagnosis of Alzheimer's dementia and vascular dementia. Dis Mon. 2007;53:148-51. [PMID: 17544644]

Item 13   Answer: C

The next step in the evaluation of this patient is a Mini–Mental State Examination. The patient's progressive loss of memory and cognitive function strongly suggests dementia. The social history is significant for the timing of the symptom recognition. With the death of his wife, he lost his caregiver who may have been compensating for these deficits. A recent U.S. Preventive Services Task Force guideline concluded that evidence is insufficient to recommend routine screening for dementia in older adults. There are not yet any randomized, prospective studies showing the benefits of routine screening for dementia, but case series and clinical experience indicate its usefulness. Screening should be pursued in patients, such as this patient, with symptoms of dementia. The Mini–Mental State Examination, a 30-point questionnaire, is a brief

screening test with a sensitivity of 87% and specificity of 82% for detecting Alzheimer's disease.

The other tests may help determine the cause of dementia after the diagnosis is established. The results of a basic metabolic profile may help distinguish some of the reversible causes of memory loss, including metabolic abnormalities, infection, and endocrinopathies. Numerous expert consensus statements recommend that neuroimaging be done in patients with dementia to detect clinical findings not suspected from the history and physical examination. However, the benefit of detecting these unsuspected lesions is not always clear. Lumbar puncture and electroencephalography, although not part of the routine evaluation of the patient with dementia, may help establish a diagnosis in some patients. For example, in patients with clouding of consciousness or delirium, the lumbar puncture would be helpful in identifying meningitis. Toxicology screening should be directed by clinical clues in the history or physical examination and is not part of the routine evaluation of the patient with likely dementia.

KEY POINT

• The Mini–Mental State Examination is the most well known and validated screening test for dementia, with a sensitivity of 87% and specificity of 82% in discriminating patients with Alzheimer's disease from normal controls.

Bibliography

1. **Karlawish JH, Clark CM.** Diagnostic evaluation of elderly patients with mild memory problems. Ann Intern Med. 2003;138:411-9. [PMID: 12614094]

Item 14   Answer: A

This patient has symptoms consistent with progressive dementia, most likely Alzheimer's dementia. Clinical trials of cholinesterase inhibitors (including galantamine, donepezil, and rivastigmine) in patients with mild to moderate Alzheimer's disease consistently demonstrate a modest efficacy on cognitive and global function scales. Cholinesterase inhibitors may also alleviate psychiatric symptoms, including agitation, apathy, and hallucinations, although there is no evidence that these agents delay the natural history of Alzheimer's disease.

Although some evidence suggests that vitamin E and selegiline delay the progression of Alzheimer's disease, these agents do not directly relieve cognitive or psychiatric symptoms. Ginkgo biloba probably exerts modest effects on cognitive symptoms in patients with Alzheimer's disease, but has not been shown to improve global or psychiatric function. In addition, no standard preparation of Ginkgo biloba is available, and it is therefore not the agent of choice in patients with mild to moderate Alzheimer's disease.

Memantine has been shown to be effective for relief of cognitive symptoms in patients with moderate to severe, but not mild, Alzheimer's disease. Estrogen replacement therapy in postmenopausal women with Alzheimer's dementia has not been shown to have any benefit for cognitive symptoms or disease progression.

- Cholinesterase inhibitors have modest efficacy on cognitive and global function in mild to moderate Alzheimer's disease.

Bibliography

1. **Farlow MR, Cummings JL.** Effective pharmacologic management of Alzheimer's disease. Am J Med. 2007;120:388-97. [PMID: 17466645]

Item 15   Answer: D

The most likely diagnosis is herpes simplex virus encephalitis that is causing focal neurologic findings of the temporal lobe. Herpes encephalitis is the most common cause of fatal sporadic encephalitis in the United States. Herpes encephalitis is characterized by the rapid development of fever, headache, seizures, focal neurologic signs, and impaired consciousness. The cerebrospinal fluid typically shows a lymphocytic pleocytosis, increased number of erythrocytes, and elevated protein; glucose is usually normal. Acyclovir should be started immediately, and cerebrospinal fluid polymerase chain reaction for herpes simplex virus DNA should be obtained. MRI of the head should also be performed. An abnormality in the temporal lobe (e.g., a hemorrhagic lesion) is a poor prognostic sign for neurologic recovery.

Although cytomegalovirus, Epstein–Barr virus, and echovirus can cause the same syndrome, infection due to these viruses would be exceedingly rare in a 45-year-old immunocompetent patient. West Nile virus infection is more frequently associated with a poliomyelitis syndrome (muscle weakness and flaccid paralysis). Furthermore, vector-borne diseases such as West Nile virus infection are unlikely events during a Minnesota winter.

- Herpes encephalitis is the most common cause of fatal sporadic encephalitis in the United States.

- Herpes encephalitis is characterized by the rapid development of fever, headache, seizures, focal neurologic signs, and impaired consciousness.

Bibliography

1. **Kennedy PG.** Viral encephalitis. J Neurol. 2005;252:268-72. Epub 2005 Mar 11. [PMID: 15761675]

Item 16   Answer: B

The most appropriate empiric therapy for this patient is ampicillin, ceftriaxone, and vancomycin. The cerebrospinal fluid findings support a diagnosis of meningitis, but the causative organism is unknown. Empiric vancomycin and ceftriaxone generally are recommended for treatment of meningitis in patients 2 to 50 years of age. This regimen covers *Streptococcus pneumoniae* and *Neisseria meningitidis*, the most common organisms responsible for meningitis in this age group. However, this patient also is at increased risk for meningitis secondary to *Listeria monocytogenes* because of his history of kidney transplantation and use of immunosuppressive agents, including corticosteroids. Therefore, ampicillin (or penicillin) should be added to ceftriaxone and vancomycin.

Listeria infection also is associated with extremes of age (neonates and patients older than 50 years), alcoholism, malignancy, diabetes mellitus, hepatic failure, renal failure, iron overload, collagen vascular disorders, and HIV infection. In addition, although this patient does not have a recent history of gastroenteritis, ingestion of contaminated dairy and meat products is a potential source of *L. monocytogenes* infection.

Diagnosis of *Listeria* meningitis can be difficult, and the presence of risk factors or other epidemiologic considerations should guide the selection of empiric therapy. Cerebrospinal fluid (CSF) analysis in patients with meningitis often does not reveal gram-positive rods but typically shows pleocytosis and may demonstrate a significant number of lymphocytes in addition to neutrophils. Patients also usually have elevated CSF protein levels; however, decreased CSF glucose levels are found less commonly with *Listeria* meningitis than with other, more common causes of bacterial meningitis.

Ceftriaxone and vancomycin are effective therapy for *S. pneumoniae* and *N. meningitidis* meningitis but are not effective against *L. monocytogenes*. The fluoroquinolone moxifloxacin has not been adequately evaluated in treating *Listeria* meningitis.

- Risk factors for *Listeria* meningitis include immunosuppression, neonate status or age >50 years, alcoholism, malignancy, diabetes mellitus, hepatic failure, renal failure, iron overload, collagen vascular disorders, and HIV infection.

Bibliography

1. **Wing EJ, Gregory SH.** *Listeria monocytogenes*: clinical and experimental update. J Infect Dis. 2002;185:S18-24. [PMID: 11865436]

Item 17   Answer: D

This patient has meningitis caused by *Streptococcus pneumoniae* that most likely originated in her middle ear. A diagnosis of *S. pneumoniae* meningitis can be made presumptively based on the positive cerebrospinal fluid Gram stain, as in this patient, and antimicrobial therapy should be targeted towards that organism. Pending in vitro susceptibility testing, empiric antimicrobial therapy for pneumococcal meningitis includes vancomycin plus a third-generation cephalosporin (either cefotaxime or ceftriaxone). This combination is recommended based on data from experimental animal models that show that these drugs are synergistic in killing resistant pneumococci. The patient should also receive adjunctive dexamethasone, administered concomitant with or just prior to the first dose of antimicrobial therapy, as data have shown improved morbidity and mortality in adult patients who are given this adjunctive agent.

If the organism is highly resistant to penicillin or cephalosporins, treatment with either penicillin or ceftriaxone alone may not achieve adequate cerebrospinal fluid concentrations to kill the pathogen. Although vancomycin has good in vitro activity against resistant pneumococci, it should not be used alone in the treatment of pneumococcal meningitis because of its unreliable cerebrospinal fluid penetration.

KEY POINT

- The most appropriate empiric therapy for *Streptococcus pneumoniae* meningitis is vancomycin plus ceftriaxone and dexamethasone.

Bibliography
1. van de Beek D, de Gans J, Tunkel AR, Wijdicks EF. Community-acquired bacterial meningitis in adults. N Engl J Med. 2006;354:44-53. [PMID: 16394301]

Item 18   Answer: B

This patient is in a "locked-in" state. The locked-in state is due to a lesion of the base of the pons, usually from pontine infarction that may be due to a basilar artery occlusion. Patients with the locked-in syndrome are not comatose; they are quadriplegic, have paralysis of horizontal eye movements and bulbar muscles, and can communicate only by moving their eyes vertically or blinking. In this patient, the spontaneous brisk downward eye movements are consistent with ocular bobbing, a movement typical of large pontine lesions, and her pinpoint pupils are also typical of a pontine stroke. In addition, the extensor posturing is suggestive of a brainstem lesion.

Cerebral anoxia, such as from a cardiac arrest, typically causes diffuse cerebral hemispheric dysfunction that often spares the brainstem and would not explain this patient's eye movements or the intact alertness in the presence of quadriplegia. Nonconvulsive status epilepticus should be considered in the differential diagnosis of a comatose patient. However, this patient is not comatose but rather shows intact alertness and cortical function because of her ability to blink on command. Thiamine deficiency can cause impairment of eye movements but would not explain the patient's prominently preserved vertical eye movements, the spontaneous extensor posturing, or acute onset of quadriplegia.

KEY POINT

- Patients with the locked-in syndrome are quadriplegic, have paralysis of horizontal eye movements and bulbar muscles, and can communicate only by moving their eyes vertically or blinking.

Bibliography
1. Smith E, Delargy M. Locked-in syndrome. BMJ. 2005;330:406-409. [PMID: 15718541]

Item 19   Answer: D

This patient has an intracerebral (intraparenchymal) hemorrhage with extensive subarachnoid hemorrhage, which is the hallmark of a ruptured arteriovenous malformation, but can occasionally occur with a ruptured middle cerebral artery aneurysm. Both of these entities require conventional cerebral angiography for establishing the diagnosis and planning either surgical or endovascular treatment.

Cerebral artery embolism and carotid artery stenosis both cause ischemic infarction and are not associated with blood in the subarachnoid space. Cerebral amyloid angiopathy is a cause of lobar hemorrhage in elderly patients and is occasionally associated with dementia. The patient's age, location of the intracerebral hemorrhage, and extensive subarachnoid bleeding make amyloid angiopathy unlikely.

KEY POINT

- Intracerebral hemorrhage with extensive subarachnoid hemorrhage is the hallmark of a ruptured arteriovenous malformation.

Bibliography
1. Brown RD Jr, Flemming KD, Meyer FB, Cloft HJ, Pollock BE, Link ML. Natural history, evaluation, and management of intracranial vascular malformations. Mayo Clin Proc. 2005;80:269-81. [PMID: 15704783]

Item 20   Answer: D

This patient has an ischemic stroke (cerebral infarction) in the territory of the vertebral artery. The symptoms and signs (dysphagia, dysarthria) involve multiple lower cranial nerves, crossed sensory deficits, and cerebellar ataxia, which suggest a left lateral medullary localization, possibly also involving the left cerebellum. The sudden onset of symptoms suggests that stroke is the cause. Blood is supplied to this area by the posterior inferior cerebellar artery, a major branch of the vertebral artery. In a previously healthy young person, the less common causes of stroke must be considered, such as vertebral artery dissection, which often occurs spontaneously without trauma or typical vascular risk factors. Typical symptoms of vertebral artery dissection include neck or posterior head pain, Horner's syndrome (ptosis and miosis), dysarthria, dysphagia, decreased pain and temperature sensation of the face and contralateral body, dysmetria, ataxia, and vertigo.

A stroke in the territory of the anterior cerebral artery is most likely to present as contralateral leg weakness. A stroke in the territory of the middle cerebral artery will manifest as contralateral face and arm weakness greater than leg weakness, sensory loss, visual field deficit, and either aphasia due to left hemispheric stroke or hemi-inattention (neglect) due to right hemispheric stroke. Posterior cerebral artery ischemia presents primarily as a contralateral visual field deficit.

KEY POINT

- Vertebral artery stroke presents with Horner's syndrome, dysarthria, dysphagia, decreased pain and temperature sensation, dysmetria, ataxia, and vertigo.

Bibliography
1. **Savitz SI, Caplan LR.** Vertebrobasilar disease. N Engl J Med. 2005;352:2618-26. [PMID: 15972868]

Item 21   Answer: B

This patient had an acute ischemic stroke in the right middle cerebral artery territory. The time of onset is unknown, but he was last known to be well at midnight, and he is therefore not eligible for intravenous thrombolytic therapy, which is indicated if therapy is started within 3 hours of onset of stroke symptoms or when the patient was last known to be well (in this case, when the patient went to bed). Patients often do not recognize stroke symptoms, and at-risk patients should be educated about these symptoms. Early administration of aspirin, 160 to 325 mg daily, results in a modest reduction in the risk of recurrent stroke in the short term and slightly less death and disability in the long term.

Early administration of parenteral anticoagulants has no benefit for patients with acute stroke and may cause harm. Early blood pressure lowering is not recommended for most patients with acute stroke unless they are being considered for thrombolytic therapy or have a concomitant myocardial infarction or aortic dissection. In such patients, some experts aim for a target mean arterial pressure of 140 mm Hg, although there is no definitive evidence that this is beneficial. Elevated blood pressure is common at the time of stroke, even among patients without chronic hypertension. Rapid lowering of the blood pressure may further impair cerebral blood flow and worsen the ischemic injury. Elevated blood pressure will often spontaneously and gradually improve during the first days after the stroke.

KEY POINT

• In patients with acute stroke, thrombolytic therapy must be started within 3 hours of the onset of symptoms or at the time the patient was last known to be well.

Bibliography
1. **van der Worp HB, van Gijn J.** Clinical practice. Acute ischemic stroke. N Engl J Med. 2007;357:572-9. [PMID: 17687132]

Item 22   Answer: A

The intravenous thrombolytic agent alteplase (recombinant tissue-type plasminogen activator or rtPA) increases chances of recovery when administered within 3 hours of onset of symptoms in patients with ischemic stroke. Alteplase therapy increases the percentage of patients who recover completely after stroke from about 35% to about 50%. The number needed to treat to render one additional patient completely recovered is 7 to 8. The risk of symptomatic hemorrhage after intravenous rtPA therapy is approximately 6%. However, the risk of death or severe disability from rtPA-induced hemorrhage is less than that from severe untreated stroke. Alteplase is contraindicated in patients with mean arterial pressure >130 mm Hg or blood pressure >185/110 mm Hg. Alteplase and antiplatelet agents are the only therapies shown to improve outcome in patients with acute ischemic stroke.

Antiplatelet agents (aspirin, dipyridamole/aspirin, or clopidogrel) reduce the risk of subsequent stroke, but they are not given within 24 hours of administration of alteplase because of the risk of hemorrhage and death. Hypertension is one of the most important modifiable risk factors for stroke in the long term; however, in the acute setting, antihypertensive agents such as metoprolol may cause hypoperfusion, and are used only in patients with systolic blood pressure >220 mm Hg, diastolic blood pressure >120 mm Hg, or if pressure rises above 185/110 mm Hg after the administration of alteplase. Although anticoagulation is typically used in patients with thromboembolic stroke, neither unfractionated heparin nor low-molecular-weight heparin has been shown to be beneficial in patients with ischemic stroke. In addition, even in patients with ischemic stroke who have a potential source of cerebral emboli, cerebral perfusion should first be restored with alteplase; anticoagulation should then be started 24 to 48 hours after the administration of alteplase. Warfarin is not indicated in acute ischemic stroke; it is administered only for deep venous thrombosis or thromboembolic stroke after effective anticoagulation with heparin.

KEY POINTS

• The thrombolytic agent alteplase (recombinant tissue-type plasminogen activator or rtPA) increases chances of recovery when administered within 3 hours of the onset of symptoms in patients with ischemic stroke.

• In patients with ischemic stroke treated with thrombolytic agents, antiplatelet agents and anticoagulants should be withheld for 24 to 48 hours following thrombolysis.

Bibliography
1. **Adams HP Jr, Adams RJ, Brott T, del Zoppo GJ, Furlan A, Goldstein LB, Grubb RL, Higashida R, Kidwell C, Kwiatkowski TG, Marler JR, Hademenos GJ; Stroke Council of the American Stroke Association.** Guidelines for the early management of patients with ischemic stroke: A scientific statement from the Stroke Council of the American Stroke Association. Stroke. 2003;34:1056-83. [PMID: 12677087]

Item 23   Answer: C

This patient requires a lumbar puncture. She had a very severe headache 1 week before presentation with left hemispheric dysfunction, findings that are suggestive of subarachnoid hemorrhage (SAH). A CT scan is only about 90% sensitive for detecting SAH, which is most likely to be missed when there is a delay in the presentation, as in this patient. In such patients, lumbar puncture is required to look for xanthochromic staining of the cerebrospinal fluid, which can be detected up to 14 days after the hemorrhage, or gross blood in the fluid.

This patient's symptoms 7 days after the so-called "sentinel" hemorrhage are due to SAH-induced vasospasm with localized cerebral ischemia. Magnetic resonance angiography may detect an aneurysm but would not detect subarachnoid blood as accurately as lumbar puncture. Carotid duplex ultrasonography and echocardiography would not be helpful in diagnosing the SAH. Carotid duplex ultrasonography is useful in diagnosing carotid artery disease, and echocardiography is helpful in locating a source of cerebral emboli, but neither are considerations in this patient.

KEY POINT

- In patients with suspected subarachnoid hemorrhage but normal CT scan of the head, a lumbar puncture should be obtained to detect cerebrospinal fluid blood or xanthochromia.

Bibliography

1. van Gijn J, Kerr RS, Rinkel GJ. Subarachnoid haemorrhage. Lancet. 2007;369:306-18. [PMID: 17258671]

Item 24   Answer: A

This patient requires carotid duplex ultrasonography. She had two episodes of transient left monocular blindness consistent with retinal ischemia, possibly due to left carotid artery stenosis. If she has a >50% stenosis of the extracranial left internal carotid artery, she may be considered for carotid endarterectomy.

While MRI is more sensitive than CT in detecting acute infarction and can determine whether there is evidence of prior cerebrovascular disease or other disorders, it does not diagnose carotid artery disease. Electroencephalography is useful in the evaluation of seizures, but seizures cannot cause monocular loss of vision. Lumbar puncture is used to evaluate subarachnoid hemorrhage or central nervous system infections, but these disorders do not cause a transient ischemic attack.

KEY POINT

- In a patient with a transient ischemic attack, carotid artery ultrasonography showing a >50% stenosis of the internal carotid artery is an indication for carotid endarterectomy.

Bibliography

1. Meschia JF, Brott TG, Hobson RW 2nd. Diagnosis and invasive management of carotid atherosclerotic stenosis. Mayo Clin Proc. 2007;82:851-8. [PMID: 17605967]

Item 25   Answer: C

This patient's signs and symptoms are most consistent with Guillain–Barré syndrome. Guillain–Barré syndrome is an immune-mediated demyelinating polyneuropathy characterized by proximal and distal weakness, distal sensory loss, autonomic symptoms, cranial nerve involvement, and respiratory failure in 25% of patients. Up to 75% of cases are preceded by an infection, immunization, or surgical procedure. Symptoms typically evolve over 2 to 4 weeks. Treatment consists of either intravenous immune globulin or plasmapheresis, which have been shown in clinical studies to be equally effective. The key

to the diagnosis is recognition of a symmetrical, rapidly progressive ascending paralysis.

Amyotrophic lateral sclerosis causes symptoms related to upper motor neuron degeneration and includes loss of dexterity, slowed movements, muscle weakness, and stiffness. Physical examination findings include hyperreflexia, spasticity, weakness, muscle atrophy, and fasciculations. Muscle weakness begins distally and asymmetrically. The finding of both upper and lower motor neuron disease, the initial asymmetry, and more gradual onset distinguish amyotrophic lateral sclerosis from Guillain–Barré syndrome.

Myasthenia gravis is an autoimmune disease affecting the acetylcholine receptors and is characterized by fatigable weakness (weakness that worsens with use of muscles) with a predilection for ocular, bulbar, neck, and proximal extremity muscles. Diabetic lumbosacral polyradiculopathy (diabetic amyotrophy) is a specific condition characterized by severe thigh pain followed by lower-extremity weakness that affects the proximal muscles more than the distal muscles. It progresses slowly over a period of months.

KEY POINT

- Guillain–Barré syndrome is characterized by proximal and distal weakness, autonomic symptoms, cranial nerve involvement, and respiratory failure.

Bibliography

1. Hughes RA, Cornblath DR. Guillain-Barre syndrome. Lancet. 2005;366:1653-66. [PMID: 16271648]

Item 26   Answer: A

This patient has signs and symptoms consistent with chronic inflammatory demyelinating polyneuropathy. Patients with this disorder present with progressive, relatively symmetric proximal and distal weakness in all extremities. Although sensory symptoms (such as numbness or tingling) are common, motor symptoms usually predominate. The clinical manifestations develop over several months and may follow a progressive or relapsing and remitting course. Physical examination confirms relatively symmetric weakness of proximal and distal muscles. Deep tendon reflexes are usually diminished or absent, and there is preferential loss of vibration and joint position sense. Nerve conduction studies show evidence of a demyelinating neuropathy with widespread decreases in motor and sensory nerve conduction velocities. Clinical manifestations usually improve with immunosuppressive therapy (corticosteroids, intravenous immune globulin, or plasmapheresis). Chronic inflammatory demyelinating polyneuropathy is important to recognize because it is one of the few peripheral neuropathies amenable to treatment.

A hemispheric stroke will lead to the abrupt onset of unilateral signs and symptoms. Patients with polymyositis typically present with greater proximal than distal muscle weakness; deep tendon reflexes are normal, and there is no associated pain or sensory disturbances. Diabetic peripheral neuropathy is an axonal (as opposed to demyelinating) neuropathy that classically presents with symmetric sensory loss in the feet with or without burning or tingling. As the disease progresses and the sensory symptoms ascend up the legs, the fingers and hands become involved, resulting in the classic "stocking-glove" pattern. In addition to diminished vibration sensation and position sense, pinprick and light touch sensations are usually decreased as well. Although absent ankle reflexes and mild weakness in the feet often occur early in the course of diabetic peripheral neuropathy, more widespread loss of reflexes and motor weakness are late findings that would be extremely unusual in a patient with a relatively short history of well-controlled diabetes, making this diagnosis unlikely.

KEY POINT

- The combination of symmetric proximal and distal muscle weakness, decreased deep tendon reflexes, and distal loss of vibration and position senses is characteristic of a demyelinating polyneuropathy.

Bibliography

1. Koller H, Kieseier BC, Jander S, Hartung HP. Chronic inflammatory demyelinating polyneuropathy. N Engl J Med. 200531;352:1343-56. [PMID: 15800230]

Chapter 9

Oncology

Oncology contains self-assessment items that correspond to the following chapters in the *Internal Medicine Essentials for Clerkship Students 2* textbook:

Breast Cancer
Colon Cancer
Lung Cancer
Prostate Cancer
Cervical Cancer
Skin Cancer
Pain Management

Oncology contains self assessment items that correspond to the following Training Problems in the *Core Medicine Clerkship Guide*:

Common Cancers

Chapter 9

Oncology

Questions

Item 1

A 30-year-old woman is evaluated in the office during a routine examination. Her medical history is significant for Hodgkin's lymphoma that was treated successfully with radiation therapy to the chest and abdominal lymph node sites 10 years ago; she never received chemotherapy. The patient has never smoked, has no family history of cancer, and has no current medical problems. Her physical examination is normal.

The patient is at the most increased risk for developing which of the following cancers?

(A) Acute myeloid leukemia
(B) Breast cancer
(C) Hodgkin's lymphoma
(D) Lung cancer
(E) Non-Hodgkin's lymphoma

Item 2

A 28-year-old woman is evaluated in the office for a lump in the right side of her neck that has grown large over the past month. She has not had fever, soaking night sweats, weight loss, or recent illness. She does not smoke cigarettes and takes no medications. The remainder of the history is noncontributory.

On physical examination, a 3.5-cm right anterior cervical lymph node and a 1-cm right supraclavicular lymph node are palpable. Laboratory studies, including complete blood count, comprehensive metabolic profile, lactate dehydrogenase concentration, and heterophile antibody assay, are normal. Chest radiograph is unremarkable.

Which of the following is the most appropriate management for this patient?

(A) Bone marrow aspirate and biopsy
(B) Empiric antibiotic therapy and re-evaluation in 2 weeks
(C) Lymph node excision
(D) Observation for 3 months

Item 3

A 78-year-old man is evaluated in the office because of a 6-week history of abdominal pain, diarrhea, and weight loss of 11 kg (25 lb). Physical examination reveals evidence of jaundice and weight loss. Abdominal examination is normal except for a palpable gallbladder. A stool specimen is negative for occult blood.

Laboratory studies:

Total bilirubin	3.4 mg/dL
Aspartate aminotransferase	18 U/L
Alanine aminotransferase	28 U/L
Alkaline phosphatase	110 U/L

Abdominal ultrasonography shows a dilated common bile duct and distended gallbladder but no stones. The pancreas cannot be visualized.

Which of the following is the most likely diagnosis?

(A) Choledocholithiasis
(B) Cholangiocarcinoma
(C) Pancreatic adenocarcinoma
(D) Primary sclerosing cholangitis

Item 4

A 70-year-old woman is hospitalized because of acute-onset mid-abdominal pain. The patient has lost approximately 11 kg (25 lb) over the past 2 months. She has stable coronary artery disease and underwent cholecystectomy many years ago.

Physical examination discloses decreased bowel sounds and guarding but no peritoneal signs. Serum amylase is 1200 U/L. Liver chemistry studies are normal. A helical CT scan of the abdomen shows a dilated biliary tree and pancreatic duct and a solid mass confined to the head of the pancreas. No other lesions are seen.

Which of the following therapeutic options is most likely to provide a chance for cure for this patient?

(A) Choledochojejunostomy (biliary bypass procedure)
(B) Endoscopic retrograde cholangiopancreatography with brachytherapy
(C) Gemcitabine and radiation therapy
(D) Pancreaticoduodenectomy (Whipple procedure)

Item 5

A 46-year-old woman is evaluated in the office for fatigue, intermittent fever, and dyspnea for the past 4 weeks with an 11-kg (25-lb) weight loss over the past 12 months. She does not have chest pain, palpitations, orthopnea, or peripheral edema. There is no history of recent cough, myalgias, or upper respiratory tract infection, and the patient does not smoke cigarettes.

On physical examination, BMI is 16. Heart rate is 90/min and blood pressure is 110/60 mm Hg. Breast examination shows a 2-cm firm mass in the upper outer quadrant of the left breast. No lymphadenopathy is noted. Jugular venous pressure is 8 cm H_2O. Lungs are clear. Cardiac examination shows distant heart sounds and no murmurs. There is no peripheral edema.

An electrocardiogram shows diffuse low voltage. Chest radiograph shows an enlarged cardiac silhouette and normal pulmonary parenchyma. Transthoracic echocardiography shows a 4- × 3-cm mass lateral to the left ventricular epicardial wall. A moderate-sized circumferential pericardial effusion is seen.

Which of the following is the most likely cause of the pericardial effusion and pericardial mass in this patient?

(A) Breast cancer
(B) Lung cancer
(C) Melanoma
(D) Mesothelioma
(E) Uterine cancer

Item 6

A 46-year-old woman is evaluated in the office for a 6-month history of increasing back pain, fatigue, and an 11-kg (25-lb) weight loss from baseline. She does not smoke cigarettes. The remainder of her medical history is noncontributory, and her family history is unremarkable.

On physical examination, there is bone tenderness in the midthoracic spine and the right anterior sixth rib. The remainder of the examination, including evaluation of the pelvis and breasts, is normal.

Laboratory studies include a hemoglobin of 11.1 g/dL with a mean corpuscular volume of 92 fL. Results of mammography are normal. A CT scan of the chest, abdomen, and pelvis is unremarkable except for bone abnormalities; a bone scan reveals multiple areas of increased radioisotope uptake in the lumbar and thoracic spine and in multiple ribs. A poorly differentiated tumor is identified by needle biopsy of a large sixth rib lesion.

Which of the following is the most appropriate next diagnostic step?

(A) Breast biopsy
(B) Colonoscopy
(C) Immunohistochemical staining of the tumor biopsy specimen
(D) Positron emission tomography

Item 7

A 55-year-old postmenopausal woman (G2P2) is evaluated in the office after a recent diagnosis of breast cancer. A preoperative mammogram of the affected breast shows a 2.5-cm spiculated mass with associated calcifications; the contralateral breast is normal. The tumor is excised and is an estrogen receptor–/progesterone receptor–positive, *HER2*-negative infiltrating ductal carcinoma of the breast. The surgical margins are free of tumor; a sentinel node is also free of tumor.

Which of the following is the most appropriate next step in management?

(A) Bilateral mastectomy
(B) Ipsilateral mastectomy
(C) Oophorectomy
(D) Radiation therapy

Item 8

A 55-year-old woman (G5P5) is evaluated in the office for a firm and tender 2-cm mass in the upper outer quadrant of the left breast. No other masses or axillary lymphadenopathy is noted. The patient began menopause at age 49 years. She is otherwise healthy and takes no medications. There is no family history of breast cancer; her mother died of colon cancer at age 72 years. A mammogram is normal.

Which of the following is the most appropriate next step in the management of this patient?

(A) Breast biopsy
(B) Radiation therapy and tamoxifen
(C) Repeat mammogram in 1 year
(D) Screening for *BRCA1* and *BRCA2* genes

Item 9

An 83-year-old woman is evaluated in the office for a 4-month history of weight loss and fatigue. She is a former cigarette smoker, but quit smoking 10 years ago. She is otherwise well and does her own cooking, cleaning, and grocery shopping. Diagnostic studies show a 5-cm left perihilar mass and metastatic disease involving her skeleton and liver. Biopsy reveals small-cell lung cancer.

Which of the following is the best treatment option for this patient?

(A) Chemotherapy
(B) Chemotherapy and radiation therapy
(C) Chemotherapy and surgery
(D) Palliative care only
(E) Radiation therapy

Item 10

A 63-year-old man is found to have a 1.5-cm spiculated, noncalcified nodule in the right upper lobe of the lung on chest radiograph performed before elective resection of the sigmoid colon for recurrent diverticulitis. There is no lymphadenopathy or evidence of calcified lymph nodes. A chest radiograph obtained 15 years ago does not show the nodule. The patient is a life-long nonsmoker and has no occupational risks for lung disease. Other than recurrent diverticulitis, he is healthy and takes no medication.

Which of the following is the best management option for the pulmonary nodule?

(A) Biopsy of the nodule
(B) Positron emission tomography of the chest
(C) Repeat chest radiography in 6 months
(D) Spiral CT scan of the chest

Item 11

A 35-year-old Jewish woman of Ashkenazi descent is evaluated in the office during a routine examination. Her medical history is noncontributory. The family history includes a paternal grandmother who had bilateral breast cancer at ages 42 and 50 years and died of metastatic breast cancer at age 53 years and a paternal great aunt who had ovarian cancer at age 45 years and breast cancer at age 51 years. Her two sisters, mother, and mother's relatives have not had breast or ovarian cancer, and her father is healthy without any cancer.

Physical examination, including breast and pelvic examination, is normal.

Which of the following is the most appropriate next step in management?

(A) Genetic counseling
(B) Low-fat diet
(C) Prophylactic bilateral mastectomy
(D) Prophylactic oophorectomy
(E) Tamoxifen

Item 12

A 65-year-old woman is evaluated in the office during a routine examination. Her medical history is significant for severe, debilitating hot flushes and sexual dysfunction that she experienced when she underwent natural menopause at age 52 years. Her symptoms have been successfully controlled since that time with combination hormone replacement therapy, consisting of conjugated equine estrogen and progesterone, which she is still taking.

For which of the following diseases is this patient most likely to be at increased risk?

(A) Breast cancer
(B) Colorectal cancer
(C) Melanoma
(D) Ovarian cancer
(E) Uterine cancer

Item 13

A 47-year-old white premenopausal woman is evaluated in the office during a routine examination. She had her first menstrual period at 14 years of age, and her first live birth at age 32 years. Results of two previous breast biopsies were benign. Her family history includes a mother who had *BRCA1/BRCA2*-negative breast cancer. Physical examination is normal.

The patient is concerned about developing breast cancer and wants to know if there is anything she can do to reduce her risk for this disease. The National Cancer Institute's online breast cancer risk prediction tool (www.cancer.gov/bcrisktool) is used to determine that her breast cancer risk over the next 5 years is 3.5%.

Which of the following is the most appropriate intervention for lowering this patient's breast cancer risk?

(A) Bilateral prophylactic mastectomy
(B) Chemotherapy
(C) Conjugated equine estrogen
(D) Tamoxifen

Item 14

A 78-year-old woman is evaluated at her home for worsening symptoms of metastatic colorectal cancer. At diagnosis 5 months ago, she had an 11-cm hepatic lesion, extensive large pulmonary nodules, and a 5-cm sigmoid mass. She underwent resection of the primary tumor to relieve obstructive symptoms. Despite chemotherapy, she had disease progression after 8 weeks of therapy. Currently, she is bedbound and cannot care for herself because of cancer-related symptoms of weakness and fatigue. She has minimal pain that is easily controlled with nonsteroidal anti-inflammatory drugs and small doses of narcotics.

Which of the following is the most appropriate next step in management?

(A) Cryotherapy
(B) Irinotecan chemotherapy
(C) Palliative care
(D) Radiation therapy

Item 15

A 40-year-old woman has an 18-year history of ulcerative colitis that is limited to the left side and has responded well to mesalamine and occasional corticosteroid enemas. Recent surveillance colonoscopy with biopsies showed low-grade dysplasia.

Which of the following is the most appropriate next step in managing this patient?

(A) Administer a low-dose corticosteroid
(B) Administer sulindac
(C) Refer for colectomy
(D) Repeat colonoscopy in 1 to 2 years

Item 16

A 48-year-old man is evaluated in the office during a general physical examination. He feels well and is asymptomatic. Medical history is significant only for hypertension treated with atenolol. He takes no other medications or over-the-counter drugs. Family history is unremarkable.

Physical examination is normal. Results of routine laboratory studies are also normal, including a hemoglobin level of 14.8 g/dL. One of three stool samples submitted for fecal occult blood testing is positive.

Which of the following is the most appropriate next step in evaluating this patient?

(A) Colonoscopy
(B) Double-contrast barium enema examination
(C) Flexible sigmoidoscopy
(D) Repeat fecal occult blood test
(E) Repeat fecal occult blood test and flexible sigmoidoscopy

Item 17

A 75-year-old man is evaluated in the office for cough and recent weight loss. On physical examination, the patient appears cachectic, and there is obvious right supraclavicular lymphadenopathy. Chest radiograph shows a 7-cm mass in the right lower pulmonary lobe. CT scan of the chest shows the lung mass, several enlarged mediastinal lymph nodes, three small contralateral lung nodules, and a 4-cm right adrenal mass. MRI of the brain shows a 1-cm posterior fossa lesion with edema, consistent with a single brain metastasis.

Which of the following is most appropriate for managing this patient?

(A) Biopsy of the brain
(B) Biopsy of the right adrenal gland
(C) Biopsy of the supraclavicular lymph node
(D) Mediastinoscopy
(E) Positron emission tomography

Item 18

A 72-year-old man is evaluated in the office for a 4-month history of hemoptysis, weakness, and 15% loss of baseline weight. He is wheelchair-bound because of his severe weakness and has been bedbound for more than 1 week. The patient has an 85-pack-year smoking history.

On physical examination, heart rate is 72/min, respiration rate is 16/min, and blood pressure is 120/82 mm Hg. Cardiopulmonary and abdominal examinations are normal.

CT scans of the head, chest, abdomen, and pelvis show a 12-cm right hilar lymph node mass, multiple liver metastases, and three brain metastases. A bone scan indicates bone metastases too numerous to count. Small-cell lung cancer is confirmed by bronchoscopic biopsy.

Which of the following is the most appropriate next step in the management of this patient?

(A) Chemotherapy and brain radiation therapy
(B) Chest and brain radiation therapy
(C) Hospice referral
(D) Lung tumor resection and chemotherapy

Item 19

A 68-year-old man is evaluated in the emergency department for hemoptysis, increasing weakness, and a 13.5-kg (30-lb) weight loss over 4 months. He is wheelchair-bound because of his severe weakness and has been bedbound for 1 week. He has an 80-pack-year smoking history.

On physical examination, heart rate is 72/min, respiration rate is 18/min, and blood pressure is 120/80 mm Hg. Abdominal and cardiopulmonary examinations are normal. Radiographs and CT scans of the head, chest, abdomen, and pelvis show a 10-cm right perihilar lymph node mass with involvement of multiple mediastinal lymph nodes and more than 10 hepatic metastases, but no brain metastases. Bone metastases too numerous to count are shown on bone scan. Squamous cell carcinoma is confirmed by bronchoscopic biopsy.

Which of the following is the most appropriate next step in the management of this patient?

(A) Chemotherapy and bisphosphonate therapy
(B) Chemotherapy, radiation therapy, and bisphosphonate therapy
(C) Hospice referral
(D) Lung tumor resection, chemotherapy, radiation therapy, and bisphosphonate therapy
(E) Radiation therapy and bisphosphonate therapy

Item 20

A 51-year-old asymptomatic man is evaluated in the office during a routine physical examination. His family history includes an uncle with prostate cancer. He has no known allergies and takes no medications.

A detailed physical examination is normal, although he declines a digital rectal examination. At the end of the examination, the patient requests a screening prostate-specific antigen (PSA) blood test for prostate cancer. After a discussion of the benefits and risks of prostate cancer screening, a PSA blood test is obtained.

One week later, the PSA test is returned and is elevated to 13.5 ng/mL.

Which of the following is the next best step in this patient's management?

(A) CT scan of the chest, abdomen, and pelvis; bone scan
(B) Measurement of free PSA
(C) Repeat PSA measurement in 3 to 6 months
(D) Transrectal ultrasound-guided biopsy of the prostate gland
(E) Reassurance

Item 21

A 58-year-old man is evaluated in the office during a routine examination. He is healthy but seeks advice on how to avoid developing prostate cancer because his father was recently diagnosed with this disease. The remainder of his medical and family history is noncontributory. The physical examination is normal.

Which of the following interventions would be most likely to decrease this patient's risk for prostate cancer?

(A) Annual digital rectal examination
(B) Annual prostate-specific antigen measurement
(C) Finasteride
(D) Five servings of fruits and vegetables daily

Item 22

A 35-year-old asymptomatic woman has a routine Pap smear that reveals atypical squamous cells of undetermined significance. She regularly undergoes routine Pap smear screening, and results of these studies have always been normal. Her most recent Pap smear was 3 years ago. She has been in a monogamous sexual relationship for 10 years and takes no medications. Serologic studies for HIV 1 year ago were negative. A physical examination, including pelvic examination, 1 week ago was normal.

Which of the following is the most appropriate management for this patient?

(A) Repeat Pap smear in 1 month
(B) Repeat Pap smear in 1 year
(C) Testing for human papillomavirus
(D) Reassurance

Item 23

A 65-year-old man is evaluated in the office for a facial lesion on his left cheek. The medical history is noncontributory. The lesion is shown (*see Figure 32 in Color Plates*).

Which of the following is the most likely diagnosis?

(A) Basal cell carcinoma
(B) Dermatofibroma
(C) Keratoacanthoma
(D) Squamous cell carcinoma

Item 24

A 58-year-old man is evaluated in the office for an enlarging dark mole on his back. One of its borders bleeds occasionally. He feels well and has no history of rash, trauma to that area, or skin cancer. The skin examination findings are shown (*see Figure 33 in Color Plates*).

Which of the following is the most appropriate next step in management?

(A) Electrodesiccation
(B) Excisional biopsy
(C) Liquid nitrogen
(D) Superficial shave biopsy

Item 25

A 30-year-old woman is evaluated in the office during a routine examination. Her medical history is noncontributory, and her family history is unremarkable. Physical examination is normal.

The patient is fair skinned and freckled and seeks advice on how to avoid developing skin cancer.

Which of the following interventions is most likely to reduce this patient's risk for malignant melanoma?

(A) β-Carotene
(B) Selenium
(C) Sun-avoidance strategies
(D) Sunscreen with sun-protection factor >30

Item 26

A 64-year-old man with end-stage metastatic prostate cancer is experiencing worsening skeletal pain throughout his back and bilateral lower extremities. He has already experienced disease progression despite anti-hormonal therapy, has refused further chemotherapy, and has received the maximal dose of radiation to the spine and metastatic lesions. He had been controlling his pain with regular use of nonsteroidal anti-inflammatory drugs but now requires short-acting narcotics almost every 4 to 6 hours.

On physical examination, no focal neurologic findings are noted. Results of renal function and liver chemistry tests are normal.

Which of the following is the most cost-effective choice for long-acting analgesic medication in this patient?

(A) Duloxetine
(B) Long-acting morphine
(C) Long-acting oxycodone
(D) Transdermal fentanyl

Chapter 9

Oncology
Answers and Critiques

Item 1   Answer: B

Hodgkin's lymphoma survivors who receive extended-field radiation therapy have a 1% risk/year for developing solid tumors. Young women are particularly prone to developing breast cancer in this setting, with an actuarial lifetime risk for a 20-year-old patient treated with mediastinal radiation therapy of 50% to 60%.

If this patient were a smoker, her history of radiation therapy would put her at increased risk for lung cancer. After 10 years, this patient's risk for developing recurrent Hodgkin's lymphoma is very low (2% lifetime risk). Radiation therapy does not increase the risk for acute myeloid leukemia, but alkylating-agent chemotherapy does. Finally, this patient's lifetime risk for developing non-Hodgkin's lymphoma after a previous diagnosis of Hodgkin's lymphoma is low (5%), and its occurrence would probably be unrelated to prior therapy.

KEY POINT

- Hodgkin's lymphoma survivors who receive extended-field radiation therapy have a 1% risk/year for developing solid tumors.

Bibliography

1.   **Dores GM, Metayer C, Curtis RE, et al**. Second malignant neoplasms among long-term survivors of Hodgkin's disease: a population-based evaluation over 25 years. J Clin Oncol. 2002;20:3484-94. [PMID: 12177110]

Item 2   Answer: C

The rapid onset of enlarged lymph nodes over the course of 1 month and size >2 cm are symptoms suspicious for infectious or malignant disease. Lymphadenopathy in the supraclavicular region almost always indicates an infectious or neoplastic cause and requires an immediate diagnostic procedure. This young patient, who does not smoke, most likely has Hodgkin's or non-Hodgkin's lymphoma. A complete lymph node excision is always preferred over a percutaneous needle biopsy in this setting because an adequate amount of tissue and preserved lymph node architecture can ensure a proper histologic diagnosis.

Observation for 3 months would be appropriate only in patients with smaller cervical lymph nodes (<2 cm). Antibiotic trials are never of value in the absence of signs, symptoms, or cultures suggesting infection. Bone marrow biopsies or aspirates are not optimal for establishing a primary diagnosis of lymphoma because of the lack of lymph node architecture

present in this type of specimen; however, this test is the preferred diagnostic approach when lymphoma is suspected but no tissue from a peripheral enlarged lymph node is available for biopsy.

KEY POINT

- Lymphadenopathy in the supraclavicular region almost always indicates an infectious or neoplastic cause and requires an immediate diagnostic procedure.

Bibliography

1.   **Huntington MK, Sewall BO.** Neck mass: how would you treat? J Fam Pract. 2007;56:116-20.[PMID: 17270117]

Item 3   Answer: C

This patient has most likely has pancreatic adenocarcinoma with biliary obstruction. Symptoms of pancreatic cancer may be nonspecific and mimic other intra-abdominal benign or malignant conditions. The type of symptoms that initially develop tends to vary, depending on the location of the pancreatic tumor. Pain and weight loss occur primarily in patients with cancers of the pancreatic body and tail. Patients with cancers of the head of the pancreas tend to have obstructive jaundice, steatorrhea, and weight loss. This patient's palpable gallbladder and evidence of gallbladder and common bile duct dilatation support a diagnosis of distal obstruction, and the patient's 6-week history of diarrhea and weight loss is most compatible with a malignancy.

Choledocholithiasis can also cause common bile duct dilatation but is not typically associated with a 6-week course of symptoms. Choledocholithiasis more typically causes severe, acute right upper quadrant abdominal pain, and this diagnosis would not explain this patient's weight loss or other systemic symptoms. In addition, most patients with choledocholithiasis have cholelithiasis. The key to the diagnosis of primary sclerosing cholangitis is the recognition of laboratory results compatible with cholestatic liver disease, including a high alkaline phosphatase concentration, normal or minimally elevated bilirubin level, and modestly elevated aminotransferase values. Dilatation of the peripheral bile ducts on ultrasonography without evidence of apparent obstruction in the common bile duct is also an important clue to diagnosing primary sclerosing cholangitis, which is not present in this patient. While jaundice and weight loss are suggestive of cholangiocarcinoma, most patients with this disorder have sclerosing cholangitis. Finally, cholangiocarcinoma is associated with a moderate dilatation of the intrahepatic bile ducts rather than the gallbladder and common bile duct dilatation seen in this patient.

KEY POINT

• In patients with pancreatic carcinoma, pain and weight loss occur primarily in cancers of the pancreatic body and tail and obstructive jaundice and weight loss occur primarily in cancers of the pancreatic head.

Bibliography

1. **Freelove R, Walling AD.** Pancreatic cancer: diagnosis and management. Am Fam Physician. 2006;73:485-92. [PMID: 16477897]

Item 4   Answer: D

A small subset of patients (<10%) who have pancreatic cancer will present with pancreatitis. This elderly patient with an unexplained episode of pancreatitis and weight loss is found to have a pancreatic mass and "double duct" sign (dilatation of the pancreatic duct and bile duct) on CT scanning. Although long-term survival rates are poor, the best chance for cure is a pancreaticoduodenectomy (Whipple procedure).

Endoscopic retrograde cholangiopancreatography with brachytherapy can provide palliation but is not curative. Although chemotherapy and radiation therapy can be used for neoadjuvant therapy or treatment of unresectable or residual disease, only surgery offers the best chance for cure. A biliary bypass procedure such as choledochojejunostomy would provide relief of the jaundice due to biliary obstruction but would not treat the underlying tumor.

KEY POINT

• Pancreaticoduodenectomy (Whipple procedure) offers the best chance of cure for a patient with cancer of the head of the pancreas.

Bibliography

1. **Lockhart AC, Rothenberg ML, Berlin JD.** Treatment for pancreatic cancer: current therapy and continued progress. Gastroenterology. 2005;128:1642-54.[PMID: 15887156]

Item 5   Answer: A

The finding of a pericardial mass and pericardial effusion on transthoracic echocardiography in a female patient with a history of substantial weight loss and a breast mass should raise the suspicion of metastatic pericardial disease from breast cancer. Because of their greater prevalence, cancers of the lung and breast are the most frequent metastatic tumors to involve the heart. Lung and breast cancers may reach the heart by direct extension. This patient has no history of tobacco abuse nor is there radiographic evidence of a pulmonary mass, so lung cancer would be unlikely.

Although melanoma, uterine cancer, and mesothelioma may metastasize to the heart, in this patient with pericardial involvement and a breast mass, metastasis from the breast is more likely.

KEY POINT

• Breast and lung cancers are the most common causes of malignant pericardial disease.

Bibliography

1. **Bussani R, De-Giorgio F, Abbate A, Silvestri F.** Cardiac metastases. J Clin Pathol. 2007;60:27-34. Epub 2006 Nov 10. [PMID: 17098886]

Item 6   Answer: C

In patients with adenocarcinoma of an unknown primary site, the workup should be guided by the patient's history and physical and laboratory findings. In this patient, immunohistochemical staining of the tumor for the presence of the *HER2-Neu* oncogene and estrogen and progesterone receptor expression (i.e., tumor markers for breast cancer) may be useful in making therapeutic decisions.

Colonoscopy would be indicated in this patient only if her history or physical or laboratory findings suggest the likelihood for the colon as the primary site and immunohistochemical staining and hormone receptor expression tests were not helpful.

In small trials, positron emission tomography has been found to detect the source of cancer in 20% to 30% of patients with an unknown primary site; however, larger trials are needed to confirm these results and demonstrate the usefulness of this detection method in various clinical scenarios. A breast biopsy should not be performed in this patient because there are no radiographic or physical findings suggestive of a breast primary tumor.

KEY POINT

• In women with adenocarcinoma of unknown primary site, immunohistochemical staining of the tumor for the presence of the *HER2-Neu* oncogene and estrogen and progesterone receptor expression may be useful in making therapeutic decisions.

Bibliography

1. **Varadhachary GR, Abbruzzese JL, Lenzi R.** Diagnostic strategies for unknown primary cancer. Cancer. 2004;100:1776-85. [PMID: 15112256]

Item 7   Answer: D

This patient needs radiation therapy. Several prospective randomized clinical trials, some with 25- to 30-year follow-up, have demonstrated that breast-conserving therapy (lumpectomy and radiation therapy) results in similar, if not superior, survival for patients with early-stage (stage I or II) breast cancer, regardless of patient age, compared with mastectomy. Recent studies have suggested that breast radiation therapy may not be necessary for older (>65 years) women with small (<2 cm), estrogen receptor–positive tumors, clear margins, and no lymph node involvement; however, the standard of care for younger patients includes radiation therapy to the breast, and usually, to the axillary lymph nodes.

A prophylactic mastectomy is not indicated in this patient. She has nongenetic, sporadic breast cancer, and her risk for a subsequent primary tumor, although approximately twofold higher than that of age-matched, unaffected women, is not sufficiently high to warrant such a strategy. Furthermore, if she receives adjuvant endocrine therapy, her risk for a subsequent second primary tumor will be equal to that of average-risk, unaffected women.

Many patients with early-stage breast cancer will likely benefit from adjuvant systemic therapy with hormonal therapy, chemotherapy, or both, in terms of both disease-free and overall survival. Some *HER2*-positive patients (node positive and high-risk node negative) may benefit from trastuzumab. Ovarian ablation may be considered in premenopausal patients who wish to avoid chemotherapy, but such therapy is not considered standard of care. Depending upon the clinical circumstances and patient preferences, the following ovarian ablation options are available: oophorectomy (irreversible), pelvic irradiation (irreversible), and a luteinizing hormone–releasing hormone agonist for 2 to 5 years (reversible). This patient is postmenopausal and in addition to radiation therapy, standard hormonal therapy remains the first line of treatment.

KEY POINT

- Breast-conserving surgery with radiation therapy results in similar and sometimes superior survival in patients with early-stage breast cancer regardless of patient age compared with mastectomy.

Bibliography
1. Veronesi U, Cascinelli N, Mariani L, et al. Twenty-year follow-up of a randomized study comparing breast-conserving surgery with radical mastectomy for early breast cancer. N Engl J Med. 2002;347(16):1227-32. [PMID: 12393819]

Item 8   Answer: A

This patient needs further evaluation of the breast mass despite the normal mammogram; a breast mass should always be completely evaluated and a definitive diagnosis established. Tissue examination is essential for diagnosis and therapeutic management. A tissue diagnosis should be obtained in any woman with a suspicious abnormality on mammogram or with a suspicious palpable mass even if an imaging study is normal. Tissue may be obtained by core biopsy, or a cytology specimen may be obtained by fine-needle aspiration from any suspicious breast mass or abnormal area noted on breast imaging.

Patients are not subjected to cancer treatment, including radiation or tamoxifen, until a histologic diagnosis of malignancy is made and the extent of disease known. Inherited germline

abnormalities in *BRCA1* and *BRCA2* confer a very high risk for breast and ovarian cancer (absolute risk of breast cancer greater than 50% by age 60 years). However, less than 5% of all cases of breast cancer are attributed to these germline abnormalities, and the prevalence of these abnormalities in the general population is only approximately 1/800. Testing for *BRCA1* and *BRCA2* should therefore be performed only in women who appear to have a genetic risk (multiple relatives with breast or ovarian cancer, especially with early onset of disease). Such women and their families should be referred to a genetic counselor for discussion and consideration of these complex issues.

Bibliography
1. Carlson RW, Anderson BO, Burstein HJ, Cox CE, Edge SB, Farrar WB, Goldstein LJ, Gradishar WJ, Hayes DF, Hudis C, Jahanzeb M, Ljung BM, Marks LB, McCormick B, Nabell LM, Pierce LJ, Reed EC, Silver SM, Smith ML, Somlo G, Theriault RL, Ward JH, Winer EP, Wolff AC; National Comprehensive Cancer Network. Breast cancer. J Natl Compr Canc Netw. 2005;3:238-89. [PMID: 16002000]

Item 9   Answer: A

Small-cell lung cancer, even at an advanced stage, responds to chemotherapy, and treatment markedly improves survival. Small-cell lung cancer accounts for approximately 15% of all cases of lung cancer and occurs almost exclusively in current or former smokers. It is a systemic disease, and patients almost always have concurrent micrometastases at diagnosis. The mainstay of chemotherapy for extensive disease is a combination of a platinum agent (cisplatin or carboplatin) and etoposide or irinotecan. For patients with extensive small-cell lung cancer, combination chemotherapy alone may result in a 70% to 85% overall response rate and a 20% to 30% complete response rate. Median survival is 8 to 12 months, with survival beyond 2 years rare.

Even patients with extensive disease and poor performance status (i.e.,, those who are usually bed bound) may derive significant short-term palliative benefit and improved survival from chemotherapy. This patient's performance status is good, and she will likely benefit from treatment.

At diagnosis, 30% of patients with small-cell lung cancer have visibly localized disease that can be encompassed within a radiation therapy port, usually with confinement to one hemithorax lymph node, the mediastinum, and supraclavicular lymph nodes. Such patients are designated as having limited disease. Patients with limited small-cell lung cancer have a 5% absolute improvement in 3-year survival rates after receiving combination chemotherapy and radiation therapy compared with chemotherapy alone. This patient has extensive disease, i.e., disease that extends beyond the radiation port, and the best treatment is chemotherapy alone.

Surgical resection is indicated only in patients with stage I small-cell lung cancer (small, localized tumors), and surgery is augmented with induction or adjuvant chemotherapy. The few patients who can undergo complete resection have the best prognosis. Some of these patients may actually have atypical carcinoid or well-differentiated neuroendocrine tumors, which are much less likely to metastasize but are histologically similar to and may be mistaken for small-cell lung cancer.

KEY POINT

- Treatment of extensive small-cell lung cancer with chemotherapy improves survival.

Bibliography

1. **Murray N, Turrisi AT 3rd.** A review of first-line treatment for small-cell lung cancer. J Thorac Oncol. 2006;1:270-8.[PMID: 17409868]

Item 10   Answer: A

The best management for this pulmonary nodule is immediate biopsy. The solitary pulmonary nodule—a single, discrete intrapulmonary density <3 cm in diameter completely surrounded by aerated lung—is a common finding. The differential diagnosis includes bronchogenic carcinoma, solitary metastasis to the lung, granulomas (both infectious and noninfectious), benign lung tumors (such as hamartomas), and miscellaneous lesions ranging from pulmonary arteriovenous malformations to resolving pneumonias and pulmonary infarcts. The initial management of a solitary pulmonary nodule must be individualized based on the probability of malignancy, lesion size and location, the patient's overall condition, and the patient's preferences. A 1.5-cm spiculated nodule in a 63-year-old otherwise healthy man is a moderate cancer risk. Immediate biopsy is the best option for this patient.

The probability of malignancy of a solitary pulmonary nodule varies from 10% to 70% among various patient populations, but can be crudely estimated from the smoking history, age of the patient, size of the lesion, and whether or not there is a history of malignancy. Malignant nodules tend to have spiculated margins, little or no calcification, and intermediate doubling times (between 30 and 500 days), whereas benign lesions classically have smooth margins and central, diffuse, or laminated calcification and either double within 30 days or show no growth over a 2-year period. Therefore, the patient's previous radiographs should be reviewed if possible to assess growth of the lesion over time. There is no uniformly reliable radiographic rule or technique for determining whether a solitary nodule is a malignant lesion. Even positron emission tomography (PET) scans, which show increased uptake in >90% of malignant solitary nodules >1 cm in diameter, may be falsely negative in patients with alveolar cell carcinoma or small lesions and falsely positive in those with various inflammatory lesions.

Waiting 6 months may place the patient at increased risk for developing inoperable lung cancer. Spiral CT or PET scans are unlikely to provide additional useful information that will significantly increase or decrease the probability of cancer.

KEY POINTS

- Malignant pulmonary nodules tend to have spiculated margins, little or no calcification, and intermediate doubling times (between 30 and 500 days).

- Benign pulmonary nodules classically have smooth margins; central, diffuse, or laminated calcification; and either double within 30 days or show no growth over a 2-year period.

- No radiographic rule or technique has proved uniformly reliable in distinguishing benign from malignant pulmonary nodules.

Bibliography

1. **Ost D, Fein A.** Management strategies for the solitary pulmonary nodule. Curr Opin Pulm Med. 2004;10:272-8. [PMID: 15220751]

Item 11   Answer: A

This patient's family history of breast and ovarian cancer and the constellation of disease in the affected relatives—combined with the patient's Ashkenazi Jewish descent—may increase her risk for these types of cancer. Compared with the general population, women who are of Ashkenazi Jewish descent are five times more likely to harbor *BRCA1* or *BRCA2* mutations, which confer a significantly higher risk for breast and ovarian cancer compared with persons without these mutations. Therefore, referral to a genetic counselor is appropriate for this patient and will enable her to become informed about her options for reducing cancer risk. Although women with *BRCA1/BRCA2*-positive breast or ovarian cancer do not necessarily have a worse prognosis than those without these genetic mutations, they do have a substantially higher risk for mortality simply because of the enormously increased frequency with which breast and ovarian cancers occur in these higher-risk populations.

Retrospective and prospective studies have suggested that prophylactic bilateral mastectomy in high-risk patients decreases the risks for breast cancer incidence and mortality by 90% or more. Likewise, prophylactic oophorectomy should be considered in women who have tested positive for a *BRCA1/BRCA2* mutation and who have completed childbearing. However, these are drastic approaches and not a consideration for this patient until she learns more about her degree of cancer risk by genetic counseling.

Breast cancer risk was not reduced in an unplanned, retrospective subset analysis of women who appeared likely to harbor *BRCA1* and/or *BRCA2* abnormalities and who participated in a prospective randomized clinical trial of tamoxifen versus placebo for chemoprevention. However, other studies have suggested that tamoxifen is equally effective in preventing breast cancer regardless of *BRCA1* and/or *BRCA2* status. Nonetheless, tamoxifen therapy would be premature in this patient before she is determined to be at high risk for breast and/or ovarian cancer.

• Patients with a family history suggestive of germline-susceptibility cancer should be referred for genetic counseling.

Bibliography
1. U.S. Preventive Services Task Force. Genetic risk assessment and BRCA mutation testing for breast and ovarian cancer susceptibility: recommendation statement. Ann Intern Med. 2005;143:355-61. Erratum in: Ann Intern Med. 2005;143:547. [PMID: 16144894]

Item 12   Answer: A

Estrogen replacement therapy increases the risk of breast cancer. Before the release of the results of the prospective randomized clinical trials conducted by the Women's Health Initiative (WHI), results from observational studies strongly suggested that the relative risk for breast cancer in women taking hormone replacement therapy was 1.2 to 1.5. These data were confirmed by the WHI trials, but, surprisingly, this increased risk was observed only in women who took combination hormone therapy. For women with a prior hysterectomy who were randomly assigned to receive conjugated equine estrogen alone, breast cancer risk was not increased and may have even decreased (relative risk = 0.77).

Observational studies and the WHI suggest a protective effect of combination hormonal therapy against colorectal cancer, which was not observed in women taking conjugated equine estrogen alone. Other observational studies have suggested that unopposed estrogen therapy increases the risk for uterine cancer by two- to threefold, but this risk is abrogated by concurrent administration of progestational agents. The data regarding estrogen use and ovarian cancer are mixed. Oral contraceptives appear to decrease ovarian cancer risk, whereas estrogen therapy, with or without progestin, does not appear to confer any identifiable risk for ovarian cancer. Likewise, the risk for melanoma does not appear to be increased or decreased in women taking hormone replacement therapy. The United States Preventive Services Task Force concluded that the harmful effects of combined hormone replacement therapy exceed its chronic disease prevention benefits in most women. Women who do require hormone replacement therapy to control menopausal symptoms should receive it for the shortest possible period and at the lowest possible dose to control symptoms.

• Combination hormone replacement therapy increases the risk for breast cancer.

Bibliography
1. Stefanick ML. Estrogens and progestins: background and history, trends in use, and guidelines and regimens approved by the US Food and Drug Administration. Am J Med. 2005;118:64-73. [PMID: 16414329]

Item 13   Answer: D

This patient has a substantially elevated risk for breast cancer compared with a woman of the same age who is at average risk for breast cancer (3.5% absolute risk vs. 1.1% absolute risk). Tamoxifen has been shown in randomized trials to decrease the risk for breast cancer by approximately 50% in pre- and postmenopausal women who have an absolute risk of breast cancer over the subsequent 5 years of at least 1.66% and is a reasonable intervention in this patient. Although she is likely to derive net benefits from the use of tamoxifen because of her elevated breast cancer risk, the patient must be informed of the potential harms of this therapy, including hot flushes, endometrial cancer, thromboembolic disease, and ocular problems.

In the Women's Health Initiative trial, when compared with placebo, conjugated equine estrogen was associated with a borderline-significant decreased risk for breast cancer (relative risk 0.77; 95% CI 0.59 to 1.01). However, this trial included only postmenopausal women, and the results would therefore not be applicable to this patient.

Because she is unlikely to have a mutation in a high-risk breast cancer gene considering the absence of BRCA1 and BRCA2 mutations in her only relative with breast cancer, bilateral prophylactic mastectomy is an overly extreme and unreasonable intervention in this setting. Chemotherapy is reserved for patients with established breast cancer and is never used to prevent cancer; many chemotherapeutic drugs are associated with an increased risk of secondary cancers.

• Tamoxifen decreases breast cancer risk by approximately 50% in pre- and postmenopausal women who have an elevated risk for this disease.

Bibliography
1. Newman LA, Vogel VG. Breast cancer risk assessment and risk reduction. Surg Clin North Am. 2007;87:307-16, vii-viii. [PMID: 17498528]

Item 14   Answer: C

The best management for this patient is palliative care. Although there are now many active agents for treating colorectal cancer, including 5-fluorouracil, oxaliplatin, irinotecan, bevacizumab, and cetuximab, none of these has been significantly effective in bedbound patients. The risks of chemotherapy outweigh its benefits in patients with a poor performance status (a measure of the functional status of the patient) because these patients are much less likely to respond to chemotherapy and are more likely to experience therapy-induced toxicity.

Irinotecan therapy can be effective in treating colorectal cancer; however, its toxicity in this setting would likely outweigh any potential benefits. Although cryotherapy to the liver can potentially slow the growth of hepatic tumors, it would not be effective in treating the extent of disease outside the liver in this patient or in improving her survival. Adjuvant radiation therapy can be successfully used for palliation, especially for pain control of metastases to bone, brain, and the presacral area. This patient does not currently require treatment for these conditions, and radiation therapy is therefore not indicated.

KEY POINT

• The risks of chemotherapy in bedbound patients with colorectal cancer who have a poor performance status outweigh its benefits because of poor likelihood for response and high likelihood for therapy-induced toxicity.

Bibliography

1. Meyerhardt JA, Mayer RJ. Systemic therapy for colorectal cancer. N Engl J Med. 2005;352:476-87. [PMID: 15689586]

Item 15   Answer: C

This patient requires referral for a prophylactic colectomy. The finding of low-grade dysplasia on surveillance colonoscopy is associated with concurrent adenocarcinoma or progression to high-grade dysplasia and cancer in up to 24% of patients with chronic ulcerative colitis. Current guidelines recommend colectomy for patients with chronic ulcerative colitis and dysplasia of any grade. Neither increased colonoscopic surveillance nor more aggressive medical therapy (such as administration of sulindac or a low-dose corticosteroid) has been found to reduce the risk of cancer in these patients. Repeating the colonoscopy in 1 to 2 years places this patient at increased risk for the development of colon cancer.

KEY POINT

• Patients with chronic ulcerative colitis and dysplasia of any grade detected on surveillance colonoscopy should be referred for colectomy.

Bibliography

1. Ahmadi AA, Polyak S. Endoscopy/surveillance in inflammatory bowel disease. Surg Clin North Am. 2007;87:743-62.[PMID: 17560423]

Item 16   Answer: A

This patient has a positive result on a screening test for colorectal neoplasia. Even though only one of three samples submitted for fecal occult blood testing (FOBT) was positive, this requires appropriate follow-up with a diagnostic test such as colonoscopy.

Repeating the FOBT is inappropriate because one test was already positive. Since bleeding from colorectal neoplasia can occur intermittently, a negative FOBT on subsequent testing would not rule out a neoplastic disorder. Flexible sigmoidoscopy, FOBT plus flexible sigmoidoscopy, and double-contrast barium enema examination are all considered screening studies rather than diagnostic tests and are therefore inade-

quate for determining whether this patient has colorectal neoplasia.

KEY POINT

• An asymptomatic patient with a single positive fecal occult blood test on routine screening requires follow-up with colonoscopy.

Bibliography

1. Lieberman D. Colorectal cancer screening in primary care. Gastroenterology. 2007;132:2591-4. [PMID: 17570229]

Item 17   Answer: C

This patient with advanced metastatic lung cancer requires a supraclavicular lymph node biopsy. In such patients, it is appropriate to perform a biopsy of an accessible site that will provide the diagnosis of metastatic disease with a minimum of discomfort, risk, and expense. Therefore, a supraclavicular lymph node biopsy would be preferred over adrenal or brain biopsy.

Although a 4-cm adrenal mass is highly likely to be metastatic disease, adrenal biopsy is more invasive and subject to histologic uncertainty compared with a supraclavicular lymph node biopsy. A stereotactic brain biopsy would similarly carry a higher degree of risk and invasiveness. Mediastinoscopy would likewise undoubtedly provide the correct diagnosis but would subject the patient to unnecessary discomfort and risk. Positron emission tomography would add little information, as the presence of metastatic disease in this patient is already clearly suggested by other imaging techniques.

KEY POINT

• In a patient presenting with likely advanced metastatic lung cancer, a biopsy of an accessible site should be done to confirm the diagnosis of metastatic disease with a minimum of discomfort, risk, and expense.

Bibliography

1. Dubey S, Powell CA. Update in lung cancer 2006. Am J Respir Crit Care Med. 2007;175:868-74. [PMID: 17446343]

Item 18   Answer: A

Most patients with small-cell lung cancer, even those with an extremely poor performance status and widespread metastases, respond dramatically to chemotherapy and whole-brain radiation therapy. Small-cell lung cancer is very chemosensitive compared with non–small-cell lung cancer. Although treatment in this setting is almost never curative, meaningful palliation for 1 to 2 years may be possible in 50% of patients. The addition of a bisphosphonate such as pamidronate or zoledronate has been shown to help reduce skeletal-related events in patients with metastatic lung cancer.

If this patient had non–small-cell lung cancer, hospice referral would be appropriate. Systemic chemotherapy is an essential treatment component in patients with small-cell lung cancer that prolongs life; therefore, any treatment modalities that lack chemotherapy would be inadequate.

KEY POINT

- Most patients with metastatic small-cell lung cancer respond dramatically to combination chemotherapy and whole-brain radiation therapy.

Bibliography

1. Jackman DM, Johnson BE. Small-cell lung cancer. Lancet. 2005;366:1385-96. [PMID: 16226617]

Item 19   Answer: C

This patient is best managed with a hospice referral. He has widely metastatic (stage IV) non–small-cell lung cancer of squamous cell histology, poor performance status, and a poor prognosis. Patients in this condition almost never respond to any type of therapy, and any rare responses are of exceedingly short duration; therefore, hospice referral is indicated. When patients and/or family members demand therapy even in hopeless circumstances, such as those described here, no harm should be allowed to befall the patient as a result of instituting such "futile therapy."

KEY POINT

- Patients with a poor performance status and widely metastatic non–small-cell lung cancer of squamous cell histology almost never respond to any type of therapy and require hospice care.

Bibliography

1. Molina JR, Adjei AA, Jett JR. Advances in chemotherapy of non-small cell lung cancer. Chest. 2006;130:1211-9. [PMID: 17035458]

Item 20   Answer: D

Transrectal ultrasound-guided prostate biopsy is the next best step in this patient's management. Most patients diagnosed with prostate cancer have no clinical symptoms related to their condition. Symptoms of urinary outflow obstruction may be present but are often associated with coexisting benign prostatic hyperplasia. In men who undergo biopsies, approximately 25% of those with a prostate-specific antigen (PSA) level between 4 ng/mL and 10 ng/mL and more than 50% of those with a PSA level >10 ng/mL have prostate cancer. Pathologic confirmation is needed to diagnose this condition, and transrectal ultrasound-guided biopsy is a relatively simple office procedure. Therefore, this study is indicated for all potential candidates for prostate cancer treatment and those who have a PSA level >4 ng/mL

Radiographic evaluation for metastatic disease is not indicated in the absence of a histologic diagnosis of prostate cancer. Repeat PSA measurement in 3 to 6 months is not warranted, because a PSA level >10 ng/mL is in itself highly sensitive and specific for prostate cancer. The sensitivity and specificity of free PSA measurement in the diagnosis of prostate cancer are unclear. Reassurance is not appropriate at this time because

this patient has a relatively high likelihood of having prostate cancer.

KEY POINT

- Approximately 25% of men with a prostate-specific antigen level between 4 ng/mL and 10 ng/mL and more than 50% of those with a prostate-specific antigen level >10 ng/mL have prostate cancer.

Bibliography

1. Barry MJ. Clinical practice. Prostate-specific-antigen testing for early diagnosis of prostate cancer. N Engl J Med. 2001;344:1373-7. [PMID: 11333995]

Item 21   Answer: C

A large multicenter, randomized, placebo-controlled trial showed that finasteride, an inhibitor of 5-α-reductase that converts testosterone to dihydrotestosterone, administered at a dose of 5 mg/d for 7 years, reduces the prevalence of prostate cancer by approximately 25% (absolute risk 24.4% in the placebo group vs. 18.4% in the finasteride group; number needed to treat = 17). High-grade disease (Gleason score 7 to 10) developed in more men in the finasteride group (6.4%) than in the placebo group (5.1%); however, the Gleason tumor grading system was developed for men who were not taking antiandrogen medications, and its extrapolation to men receiving finasteride is unclear. There was no difference in prostate cancer mortality rates between the two study groups. Finasteride is associated with an increase in sexual side effects compared with placebo, including a reduced volume of ejaculate (60.4% vs. 47.3%), erectile dysfunction (67.4% vs. 61.5%), and loss of libido (65.4% vs. 59.6%). Gynecomastia is also more common (4.5% vs. 2.8%). However, finasteride is also associated with a lower incidence of urinary obstructive symptoms (12.9% vs. 15.6%). Therefore, patients who are considering preventive therapy with finasteride must consider its benefits and harms before deciding whether to begin treatment.

Screening with digital rectal examination or prostate-specific antigen measurement has not been shown to decrease prostate cancer mortality rates in controlled trials and will result in an increase, rather than a decrease, in cancer incidence. Intake of fruits and vegetables has not been shown to decrease the risk for prostate cancer, although some observational studies have suggested that some dietary constituents, such as lycopenes, are associated with a lower risk for this disease; however, these data are not consistent and have not been tested in controlled trials.

KEY POINT

- Finasteride reduces prostate cancer prevalence by 25%.

Bibliography

1. D'Amico AV, Barry MJ. Prostate cancer prevention and finasteride. J Urol. 2006;176:2010-2; discussion 2012-3.[PMID: 17070238]

Item 22   Answer: C

The most appropriate management for this patient is immediate human papillomavirus (HPV) testing. Cervical cytologic studies commonly show atypical squamous cells of undetermined significance (ASCUS). Before HPV testing was available, a repeat Pap smear every 4 to 6 months until two consecutive studies for intraepithelial lesions were negative was recommended in this setting. The presence of cytologic abnormalities, including ASCUS, on a repeat Pap smear warranted referral for colposcopy. Immediate colposcopy also was an acceptable option but was not cost effective or convenient for patients. However, colposcopy is warranted if HPV testing reveals infection with a high-risk type of HPV (HPV-16 or HPV-18). Continued routine Pap smear screening is warranted even if results of HPV testing are negative.

One month is too short of an interval to wait before performing a repeat Pap smear and would increase the overall number of unnecessary Pap smears and possibly follow-up colposcopy; conversely, 1 year is most likely too long an interval to wait. In 5% to 17% of patients with ASCUS on cytologic studies, biopsy confirms the presence of grade II or III cervical intraepithelial neoplasia. Cervical intraepithelial neoplasia is characterized by a precancerous cervical lesion that, if untreated, may progress to cervical cancer. Grade III cervical intraepithelial neoplasia is the most severe type and has the greatest risk of progressing to invasive cervical cancer. Reassurance would be misleading and potentially harmful to this patient.

KEY POINT

- Human papillomavirus testing is indicated for patients with Pap smear results showing atypical squamous cells of undetermined significance.

Bibliography

1. Wright TC Jr, Cox JT, Massad LS, Twiggs LB, Wilkinson EJ. 2001 Consensus Guidelines for the management of women with cervical cytological abnormalities. JAMA. 2002;287:2120-9. [PMID: 11966387]

Item 23   Answer: A

Basal cell carcinoma is the most common malignancy in humans. Early basal cell carcinomas are small, nodular lesions with rolled borders, usually of flesh or pearly color with areas of translucency and surface telangiectasia. They usually occur on sun-exposed skin and, with time, invade locally both out and down into surrounding tissue. Often, patients describe a nonhealing sore that bleeds easily even with minimal trauma. Early identification with prompt treatment prevents the disfiguring effect of local tissue destruction from expanding tumors.

The characteristics of this patient's lesion do not coincide with those of squamous cell carcinoma. Like basal cell carcinoma, squamous cell carcinoma occurs on sun-exposed skin. It is recognized as a well-demarcated, firm, hyperkeratotic, skin colored or pink to red macule, papule, nodule, or plaque. It lacks the distinctive rolled edge and pearl-like translucency of basal cell carcinoma. Keratoacanthoma originates in the pilosebaceous glands and typically grows rapidly over a few weeks; it appears on sun-exposed areas. It is generally a solitary reddish-colored, dome-shaped papule with a smooth shiny surface and a central ulceration or keratin plug (horn). Keratoacanthoma spontaneously resolves over 4 to 6 months. A dermatofibroma is a very common benign growth appearing as a button-like nodule, typically on the extremities, but rarely, if ever, on the face. The color may be variable, from pink to dark brown. Lateral compression of a dermatofibroma will produce a depression, or dimple, that helps distinguish this lesion from other papular or nodular lesions.

KEY POINT

- Early basal cell carcinomas are small, nodular lesions with rolled borders, usually of flesh or pearly color, with areas of translucency and surface telangiectasia, frequently occurring on sun-exposed skin.

Bibliography

1. Rubin AI, Chen EH, Ratner D. Basal-cell carcinoma. N Engl J Med. 2005;353:2262-9. [PMID: 16306523]

Item 24   Answer: B

This lesion is a nodular melanoma and the preferred method to confirm the diagnosis is excisional biopsy. Melanoma is characterized by the ABCD mnemonic: Asymmetry (inability to draw a line down the middle to produce two mirror images; Border that is irregular, scalloped, or poorly circumscribed; Color (more than one color in the same lesion or very dark, black, occasionally white, red, or blue); and Diameter ≥6 mm (the size of a pencil eraser) . Patients should also be suspicious of moles that are different from others or that change, itch, or bleed. Persons who have fair skin or a family or personal history of malignant melanoma should have a thorough skin examination yearly by a dermatologist.

Destruction of suspicious lesions could not only result in the spread of malignant cells and significantly alter the prognosis, but it also makes it impossible to diagnose or stage the lesion and thereby select the correct treatment. Superficial shave biopsies, electrodesiccation, and liquid nitrogen are dangerous options for this patient.

KEY POINT

- Lesions suspicious for melanoma require an excisional biopsy.

Bibliography

1. Markovic SN, Erickson LA, Rao RD, Weenig RH, Pockaj BA, Bardia A, Vachon CM, Schild SE, McWilliams RR, Hand JL, Laman SD, Kottschade LA, Maples WJ, Pittelkow MR, Pulido JS, Cameron JD, Creagan ET; Melanoma Study Group of the Mayo Clinic Cancer Center. Malignant melanoma in the 21st century, part 1: epidemiology, risk factors, screening, prevention, and diagnosis. Mayo Clin Proc. 2007;82:364-80.[PMID: 17352373]

Item 25   Answer: C

Avoiding the direct sunlight during peak hours and wearing broad-rimmed hats, long-sleeved shirts, and long pants are associated with a decreased risk for squamous cell carcinoma and its precursors, as well as malignant melanoma. The regular use of sunscreen has been shown to decrease the risk for developing solar keratoses, the precursors to squamous cell carcinoma; however, a meta-analysis found no association between melanoma risk and sunscreen use. The exact reasons for this surprising observation are not known, but it may be that fair-skinned people who are at increased risk for melanoma wear sunscreen more frequently than those who have a lower risk for melanoma. It is also possible that sunscreen does not filter the spectrum of solar radiation most responsible for melanoma initiation or promotion. One double-blind, randomized, placebo-controlled trial offers some insight: 87 young white adults were randomly assigned to use sunscreen with a sun-protection factor (SPF) of either 10 or 30 during their vacation. Those assigned to use sunscreen with an SPF of 30 spent a longer cumulative and average daily time sunbathing over the course of their vacation than those who used sunscreen with an SPF of 10. This finding suggests that although sunscreen may protect against the rays most responsible for sunburn, it may encourage more exposure to rays associated with melanoma formation. Because of this seeming paradox between sunscreen use and melanoma, countries such as Australia that have a very high incidence of skin cancer and melanoma emphasize sun avoidance and protective clothing more than sunscreen use.

Whereas β-carotene has not been found to provide protection for the development of new skin cancer in patients with prior nonmelanoma skin cancer, selenium has been associated with a statistically significant increase in nonmelanoma skin cancer compared with placebo in patients who are at high risk for skin cancer.

KEY POINT

- Avoiding direct sunlight during peak hours and other sun-avoidance strategies are associated with a decreased risk for squamous cell carcinoma and malignant melanoma.

Bibliography

1. **Dennis LK, Beane Freeman LE, VanBeek MJ**. Sunscreen use and the risk for melanoma: a quantitative review. Ann Intern Med. 2003;139:966-78. [PMID: 14678916]

Item 26   Answer: B

This patient has chronic, progressive metastatic cancer–induced pain that is not alleviated by standard short-term pain management. He requires high-dose, escalating, long-acting narcotic analgesia, and in this setting, morphine would be appropriate. Methadone is another effective long-acting narcotic that is comparable in cost and efficacy to morphine and, therefore, would be an appropriate cost-effective alternative.

There is no evidence that any long-acting narcotic is better than another such agent. In particular, the efficacy of oxycodone is similar to that of morphine and is appropriate for use in patients with cancer-related pain. However, oxycodone is considerably more expensive than morphine, and because there is no evidence of its improved efficacy or a better side-effect profile compared with morphine, it would be appropriate to first use the lowest-cost alternative of agents with comparable efficacy. Transdermal fentanyl is also a useful long-acting narcotic but is considerably more expensive than long-acting morphine and is often used in patients who have limitations on oral intake or intolerance to other long-acting narcotics. Duloxetine is a new antidepressant drug with an approved indication for some chronic pain syndromes but would not be an appropriate alternative to long-acting narcotic analgesia for the treatment of severe, progressive, cancer-related pain. Selected antidepressants are commonly used along with narcotics as adjuvant treatment for chronic pain associated with malignancy.

KEY POINT

- Cancer patients with progressive pain that ceases to respond to short-term pain management may require high-dose, escalating, long-acting narcotic analgesia.

Bibliography

1. **Reid CM, Martin RM, Sterne JA, Davies AN, Hanks GW**. Oxycodone for cancer-related pain: meta-analysis of randomized controlled trials. Arch Intern Med. 2006;166:837-43. [PMID: 16636208]

Chapter 10

Pulmonary Medicine

Pulmonary Medicine contains self-assessment items that correspond to the following chapters in the *Internal Medicine Essentials for Clerkship Students 2* textbook:

Approach to Dyspnea
Pleural Effusion
Asthma
Chronic Obstructive Pulmonary Disease
Obstructive Sleep Apnea
Infiltrative and Fibrotic Lung Diseases
Venous Thromboembolism
Interpretation of Pulmonary Function Tests

Pulmonary Medicine contains self assessment items that correspond to the following Training Problems in the *Core Medicine Clerkship Guide*:

Dyspnea
COPD/Obstructive Airways Disease
Venous Thromboembolism

Chapter 10

Pulmonary Medicine
Questions

Item 1

A 36-year-old woman is evaluated in the office for an uncomfortable, occasionally burning feeling in her legs for the past year. The symptoms are most pronounced when she drives long distances and are relieved when she gets out of the car and starts walking. The symptoms also occur at night and interfere with her ability to fall sleep. Getting up and walking around the house help relieve the discomfort. Physical examination is normal.

Which of the following is the most likely diagnosis?

(A) Hypothyroidism
(B) Multiple sclerosis
(C) Restless legs syndrome
(D) Wilson's disease

Item 2

A 24-year-old woman is evaluated in the office for episodes of falling asleep at inappropriate times during the day. Sleepiness occurs most often after lunch or while driving a car. She goes to bed at midnight and gets up for work at 5:30 AM. Her only medication is an oral contraceptive. She has no symptoms of depression, illicit drug use, restless legs syndrome, hypothyroidism, or insomnia. She does not know whether she snores, and no one in her family has sleep problems.

Physical examination reveals a BMI of 20 and normal vital signs. The oral pharynx is normal, and there is no evidence of enlarged tonsils or crowding of the airway. The remainder of the physical examination is normal.

Which of the following is the most appropriate first step in the management of this patient?

(A) Electroencephalography
(B) Increase in sleep time
(C) Modafinil (a psychostimulant)
(D) Polysomnography

Item 3

A 64-year-old man is evaluated in the office for dyspnea that has gradually worsened over the past 6 months. He now has dyspnea with minimal exertion, such as walking from his bed to the bathroom. He does not have cough, chest pain, weight gain, or ankle edema. He is slightly more short of breath lying down, but he has no difficulty sleeping, generally feels refreshed when he awakens, and does not have daytime headache or somnolence. He has a 46-pack-year history of cigarette smoking. His medical history includes only hypertension, treated with hydrochlorothiazide and atenolol.

On physical examination, temperature is 37.0 °C (98.7 °F), blood pressure is 162/98 mm Hg, heart rate is 76/min, respiration rate is 18/min, and oxygen saturation is 90% with the patient breathing room air. BMI is 22. His jugular venous pressure is estimated to be 4 cm H_2O. Heart sounds are distant, and an S_4 is present. Lung examination reveals bilateral hyperresonance to percussion, diminished vesicular breath sounds, and a prolonged expiratory phase.

Which of the following is the most likely cause of this patient's dyspnea?

(A) Chronic obstructive pulmonary disease
(B) Heart failure
(C) Idiopathic pulmonary fibrosis
(D) Obstructive sleep apnea
(E) Pulmonary embolism

Item 4

A 68-year-old man is evaluated in the emergency department because of a 5-day history of shortness of breath. He describes falling on the ice 5 days earlier and sustaining a large bruise on his right flank. That evening, he had trouble sleeping from the pain but finally managed to rest while sitting in a recliner. Over the past 5 days, he has had progressive shortness of breath; originally it was related to exertion, but it now occurs at rest. He continues to sleep in the recliner for comfort. He does not smoke.

On physical examination, an ecchymosis is evident on his right flank. He is mildly dyspneic during conversation. BMI is 25.7. Temperature is 37.6 °C (99.8 °F), heart rate is 112/min, respiration rate is 26/min, and blood pressure is 142/72 mm Hg. Oxygen saturation is 93% with the patient breathing room air. The trachea is in the midline, and jugular venous pressure is 6 cm H_2O. The right posterior lung is dull to percussion, and there are decreased breath sounds on the right side of the chest. The cardiac point of maximal impulse is at the fifth intercostal space in the midclavicular line. No rubs, murmurs, or gallops are heard, and there is no evidence of edema.

Which of the following is the most likely diagnosis?

(A) Chylothorax
(B) Hemothorax
(C) Pneumonia
(D) Pulmonary embolism
(E) Transudative pleural effusion

Item 5

A 32-year-old woman is evaluated in the office for exertional dyspnea and bilateral pedal edema that has increased in severity over the past 6 months. She has no history of hypertension, diabetes mellitus, or hyperlipidemia and has never smoked. Her medical history is unremarkable except for Hodgkin's disease treated 14 years ago with chemotherapy and mediastinal radiation therapy with no evidence of recurrent disease.

Physical examination shows a regular heart rate of 84/min, a respiration rate of 18/min, and blood pressure of 100/60 mm Hg. Jugular venous pressure is 15 cm H_2O with prominent x and y descents. Jugular venous pressure increases with inspiration. The lungs are clear. S_1 and S_2 are normal, and no murmurs, rubs, or gallops are heard. Abdominal fullness and 2+ bilateral lower-extremity edema are present.

The electrocardiogram shows only nonspecific ST-T changes. The chest radiograph shows a normal cardiac size and clear lung fields. Echocardiography shows small ventricles with normal systolic function, aortic and mitral valve thickening with mild aortic and mitral regurgitation, normal pulmonary artery pressures, and no pericardial effusion.

Which of the following is most likely responsible for this patient's symptoms?

(A) Constrictive pericarditis
(B) Coronary artery disease
(C) Mitral valve fibrosis
(D) Myocardial fibrosis

Item 6

A 27-year-old woman with a history of cystic fibrosis and a long-standing productive cough and multiple prior exacerbations of dyspnea is evaluated in the emergency department for the acute onset of shortness of breath and left-sided pleuritic chest pain. She has had no fever.

On physical examination, she is in moderate distress. Her temperature is 36.9 °C (98.4 °F), blood pressure is 132/66 mm Hg, heart rate is 126/min, and respiration rate is 24/min. Oxygen saturation is 93% with the patient receiving oxygen, 2 L/min, by nasal cannula. Auscultation of the chest shows absent air movement throughout the left chest and crackles on the right side.

Chest radiograph shows a left-sided pneumothorax that is 3 cm from the lung margin to the chest wall (>50% size) with no mediastinal shift or diaphragmatic depression.

Which of the following is the most appropriate next step in this patient's management?

(A) Intubation and mechanical ventilation
(B) Needle aspiration of the pneumothorax
(C) 100% oxygen and observation
(D) Tube thoracostomy

Item 7

A 53-year-old woman with a 20-year history of Raynaud's phenomenon develops increasing fatigue and a 7-month history of progressive dyspnea on exertion. She now must stop and rest while making her bed. She does not have chest pain, dizziness, or palpitations. Her only medication is nifedipine, 30 mg/d.

On physical examination, heart rate is 80/min, respiration rate is 18/min, and blood pressure is 115/78 mm Hg. Jugular venous pressure is not elevated, and there are no abnormal jugular venous waves. The lungs are clear to auscultation. On cardiac examination, the pulmonic component of the S_2 is accentuated. There is a grade 2/6 holosystolic murmur heard loudest at the left lower sternal border that increases with inspiration. Abdominal examination is normal. Sclerodactyly and digital pitting are present. There is no lower-extremity edema.

Hemoglobin is 11.5 g/dL. Chest radiograph is normal. On pulmonary function testing, FVC is 82% of predicted and DL_{CO} is 48% of predicted.

Which of the following is the most likely diagnosis?

(A) Heart failure
(B) Interstitial lung disease
(C) Mitral stenosis
(D) Pulmonary hypertension

Item 8

A 40-year-old woman with muscular dystrophy is evaluated in the office for daytime sleepiness, disturbed sleep, and morning headaches. Physical examination shows decreased air movement bilaterally. In the supine position, her abdomen moves inward with inspiration.

Pulmonary function testing shows a reduction in the FEV_1 and a low FVC. The ratio of FEV_1/FVC is normal. In the supine position, the FVC decreases by 30% compared with the FVC in the upright position (normal <10% reduction). The maximum negative inspiratory force is –40 cm H_2O (normal, <–80 cm H_2O). Measurement of arterial blood gases with the patient breathing room air shows pH 7.38, PCO_2 49 mm Hg, and PO_2 84 mm Hg.

Which of the following is the most likely cause of this patient's pulmonary disorder?

(A) Asthma
(B) Neuromuscular weakness
(C) Pulmonary fibrosis
(D) Tracheal stenosis

Item 9

A 63-year-old man is evaluated in the office for a 2-week history of cough, fever, and increasing shortness of breath. The patient has a 45-pack-year smoking history and a long history of heavy alcohol consumption; he also has poorly controlled type 2 diabetes mellitus.

On physical examination, the temperature is 38.9 °C (102 °F), blood pressure is 96/60 mm Hg, heart rate is 120/min, and respiration rate is 26/min. Oxygen saturation is 85% with the patient breathing oxygen, 2 L/min, by nasal cannula. He has poor oral hygiene. There is decreased respiratory excursion on the right side with decreased breath sounds and egophony. Tubular bronchial breathing is heard in the right mid-chest posteriorly.

Chest radiograph shows a moderate-sized right pleural effusion. A right lateral decubitus film shows the effusion to be large (>3 cm from the chest wall to the lung margin), free flowing, and associated with a right lower lobe infiltrate. Thoracentesis is performed, and 1 L of foul-smelling turbid fluid is aspirated. Gram stain reveals gram-positive cocci and gram-negative rods. Pleural fluid analysis is as follows.

Cell count	Erythrocytes 1200/μL, leukocytes 2495/μL with 80% neutrophils, 15% lymphocytes, 2% mesothelial cells, and 3% eosinophils
Total protein	5.5 mg/dL
Lactate dehydrogenase	3200 U/L
Glucose	25 mg/dL
pH	6.95

In addition to broad-spectrum intravenous antibiotics, which of the following is the most appropriate next step in the management of this patient?

(A) No additional therapy
(B) Intrapleural streptokinase therapy
(C) Repeated thoracentesis as necessary
(D) Tube thoracostomy
(E) Video-assisted thoracoscopy

Item 10

A 50-year-old man is evaluated in the emergency department for a 3-day history of productive cough, fever, chills, pleuritic chest pain, and difficulty breathing. His only medical problem is heart failure after a myocardial infarction 2 years ago, and his medications are metoprolol, enalapril, furosemide, and aspirin.

On physical examination, temperature is 38.9 °C (102 °F), blood pressure is 130/78 mm Hg, heart rate is 80/min, and oxygen saturation is 89% with the patient breathing oxygen, 2 L/min, by nasal cannula. There are decreased breath sounds and dullness to percussion at the left lower lung base. Cardiac examination reveals no murmurs or extra sounds.

Chest radiograph shows a pleural effusion that occupies one third of the left lung. A lateral decubitus chest radiograph shows a 1.5-cm layer of pleural fluid.

Which of the following is the most appropriate next step in the management of this patient?

(A) CT scan of the chest
(B) Pleural biopsy
(C) Thoracentesis
(D) Tube thoracostomy

Item 11

A 75-year-old man with an 80-pack-year smoking history is evaluated in the office for a 3-month history of night sweats, weight loss, and progressive shortness of breath. He has a dull ache in his left chest. He also has an occasional cough with mucoid sputum production and becomes dyspneic with minimal exertion.

On physical examination, his temperature is 36.8 °C (98.2 °F), heart rate is 112/min, respiration rate is 26/min, and systolic blood pressure is 96 mm Hg. The trachea is shifted to the right. He has dullness to percussion and decreased breath sounds on examination of the left hemithorax. The abdomen is scaphoid with no organomegaly. There is no peripheral edema.

Laboratory tests show a leukocyte count of 6800/μL, serum total protein of 5.0 g/dL, and lactate dehydrogenase of 188 U/L. Chest radiograph shows complete opacification of the left hemithorax with a mediastinal shift to the right. Thoracentesis is performed, and pleural fluid analysis is as follows.

Cell count	Erythrocytes 150,000/μL; leukocytes 980/μL with 20% neutrophils, 55% lymphocytes, 10% mesothelial cells, and 15% eosinophils
Total protein	4.5 mg/dL
Lactate dehydrogenase	1200 U/L
Glucose	45 mg/dL
pH	7.2

Pleural fluid Gram stain is negative; results of cytologic testing are pending.

Which of the following is the most likely diagnosis?

(A) Malignant pleural effusion
(B) Parapneumonic pleural effusion
(C) Pleural effusion associated with esophageal rupture
(D) Transudative pleural effusion

Item 12

A 53-year-old woman with a long-standing history of moderate persistent asthma is evaluated in the office for increasing shortness of breath and exercise intolerance over the preceding 3 months. She does not have cough, fever, or sputum production and has been compliant with her asthma medications, which consist of inhaled salmeterol and fluticasone with albuterol as a rescue medication. In addition to asthma, she has hypertension, hyperlipidemia, and type 2 diabetes mellitus; her medications for these disorders are metformin, glipizide, lisinopril, atenolol, and simvastatin. The patient responds to these medications, but at a previous office visit, the dosages were increased to achieve better disease control. She is allergic to aspirin.

Which of the following medications is the most likely cause of the exacerbation of the patient's asthma?

(A) Atenolol
(B) Glipizide
(C) Lisinopril
(D) Metformin
(E) Simvastatin

Item 13

A 47-year-old man is evaluated in the office for a 6-month history of cough. He does not smoke cigarettes. The cough is episodic and worse at night and after exposure to cold air. At times it is brought on by taking deep breaths or by laughter. He has no postnasal drip, wheezing, or heartburn. There is a family history of allergies.

Physical examination, chest radiograph, and spirometry are normal. A 3-month trial of acid suppression therapy, intranasal corticosteroids, and antihistamines is not beneficial.

Which of the following would likely provide the diagnosis of this patient's chronic cough?

(A) Bronchoscopy
(B) CT scan of the chest
(C) CT scan of the sinuses
(D) 24-Hour esophageal pH testing
(E) Trial of inhaled albuterol

Item 14

An 18-year-old male high school football player is evaluated in the office for recurrent episodes of dyspnea, chest tightness, and cough that have occurred during a game and limited his ability to participate. The symptoms resolve spontaneously in 20 to 30 minutes. The patient's father has allergies but no lung disease.

On physical examination, the patient is a healthy young man; the lungs are clear on auscultation. Office spirometry shows an FEV_1 of 90% of predicted, FVC of 88% of predicted, and FEV_1/FVC of 80%.

Which of the following is the most appropriate next step in the evaluation of this patient?

(A) Allergy skin testing
(B) Exercise challenge test
(C) Measurement of lung volumes and DL_{CO}
(D) Physical conditioning program

Item 15

A 46-year-old female nurse is evaluated in the office for a 2-year history of episodic cough and wheezing. She says that these changes began after a severe respiratory tract infection. This past spring, she experienced similar symptoms requiring her to seek medical attention. She was placed on a short-acting β-agonist, but she is not certain if it consistently helped. The patient feels well and has had no symptoms for several weeks; she is not taking any medications. Physical examination shows no abnormalities, and spirometry is normal before and after administration of inhaled bronchodilators.

Which of the following is the most appropriate test to evaluate this patient's condition?

(A) Bronchoscopy
(B) CT scan of the sinuses
(C) Exercise echocardiography
(D) Methacholine challenge testing

Item 16

A 42-year-old man is evaluated in the office after a recent visit to the emergency department because of a 4-week history of steadily progressive shortness of breath and wheezing. New-onset asthma was diagnosed, an albuterol inhaler was prescribed, and he was advised to follow-up with his physician. His medical history prior to this diagnosis was negative for asthma, urticaria, eczema, aspirin sensitivity, and allergies. The work history includes a job as a spray painter in an automobile body shop that began 4 months ago. The patient indicates that his symptoms are worse while he is at work, beginning as soon as he starts painting, and that he feels better on the weekends. The albuterol inhaler provides some relief of his symptoms.

On physical examination, vital signs are normal. Only occasional wheezing is heard on auscultation of the lungs.

Which of the following is the most appropriate next diagnostic test in evaluating this patient's asthma?

(A) Bronchoprovocation testing with isocyanate
(B) Bronchoprovocation testing with methacholine
(C) Peak expiratory flow rate measurements at work and at home
(D) Radioallergosorbent test for IgE antibodies to isocyanate

Item 17

A 45-year-old woman is evaluated in the emergency department for an asthma exacerbation. She developed an upper respiratory tract infection 4 days ago, and 2 days later she noted increased cough, sputum production, wheezing, and chest tightness. She has used her albuterol inhaler many times over the past 2 days with limited benefit.

On physical examination, she is alert but anxious; her temperature is 37 °C (98.6 °F), blood pressure is 140/85 mm Hg, heart rate is 115/min, and respiration rate is 32/min. Oxygen saturation is 93% with the patient receiving low-flow supplemental oxygen. Examination of the chest shows reduced breath sounds over both lung fields with prolonged expiration and minimal wheezing.

Spirometry shows an FEV_1 of 0.96 L (31% of predicted). After the patient is given nebulized albuterol/ipratropium bromide, only minimal improvement is noted. On repeat physical examination, the heart rate is 130/min and the respiration rate is 24/min. Examination of the lungs shows decreased air entry and minimal wheezing; spirometry shows an FEV_1 of 1.05 L (34% of predicted). Chest radiograph shows evidence of hyperinflation.

Which of the following is the most appropriate next step in the evaluation of this patient?

(A) Complete blood count
(B) Electrocardiography
(C) Measurement of arterial blood gases
(D) Measurement of peak expiratory flow rate

Item 18

A 38-year-old woman is evaluated in the office for worsening control of mild-persistent asthma. Her disease had been under good control on therapy with moderate-dose inhaled corticosteroids plus as-needed inhaled albuterol until 6 weeks ago when she had an acute respiratory tract infection. Since then, she has had significant worsening of her symptoms, with nightly cough and wheezing and use of an albuterol rescue inhaler six to eight times per day. She is able to demonstrate proper use of the inhaled medications.

Which of the following is the most appropriate therapy for this patient?

(A) Fluoroquinolone antibiotic
(B) Leukotriene receptor antagonist
(C) Nebulized albuterol/ipratropium bromide
(D) Oral corticosteroid therapy

Item 19

A 23-year-old woman with a long history of asthma and previous exacerbations requiring intubation is evaluated in the emergency department for a 2-day history of increasing wheezing and dyspnea after the onset of a sore throat. She has a cough productive of small amounts of whitish mucus with some plugs. She has no fever or chills and says that she has used her albuterol inhaler many times in the past day. She had been taking montelukast daily but had not been using her corticosteroid inhaler because she had previously felt well.

On physical examination, she is alert and cooperative but in severe respiratory distress; the blood pressure is 160/80 mm Hg, heart rate is 140/min, and respiration rate is 36/min. She is using accessory muscles of breathing. She has nasal flaring, and chest examination reveals diffuse inspiratory and expiratory wheezes.

Peak expiratory flow rate is 110 L/min; leukocyte count is 16,500/μL. Measurement of arterial blood gases shows a pH of 7.32, P_{CO_2} of 44 mm Hg, and P_{O_2} of 76 mm Hg with the patient breathing oxygen, 5 L/min by nasal cannula. Chest radiograph shows hyperinflation but is otherwise normal.

Intravenous corticosteroid therapy is begun.

Which of the following is the most appropriate next step in this patient's management?

(A) An anticholinergic agent and a short-acting β-agonist
(B) Helium combined with oxygen (Heliox)
(C) Intravenous or inhaled magnesium sulfate
(D) Prompt intubation

Item 20

A 75-year-old woman with a long-standing history of asthma is evaluated in the office for increased nocturnal asthma symptoms and the frequent need to use an albuterol inhaler. Her treatment regimen now consists of daily moderate-dose inhaled corticosteroids. She has no other medical problems.

On physical examination, she has occasional wheezing; the examination is otherwise unremarkable. Office spirometry shows an FEV_1 of 2.2 L (75% of predicted).

Which of the following is the most appropriate adjustment to this patient's asthma therapy?

(A) Add a leukotriene receptor antagonist
(B) Add a long-acting β-agonist
(C) Add anti-IgE antibody
(D) Add theophylline
(E) Double the inhaled corticosteroid dose

Item 21

A 46-year-old woman with persistent asthma is evaluated in the office during a scheduled follow-up visit. Since her most recent visit 6 months ago, her disease has been stable on high-dose inhaled corticosteroids (beclomethasone, 800 μg/d) plus a long-acting β-agonist and an as-needed albuterol inhaler, which she uses approximately once every 2 weeks. The patient is pleased with the current therapy, except for the occasional problem with oral thrush.

In addition to continuing the as-needed albuterol, which of the following is the most appropriate next step in treating this patient?

(A) Continue current program
(B) Continue the long-acting β-agonist and reduce the dose of inhaled corticosteroids
(C) Discontinue inhaled corticosteroids and the long-acting β-agonist
(D) Discontinue the long-acting β-agonist and reduce the dose of inhaled corticosteroids

Item 22

A 76-year-old woman is evaluated in the office in October after an acute exacerbation of chronic obstructive pulmonary disease 10 days ago that was treated with ampicillin. She is now doing well. The patient also has a 10-year history of type 2 diabetes mellitus and hypertension. She does not currently smoke. Medications are albuterol, salmeterol, metformin, glyburide, hydrochlorothiazide, enalapril, pravastatin, and aspirin. She also uses oxygen, 2 L/min by nasal cannula, at home. Her most recent pneumococcal vaccination was 12 years ago; her most recent influenza vaccination was 1 year ago.

On physical examination, vital signs are normal. Examination of the chest reveals diminished breath sounds and occasional end-expiratory wheezing, findings similar to her baseline findings. Cardiac examination is normal.

Which of the following is the most appropriate management for this patient at this time?

(A) Influenza vaccination
(B) Pneumococcal vaccination
(C) Influenza and pneumococcal vaccinations
(D) Long-term ampicillin prophylaxis
(E) Long-term trimethoprim–sulfamethoxazole prophylaxis

Item 23

A 55-year-old man is evaluated in the office for a 2-week history of nasal congestion and cough. The cough was initially nonproductive but over the past week has become productive of greenish-yellow sputum. He also states that his anterior chest is sore, especially when he coughs. He has not had fevers, chills, or dyspnea. The patient is otherwise healthy.

The physical examination, including vital signs, is normal.

The presence of which of the following medical conditions would be an indication for antibiotic treatment in this patient?

(A) Asthma
(B) Chronic obstructive pulmonary disease
(C) Diabetes mellitus
(D) Heart failure
(E) Renal failure

Item 24

A 67-year-old woman with emphysema is evaluated in the office for worsening dyspnea. She also has increased ankle edema and is less responsive to a regimen of long-acting bronchodilators, inhaled corticosteroids, and theophylline along with continuous supplemental oxygen. She has difficulty managing her activities of daily living because of dyspnea.

On physical examination, she uses accessory muscles for breathing. Vital signs are normal except for a respiration rate of 16/min. There is no jugular venous distention, and heart sounds are distant. Breath sounds are distant without wheezes or crackles.

Chest radiograph shows hyperinflation with decreased pulmonary markings. High-resolution CT scan of the chest shows widespread homogeneous emphysema. The FEV_1 is 0.6 L (approximately 19% of predicted) and the DL_{CO} is <20%. Her 6-minute walk distance is 250 m. Measurement of arterial blood gases on oxygen 2 L/min by nasal canula shows a pH of 7.40, P_{CO_2} of 42 mm Hg, and P_{O_2} of 62 mm Hg.

Which of the following is the most appropriate management for this patient?

(A) Lung transplantation
(B) Lung volume reduction surgery
(C) Noninvasive positive pressure ventilation
(D) Pulmonary rehabilitation

Item 25

A 54-year-old man is evaluated during a routine follow-up office visit for poorly controlled hypertension. He is accompanied by his daughter, who states that he has fallen asleep while driving. The patient adds that he rarely feels refreshed on awakening and frequently awakens with a headache. He has no nasal congestion or postnasal drip. His medications are maximal-dose lisinopril, hydrochlorothiazide, and metoprolol.

On physical examination, blood pressure is 150/94 mm Hg, heart rate is 50/min, and respiration rate is 12/min. BMI is

32. Oxygen saturation is 98% with the patient breathing room air. The posterior pharynx is small because of redundant soft tissue and enlargement of the tonsils and uvula. Breath sounds are distant but clear; there is no wheezing. Cardiac examination reveals an S_4 and increased intensity of the pulmonic sound (P_2); there are no murmurs. A sleep study is done, and a representative polysomnogram is shown (*see Figure 34 in Color Plates*).

Which of the following is the most appropriate management for this patient?

(A) Counseling to improve sleep hygiene
(B) Inhaled corticosteroids
(C) Nocturnal continuous positive airway pressure
(D) Tongue and mandibular repositioning device

Item 26

A 33-year-old woman is evaluated in the office for progressive dyspnea. She has no constitutional symptoms or significant environmental exposures and has never smoked. She had a small pneumothorax 3 year ago treated with needle drainage.

On physical examination, she has a prolonged expiratory phase and a few basilar crackles in both lower lobes. Cardiovascular examination is normal. She has trace edema of the lower extremities.

Chest radiograph shows diffuse reticulonodular infiltrates. Pulmonary function testing shows a decreased TLC, FVC, and FEV_1; an increased FEV_1/FVC ratio; and a decreased DL_{CO}.

Which of the following is the most likely diagnosis?

(A) Asthma
(B) Idiopathic cardiomyopathy
(C) Interstitial lung disease
(D) Pulmonary embolism

Item 27

A 48-year-old man is evaluated in the office for progressive exertional dyspnea and a nonproductive cough. He is an ex-smoker (30-pack-years) and has gastroesophageal reflux disease, hypertension, and hypothyroidism. His medications are a proton pump inhibitor, an angiotensin-converting enzyme inhibitor, and thyroid hormone replacement.

On physical examination, blood pressure is 140/88 mm Hg, heart rate is 86/min, and respiration rate is 16/min. The skin on the hand is shown (*see Figure 35 in Color Plates*). He has localized areas of skin thickening on the arms and chest. Bibasilar mid- to late-inspiratory crackles are audible. There is no peripheral edema.

High-resolution CT scan of the chest shows reticular lines that are most prominent in the periphery of the lower lobes, accompanied by patchy, ground-glass opacities. Pulmonary function testing shows an FEV_1 84% of predicted, an FVC 78% of predicted, and a DL_{CO} 39% of predicted. Antinuclear antibody titer is 1:160.

Which of the following is the most likely diagnosis?

(A) Hypersensitivity pneumonitis
(B) Idiopathic pulmonary fibrosis
(C) Systemic sclerosis (scleroderma)
(D) Systemic lupus erythematosus

Item 28

A 70-year-old man is evaluated in the office for dyspnea on exertion. He reports feeling well until about 8 months ago, when he developed slowly progressive shortness of breath. He also developed an intermittent dry cough. He does not have chest pain, fever, or chills. He has no other medical problems, has never smoked cigarettes, and takes no medications other than an occasional aspirin. He is a retired professor and has never worked outside of academia. His hobbies include golf and fishing.

On physical examination, the patient is dyspneic at rest and has digital clubbing. Temperature is 37 °C (98.6 °F), blood pressure is 130/82 mm Hg, heart rate is 90/min, respiration rate is 16/min, and oxygen saturation is 88% with the patient breathing room air. Pulmonary auscultation reveals bilateral basilar end- inspiratory Velcro-like crackles. Cardiac examination is normal.

Routine serologic studies and urinalysis are normal. Chest radiograph shows diffuse, predominantly basilar bilateral infiltrates.

Which of the following is the most likely diagnosis?

(A) Asbestosis
(B) Chronic obstructive pulmonary disease
(C) Cryptogenic organizing pneumonia
(D) Idiopathic pulmonary fibrosis
(E) Sarcoidosis

Item 29

A 22-year-old woman is referred by her ophthalmologist for evaluation of skin nodules. Two days ago, she saw the ophthalmologist for acute onset of pain and redness in the left eye with decreased visual acuity. Her eye symptoms have improved since starting the eye drops prescribed by the ophthalmologist. History includes bilateral knee and ankle pain that developed 6 weeks ago and has improved with ibuprofen. Three weeks ago, she developed painful nodules on the anterior surfaces of both legs. She has no other symptoms and is otherwise healthy.

On physical examination, temperature is 37 °C (98.6 °F) and blood pressure is 124/78 mm Hg. She has three red to violaceous subcutaneous nodules measuring 1 to 2 cm in diameter on the anterior surfaces of her legs; they are not warm but are painful to palpation. Her left eye has redness located primarily around the iris; the pupil responds normally to light and accommodation. Lungs are clear, and cardiac examination is normal. There is mild, symmetric ankle swelling.

Chest radiograph is shown. Blood tests are ordered.

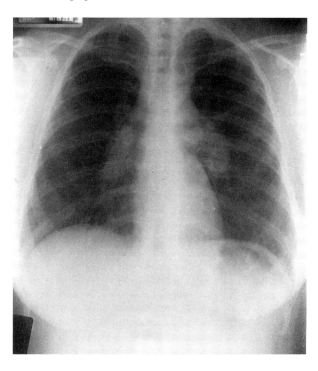

Which of the following is the most likely diagnosis?

(A) Hodgkin's lymphoma
(B) Sarcoidosis
(C) Systemic lupus erythematosus
(D) Tuberculosis

Item 30

A 65-year-old man is evaluated in the emergency department for dyspnea and pleuritic chest pain that began 60 minutes ago. The patient underwent a total knee replacement 2 weeks ago and had been sedentary since the operation. He is otherwise healthy and takes no medications; he has no known allergies and does not use alcohol, tobacco, or illicit drugs.

On physical examination, the patient is obese (BMI 31). The temperature is 37.7 °C (100 °F), blood pressure is 128/86 mm Hg, heart rate is 120/min, respiration rate is 30/min, and oxygen saturation is 90% with the patient receiving oxygen, 2 L/min, by nasal cannula,. There are crackles and dullness to percussion in the right lower lung field. Cardiac rhythm is regular, heart sounds are normal without murmurs, and there is an S_4 at the cardiac apex.

Laboratory tests, including hemoglobin, electrolytes, creatinine, and initial cardiac enzyme measurements, are normal; D-dimer is 2.5 µg/mL (normal, <0.5 µg/mL). Chest radiograph shows atelectasis and a small pleural effusion in the right lower lung field. Other than sinus tachycardia, the electrocardiogram is normal.

Which of the following is the most appropriate next test for this patient?

(A) Contrast-enhanced helical CT scan of the chest
(B) Echocardiography
(C) Exercise electrocardiographic stress test
(D) Telemetry, serial measurement of cardiac enzymes, and serial electrocardiograms

Item 31

A 65-year-old woman is evaluated in the emergency department for an episode of syncope that occurred after she took a 24-hour plane flight home from Australia. Her medical history is noncontributory, and she has no other medical problems.

On physical examination, the patient is in moderate respiratory distress. The heart rate is 110/min and weak, respiration rate is 16/min, and blood pressure is 90/60 mm Hg. Cardiopulmonary examination reveals soft heart sounds and clear lungs.

Which of the following physical findings will be most helpful in ruling out massive pulmonary embolism as the cause of the patient's hypotension?

(A) Flat neck veins
(B) Holosystolic murmur over the epigastrium that is louder on inspiration
(C) Left parasternal precordial heave
(D) Palpable and accentuated S_2 over the second left parasternal space
(E) Presystolic low-pitched extra sound over the subxiphoid area

Item 32

A previously healthy 24-year-old man is evaluated in the emergency department after he develops shortness of breath 4 days into a cross-country automobile trip. A ventilation/perfusion scan shows unmatched perfusion defects in his right lower lobe and left lower lobe, accounting for about 25% of total perfusion. He is hospitalized and treated with intravenous heparin and warfarin. One week later, the symptoms have resolved, and the INR is in the range of 2 to 3 for 2 consecutive days. However, because of residual chest pain and shortness of breath, a repeat ventilation/perfusion scan is obtained that shows persistent localized perfusion defects, accounting for about 20% of total perfusion.

Which of the following is the most appropriate next step in the management of this patient?

(A) Continue heparin
(B) CT angiography
(C) Discharge on warfarin
(D) Measure pulmonary artery pressures

Item 33

A previously healthy 54-year-old man is admitted to the intensive care unit with severe community-acquired pneumonia. He requires endotracheal intubation and mechanical ventilation. He has a right subclavian vein catheter, through which he is receiving antibiotics, vasopressors, and analgesic and sedating agents.

On physical examination, temperature is 38 °C (100.4 °F), blood pressure is 110/70 mm Hg, and heart rate 110/min on vasopressors.

Which of the following is the most appropriate prophylaxis for venous thromboembolism in this patient?

(A) Aspirin
(B) Low-dose heparin
(C) Warfarin adjusted to an INR of 2 to 3
(D) No prophylaxis required

Item 34

A 72-year-old man is hospitalized with pneumonia and treated with intravenous antibiotics. His medical history is significant for a right hip replacement 1 year ago, complicated by heparin-induced thrombocytopenia and subsequent deep venous thrombosis in his left popliteal vein. He takes no regular medications.

Which of the following is the most appropriate next step in reducing this patient's risk for venous thromboembolism?

(A) Aspirin
(B) Intermittent pneumatic compression
(C) Low-molecular-weight heparin
(D) Unfractionated heparin

Item 35

A 58-year-old woman is diagnosed with bilateral pulmonary emboli and metastatic uterine adenocarcinoma to the liver. Two years ago, she had a right lower-extremity deep venous thrombosis at the time of her diagnosis of uterine cancer. She underwent anticoagulation therapy with warfarin for 6 months following surgery.

After an initial 7-day course of low-molecular-weight heparin, which of the following is most appropriate for preventing recurrent venous thromboembolism in this patient?

(A) Continue low-molecular-weight heparin
(B) Place an inferior vena cava filter
(C) Transition to warfarin with a target INR of 2 to 3
(D) Transition to warfarin with a target INR of 3 to 4

Item 36

A 46-year-old woman (G0P0) is evaluated in the office for follow-up monitoring of pulmonary emboli that developed 13 months ago. The thrombotic event was unprovoked, and anticoagulation was discontinued after 6 months of therapy. The family history is negative for thrombosis.

Genetic analysis performed 3 weeks after the discontinuation of warfarin therapy indicated that she is heterozygous for the factor V Leiden mutation. Five weeks after therapy was discontinued, the patient experienced left lower-extremity pain and swelling in the absence of transient risk factors. A nonocclusive thrombus in the popliteal vein was shown on ultrasonography for which she underwent anticoagulation therapy with low-molecular-weight heparin followed by warfarin for 6 months.

Which of the following is the most appropriate management of this patient's thrombophilic disorder?

(A) Daily aspirin therapy
(B) Long-term unfractionated heparin
(C) Long-term low-molecular-weight heparin
(D) Long-term warfarin

Item 37

A 26-year-old-woman who is 20 weeks pregnant is hospitalized for acute shortness of breath with pleuritic chest pain. Her chest radiograph is normal. A ventilation/perfusion scan is interpreted as high probability for pulmonary embolism. She has no pertinent medical history and takes no medications.

Which of the following is the most appropriate management for this patient?

(A) Intravenous thrombolytic therapy
(B) Low-molecular-weight heparin followed by warfarin
(C) Unfractionated heparin or a low-molecular-weight heparin
(D) Warfarin

Item 38

A 50-year-old woman is evaluated in the office for intermittent cough and dyspnea on exertion of 3 months' duration. There is no significant sputum production, and she does not have wheezing, chest pain or tightness, or peripheral edema. She has a 30-pack-year history of cigarette smoking. She has no other medical problems and takes no medications.

On physical examination, she is resting comfortably. Blood pressure is 134/82 mm Hg, heart rate is 60/min, respiration rate is 12/min, and oxygen saturation is 96% with the patient breathing room air. Breath sounds are normal with no adventitious sounds. Chest radiograph is normal.

Pulmonary function studies:

Forced vital capacity (FVC)	78% of predicted
Forced expiratory volume in 1 sec (FEV_1)	76% of predicted
FEV_1/FVC ratio	65% (0.65)
Diffusing capacity for carbon monoxide (DL_{CO}) (single breath; corrected to hemoglobin)	Normal

Which of the following is the most likely diagnosis?

(A) Asthma
(B) Chronic bronchitis
(C) Emphysema
(D) Interstitial lung disease
(E) Pulmonary embolism

Chapter 10

Pulmonary Medicine
Answers and Critiques

Item 1   Answer: C

Abnormal sensations in the legs and restlessness relieved by movement are consistent with restless legs syndrome, a neurologic movement disorder that is often associated with a sleep complaint. The diagnosis of restless legs syndrome is based primarily on the patient's history of a compelling urge to move the limbs, usually associated with paresthesias/dysesthesias accompanied by motor restlessness associated with activities such as floor pacing, tossing in bed, and rubbing the legs. Symptoms are worse or exclusively present at rest with variable and temporary relief by activity. Symptoms are worse in the evening and at night. The disorder is treated with dopamine agonists, but it is essential before initiating treatment to check serum iron levels. Oral iron therapy can alleviate symptoms and is recommended if serum ferritin levels are <50 ng/mL. Nerve conduction velocity studies can be performed and at times can be consistent with peripheral neuropathy but are not essential to make the diagnosis.

The clinical presentation of this patient is not consistent with Wilson's disease or hypothyroidism. Wilson's disease is characterized by fatigue, anorexia, abdominal pain, tremors, poor coordination, spastic dystonia, and psychiatric or behavioral disorders. Hypothyroidism can present with a wide range of clinical symptoms, including fatigue, weakness, and paresthesias, but not leg dysesthesias that improve with movement. Multiple sclerosis is associated with highly variable signs and symptoms and can overlap with a number of other conditions. Generally, neurologic symptoms develop over hours to days, sometimes years, can spontaneously remit, and are not relieved by movement. Common symptoms and signs of multiple sclerosis include diplopia, hemiparesis, hemisensory deficit, urinary retention or hesitancy, cognitive problems, and fatigue. Many patients also have a history of painful optic neuritis.

KEY POINT
- The restless legs syndrome consists of abnormal sensations in the legs and restlessness relieved by movement.

Bibliography
1. **Kushida CA.** Clinical presentation, diagnosis, and quality of life issues in restless legs syndrome. Am J Med. 2007;120:S4-S12. [PMID: 17198769]

Item 2   Answer: B

Inadequate amount of sleep is the most common cause of excessive daytime sleepiness in young patients, and the first step in managing patients without other apparent causes of a sleep disorder is counseling about increasing the quality and amount of night-time sleep. Research suggests that most people require approximately 8 hours of sleep nightly, but this patient is only getting 5.5 hours. Each day the patient's sleep debt is carried over to the next night, resulting in symptoms of sleep deprivation and excessive sleepiness during the day, psychomotor deterioration, and accidents. She needs to increase the number of hours she is sleeping.

This patient does not have risk factors for sleep apnea, which include obesity and craniofacial and upper airway anatomic abnormalities such as enlarged tonsils. Therefore, polysomnography would likely not be helpful. Narcolepsy could be considered if her symptoms did not improve after adequate nocturnal sleep patterns had been established; therefore, electroencephalography would not be indicated initially. Because the diagnosis of narcolepsy is not likely at this point, prescribing a psychostimulant such as modafinil would be premature.

KEY POINT
- Inadequate amount of sleep is the most common cause of daytime somnolence in young adults.

Bibliography
1. **Lee-Chiong TL Jr.** Sleep and sleep disorders: an overview. Med Clin North Am. 2004;88:xi-xiv. [PMID: 15087216]

Item 3   Answer: A

This patient most likely has chronic obstructive pulmonary disease (COPD). The physical findings of hyperresonance and diminished breath and heart sounds suggest air trapping, and the prolonged expiratory phase indicates air flow obstruction. The 46 pack-year smoking history is a significant risk factor for COPD. The use of atenolol, a β_2-selective blocker, may also contribute to his dyspnea; β_2 selectivity is not absolute protection against bronchospasm, particularly if β_2-selective drugs are used at higher doses.

Although heart failure may cause worsening dyspnea and the patient's poorly controlled hypertension is a risk factor for heart failure, there are no supportive physical findings for this diagnosis, such as increased jugular venous pressure, crackles, an S₃ gallop, or peripheral edema. Idiopathic pulmonary fibrosis would cause diminished lung volumes, late inspiratory Velcro-like crackles, and sometimes clubbing. Chest radiography and pulmonary function testing clearly differentiate between obstructive pulmonary disease and pulmonary fibrosis. The patient has no findings to suggest obstructive sleep apnea, such as obesity, daytime headache, or somnolence. Furthermore, obstructive sleep apnea is not likely to cause exertional dyspnea. Pulmonary embolism would more commonly present as acute dyspnea and often pleuritic chest pain, although recurrent or unresolved emboli can cause chronic dyspnea due to pulmonary hypertension. This patient does not have any physical findings of pulmonary hypertension, such as increased jugular venous pressure, a right ventricular heave, a right-sided S₃ that increases with inspiration, an increased pulmonic sound (P₂), or a tricuspid regurgitant murmur.

KEY POINT

• Chronic dyspnea with hyperinflated lungs and a prolonged expiratory phase is characteristic of chronic obstructive pulmonary disease, especially when associated with a history of cigarette smoking.

Bibliography
1. Dyspnea. Mechanisms, assessment, and management: a consensus statement. American Thoracic Society. Am J Respir Crit Care Med. 1999;159:321-40. [PMID: 9872857]

Item 4   Answer: B

The patient's history of trauma and the evidence of significant injury point to hemothorax as the most likely cause of his dyspnea. Hemothorax is most commonly due to trauma, either blunt or penetrating (including iatrogenic). Examination should include auscultation and percussion of the chest with the patient in the upright position. (Examination of the patient in the supine position will obscure findings.) Nontraumatic causes of blood in the pleural space are less common. They include malignancy, blood dyscrasias, pulmonary embolism, bullous emphysema, and necrotizing infections, including tuberculosis. Cases have been reported of endometriosis causing hemothorax.

Pneumonia usually presents with cough and evidence of infection (fever, chills, or sweats). Chest pain is common, as is abdominal pain in patients with lower-lobe pneumonias. Cough is also a strong clinical factor in patients with atypical pneumonias. This patient describes primarily dyspnea and orthopnea and shows no other evidence of pneumonia or infection. Pulmonary embolism must be considered in all patients with dyspnea and could have a similar presentation. However, this patient's symptoms began the night of the injury and progressively worsened, and he does not have the marked hypoxia associated with pulmonary embolism. This patient also has no known predisposing factors for pulmonary embolism (obesity, immobilization, recent surgery, or known cancer). Pleural effusion as a result of heart failure (transuda-

tive pleural effusion) must be considered because of the patient's orthopnea. However, his examination does not support such a diagnosis because of the absence of an S₃ gallop, crackles, and elevated jugular venous pressure. Chylothorax is drainage of lymphatic fluid into the pleural space secondary to disruption or blockage of the thoracic duct. It is usually associated with malignancy (non-Hodgkin's lymphoma accounts for almost 60% of cases), but it can also be idiopathic or due to cirrhosis, tuberculosis, or filariasis. About 25% of cases of chylothorax are preceded by cardiothoracic procedures. Nonsurgical traumatic chylothorax is rare and not consistent with this patient's history of trauma followed by dyspnea.

KEY POINT

• Hemothorax is most commonly due to trauma, either blunt or penetrating (including iatrogenic).

Bibliography
1. Miller LA. Chest wall, lung, and pleural space trauma. Radiol Clin North Am. 2006;44:213-24, viii. [PMID: 16500204]

Item 5   Answer: A

This patient has a history of mediastinal radiation therapy, and the physical examination findings suggest the possibility of constrictive pericarditis. Increasing fatigue, dyspnea, peripheral edema, and ascites are common, albeit nonspecific, signs and symptoms associated with chronic constrictive pericarditis. Jugular venous pressure is elevated in nearly all patients with constrictive pericarditis, and prominent x and y descents are typical as a result of the rapid right atrial filling in systole and diastole. Kussmaul's sign, a paradoxical increase in jugular venous pressure with inspiration, is seen in only a minority of patients with constrictive pericarditis. Pericardial thickening, a sensitive sign of constrictive pericarditis, is often best identified with a CT scan of the chest.

In addition to constrictive pericarditis, radiation-induced heart diseases include myocardial fibrosis, valve dysfunction, and premature coronary artery disease. None of these entities can explain the jugular venous abnormalities seen in this patient or are compatible with the echocardiography findings. In patients with a history of mediastinal radiation therapy, accelerated atherosclerosis results in premature coronary artery disease. The relative risk of cardiovascular death is 3.1 at 10 years in patients who have undergone radiation therapy for Hodgkin's disease, with most of those deaths related to coronary artery disease. Mediastinal irradiation may also result in myocardial fibrosis, which causes symptoms of diastolic dysfunction and complicates the perioperative management of patients with prior radiation therapy who must undergo surgery.

KEY POINT

• Jugular venous pressure is elevated in nearly all patients with constrictive pericarditis, and prominent x and y descents are due to the characteristic rapid right atrial filling in systole and diastole.

Bibliography

1. **Nishimura RA.** Constrictive pericarditis in the modern era: a diagnostic dilemma. Heart. 2001;86:619-23.[PMID: 11711451]

Item 6   Answer: D

This patient has a symptomatic pneumothorax and requires immediate chest tube placement (tube thoracostomy). Approximately 16% to 20% of adult patients with cystic fibrosis have an episode of pneumothorax at some time in their lives. Secondary spontaneous pneumothorax (due to underlying lung disease) is more serious than primary spontaneous pneumothorax (no underlying lung disease) because pulmonary function is already compromised and secondary spontaneous pneumothorax can be life threatening. Rapid chest tube placement is needed to quickly alleviate the patient's symptoms and manage the pneumothorax.

Needle aspiration in patients with a secondary pneumothorax is less likely to be successful than in patients with a primary spontaneous pneumothorax. The size of the pneumothorax and the patient's presentation (significant shortness of breath and severe underlying lung disease) suggest that aspiration alone would not be adequate initial treatment. Needle aspiration should be reserved for patients with minimal dyspnea who are under the age of 50 years and have small pneumothoraces (<2 cm from the lung margin to the chest wall), and some authorities would not use needle aspiration in any patient with significant underlying lung disease.

Observation will result in absorption of a pneumothorax at the rate of 1.25% per day. Therefore, a 50% pneumothorax will take about 40 days to absorb, assuming there is no continued air leak. While administration of oxygen is an important adjunctive therapy and will increase the rate of absorption of the pneumothorax six-fold, this option is not adequate as initial therapy for a pneumothorax of this size, particularly in a patient with acute-onset shortness of breath and significant underlying lung disease. Intubation and mechanical ventilation are likely to worsen the patient's pneumothorax if there is a continued air leak to the pleural space, potentially resulting in tension pneumothorax.

KEY POINT
- Tube thoracostomy is the preferred treatment for secondary pneumothorax.

Bibliography

1. **Henry M, Arnold T, Harvey J.** BTS guidelines for the management of spontaneous pneumothorax. Thorax. 2003;58 Suppl 2:ii39-52. [PMID: 12728149]

Item 7   Answer: D

This patient with a long history of Raynaud's phenomenon and limited cutaneous scleroderma has evidence of pulmonary hypertension on cardiovascular examination (increasing dyspnea, normal pulmonary examination, increased pulmonic component of the S_2, evidence of tricuspid regurgitation, and abnormal DLCO). Patients with diffuse cutaneous scleroderma have an increased risk for developing pulmonary vascular disease as well, but the risk is higher in those with limited disease.

There are no findings on pulmonary examination to suggest interstitial lung disease. Crackles or "Velcro rales" are commonly heard in patients with interstitial lung disease and almost always precede the development of secondary pulmonary hypertension. A diagnosis of heart failure is unlikely in a patient without an elevated jugular venous pressure or an S_3 and a normal chest radiograph. Mitral stenosis may cause pulmonary hypertension and exertional dyspnea, but the patient's heart murmur is a systolic, not a diastolic, murmur that increases with inspiration, indicating that it is a right-sided heart murmur.

KEY POINT
- Patients with a long history of Raynaud's phenomenon and diffuse or limited cutaneous scleroderma are at risk for pulmonary vascular disease.

Bibliography

1. **Ramirez A, Varga J.** Pulmonary hypertension in systemic sclerosis: Clinical manifestations, pathophysiology, evaluation and management. Treat Respir Med. 2004;3:339-52. [PMID: 15658881]

Item 8   Answer: B

The patient has chronic ventilatory failure due to neuromuscular weakness. Patients with neuromuscular syndromes causing respiratory failure may present with acute or gradual decompensation. The major groups of muscles involved include the following: inspiratory (diaphragm, intercostal, and accessory muscles) that provide the ability to ventilate; expiratory (abdominal and intercostal muscles) that generate pressure for an effective cough; and bulbar (muscles of speech and glutition) that protect the airway. Clues to this diagnosis include the paradoxical abdominal motion with inspiration and the excessive fall in FVC in the supine position, indicating the presence of bilateral diaphragmatic paralysis, and the poor inspiratory force.

The patient's physical findings and pulmonary function test results do not support a diagnosis of either asthma or pulmonary fibrosis. Asthma is unlikely because there is no evidence of wheezing on examination, and spirometry does not show obstruction. Pulmonary fibrosis is an unlikely because of the absence of late inspiratory crackles and the low inspiratory force. Upper airway obstruction can mimic asthma. Symptoms are usually shortness of breath with wheezing or stridor, which may be both inspiratory and expiratory if the obstruction is due to tracheal stenosis. A flow-volume loop may show a characteristic expiratory or inspiratory plateau or both. Diagnosis usually requires CT or MRI scan and direct visualization of the affected airway by endoscopy. Since the physical examination does not reveal wheezing or stridor and the pulmonary function test results do not demonstrate an obstructive pattern, tracheal stenosis is unlikely.

KEY POINT

- Neuromuscular respiratory failure is characterized by paradoxical abdominal motion, an excessive decrease in forced vital capacity in the supine position, and poor inspiratory force.

Bibliography

1. **Laghi F, Tobin MJ.** Disorders of the respiratory muscles. Am J Respir Crit Care Med. 2003;168:10-48. [PMID: 12826594]

Item 9   Answer: D

This patient has an anaerobic pleural effusion with characteristics that suggest the probability of subsequent loculation if chest tube drainage (tube thoracostomy) is not done in conjunction with institution of antibiotic therapy. Pleural infections often resolve with antibiotic therapy alone, but fibrinous organization and lung entrapment require invasive treatment in about 10% of parapneumonic effusions. Effusions at risk for loculation are called complicated parapneumonic effusions. Because clinical prediction is unreliable, thoracentesis should be done to assess the need for invasive treatment if the effusion is >10 mm on either a lateral decubitus chest film or ultrasound examination. Chest tube drainage should be instituted if pus or gram-positive fluid is detected or if the pleural fluid pH is <7.0. While some authorities advocate institution of antibiotics and serial thoracenteses when the pH is ≥7.2, others favor these measures when the pH is between 7.0 and 7.2 if the Gram stain and culture are negative, since some complicated effusions will resolve with antibiotics alone. This patient has both gram-positive fluid and a pleural fluid pH <7.0; therefore, chest tube drainage is indicated.

A multicenter trial showed that streptokinase did not improve mortality or surgical or length-of-hospital-stay outcomes, challenging the use of routine fibrinolytic therapy for empyema. Early video-assisted thoracoscopy or thoracotomy is the generally preferred approach for patients who are candidates for surgery and who have persistent sepsis and loculation despite chest tube drainage; it is too premature to consider this treatment for this patient. Repeated thoracentesis is not adequate therapy for complicated parapneumonic effusions, and chest tube drainage is preferred.

KEY POINT

- Chest tube drainage (tube thoracostomy) of a parapneumonic effusion should be instituted if pus or gram-positive pleural fluid is detected or if the pleural fluid pH is <7.0.

Bibliography

1. **Davies CW, Gleeson FV, Davies RJ.** BTS guidelines for the management of pleural infection. Thorax. 2003;58:ii18-28. [PMID: 12728147]

Item 10   Answer: C

Thoracentesis is the appropriate next step in the evaluation of this patient. His pleural effusion is most likely a parapneumonic effusion secondary to community-acquired pneumonia. Thoracentesis is indicated because of the presence of free-flowing pleural fluid that is >10 mm in height on a lateral decubitus chest radiograph in the setting of pneumonia. Thoracentesis results will help guide further management.

Chest tube drainage (tube thoracostomy) is indicated for complicated parapneumonic effusions. The criteria for a complicated parapneumonic effusion include the presence of pus or Gram stain–positive pleural fluid or a pleural fluid pH <7.0. Pleural effusions not meeting these criteria are managed with intravenous antibiotics and observation. It would be premature to insert a chest tube without first analyzing the pleural fluid. A CT scan of the chest, which may show signs of loculated fluid or suggest an empyema (thickened pleura) may be indicated if free-flowing fluid is not readily apparent on a chest radiograph. Only a thoracentesis can diagnose a complicated parapneumonic effusion that predicts a high risk for future loculation and the need for immediate chest tube insertion. Pleural biopsy is indicated for undiagnosed pleural effusions following thoracentesis and pleural fluid analysis. Pleural biopsy may be most helpful in the diagnosis of tuberculous pleurisy.

KEY POINTS

- In the setting of pneumonia, thoracentesis is indicated in the presence of free-flowing pleural fluid >10 mm in height on a lateral decubitus chest radiograph.

- Chest tube drainage is indicated for complicated parapneumonic effusions, defined as the presence of pus or Gram stain–positive pleural fluid or a pleural fluid pH that is <7.0.

Bibliography

1. **Colice GL, Curtis A, Deslauriers J, Heffner J, Light R, Littenberg B, Sahn S, Weinstein RA, Yusen RD.** Medical and surgical treatment of parapneumonic effusions : an evidence-based guideline. Chest. 2000;118:1158-71. Erratum in: Chest 2001;119:319. [PMID: 11035692]

Item 11   Answer: A

This patient's history is consistent with a chronic illness, with an underlying indolent infection or neoplasm being prominent considerations in the differential diagnosis. Malignant pleural effusion is most likely. The patient has a large left-sided pleural effusion on physical examination that is confirmed by chest radiograph. The effusion is serosanguineous, exudative, and predominantly lymphocytic with a relatively low pH and glucose and negative Gram stain. The biochemical analyses confirm that the effusion is exudative, based on Light's criteria (exudative effusion is characterized by a pleural fluid to serum total protein ratio >0.5; pleural fluid to serum lactate dehydrogenase (LDH) ratio >0.6; or pleural fluid LDH value >two thirds of the serum value). Malignant pleural effusions are usually exudative. Transudative effusions in patients with thoracic malignancies may occur as a result of hypoproteinemia, atelectasis, or concurrent congestive heart failure. Malignant effusions may be hemorrhagic. Pleural fluid erythrocyte counts >100,000/μL, when not associated with trauma or pulmonary infarction, are suggestive of pleural malignancy. The pleural fluid leukocyte count is usually low (<4000/μL) and the distribution of pleural fluid leukocytes is lymphocytic. In malignant pleural effusions, a pleural fluid glucose <60 mg/dL portends a poor prognosis (survival <6 months). A pH of <7.3 likewise indicates a poor prognosis. Malignant effusions uncommonly involve the entire hemithorax (10% of patients), but when they do, the massive size of the effusion itself suggests the likelihood of an underlying malignancy.

A massive parapneumonic effusion would likely be accompanied by a neutrophilic pleocytosis, and the patient would likely be febrile. The pleural fluid pH could approach or fall below 7.2, as occurs in this case, but the patient would be acutely ill. Esophageal rupture may be associated with an exudative effusion with a very low pH (<6.0). Pleural fluid amylase is usually markedly elevated. Cytologic analysis typically demonstrates squamous cells in the pleural fluid. The history is characterized by retching and vomiting with the acute onset of left-sided chest pain. The effusion in these instances is usually small.

KEY POINTS

- Malignant pleural effusions are typically lymphocytic and are usually exudative.

- Pleural fluid erythrocyte counts >100,000/μL, when not associated with trauma or pulmonary infarction, are suggestive of pleural malignancy.

Bibliography

1. **Maskell NA, Butland RJ.** BTS guidelines for the investigation of a unilateral pleural effusion in adults. Thorax. 2003;58 Suppl 2:ii8-17. [PMID: 12728146]

Item 12   Answer: A

This patient's asthma was most likely exacerbated by higher doses of the selective β-blocker atenolol. β-Adrenergic receptors (β$_1$ and β$_2$) are widely distributed in the cardiovascular and respiratory systems. β$_2$ receptors are more prevalent in the lungs, whereas β$_1$ receptors are more common in the heart. In almost all patients with asthma, nonselective β-blockade causes bronchoconstriction. Regular use of nonselective β-blockers causes a 13.5% reduction in FEV$_1$, which can be significant in patients with asthma. β$_2$ selectivity is not absolute protection against bronchospasm, particularly if β$_2$-selective drugs (e.g., atenolol, metoprolol) are used at higher doses. Drugs with combined β- and α-blockade (e.g., labetalol, carvedilol) may be better tolerated than nonselective agents, but if used at all, they should be used cautiously and at low dosages. Severe bronchoconstriction and even death have been reported with use of topical β-blockers to treat glau-

coma. Ipratropium bromide is used to treat β-blocker–induced bronchoconstriction. Other agents such as β$_2$-agonists, atropine, aminophylline, corticosteroids, and glucagon can also be used to reverse the β-blockade effects.

Use of angiotensin-converting enzyme (ACE) inhibitors (such as lisinopril) is associated with a cough in 10% to 20% of patients. Asthma does not seem to increase the risk of this side effect. Furthermore, studies have failed to show a reduction in FEV$_1$ with ACE inhibitors, and they are generally considered safe to use in patients with asthma. There have been a few case reports of significant respiratory compromise with ACE inhibitors, but this effect seems to be rare. Biguanides such as metformin, statins such as simvastatin, and sulfonylureas such as glipizide have not been associated with bronchoconstriction.

KEY POINTS

- Nonselective β-blockers should not be used in patients with asthma.

- If selective β-blockers or combined α- and β-blockers must be used in patients with asthma, they should be used cautiously and at low dosages.

Bibliography

1. **Covar RA, Macomber BA, Szefler SJ.** Medications as asthma triggers. Immunol Allergy Clin North Am. 2005;25:169-90. [PMID: 15579370]

Item 13   Answer: E

The patient has cough-variant asthma. A trial of inhaled albuterol could help control his symptoms and confirm the diagnosis. The three most common causes of chronic cough are postnasal drip syndrome, asthma, and gastroesophageal reflux disease (GERD). The diagnosis of cough-variant asthma is suggested by the presence of airway hyperresponsiveness and confirmed when the cough resolves with asthma therapy. Sensitivity to cold air is a clinical marker of airway hyperresponsiveness that can be confirmed with methacholine challenge testing. The methacholine challenge test has a negative predictive value of nearly 100%, in the context of cough; this test is extremely useful in ruling out asthma.

There is little about the characteristics and timing of chronic cough due to GERD that distinguishes it from other conditions; in addition, GERD often can be "silent" from a gastrointestinal standpoint. However, this patient failed to benefit from 3 months of empiric therapy for GERD; therefore it is reasonable to rule out cough-variant asthma before doing 24-hour esophageal pH testing. In patients who have a history strongly suggestive of hyperresponsive airways, bronchoscopy and CT scans of the chest and sinuses have no role as first-line diagnostic tests.

- The diagnosis of cough-variant asthma is suggested by the presence of airway hyperresponsiveness and confirmed when cough resolves with asthma therapy.

Bibliography

1. **Dicpinigaitis PV.** Chronic cough due to asthma: ACCP evidence-based clinical practice guidelines. Chest. 2006;129:75S-79S. [PMID: 16428696]

Item 14   Answer: B

Exercise-induced asthma is a common manifestation of asthma and can be confirmed with an exercise challenge test. Nearly 90% of patients with asthma have exercise-induced asthma if exercise is sufficiently intense. Cold, dry air can enhance its occurrence. Exercise challenge testing (to >85% of maximal predicted heart rate) with post-exercise spirometry showing a reduction in FEV_1 confirms the diagnosis of exercise-induced asthma. An exercise challenge test has a high specificity for the diagnosis when the post-exercise reduction in FEV_1 is $\geq 20\%$. Airway obstruction after exercise peaks in 5 to 15 minutes and resolves in 20 to 30 minutes. Treatment with short-acting inhaled β-agonists 5 to 10 minutes before exercise prevents exercise-induced asthma in >80% of patients. With appropriate management, patients can engage in physical activities and do not need to limit or stop their involvement in sports.

Measurement of lung volumes and DLco is helpful in evaluating patients with suspected parenchymal lung diseases but is not likely to be useful in this patient. Although patients with parenchymal lung disease have dyspnea on exertion, their symptoms are typically progressive rather than intermittent. Allergy skin testing could be done in this patient, but positive results would not explain his symptoms and would not change his management. Deconditioning manifests as dyspnea on exertion but is not typically associated with cough or chest tightness; therefore, a physical conditioning program would not be very helpful in this patient.

- Exercise-induced asthma is confirmed by exercise challenge testing with post-exercise spirometry showing a $\geq 20\%$ fall in FEV_1.

- Treatment with short-acting inhaled β-agonists 5 to 10 minutes before exercise prevents exercise-induced asthma in >80% of patients.

Bibliography

1. **Parsons JP, Mastronarde JG.** Exercise-induced bronchoconstriction in athletes. Chest. 2005;128:3966-74. [PMID: 16354868]

Item 15   Answer: D

This patient's history is consistent with asthma, and the diagnosis can be supported by a positive methacholine challenge test. Because asthma can be an episodic disease, the baseline spirometry findings may be normal. Methacholine challenge testing can be helpful in this setting. The test is done by giving the patient increasing concentrations of methacholine by nebulization and performing spirometry after each dose until there is a >20% fall in FEV_1 compared with baseline. The methacholine dose that leads to a 20% decrease in the FEV_1, known as the provocative concentration 20 (PC_{20}), is calculated from a dose response curve. In general, a PC_{20} of <4 mg/mL is consistent with asthma. A PC_{20} between 4 and 16 mg/mL suggests some bronchial hyperreactivity and is less specific for the diagnosis of asthma. A PC_{20} >16 mg/mL is considered normal. The sensitivity of a positive methacholine challenge test is in the range of 85% to 95%. False-positive results can occur in patients with allergic rhinitis, chronic obstructive pulmonary disease, congestive heart failure, cystic fibrosis, or bronchitis. A normal bronchoprovocation test will almost always rule out a diagnosis of asthma.

Bronchoscopy to evaluate the trachea could be helpful if an anatomic lesion is suspected. However, the symptoms in patients with anatomic lesions are persistent or progressive rather than intermittent. Since this patient has intermittent symptoms, bronchoscopy is not indicated. Exercise echocardiography could help determine the presence of cardiac ischemia or myocardial dysfunction. The typical symptoms are dyspnea on exertion, chest tightness, or pain. However, cough and wheezing are not typical findings in patients with coronary artery disease. CT scan of the sinuses is not indicated in the absence of upper airway symptoms to suggest sinusitis.

- Methacholine challenge testing is most useful in evaluating patients with suspected asthma who have episodic symptoms and normal baseline spirometry.

Bibliography

1. **Dicpinigaitis PV.** Chronic cough due to asthma: ACCP evidence-based clinical practice guidelines. Chest. 2006;129:75S-79S.[PMID: 16428696]

Item 16   Answer: C

This patient's presenting symptoms and exposure to paints are suggestive of occupational asthma without latency. Latency refers to the period of time between exposure to the antigen and the onset of symptoms. Polyurethane paints contain isocyanate compounds, which are potent sensitizers that can cause asthma in workers exposed to as little as 0.001 ppm. Both immediate and dual (early and late) asthmatic responses have been described after inhalation challenges with isocyanates in sensitized workers.

The diagnosis of occupational asthma is a step-wise process that begins with clues suggesting a relationship between asthma and work, such as improved symptoms when a patient is away from work. Serial peak expiratory flow rate measurement has been demonstrated to be highly sensitive and specific for diagnosing occupational asthma, is relatively inexpensive and easy to perform, and is the first step in evaluating the cause of this patient's asthma. Bronchial challenge with methacholine can confirm nonspecific bronchial hyperreactivity in patients who do not demonstrate reversible airway obstruction on spirometry; however, bronchoreactivity testing does not provide a specific cause for asthma, and a normal test is not sufficiently specific to exclude occupational asthma in clinical practice. Blood tests for specific IgE antibodies confirm sensitization to occupational-agent exposure; however, there are few standardized allergens commercially available for this type of testing. Specific bronchoprovocation testing with the suspected causal agent is usually considered the gold standard for diagnosing occupational asthma, but it is not universally available, is time-consuming, and is not always necessary.

KEY POINT

• An occupational history and comparative serial peak expiratory flow rate measurements help establish a diagnosis of occupational asthma.

Bibliography

1. Beach J, Russell K, Blitz S, Hooton N, Spooner C, Lemiere C, Tarlo SM, Rowe BH. A systematic review of the diagnosis of occupational asthma. Chest. 2007;131:569-78. [PMID: 17296663]

Item 17   Answer: C

This patient has status asthmaticus and requires measurement of arterial blood gases as the next step in her evaluation. She has not responded well to bronchodilator therapy and is heading toward respiratory failure. Determination of oxygen saturation by pulse oximetry is a good screening and monitoring tool but is not a substitute for obtaining arterial blood gas measurements. Measuring blood gases is essential to evaluate her ventilation and direct management because decreased alveolar ventilation (elevated P_{CO_2}) may not be reflected on pulse oximetry. In mild acute asthma exacerbations, the P_{CO_2} is decreased. With increasing severity of the attack, P_{CO_2} increases and reaches normal levels in moderate to severe attacks. Elevated P_{CO_2} is an ominous sign, indicating severe obstruction and risk of sudden respiratory arrest.

Measurement of peak expiratory flow rate is unlikely to add useful information beyond what is gained from spirometry, which was already done. Electrocardiography is likely to show only sinus tachycardia and would not be expected to help in the management of this patient. Complete blood count with differential is not expected to change the management in most patients with acute asthma.

KEY POINT

• In patients in status asthmaticus, pulse oximetry is a good monitoring tool but is not a substitute for determining actual oxygenation by measuring arterial blood gases.

Bibliography

1. McFadden ER Jr. Acute severe asthma. Am J Respir Crit Care Med. 2003;168:740-59. [PMID: 14522812]

Item 18   Answer: D

This patient will do better with a short course of oral corticosteroid therapy. Her asthma was well controlled on moderate-dose inhaled corticosteroid therapy, and she now has "loss of control" after a respiratory tract infection. A short burst of an oral corticosteroid (e.g., prednisone, 0.5 mg/kg/d, for 5 to 7 days) can provide rapid resolution of asthma symptoms and allow the patient to regain control. Doubling the dose of the inhaled corticosteroid has also been recommended in such patients, but evidence to support the efficacy of this approach is mixed.

Antibiotics are not recommended for acute respiratory tract infections in patients with asthma because most of these infections are viral. Adding a leukotriene receptor antagonist can be considered in patients who cannot (or will not) take oral corticosteroids; however, they are less potent anti-inflammatory agents than corticosteroids and may not be effective in patients with significant exacerbations. Nebulized bronchodilator therapy should be reserved for patients who cannot use a metered-dose inhaler appropriately, but there is no indication that this patient cannot use an inhaler. Nebulized bronchodilator therapy should not be used as a substitute for corticosteroid therapy in patients with asthma exacerbations.

KEY POINT

• A short course of oral corticosteroids will restore asthma control in previously well-controlled patients following a respiratory tract infection.

Bibliography

1. Mallia P, Johnston SL. How viral infections cause exacerbation of airway diseases. Chest. 2006;130:1203-10. [PMID: 17035457]

Item 19   Answer: A

Prompt administration of bronchodilators is the therapy of choice for this patient, who may respond quite rapidly. The other choices may be considered depending on the initial response. If she fails to respond to bronchodilators administered every 20 minutes (or continuously) for the first hour (or less if she continues to deteriorate), then magnesium sulfate (intravenous or inhaled) has been shown to enhance bronchodilatation. Helium combined with oxygen has not been adequately studied, and the combination has not been proved beneficial in randomized controlled trials. However, its use is supported by some evidence. Helium plus oxygen could therefore be tried to avoid intubation in a failing patient, but extreme caution should be exercised to avoid a respiratory arrest.

- In a patient with acute severe asthma, prompt administration of bronchodilators is indicated after systemic corticosteroid therapy is started.

Bibliography

1. Beveridge RC, Grunfeld AF, Hodder RV, Verbeek PR. Guidelines for the emergency management of asthma in adults. CAEP/CTS Asthma Advisory Committee. Canadian Association of Emergency Physicians and the Canadian Thoracic Society. CMAJ. 1996;155:25-37. [PMID: 8673983]

Item 20   Answer: B

The patient requires the addition of a long-acting β-agonist to her medical program. Having asthma symptoms 2 or more days per week (or 2 or more nights per month) indicates that the patient has persistent asthma. All patients with persistent asthma should be treated with daily inhaled corticosteroids. When asthma is not adequately controlled on low- or moderate-dose inhaled corticosteroids, adding a long-acting β-agonist has been shown to be superior to doubling the corticosteroid dose in terms of improving asthma control and the patient's quality of life.

Although the benefits of long-acting β-agonists in asthma are well established, concerns about increased asthma-related deaths in patients using these agents have prompted a re-evaluation of their use in these patients. The Food and Drug Administration has mandated including a "black box" warning in the package insert for these drugs to warn patients about this possible risk. The majority of patients with asthma-related deaths were not taking concomitant inhaled corticosteroids, and these findings may not apply to combination therapy with inhaled corticosteroids and long-acting β-agonists. The National Asthma Education and Prevention Program (NAEPP) Expert Panel is revising their asthma treatment guidelines and is expected to address the proper placement of long-acting β-agonists in the step-wise approach to treatment of asthma.

Theophylline and leukotriene receptor antagonists are third-line drugs and should be considered in patients who are still symptomatic after adding a long-acting β-agonist. Anti-IgE antibody therapy should be reserved for patients who have elevated IgE levels and uncontrolled symptoms despite high-dose inhaled corticosteroids and a long-acting β-agonist.

- In patients with persistent asthma not adequately controlled with daily low- or moderate-dose inhaled corticosteroids, adding a long-acting β-agonist improves asthma control and quality of life.

Bibliography

1. Salpeter SR, Buckley NS, Ormiston TM, Salpeter EE. Meta-analysis: effect of long-acting beta-agonists on severe asthma exacerbations and asthma-related deaths. Ann Intern Med. 2006;144:904-12. [PMID: 16754916]

Item 21   Answer: B

This patient can continue the long-acting β-agonist and reduce the dose of inhaled corticosteroids. Inhaled corticosteroids are generally safe in patients with asthma; however, their long-term use, especially at high doses, can be associated with such side effects as osteoporosis, glaucoma, cataract, easy bruising, and suppression of the hypothalamic–adrenal axis. For many asthma outcome measures, the dose-response curve for inhaled corticosteroids is relatively flat above a dose of 400 µg/d. Therefore, when patients taking high-dose inhaled corticosteroids are stable, lowering the dose should be considered. This patient should go from a high to a moderate dose and continue the long-acting β-agonist. Asthma control is better with the combination of moderate-dose inhaled corticosteroids and a long-acting β-agonist than with high-dose inhaled corticosteroids without a β-agonist. Although the benefits of long-acting β-agonists in asthma are well established, concerns about increased asthma-related deaths in patients using these agents have prompted a re-evaluation of their use. The Food and Drug Administration has mandated including a "black box" warning in the package insert for these drugs to notify patients about this possible risk. The majority of patients with asthma-related deaths were not taking concomitant inhaled corticosteroids, and these findings may not apply to combination therapy with inhaled corticosteroids and long-acting β-agonists. The National Asthma Education and Prevention Program (NAEPP) Expert Panel is revising its asthma treatment guidelines and is expected to address the proper placement of long-acting β-agonists in the step-wise approach to treatment of asthma.

- In a patient taking high-dose inhaled corticosteroids for stable persistent asthma, reducing the dose of corticosteroids should be considered to prevent therapy-related side effects.

Bibliography

1. Panettieri RA Jr. In the clinic. Asthma. Ann Intern Med. 2007;146:ITC6-1-ITC6-16. [PMID: 17548407]

Item 22   Answer: C

This patient should receive both influenza and pneumococcal vaccinations. These two vaccines have been shown to reduce pneumonia and cardiac hospitalizations in the elderly by 30% to 40%. The influenza vaccine is offered annually to persons at risk for complications of influenza, including persons older than 65 years, patients with chronic disease, those who are immunosuppressed, and pregnant women whose last two trimesters coincide with the influenza season (late December through mid-March). Influenza vaccine can reduce the incidence of serious illness and death in patients with chronic obstructive pulmonary disease (COPD) by about 50% and should be given in the autumn of each year. Patients with documented fever, a known prior severe reaction, or an allergy to eggs should not be immunized. The primary vaccine used in the United States is a trivalent inactivated virus, but an intranasally administered vaccine from a trivalent live-attenuated virus is also available for patients 5 to 49 years old. The live vaccine is contraindicated in immunosuppressed patients and pregnant women, and its use should be delayed in patients who have received any antibody-containing products.

The pneumococcal polysaccharide vaccine (PPV23) consists of polysaccharides from 23 antigen types of streptococcal pneumonia. It is recommended for persons 65 years of age and older, patients with chronic disease (particularly diabetes mellitus and alcoholic cirrhosis), immunosuppressed hosts, patients with sickle cell disease, and in those who have had a splenectomy. The vaccine is 60% effective in protecting against bacteremic disease, the most common cause of morbidity in patients with pneumococcal disease. Immunity likely wanes 5 or more years after initial vaccination, and a single booster dose is recommended for patients continually at risk and those vaccinated before age 65 years.

Antibiotic therapy is essential for the treatment of COPD exacerbations, but it is not recommended for prophylaxis in COPD; therefore, neither long-term trimethoprim–sulfamethoxazole nor long-term ampicillin is indicated for this patient.

KEY POINTS

• Influenza and pneumococcal vaccines have been shown to reduce all-cause pneumonia and cardiac hospitalizations in the elderly by 30% to 40%.

• Influenza vaccine can reduce the incidence of serious illness and death in patients with chronic obstructive pulmonary disease by about 50%.

Bibliography
1. **Advisory Committee on Immunization Practices; Smith NM, Bresee JS, Shay DK, Uyeki TM, Cox NJ, Strikas RA.** Prevention and Control of Influenza: recommendations of the Advisory Committee on Immunization Practices (ACIP). MMWR Recomm Rep. 2006;55(RR-10):1-42. Erratum in: MMWR 2006;55(29):800. [PMID: 16874296]
2. **Kroger AT, Atkinson WL, Marcuse EK, Pickering LK; Advisory Committee on Immunization Practices (ACIP) Centers for Disease Control and Prevention (CDC).** General recommendations on immunization: recommendations of the Advisory Committee on Immunization Practices (ACIP). MMWR Recomm Rep. 2006;55(RR-15):1-48. Erratum in: MMWR 2006;55(48):1303. MMWR 2007;56(11):256. [PMID: 17136024]

Item 23   Answer: B

The presence of chronic obstructive pulmonary disease (COPD) is an indication for antibiotic treatment of acute bronchitis. Most cases of acute bronchitis are caused by viruses, such as influenza, parainfluenza, and coronaviruses. There has been a robust effort to reduce inappropriate antibiotic use in patients with acute bronchitis. With the exception of acute bronchitis in patients with underlying COPD, the only bacterial infection requiring antibiotic therapy is *Bordetella pertussis* (macrolides are first-choice agents in this set-

ting), which is typically characterized by a barking or paroxysmal cough in the setting of prolonged upper respiratory tract infection symptoms (>2 weeks). Antibiotics should be administered to patients with *B. pertussis* infection primarily to hasten clearance of the organism and limit transmission to susceptible contacts. There is no evidence to support the use of antibiotics in patients with acute bronchitis with concomitant heart failure, diabetes mellitus, asthma, or renal failure.

KEY POINT

• The presence of chronic obstructive pulmonary disease (COPD) is an indication for antibiotic treatment of acute bronchitis.

Bibliography
1. **Wenzel RP, Fowler AA 3rd.** Clinical practice. Acute bronchitis. N Engl J Med. 2006;355:2125-30. [PMID: 17108344]

Item 24   Answer: D

Pulmonary rehabilitation does not increase survival in patients with chronic obstructive pulmonary disease but does improve symptoms, exercise endurance, and quality of life and would therefore be indicated in this patient. Consider pulmonary rehabilitation in patients who experience anxiety with activity, breathlessness and limitations with exercise, and loss of independence and who are willing to undergo an intensive education and exercise program.

Lung volume reduction surgery (LVRS) increases the chance of improved exercise capacity, lung function, dyspnea, and quality of life but does not confer a survival advantage compared with medical therapy alone. A subgroup of patients with predominantly upper-lobe emphysema and low baseline exercise capacity may have improved survival. Long-term outcomes beyond 24 months are not well defined at this time. Consider LVRS for patients whose initial clinical criteria include CT scan evidence of bilateral emphysema; postbronchodilator total lung capacity and residual volume $\geq 100\%$ and 150% of predicted, respectively; maximum $FEV_1 \leq 45\%$ of predicted; $PCO_2 \leq 60$ mm Hg; and $Po2 \geq 45$ mm Hg. Patients should also complete a pulmonary rehabilitation program. Do not consider LVRS for patients whose clinical criteria include an $FEV_1 \leq 20\%$ of predicted and either homogeneous emphysema or $DLCO \leq 20\%$ of predicted; non–upper-lobe emphysema; and high baseline exercise capacity. This patient's low $DLCO$ and FEV_1 and the presence of homogeneous emphysema make her an unsuitable candidate for LVRS. Her age makes her an unlikely candidate for lung transplantation.

Noninvasive positive pressure ventilation (NPPV) consists of the provision of positive pressure ventilation without the need for an invasive airway. Consisting of a ventilator that delivers pressurized gas to the upper airway via tubing attached to a mask strapped to the face, NPPV has assumed an important role in the management of acute respiratory failure. NPPV is not effective in stable outpatients, especially those with a normal PCO_2.

Pulmonary Medicine • 285

**KEY POINT**

- In patients with end-stage chronic obstructive pulmonary disease, pulmonary rehabilitation improves symptoms, exercise endurance, and quality of life.

Bibliography

1. **Currie GP, Douglas JG.** ABC of chronic obstructive pulmonary disease. Non-pharmacological management. BMJ. 2006;332:1379-81. [PMID: 16763252]

Item 25   Answer: C

This patient has obstructive sleep apnea, and the most appropriate management is nocturnal continuous positive airway pressure (CPAP). Patients with this condition often do not identify related symptoms themselves. Resistant hypertension, obesity, daytime sleepiness, morning headache, and awakening without feeling refreshed should raise suspicion for obstructive sleep apnea. A polysomnogram showing cessation of airflow in the presence of continuing respiratory effort manifested by chest and abdominal motion confirms the diagnosis in this patient. CPAP is the treatment of choice in most symptomatic patients with obstructive sleep apnea and is believed to function as a pneumatic splint to prevent narrowing or collapse of the nasopharyngeal airway. In patients with obstructive sleep apnea, CPAP therapy has been shown to improve quality of life, cognitive function, symptoms of daytime sleepiness, blood pressure, and cardiac function; it also has a beneficial effect on mortality.

Optimal sleep hygiene is indicated for patients with obstructive sleep apnea. Avoidance of alcohol and/or sedatives 3 to 4 hours before bedtime is recommended in these patients, and it is important to exclude sleep deprivation as a cause of similar symptoms. However, CPAP therapy is indicated for a highly symptomatic patient with confirmed obstructive sleep apnea not only to improve blood pressure control but also to prevent long-term sequelae of this condition, such as stroke, myocardial infarction, and heart failure.

Inhaled corticosteroids would not benefit a patient who has no signs of airway hyperresponsiveness. Tongue and mandibular repositioning devices may be helpful in patients with mild obstructive sleep apnea or who are intolerant of CPAP but are less reliably effective than CPAP.

KEY POINTS

- Resistant hypertension, obesity, daytime sleepiness, morning headache, and awakening without feeling refreshed are suggestive of obstructive sleep apnea.

- In patients with obstructive sleep apnea, continuous positive airway pressure therapy has been shown to improve quality of life, cognitive function, symptoms of daytime sleepiness, blood pressure, and cardiac function, and to have a positive effect on mortality.

Bibliography

1. **Guilleminault C, Abad VC.** Obstructive sleep apnea syndromes. Med Clin North Am. 2004;88:611-30, viii. [PMID: 15087207]

Item 26   Answer: C

This patient's presentation suggests interstitial lung disease with an abnormal auscultatory examination, a diffusely abnormal chest radiograph, and a restrictive physiologic defect with a low DLco. The next step in her evaluation should be a high-resolution CT scan of the chest, which is more sensitive than plain chest radiographs in identifying the presence of interstitial lung disease as well as more specific for providing the potential diagnosis. In the correct clinical setting, distinctive radiographic patterns aid in identifying the underlying diagnosis.

While asthma could explain this patient's symptoms, the pulmonary function studies are not compatible with the pattern of airflow obstruction seen with asthma; furthermore, the presence of the abnormal parenchyma on the chest radiograph and the low DLco both argue against asthma as the diagnosis. Cardiomyopathy is also unlikely because there are no physical examination findings supporting this diagnosis as a cause of dyspnea (e.g., elevated jugular venous pressure, displaced cardiac apex, or an S_3). In addition, cardiomyopathy cannot explain the previous pneumothorax, abnormal chest radiograph, and restrictive physiologic defect. A pulmonary embolism is also excluded because it does not explain the patient's radiographic findings and pulmonary physiology. Pulmonary embolism is most typically associated with a normal chest radiograph; lung volumes and airflow tend to be normal but the DLco may be depressed.

KEY POINTS

- Interstitial lung disease is typically associated with an abnormal auscultatory examination, a diffusely abnormal chest radiograph, and a restrictive physiologic defect with a low DLco.

- High-resolution CT scanning is more sensitive than plain chest radiography for detecting interstitial lung disease and more specific for establishing the potential diagnosis.

Bibliography

1. **Wells AU, Hogaboam CM.** Update in diffuse parenchymal lung disease 2006. Am J Respir Crit Care Med. 2007;175:655-60. [PMID: 17384327]

Item 27   Answer: C

In patients with systemic sclerosis (scleroderma), the lung is commonly involved, and lung disease is now the most common cause of scleroderma-related morbidity and mortality. Scleroderma is suggested by the typical skin findings. Pigment changes appear first, followed by skin thickening, digital pitting, and ulceration. Skin changes can extend proximally; patients with skin findings proximal to the elbows have diffuse scleroderma, as does this patient. In patients with scleroderma, both interstitial lung disease and pulmonary hypertension can develop (either independently or together) and have an adverse impact on outcome. Pulmonary disease can also be the initial clinical manifestation of scleroderma and is most commonly associated with diffuse scleroderma. Pulmonary hypertension is more commonly associated with limited scleroderma (CREST syndrome: calcinosis, Raynaud's phenomenon, esophageal dysmotility, sclerodactyly, and telangiectasia). A comprehensive history and physical examination are necessary to identify and confirm the underlying cause. In this patient, the presence of gastroesophageal reflux disease, sclerodactyly, proximal skin findings, late crackles on examination, abnormal high-resolution CT scan findings, a restrictive pulmonary physiologic defect, and the positive antinuclear antibody titer suggest the presence of scleroderma-related interstitial lung disease.

Idiopathic pulmonary fibrosis is an idiopathic interstitial pneumonia (i.e., it occurs in the absence of other explanations for the lung disease). The presence of features suggestive of scleroderma excludes this diagnosis. Various intrathoracic complications occur in patients with systemic lupus erythematosus; however, classic interstitial lung disease is uncommon. The clinical diagnosis of hypersensitivity pneumonitis requires a specific exposure that is temporally related to the development of the lung disease, and the high- resolution CT scan pattern is generally one of centrilobular nodules with areas of focal air-trapping. In addition, hypersensitivity pneumonitis cannot explain the patient's skin findings and gastroesophageal reflux disease.

KEY POINTS

- Lung disease is the most common cause of morbidity and mortality in patients with systemic sclerosis (scleroderma).

- In systemic sclerosis, both interstitial lung disease and pulmonary hypertension can develop (independently or together) and have an adverse effect on outcome.

Bibliography
1. **Steen VD.** The lung in systemic sclerosis. J Clin Rheumatol. 2005;11:40-6. [PMID: 16357695]

Item 28   Answer: D

This patient most likely has idiopathic pulmonary fibrosis, which is a specific form of chronic fibrosing interstitial pneumonia of unknown cause limited to the lung. It is characterized by predominantly basilar infiltrates on chest radiograph, restrictive physiology, and evidence of impaired gas exchange. Most patients with this disorder are more than 50 years old and develop progressive dyspnea and nonproductive cough, with many patients reporting symptoms of more than 6 months' duration before medical evaluation. Fever is rare, and when present, suggests an alternative diagnosis. Weight loss, fatigue, and malaise may be present. More than 80% of patients have bibasilar end-inspiratory dry crackles that have a Velcro-like quality. Cardiac examination may be normal or, in the case of advanced disease, show evidence of cor pulmonale. Digital clubbing occurs in 25% to 50% of patients. The next diagnostic steps in this patient include chest CT to evaluate the type of infiltrate and complete pulmonary function testing to confirm the presence of restrictive pulmonary

disease with evidence of impaired gas exchange. Lung biopsy is often needed to establish the diagnosis.

Asbestosis is the best characterized of the occupational lung diseases and may present similarly to pulmonary fibrosis. Although asbestosis typically involves the lung bases, it is unlikely in the absence of an exposure history. On high-resolution CT scan, more than 90% of patients with asbestosis show some pleural abnormality such as pleural plaques or thickening. Chronic obstructive pulmonary disease is unlikely in a nonsmoker and in the absence of other irritant exposures. Additionally, this patient's chest radiograph is not consistent with chronic obstructive pulmonary disease, which typically includes hyperinflation, flattened diaphragms, and increased anterior-posterior diameter. Cryptogenic organizing pneumonia is characterized by a preceding flu-like illness in 40% of patients, with most patients reporting fewer than 3 months of symptoms before medical evaluation. This disorder may be associated with collagen vascular diseases, neoplasms, and viral illnesses. Chest radiograph may show unilateral or bilateral consolidation, with nodules in 10% to 50% of patients. High-resolution CT scan shows patchy air space consolidation in the periphery of the lung and often in the lower lung zones. This disorder often presents like a community-acquired pneumonia and is not compatible with this patient's slowly progressive disease. Sarcoidosis typically presents with bilateral hilar lymphadenopathy with or without infiltrates and may include extrapulmonary manifestations such as liver involvement, uveitis, or arthritis. High-resolution CT scan may show nodules along bronchovascular bundles with bilateral hilar and mediastinal lymphadenopathy.

KEY POINTS

- Idiopathic pulmonary fibrosis is characterized by basilar-predominant infiltrates on chest radiography, restrictive lung physiology, and evidence of impaired gas exchange.

- Physical examination clues compatible with idiopathic pulmonary fibrosis include digital clubbing and bibasilar end-inspiratory crackles with a Velcro-like quality.

Bibliography
1. **Martinez FJ, Safrin S, Weycker D, Starko KM, Bradford WZ, King TE Jr, Flaherty KR, Schwartz DA, Noble PW, Raghu G, Brown KK; IPF Study Group.** The clinical course of patients with idiopathic pulmonary fibrosis. Ann Intern Med. 2005;21;142:963-7. Summary for patients in: Ann Intern Med. 2005;142:I23. [PMID: 15968010]

Item 29   Answer: B

This patient most likely has sarcoidosis. Patients with sarcoidosis may be asymptomatic, have nonspecific constitutional symptoms, or have symptoms referable to the skin, eyes, joints, or lungs. Ocular involvement typically presents as uveitis; however, any part of the eye or orbit may be affected. The patient's skin lesions are most likely erythema nodosum. More than 90% of patients with sarcoidosis have lung involvement. Pulmonary function tests usually demonstrate restrictive disease, although airway obstruction is seen in some patients. Chest radiograph results are staged as follows: stage 0, normal; stage I, hilar lymphadenopathy alone; stage II, lymphadenopathy plus infiltrates; stage III, infiltrates alone; and stage IV, fibrosis.

As in this patient, sarcoidosis may present acutely with bilateral hilar lymphadenopathy, polyarthralgias, and erythema nodosum. This triad of symptoms, known as Löfgren's syndrome, is seen in 25% to 50% of patients, primarily women, with acute sarcoidosis. In addition to recognition of the typical clinical or radiographic findings of sarcoidosis, the diagnosis requires histologic evidence of noncaseating granulomas as well as exclusion of infection.

Lymphoma can be associated with asymptomatic, bulky hilar lymphadenopathy without pulmonary infiltrates, but lymphoma cannot explain the patient's uveitis or erythema nodosum. Patients with systemic lupus erythematosus may have skin and pulmonary lesions, but the pulmonary lesions are usually due to pulmonary hemorrhage or fibrosis, and hilar lymphadenopathy is not found. Skin lesions in lupus are typically limited to the face. Reactivation tuberculosis usually is characterized by a pulmonary infiltrate and unilateral hilar lymphadenopathy. The patient's lack of fever, constitutional symptoms, and pulmonary infiltrate makes tuberculosis unlikely. Furthermore, tuberculosis cannot explain the patient's other findings.

KEY POINTS

• Patients with sarcoidosis may be asymptomatic, have nonspecific constitutional symptoms, or have symptoms referable to the skin, eyes, joints, or lungs.

• Pulmonary involvement occurs in more than 90% of patients with sarcoidosis.

Bibliography
1. Cox CE, Davis-Allen A, Judson MA. Sarcoidosis. Med Clin North Am. 2005;89:817-28. [PMID: 15925652]

Item 30   Answer: A

A contrast-enhanced helical CT scan of the chest is a preferred method to diagnose pulmonary embolism in a patient with normal renal function and an abnormal chest radiograph. The first step in this patient is to estimate the pretest probability of pulmonary embolism based on the initial assessment before pulmonary imaging. According to the modified Wells' criteria, the clinical pretest probability of pulmonary embolism can be classified as high (very likely), intermediate (possible or probable), or low (unlikely) according to risk factors, symptoms, and radiographic and electrocardiographic findings. This patient has a high pretest probability of pulmonary embolism based on his recent knee replacement surgery and subsequent lack of activity; sudden onset of dyspnea and pleuritic chest pain; tachypnea and tachycardia; atelectasis and pleural effusion on the chest radiograph; and elevated D-dimer

level. The next step is a diagnostic test, such as a contrast-enhanced helical CT scan of the chest. Post-test probability depends on the pretest clinical probability and the result of pulmonary imaging.

Transthoracic or transesophageal echocardiography may rarely identify central pulmonary artery emboli or intracardiac thrombi. The finding of right ventricular dysfunction is nonspecific for pulmonary embolism but has prognostic implications. Echocardiography is most useful to help diagnose or exclude pericardial tamponade, aortic dissection, myocardial ischemia or infarction, valvular dysfunction, and myocardial rupture but is not the first test for a patient at high probability for pulmonary embolism. An exercise electrocardiographic stress test is useful for evaluating chest pain in patients with an intermediate pretest probability for ischemic heart disease. The pleuritic nature of the chest pain, chest radiograph findings, and initial normal cardiac enzyme values make acute coronary syndrome less likely than pulmonary embolism in this patient. Similarly, telemetry and serial measurement of cardiac enzymes and serial electrocardiography may be a reasonable option only after pulmonary embolism has been excluded.

KEY POINT

• Contrast-enhanced helical CT scan of the chest is a preferred method to diagnose pulmonary embolism in a patient with clinical risk factors for pulmonary embolism, normal renal function, and an abnormal chest radiograph.

Bibliography
1. Chunilal SD, Eikelboom JW, Attia J, Miniati M, Panju AA, Simel DL, Ginsberg JS. Does this patient have pulmonary embolism? JAMA. 2003;290:2849-58. [PMID: 14657070]

Item 31   Answer: A

Flat neck veins are unlikely in a patient with acute right-sided heart failure (acute cor pulmonale) and would effectively rule out the diagnosis of massive pulmonary embolism as the cause of hypotension in this patient. In fact, jugular venous distention has been described in 80% of patients with massive pulmonary embolism and no preexisting cardiopulmonary disease. Physical examination findings supporting pulmonary embolism include a palpable and accentuated S_2 over the second left parasternal space, a left parasternal precordial heave, a holosystolic murmur over the epigastrium that is louder on inspiration, and a presystolic low-pitched extra sound over the subxiphoid area. These findings are each associated with massive pulmonary embolism with varying degrees of frequency and therefore are not useful in excluding this diagnosis.

KEY POINT

• Flat neck veins argue against right-sided circulatory collapse.

Bibliography
1. Chunilal SD, Eikelboom JW, Attia J, Miniati M, Panju AA, Simel DL, Ginsberg JS. Does this patient have pulmonary embolism? JAMA. 2003;290:2849-58. [PMID: 14657070]

Item 32 Answer: C

This patient is progressing as expected, and discharge from the hospital on warfarin is the best course of action. In most patients treated with heparin for pulmonary embolism, a substantial portion of their perfusion defects resolve within the first week, although complete resolution occurs in only a minority of patients within this time. In this patient, only a relatively small portion of his defect has resolved, but it is still very early in treatment. Although he does have a 3% to 4% risk of developing chronic thromboembolic pulmonary hypertension, no intervention is required at this time beyond anticoagulation and follow-up.

There is no indication that anticoagulation was ineffective and certainly no indication that low-molecular-weight heparin would be more effective. Pulmonary hypertension would be very unlikely to develop this early after an acute pulmonary embolism; therefore, measurement of his pulmonary artery pressures is not necessary. CT scanning to follow the resolution of pulmonary embolism is not well standardized and would add little to the work-up for this patient.

KEY POINT

• In most patients treated with heparin for pulmonary embolism, a substantial portion of their perfusion defects resolve within the first week.

Bibliography

1. Nijkeuter M, Hovens MM, Davidson BL, Huisman MV. Resolution of thromboemboli in patients with acute pulmonary embolism: a systematic review. Chest. 2006;129:192-7. [PMID: 16424432]

Item 33 Answer: B

The best prophylaxis for this patient is low-dose heparin. Venous thromboembolism occurs in 13% to 30% of patients in intensive care units who have not received prophylaxis. Unfractionated heparin and low-molecular-weight heparin (LMWH) have been shown in large clinical trials to reduce the risk of clinically important venous thromboembolism in critically ill by patients by up to 60%. In a meta-analysis, there was no significant difference in rates of venous thromboembolism when either unfractionated heparin or LMWH was used, but there were fewer episodes of major bleeding with LMWH. These agents are highly recommended for patients at moderate or high risk for venous thromboembolism.

Warfarin, especially at "therapeutic doses," is not recommended for prophylactic use in medical patients. Its long duration of action may be especially detrimental in patients in the intensive care unit, who may need multiple invasive procedures. Aspirin is not commonly recommended for the prevention of venous thromboembolism and has not been demonstrated by clinical trials to reduce the incidence of thromboembolism in most populations at risk.

KEY POINT

• Unfractionated and low-molecular-weight heparins reduce the risk of clinically important venous thromboembolism in critically ill patients by up to 60%.

Bibliography

1. Francis CW. Clinical practice. Prophylaxis for thromboembolism in hospitalized medical patients. N Engl J Med. 2007;356:1438-44. Erratum in: N Engl J Med. 2007;357:203. [PMID: 17409325]

Item 34 Answer: B

The best option for this patient is intermittent pneumatic compression. Although the clinical evidence for reducing the risk for venous thromboembolism with intermittent pneumatic compression is not as strong as that for unfractionated heparin and low-molecular-weight heparin, mechanical compression has a very low risk of causing adverse effects and has been associated with substantial reductions in the incidence of thromboembolism in populations at risk. Intermittent pneumatic compression is recommended for patients at moderate to high risk in whom unfractionated heparin and low-molecular-weight heparin are contraindicated.

This patient's history of heparin-induced thrombocytopenia with thrombosis (HITT) is a contraindication for the use of unfractionated heparin and all low-molecular-weight heparins because the antibodies responsible for HITT cross-react with both medication classes. Aspirin alone is ineffective for prophylaxis against venous thromboembolism.

KEY POINT

• Intermittent pneumatic compression is effective prophylaxis in patients at moderate to high risk for venous thromboembolism in whom heparin and low-molecular-weight heparin are contraindicated.

Bibliography

1. Geerts WH, Pineo GF, Heit JA, Bergqvist D, Lassen MR, Colwell CW, et al. Prevention of venous thromboembolism: the Seventh ACCP Conference on Antithrombotic and Thrombolytic Therapy. Chest. 2004;126:338S-400S. [PMID: 15383478]

Item 35 Answer: A

This patient should be maintained on low-molecular-weight heparin. Patients with acute venous thromboembolism in association with metastatic cancer are at higher risk for recurrent venous thrombosis than those without malignancy. In such patients, it has been demonstrated that chronic low-molecular-weight heparin at therapeutic doses reduces the risk for "on-treatment" recurrence by approximately 50% at 6 months when compared with standard-intensity anticoagulant therapy (target INR, 2 to 3). High-intensity warfarin (target INR, 3 to 4) would not be appropriate in this setting because it has not been shown to be more effective in preventing recurrent venous thromboembolism than standard-intensity warfarin (target INR, 2 to 3). Retrospective studies have also shown that patients with venous thrombosis and active cancer are at increased risk for major bleeding while receiving standard-intensity warfarin.

Placement of an inferior vena cava (IVC) filter in patients with venous thrombosis without anticoagulation is associated with an increased risk for recurrent venous thrombosis. IVC filter placement is generally reserved for patients at high risk for recurrent thrombosis who have sustained major bleeding and cannot undergo anticoagulation.

KEY POINT

- Chronic low-molecular-weight heparin at therapeutic doses reduces the risk for recurrent venous thromboembolism compared with standard-intensity warfarin in patients with cancer.

Bibliography

1. Bergqvist D, Caprini JA, Dotsenko O, Kakkar AK, Mishra RG, Wakefield TW. Venous thromboembolism and cancer. Curr Probl Surg. 2007;44:157-216. [PMID: 17437761]

Item 36   Answer: D

This patient requires long-term therapy with warfarin. Although heterozygosity for the factor V Leiden mutation is a risk factor for the development of an initial episode of venous thrombosis, the risk for recurrent venous thrombosis in such patients is not typically greater than that in persons without an underlying thrombophilic abnormality. Given that this patient developed two unprovoked venous thrombotic events over a relatively short period and that she has no risk factors that increase her risk for bleeding during warfarin therapy, she should receive long-term warfarin therapy at a target INR of 2 to 3. Aspirin has not been shown to be effective for the secondary prevention of venous thromboembolism. Long-term heparin therapy is unnecessary, as it provides no increase in protection but does increase cost and inconvenience.

KEY POINT

- Patients heterozygous for factor V Leiden mutation with recurrent thrombosis should receive long-term anticoagulation therapy with warfarin.

Bibliography

1. Segal JB, Streiff MB, Hofmann LV, Thornton K, Bass EB. Management of venous thromboembolism: a systematic review for a practice guideline. Ann Intern Med. 2007;146:211-22. Epub 2007 Jan 29. Summary for patients in: Ann Intern Med. 2007;146:I43. [PMID: 17261856]

Item 37   Answer: C

This patient should be treated with either unfractionated heparin or low-molecular weight heparin during her pregnancy and for 6 weeks postpartum. During pregnancy, women have a 5-fold increased risk for venous thromboembolism as compared with nonpregnant women. Clinicians should avoid vitamin K antagonists, such as wafarin, in pregnant women because these drugs cross the placenta and are associated with embryopathy between 6 and 12 weeks' ges-

tation, as well as fetal bleeding (including intracranial hemorrhage) at delivery. Neither unfractionated heparin nor low-molecular-weight heparin crosses the placenta, and neither is associated with embryopathy or fetal bleeding. This patient is not a candidate for thrombolytic therapy because she is hemodynamically stable and thrombolytics are contraindicated during pregnancy.

KEY POINT

- Pregnant women with deep venous thromboembolism or pulmonary embolism are treated with either unfractionated heparin or a low-molecular-weight heparin during the pregnancy.

Bibliography

1. Snow V, Qaseem A, Barry P, Hornbake ER, Rodnick JE, Tobolic T, Ireland B, Segal JB, Bass EB, Weiss KB, Green L, Owens DK; American College of Physicians; American Academy of Family Physicians Panel on Deep Venous Thrombosis/Pulmonary Embolism. Management of venous thromboembolism: a clinical practice guideline from the American College of Physicians and the American Academy of Family Physicians. Ann Intern Med. 2007;146:204-10. Epub 2007 Jan 29. [PMID: 17261857]

Item 38   Answer: A

The patient's short duration of symptoms, lack of increased sputum production, obstructive pattern on pulmonary function testing, and normal diffusing capacity for carbon monoxide (DLCO) are most compatible with the diagnosis of asthma. Spirometry values >80% of predicted are categorized as normal. A FEV_1/FVC ratio of <70% (0.70) is indicative of obstructive lung disease. Obstructive lung disease also causes a decrease in vital capacity and an increase in residual lung volumes because of air trapping. If initial spirometry results are abnormal and suggest obstructive disease, the test is repeated after administration of an inhaled bronchodilator. An increase ≥12% in either the FEV_1 or FVC and an increase of 200 mL or more from baseline in either parameter constitute a significant response and are compatible with reversible airways obstruction (i.e., asthma).

The DLCO reflects the integrity of the alveolar-capillary membrane. Patients with emphysema have a reduced DLCO because of loss of lung parenchyma and less surface area for diffusion and those with pulmonary embolism have a reduced DLCO because of decreased blood flow through the pulmonary vasculature. Interstitial lung disease typically causes a diffusion barrier and is also associated with abnormal findings on chest radiograph or high-resolution CT scan. In patients with bronchitis and asthma, the alveolar-capillary membrane is intact and therefore diffusion is normal; however, bronchitis is associated with cough and increased sputum production, which are absent in this patient.

KEY POINTS

- A FEV_1/FVC ratio <70% is indicative of obstructive lung disease.

- A ≥12% increase in either the FEV$_1$ or FVC and an increase of 200 mL or more from baseline in either parameter following administration of an inhaled bronchodilator are compatible with asthma.

Bibliography

1. **Karnani NG, Reisfield GM, Wilson GR.** Evaluation of chronic dyspnea. Am Fam Physician. 2005;71:1529-37. [PMID: 15864893]

Chapter 11
Rheumatology

Rheumatology contains self-assessment items that correspond to the following chapters in the Internal *Medicine Essentials for Clerkship Students 2* textbook:

Approach to Joint Pain
Approach to Knee and Shoulder Pain
Crystalline Arthritis
Osteoarthritis
Polymyositis and Dermatomyositis
Rheumatoid Arthritis
Septic Arthritis
Systemic Lupus Erythematosus
Vasculitis

Rheumatology contains self assessment items that correspond to the following Training Problems in the *Core Medicine Clerkship Guide*:

Knee Pain
Rheumatologic Problems

Chapter 11

Rheumatology

Questions

Item 1

A 28-year-old woman is evaluated in the office for pain in her arms and legs of 7 years' duration that has recently worsened. She has a 7-year history of rheumatoid arthritis that had been well controlled with methotrexate and etanercept. She has pain in her shoulders, back, elbows, wrists, hips, and knees. She does not have fever, rash, or weight loss. The patient also has increased fatigue, particularly the day after any increased activity, such as grocery shopping.

On physical examination, there is mild interosseous muscle wasting but no synovitis, swelling, or warmth. On musculoskeletal examination, range of motion of the joints is full. Her pain is reproducible on palpation of the midpoint of the trapezius muscles, upper outer buttocks, 2 cm below the lateral epicondyles, bilateral trochanteric bursae, medial fat pads of the knees and second costochondral junctions.

Complete blood count, erythrocyte sedimentation rate, creatinine, alanine aminotransferase, aspartate aminotransferase, and thyroid-stimulating hormone values are normal.

Which of the following is the most likely diagnosis?

(A) Fibromyalgia
(B) Polymyositis
(C) Rheumatoid arthritis flare
(D) Systemic lupus erythematosus

Item 2

A 70-year-old woman is evaluated in the emergency department for a 2-day history of left knee pain. When she awoke today, the knee was warm and swollen. She also has difficulty walking due to pain. There is no history of trauma. She has a history of hypertension, type 2 diabetes mellitus, chronic renal insufficiency, and chronic venous insufficiency, and her medications are losartan, amlodipine, glyburide, furosemide, and aspirin.

On physical examination, temperature is 37.9 °C (100.2 °F), heart rate is 98/min, and blood pressure is 130/82 mm Hg. BMI is 34. The left knee is red and swollen, warm to the touch, and tender to palpation. The patella is ballottable. Passive range of motion is painful but unrestricted. There is no laxity of the joint and no joint crepitus.

Laboratory studies: leukocyte count, 11,000/µL; serum creatinine, 1.7 mg/dL; and serum uric acid, 8.2 mg/dL.

Which of the following is the most appropriate next step in this patient's management?

(A) Arthrocentesis
(B) Colchicine
(C) Ibuprofen
(D) Intravenous ceftriaxone
(E) Prednisone

Item 3

A 56-year-old man is evaluated in the office for a 2-day history of increasing pain and swelling in the right ankle. He has no history of arthritis and no recent trauma to the area. The patient has hypertension for which hydrochlorothiazide was recently started.

On physical examination, temperature is 37.2 °C (99.0 °F), blood pressure is 140/88 mm Hg, and heart rate is 70/min. The right ankle is slightly erythematous, warm to the touch, and swollen; range of motion of the ankle is limited because of pain.

Which of the following is the most appropriate next step in the evaluation of this patient?

(A) Arthrocentesis
(B) HLA-B27 testing
(C) Serum calcium measurement
(D) Serum uric acid measurement
(E) Rheumatoid factor testing

Item 4

A 64-year-old man with chronic gout is evaluated in the office for a swollen right elbow of 2 days' duration. He recalls no inciting trauma. His last attack of gout occurred 4 months ago and involved his right knee. He has a history of hypertension, hyperlipidemia, and type 2 diabetes mellitus. Medications are metformin, enalapril, atorvastatin, hydrochlorothiazide, and low-dose aspirin.

On physical examination, temperature is 38.1 °C (100.5 °F). There is no lymphadenopathy. The right elbow is warm with minimal erythema, and he holds it guardedly. Musculoskeletal examination reveals slight fullness and tenderness over the right olecranon process. Passive and active extension of the right elbow is painless, but passive flexion >90 degrees elicits pain. Rotation of the forearm is painless.

Which of the following is the most appropriate next step in this patient's management?

(A) Erythrocyte sedimentation rate
(B) Radiograph of the right elbow and forearm
(C) Right elbow joint aspiration
(D) Right olecranon bursa aspiration

Item 5

A 43-year-old woman is evaluated in the office for a 1-week history of acute left knee pain that began when she stepped down from a dock onto a sailboat and experienced a "popping sensation" and a gradual onset of knee joint swelling over the next 4 to 6 hours. She immediately applied ice to her knee and took ibuprofen with some pain relief. Over the past few days, she has continued to have moderate pain, particularly when walking up or down stairs, which has responded to ibuprofen. She reports no locking or giving way of the knee or any previous knee injury.

On physical examination, the left knee has a minimal effusion, without warmth or erythema, with full range of motion. The medial aspect of the joint line is tender to palpation. Maximally flexing the hip and knee and applying abduction (valgus) force to the knee while externally rotating the foot and passively extending the knee (McMurray's test) result in some tenderness but no crepitus. There is no palpable snap or pain.

Which of the following is the most likely diagnosis?

(A) Anserine bursitis
(B) Ligamentous tear
(C) Meniscal tear
(D) Patellofemoral pain syndrome

Item 6

A 35-year-old woman is evaluated in the office for a 12-day history of bilateral anterior knee pain. The pain is described as aching in nature; it worsens when she descends steps, and requires her get up from her chair at work every few hours to relieve stiffness and discomfort. The patient runs three times a week in the gym, but has not had any traumatic injury to the knees. She has occasionally taken ibuprofen for relief of the pain. She has no other medical problems.

On physical examination, there is no swelling, warmth, redness, or instability of the knees. Pressing the patella against the femur and moving it inferiorly and superiorly reproduces the pain.

Which of the following is the most likely cause of this patient's knee pain?

(A) Osteoarthritis
(B) Patellofemoral pain syndrome
(C) Prepatellar bursitis
(D) Referred sciatic pain

Item 7

A 48-year-old man is evaluated in the office for left knee pain that occurred after he slipped while shoveling snow yesterday. Although he did not strike his knee, he experienced the gradual onset of swelling and pain in his left knee over the next few hours, and he applied ice to the knee and took ibuprofen for pain relief. His normal activities include jogging 2 to 3 miles three times weekly without knee pain. He has not had problems with standing or walking on his left knee either immediately after his fall or currently, although the knee is sore.

On physical examination, there is a mild effusion without erythema or warmth of the left knee. The patella is ballottable, but without pain. Palpation around the knee does not produce pain at the pes anserinus, on the patella, or on the head of the fibula. He has full range of motion in both knees, although his left knee is slightly painful. He is able to bear weight with either leg. Specific maneuvers for meniscal tears are negative, and there is no evidence of laxity of the anterior cruciate, the posterior cruciate, or the medial or lateral collateral ligaments.

Which of the following is the most appropriate next step in management?

(A) Crutches and a knee brace
(B) MRI of the knee
(C) Radiograph of the knee
(D) Symptomatic treatment

Item 8

A 47-year-old man is evaluated in the office for right lateral shoulder pain. He has been pitching during batting practice for his son's Little League baseball team for the past 2 months. He has shoulder pain when lifting his right arm overhead and also when lying on the shoulder while sleeping. Acetaminophen does not relieve the pain.

On physical examination, he has no shoulder deformities or swelling. Range of motion is normal. He has subacromial tenderness to palpation, with shoulder pain elicited at 60 degrees of passive abduction. He also has pain with resisted mid-arc abduction but no pain with resisted elbow flexion or forearm supination. He is able to lower his right arm smoothly from a fully abducted position, and his arm strength for abduction and external rotation against resistance is normal.

Which of the following is the most likely diagnosis?

(A) Adhesive capsulitis
(B) Bicipital tendinitis
(C) Glenohumeral arthritis
(D) Rotator cuff tear (complete)
(E) Rotator cuff tendinitis

Item 9

A 62-year-old man is evaluated in the office for worsening right knee pain accompanied by significant swelling of 3 days' duration. He has a 5-year history of recurrent episodes of knee pain that each last several days. During these attacks, his knee becomes warm to the touch, red, and tender. Between attacks, he notes periodic stiffness and discomfort when climbing stairs.

On musculoskeletal examination of the right knee, there is moderate synovitis and a joint effusion, primarily in the supra-patellar pouch. The remainder of the examination is unremarkable. Radiograph of the knee is shown.

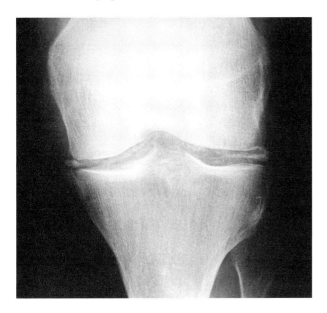

Which of the following is the most likely cause of this patient's recurrent acute attacks of knee pain?

(A) Anserine bursitis
(B) Calcium pyrophosphate dihydrate crystal deposition
(C) Gout
(D) Osteoarthritis
(E) Septic arthritis

Item 10

A 74-year-old woman with chronic hand stiffness and a 20-year history of osteoarthritis of the hands is evaluated in the office for increasingly frequent episodes of finger pain accompanied by redness and swelling. Her pain particularly involves several distal and proximal interphalangeal joints. She had been using a nonsteroidal anti-inflammatory drug to control her pain but discontinued this medication 1 year ago after an episode of gastric bleeding. She has hypertension that is well controlled with low-dose hydrochlorothiazide.

The appearance of her hand on physical examination is shown (*see Figure 36 in Color Plates*).

Which of the following is the most likely diagnosis?

(A) Inflammatory osteoarthritis
(B) Psoriatic arthritis
(C) Rheumatoid arthritis
(D) Tophaceous gout

Item 11

A 48-year-old man is evaluated in the office during an annual physical examination. He has had hypertension and tophaceous gout for several years. His last attack of gout occurred >6 months ago and promptly resolved after several doses of naproxen. Current medications are enalapril, colchicine, and low-dose allopurinol.

On physical examination, blood pressure is 126/70 mm Hg. Musculoskeletal examination reveals several nontender movable olecranon nodules and a slightly tender left first metatarsophalangeal joint with an overlying nodule. The remainder of the examination is normal. On laboratory studies, his uric acid level is 7.2 mg/dL.

Which of the following is the most appropriate next step in this patient's management?

(A) Add probenecid
(B) Discontinue colchicine
(C) Increase allopurinol
(D) Obtain 24-hour urine urate excretion

Item 12

A 55-year-old man is evaluated in the office because of a 1-year history of increasing impotence. He otherwise feels well except for mild fatigue and arthritis of both hands.

On physical examination, he is slightly overweight. Degenerative changes are noted in the metacarpophalangeal joints bilaterally. Pedal pulses are strong. The remainder of the examination is normal. Fasting glucose is 118 mg/dL, aspartate aminotransferase is 72 U/L, and alanine aminotransferase is 80 U/L.

Which of the following diagnostic studies should be done next?

(A) Measurement of ceruloplasmin
(B) Measurement of thyroid-stimulating hormone
(C) Noninvasive studies of the lower extremity vasculature
(D) Transferrin saturation

Item 13

A 53-year-old woman is evaluated in the office for a 3-month history of bilateral knee pain on ambulation. Her pain is more notable in her right knee. She has approximately 15 minutes of stiffness each morning. She has swelling of the proximal and distal interphalangeal joints. She does not have fever, rash, photosensitivity, or oral ulcers. Her sister has systemic lupus erythematosus.

Musculoskeletal examination reveals no redness or palpable synovial swelling, but she has bilateral bony hypertrophy at the third and fourth distal and proximal interphalangeal joints.

Range of motion elicits bilateral knee crepitus. There is evidence of a small right knee effusion.

Which of the following studies will be most useful in confirming this patient's diagnosis?

(A) Anti–cyclic citrullinated peptide antibody assay
(B) Antinuclear antibody assay
(C) Erythrocyte sedimentation rate
(D) Rheumatoid factor assay
(E) No additional studies

Item 14

A 53-year-old woman is evaluated in the office for a 3-day history of swelling of the right knee. Her pain is exacerbated with weight bearing and initiation of movement after inactivity. She does not have fever.

Musculoskeletal examination reveals bony hypertrophy, and the right knee has medial joint-line tenderness and a large joint effusion. Arthrocentesis is performed. Synovial fluid is clear and viscous with a leukocyte count of 1100/µL with 30% neutrophils.

Which of the following is the most likely diagnosis?

(A) Calcium pyrophosphate deposition disease
(B) Gout
(C) Osteoarthritis
(D) Septic arthritis

Item 15

A 56-year-old woman is evaluated for a 2-year history of joint pain and stiffness of the hands. The appearance of her hands on physical examination is shown (*see Figure 37 in Color Plates*).

Which of the following is the most appropriate treatment for this patient?

(A) Acetaminophen
(B) Etanercept
(C) Methotrexate
(D) Prednisolone

Item 16

A 62-year-old woman is evaluated in the office for pain in her left knee that began 1 month ago and has gradually become more intense. The patient describes the pain as a deep aching sensation that was initially present only with exertion but now is also present at rest. She has not had any trauma to the knee and is otherwise healthy and takes no medications.

On physical examination, the patient is obese (BMI 32) and has a moderate-sized left knee effusion. The knee is not erythematous but is slightly warm to touch. There is evidence of bony hypertrophy and crepitus with passive movement.

Laboratory evaluation of the synovial fluid shows a leukocyte count of 1500/µL with 60% neutrophils. No crystals are present.

Which of the following is the most likely cause of this patient's joint pain?

(A) Gout
(B) Meniscal tear
(C) Osteoarthritis
(D) Rheumatoid arthritis
(E) Septic arthritis

Item 17

A 62-year-old man is evaluated in the office for a 1-year history of progressively worsening right knee pain. Six weeks ago, he developed bleeding due to endoscopy-proven nonsteroidal anti-inflammatory drug–related gastric ulcer. He also has hypertension. Medications are atenolol, enalapril, and omeprazole.

On physical examination, the patient is obese. Musculoskeletal examination reveals bilateral knee crepitus on range of motion. There is a 4-degree valgus deviation of the right knee.

In addition to weight loss and quadriceps muscle strength training, which of the following is the most appropriate treatment for this patient?

(A) Acetaminophen
(B) Arthroscopic débridement
(C) Diclofenac
(D) Indomethacin suppositories

Item 18

A 67-year-old man is evaluated in the office for a 3-year history of right knee pain exacerbated by ambulation. Full-dose nonsteroidal anti-inflammatory drug therapy and acetaminophen, 4 g/d, do not sufficiently relieve his symptoms.

Musculoskeletal examination reveals bilateral knee crepitus and a right knee effusion that is slightly warm to the touch. However, there is no significant tenderness of the joint capsule.

Radiographs of the right knee show moderate medial joint-space narrowing with subchondral sclerosis and tibial osteophytes. Arthrocentesis of the right knee yields 30 mL of yellow fluid. Synovial fluid leukocyte count is 800/µL, and no crystals are seen.

Which of the following is the most appropriate treatment for this patient?

(A) Arthroscopic lavage
(B) Intra-articular corticosteroids
(C) Short course of prednisone
(D) Topical nonsteroidal anti-inflammatory drugs

Item 19

A 51-year-old woman is diagnosed with dermatomyositis. She has proximal muscle weakness, a periorbital heliotrope rash, and Gottron's sign. She denies stomach, abdominal, or pelvic pain; cough; a change in bowel habits; or blood in the stool or urine.

On physical examination, there is prominent proximal muscle weakness without distal involvement or atrophy. There is no swelling, warmth, or erythema of the shoulders, and range of motion is preserved and does not elicit pain.

Laboratory studies:

Hemoglobin	10 g/dL
Erythrocyte sedimentation rate	120 mm/h
Creatine kinase	3845 U/L
Urinalysis	Normal

Which of the following should be included in the patient's evaluation?

(A) Colonoscopy, mammography, and Papanicolaou smear
(B) Cystoscopy
(C) Liver biopsy
(D) Renal ultrasonography

Item 20

A 45-year-old man is evaluated in the office for a 3-month history of gradually worsening fatigue and weakness. He notes progressive difficulty getting in and out of his bathtub and his automobile. He does not have cough or shortness of breath, difficulty swallowing, nasal regurgitation and aspiration, hoarseness, or change in voice. His weight has been stable. He has no other medical problems and takes no medications.

On physical examination, vital signs are normal. He has difficulty rising from a chair without using his arms for assistance, and he has weakness of his shoulder muscles. There is no pain with palpation of the muscles and no restriction of joint movement.

Laboratory evaluation shows a normal complete blood count, serum creatine kinase of 5600 U/L, and erythrocyte sedimentation rate of 32 mm/h.

Which of following is the most likely diagnosis?

(A) Fibromyalgia
(B) Myasthenia gravis
(C) Polymyalgia rheumatica
(D) Polymyositis
(E) Syringomyelia

Item 21

A 27-year-old woman is evaluated in the office for 6 months of pain and swelling of the wrists, knuckles, and fingers bilaterally. The pain is worse in the morning, with stiffness of the joints lasting several hours. By mid-afternoon, she is exhausted and cannot continue to work. She has lost 2.2 kg (5 lb) and is very anxious.

On physical examination, temperature is 37.6 °C (99.8 °F) and blood pressure is 120/70 mm Hg. There is swelling and tenderness on palpation of the proximal interphalangeal and metacarpophalangeal joints, wrists, knees, and ankles bilaterally. A small lump is present on the extensor surface of the right ulna. There are no rashes, mucosal lesions, weakness, or neurologic findings.

Which of the following is the most likely diagnosis?

(A) Gonococcal arthritis
(B) Gout
(C) Osteoarthritis
(D) Rheumatoid arthritis

Item 22

A 45-year-old woman is evaluated in the office for an 8-month history of pain, stiffness, and swelling of the small joints of the hands and feet. She also has increasing fatigue that has caused her to miss work at least 1 day per week.

On physical examination, she is afebrile. She walks with a limp due to right knee and foot pain. Musculoskeletal examination shows symmetrical swelling, tenderness, and restricted range of motion of the wrists, second and third metacarpophalangeal joints, all proximal interphalangeal joints, knees, ankles, and forefeet. There is no sign of rash.

Hemoglobin is 11 g/dL and the erythrocyte sedimentation rate is 80 mm/h. Radiograph of one of her hands is shown.

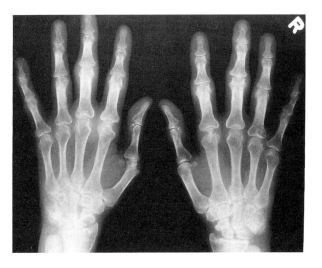

Which of the following is the most likely diagnosis?

(A) Psoriatic arthritis
(B) Rheumatoid arthritis
(C) Systemic lupus erythematosus
(D) Viral arthritis

Item 23

A 26-year-old woman in her first trimester of pregnancy is evaluated in the emergency department for an acutely painful left wrist and painful, swollen right knee. Four days ago, she developed flu-like symptoms characterized by migratory joint pains. Her pregnancy had been uncomplicated.

On physical examination, the right knee has a warm effusion and the left wrist is slightly warm but not swollen. Passive wrist motion is uncomfortable and resisted extension is extremely painful. The joint capsule of the knee is tender. On pelvic examination, there is a scant mucoid cervical discharge. The remainder of the general examination is normal.

Arthrocentesis of the knee yields 20 mL of fluid (leukocyte count, 14,000/μL; 90% neutrophils). Gram stain is negative.

Which of the following is the most appropriate next step in this patient's management?

(A) Begin ceftriaxone
(B) Begin doxycycline
(C) Begin vancomycin
(D) Perform total hemolytic complement assay

Item 24

A 25-year-old man from Hawaii is evaluated in the office for a 2-day history of severe pain in his right wrist. The patient is sexually active with multiple male partners but uses condoms only intermittently. He visited the Philippines 1 month ago, where he had unprotected sexual intercourse with several men.

On physical examination, temperature is 38.9 °C (102 °F), heart rate is 100/min, respiration rate is 16/min, and blood pressure is 110/70 mm Hg. Examination of the right wrist discloses swelling and erythema with pain on passive range of motion. Several painless papules are seen on the lower extremities. The leukocyte count is 18,000/μL; other laboratory studies are normal. An arthrocentesis of the wrist is performed, and cultures of the urethra, throat, and rectum are obtained.

Which of the following antimicrobial agents should be administered?

(A) Cefazolin
(B) Ceftriaxone
(C) Ciprofloxacin
(D) Penicillin G
(E) Trimethoprim–sulfamethoxazole

Item 25

A 65-year-old woman with rheumatoid arthritis is evaluated in the office for a 1-week history of increased pain and swelling of the proximal interphalangeal (PIP) joint of the third finger of her right hand. Current medications are prednisone and methotrexate.

On physical examination, temperature is 39.2 °C (102.5 °F); other vital signs are normal. Rheumatoid arthritis is present in all PIP and metacarpophalangeal joints of both hands. The right third PIP joint is warm and erythematous with extreme tenderness to palpation and decreased range of motion.

The leukocyte count is 15,300/μL. Examination of purulent fluid aspirated from the PIP joint is negative for crystals.

Which of the following organisms is most likely causing this patient's current findings?

(A) *Pseudomonas aeruginosa*
(B) *Salmonella enteritidis*
(C) *Staphylococcus aureus*
(D) *Streptococcus agalactiae*
(E) *Streptococcus pyogenes*

Item 26

A 62-year-old man is evaluated in the office for left anterior hip pain that began 3 days earlier. He was recently hospitalized for cystoscopic kidney stone extraction and was discharged 4 days ago. The pain is worse with activity and disturbs his sleep. He also has fever and chills. He has a history of degenerative joint disease in his hips and knees and has gout attacks in his first metatarsophalangeal joints about three times annually. There is no history of tick exposure.

On physical examination, temperature is 38.7 °C (101.7 °F), heart rate is 110/min, and blood pressure is 142/72 mm Hg. There is markedly decreased range of motion and pain in his left hip and some warmth over the lateral aspect of the hip. All other joints are normal on palpation.

A CT scan of the hip shows an effusion.

Which of the following tests is most appropriate?

(A) Antinuclear antibody assay and rheumatoid factor
(B) Bone scan
(C) Hip joint aspiration
(D) Urethral swab for *Neisseria gonorrhoeae*

Item 27

A 40-year-old woman is evaluated in the office for a 3-week history of pain over the right sternoclavicular joint. The patient has no other significant medical history and takes no medications. However, she has a recent history of illicit use of injection drugs. She is sexually active.

On physical examination, the temperature is 38.9 °C (102 °F), blood pressure is 130/78 mm Hg, and heart rate is 90/min. The right sternoclavicular joint is warm, tender, erythematous, and fluctuant. There are needle track marks on the extremities and neck. . Cardiac examination is normal. Right inguinal lymphadenopathy is present.

The hematocrit is 30%, leukocyte count is 14,400/μL, and erythrocyte sedimentation rate is 72 mm/h.

Which of the following is the most appropriate next step in the management of this patient?

(A) Aspiration of the sternoclavicular joint
(B) Empiric treatment with broad-spectrum antibiotics
(C) MRI of the sternoclavicular joint
(D) Plain radiography of the sternoclavicular joint
(E) Throat, cervical, rectal, and blood cultures

Item 28

A 38-year-old man is evaluated in the office for acute progressive left knee pain and swelling of 2 days' duration. He does not have other symptoms. He has not seen a physician since his last routine physical examination, which was normal and occurred 2 years ago. His father has gout and coronary artery disease.

On physical examination, he is afebrile. He walks with a limp because of pain. The left knee is warm, tender, and distended. The remainder of the examination is unremarkable.

Hemoglobin is 13.3 g/dL, leukocyte count is 8600/µL, and urinalysis is normal.

Aspiration of the knee joint yields 20 mL of synovial fluid (leukocyte count, 50,000/µL; 94% neutrophils). No crystals are seen on polarized light microscopy of the fluid, and Gram stain is negative. Results of mucosal, blood, and synovial fluid cultures are pending.

Which of the following is the most appropriate next step in this patient's management?

(A) Intravenous antibiotics
(B) Knee radiograph and erythrocyte sedimentation rate
(C) Nonsteroidal anti-inflammatory drugs
(D) Nonsteroidal anti-inflammatory drugs and oral antibiotics

Item 29

A 28-year-old woman develops a 2-month history of aching in the joints in her hands and knees. Her fingertips turn white and become numb with exposure to cold. In addition, she has experienced postprandial and occasional burning nocturnal chest discomfort for the past 3 months. Medical history is otherwise unremarkable, and family history is remarkable only for an aunt with systemic lupus erythematosus. The patient takes no medications.

On physical examination, heart rate is 78/min, respiration rate is 18/min, and blood pressure is 100/60 mm Hg. There is thickening of the skin of the face, chest, abdomen, arms, hands, and feet. The remainder of the physical examination is normal.

Which of the following is the most likely diagnosis?

(A) Diffuse systemic sclerosis
(B) Limited systemic sclerosis
(C) Mixed connective tissue disease
(D) Systemic lupus erythematosus

Item 30

A 24-year-old woman is evaluated in the office for a 2-month history of feeling feverish and for muscle and joint pains that all began 2 days after she got sunburned. She has also had episodes of fatigue and myalgias lasting 2 to 3 days over the past 6 months, which she attributes to emotional stress. She reports that her hand joints are swollen and painful. She has been taking up to eight ibuprofen tablets daily with only temporary relief of symptoms. She has had no major illnesses and no history of tick bites or weight loss. She is sexually active.

On physical examination, she appears ill. Temperature is 37.6 °C (99.8 °F), heart rate is 100/min, and blood pressure is 110/65 mm Hg. Her throat is injected, and there is a shallow, painless palatal ulcer; mild facial redness is present. She has bilateral synovitis of the wrists, metacarpophalangeal joints, elbows, and knees.

Which of the following is the most likely diagnosis?

(A) Behçet's disease
(B) Disseminated gonococcal arthritis
(C) Fibromyalgia
(D) Reactive arthritis
(E) Systemic lupus erythematosus

Item 31

A 32-year-old woman is evaluated in the office for an 8-month history of joint pains and rash, as well as fatigue, myalgias, and possible fever. She takes acetaminophen for these symptoms without relief. Three months ago, she was diagnosed with pleurisy and treated with ibuprofen. She has had no major medical illnesses and takes no other medications. She is not sexually active.

On physical examination, the temperature is 37.7 °C (100.0 °F), heart rate is 90/min, and blood pressure is 148/86 mm Hg. She has a rash over the bridge of her nose and cheeks, sparing the nasolabial folds and the area beneath her nose. Musculoskeletal examination reveals bilateral synovitis of the wrists and metacarpophalangeal joints.

Laboratory studies include hematocrit, 30%; reticulocyte count, 8%; leukocyte count, 2100/µL; and platelet count, 103,000/µL. Urinalysis is normal.

Which of the following blood tests will be most helpful in confirming the diagnosis?

(A) Erythrocyte sedimentation rate and C-reactive protein
(B) Serum antinuclear antibody and anti–double-stranded DNA antibody
(C) Serum rheumatoid factor and anti–cyclic citrullinated peptide antibody
(D) Serum uric acid and HLA-B27

Item 32

An 82-year-old woman is evaluated in the office for a 2-week history of severe headaches and neck pain. She has stiffness and aching in her shoulders, neck, and lower back.

On physical examination, the scalp is diffusely tender to palpation. Funduscopic examination is unremarkable, and she has carotidynia (pain over the carotid artery). On musculoskeletal examination, muscle strength testing is limited because of muscle pain. Biceps and triceps reflexes are 2+ and symmetrical. Hemoglobin is 10 g/dL, erythrocyte sedimentation rate is 50 mm/h, and creatine kinase is 150 U/L.

Which of the following is the most likely diagnosis?

(A) Carotid artery dissection
(B) Polymyalgia rheumatica
(C) Polymyalgia rheumatica and giant cell arteritis
(D) Polymyositis

Item 33

A 32-year-old woman is evaluated in the office for a 2-week history of weakness of the right arm and left leg. The initial symptom was acute right wrist drop associated with sensory loss in a radial nerve distribution and severe pain. One week later, she developed similar symptoms in the left peroneal nerve distribution. The patient has systemic lupus erythematosus, and her medications are prednisone and hydroxychloroquine.

Which of the following is the most likely diagnosis?

(A) Guillain–Barré syndrome
(B) Lyme disease
(C) Motor neuron disease
(D) Toxic neuropathy
(E) Vasculitic neuropathy

Item 34

A 65-year-old woman is evaluated in the office for a 3-month history of "tiredness." She is unable to continue her routine of walking 30 minutes each day. She has recently noted significant shoulder and hip pain, especially on awakening. She has had difficulty doing housework but identifies no exacerbating or alleviating factors. She "tosses and turns" at night because she is uncomfortable. She is otherwise healthy and takes no medications.

On musculoskeletal examination, full range of motion of the shoulders and hips elicits mild discomfort. She has tenderness to palpation of the midtrapezius, deltoid, and trochanteric areas. Strength testing is inconclusive secondary to pain. Complete blood count is normal, erythrocyte sedimentation rate is 64 mm/h, and creatine kinase is 125 U/L.

Which of the following is the most likely diagnosis?

(A) Fibromyalgia
(B) Polymyalgia rheumatica
(C) Polymyositis
(D) Rheumatoid arthritis

Item 35

A 67-year-old woman is evaluated in the office for a 6-week history of stiffness and pain, particularly around the shoulders and hips. She is unsure whether there are any exacerbating or alleviating factors or whether her pain worsens during certain times of the day but believes that it is worse in the morning. She does not have vision problems, scalp tenderness, temporal area pain, jaw claudication, or wrist or finger joint swelling.

On physical examination, she is afebrile. There are no rashes, and peripheral pulses are symmetrical and normal. There is no evidence of synovitis. On musculoskeletal examination, there is tenderness to palpation, particularly around the proximal upper and lower extremities, but muscle strength is normal. The remainder of the examination is unremarkable.

Hemoglobin is 11 g/dL, and the erythrocyte sedimentation rate is 82 mm/h.

Which of the following is the most appropriate treatment for this patient?

(A) Etanercept
(B) Hydroxychloroquine
(C) Methotrexate
(D) Prednisone

Chapter 11

Rheumatology
Answers and Critiques

Item 1   Answer: A

Generalized pain in the setting of a normal complete blood count and erythrocyte sedimentation rate and normal joint examination is consistent with fibromyalgia. Characteristic manifestations of fibromyalgia are widespread musculoskeletal pain and stiffness, nonrestorative sleep, and fatigue. On physical examination, there are multiple symmetrical painful tender points; a diagnosis of fibromyalgia may be established in patients with pain at 11 or more of 18 tender points defined by the American College of Rheumatology. Laboratory and joint examination findings are normal. Management of fibromyalgia is multimodal and includes interventions to improve sleep and conditioning with a graded aerobic exercise program. Treatment for anxiety and/or depression, if present, also is indicated. Amitriptyline effectively improves general disease activity in patients with this condition. This agent also improves sleep habits in patients with fibromyalgia with associated sleep disturbances.

Because this patient has no evidence of synovitis or muscle weakness on examination, a diagnosis of active or flaring rheumatoid arthritis or polymyositis is unlikely. While many patients with systemic lupus erythematosus (SLE) experience fatigue, other manifestations are present as well, including active synovitis, serositis, rash, aphthous ulcers, cytopenia, and an abnormal urinalysis. In the absence of these findings, SLE is unlikely.

KEY POINT

• Patients with fibromyalgia have widespread musculoskeletal pain and stiffness, nonrestorative sleep, fatigue, multiple symmetrical painful tender points, and normal laboratory evaluation.

Bibliography
1. **Chakrabarty S, Zoorob R.** Fibromyalgia. Am Fam Physician. 2007;76:247-54. [PMID: 17695569]

Item 2   Answer: A

Arthrocentesis is indicated to evaluate undiagnosed monoarticular arthritis. The differential diagnosis of monoarticular arthritis includes septic arthritis, gout, pseudogout, rheumatoid arthritis, systemic lupus erythematosus, and the spondyloarthritides. In septic arthritis, early identification and aggressive treatment are crucial to prevent joint destruction. In most patients with septic arthritis, the synovial fluid leukocyte count

is >50,000/μL (90% neutrophils). Culture results should direct antibiotic therapy, although ceftriaxone would be a reasonable empiric therapy in the absence of clinical suspicion for methicillin-resistant *Staphylococcus aureus* or *Pseudomonas aeruginosa*. Repeated drainage of the joint space also may be needed.

Crystalline and inflammatory arthropathies may closely mimic the clinical presentation of septic arthritis, presenting with pain, erythema, edema, tenderness, and fever. This patient has multiple risk factors for gout, including obesity, chronic kidney disease, diuretic use, and hyperuricemia, but synovial fluid analysis is needed to establish a diagnosis. In patients with gout, polarized light microscopy of the synovial fluid reveals needle-shaped, strongly negatively birefringent monosodium urate crystals and a leukocyte count of 2000 to 50,000/μL. Although the risk of developing gout increases as uric acid levels increase, measurement of these levels during an episode of acute monoarticular arthritis is not helpful. Treatment of gout is particularly risky for patients with chronic kidney disease, and colchicine and nonsteroidal anti-inflammatory drugs (NSAIDs) can be deleterious in this setting. Colchicine toxicity may be lethal and can develop quickly in patients with chronic renal insufficiency, whereas NSAIDs can substantially worsen renal function. Prednisone is potentially highly effective for gout but would be inappropriate in a patient with septic arthritis; gout and septic arthritis can coexist.

KEY POINTS

• Arthrocentesis is indicated to diagnose acute monoarticular arthritis.

• Aggressive, timely treatment is crucial in patients with septic arthritis.

Bibliography
1. **Sack K.** Monarthritis: differential diagnosis. Am J Med. 1997;102:30S-34S. [PMID: 9217557]

Item 3   Answer: A

Arthrocentesis with analysis of joint fluid for cell count and differential, glucose, culture, and crystal examination is essential for making a diagnosis of acute monoarticular arthritis. This patient may well have acute gout related to the recent initiation of hydrochlorothiazide, which can cause hyperuricemia. The definitive diagnosis of acute gout requires polarized microscopic detection of monosodium urate crystals in synovial fluid polymorphonuclear leukocytes. Other common causes of acute monoarticular arthritis that can be differentiated by joint aspiration and synovial fluid analysis include calcium pyrophosphate deposition disease (pseudogout) and infection. It is essential to diagnose infection with early arthrocentesis to avoid rapid joint destruction and its long-term sequelae.

Rheumatoid arthritis is an unlikely diagnosis in this patient and should not be considered until crystal-induced and septic arthritis are excluded. Furthermore, detecting rheumatoid factor without characteristic historical and clinical findings does not establish the diagnosis of rheumatoid arthritis. The serum uric acid level is not diagnostic even if elevated, and at the time of an acute attack of gout, the level may not be indicative of baseline levels. HLA-B27–positive persons are at increased risk for ankylosing spondylitis and reactive arthritis (which may present as monoarthritis), but HLA-B27 testing is not a particularly useful diagnostic study because significant proportions of the population are HLA-B27 positive and only a few percent ever develop manifestations of spondyloarthritis or reactive arthritis. Measuring serum calcium may be very useful if the patient has calcium pyrophosphate crystals in the synovial fluid, but an elevated serum calcium level will not itself define the nature of the monoarthritis nor obviate the need for a joint aspiration.

KEY POINT

- Aspiration and joint fluid analysis for cell count and differential, glucose, culture, and crystal examination are essential for making a diagnosis in acute monoarticular arthritis.

Bibliography
1. **Agudelo CA, Wise CM.** Gout: diagnosis, pathogenesis, and clinical manifestations. Curr Opin Rheumatol. 2001;13:234-9. [PMID: 11333355]

Item 4   Answer: D

Immediate aspiration of the right olecranon bursa is indicated for this patient. There is a strong clinical suspicion for olecranon bursitis, which may be infectious, crystalline, or traumatic. Synovial fluid analysis will help guide therapy in this setting. Acute crystalline or infectious synovitis usually is associated with extreme pain on passive joint motion. This patient has pain only on full flexion of the joint, most likely because this movement causes tautness of the bursa and surrounding soft tissue.

Joint aspiration is not indicated in the absence of convincing evidence that the joint itself is the source of the problem. Radiography is useful in evaluating traumatic causes of acute pain near a joint but would not help to differentiate between crystalline and infectious arthritis or to diagnose bursitis. Nuclear scanning and MRI are similarly not particularly useful in establishing a diagnosis among these conditions, and measurement of the erythrocyte sedimentation rate will not help to distinguish between crystal-induced arthritis and infection.

KEY POINT

- Olecranon bursitis is typically associated with painful full elbow flexion; acute crystalline or infectious synovitis is usually associated with pain on any passive joint motion

Bibliography
1. **Cardone DA, Tallia AF.** Diagnostic and therapeutic injection of the elbow region. Am Fam Physician. 2002;66:2097-100. [PMID: 12484691]

Item 5   Answer: C

The patient's history is suspicious for a meniscal tear. Patients describe a twisting injury with the foot in a weight-bearing position in which a popping or tearing sensation is often felt, followed by severe pain. Swelling occurs over several hours, in contrast to ligamentous injuries, in which swelling is immediate. Walking up and down stairs is difficult and squatting may be painful in patients with meniscal damage. Patients with meniscal tears may report a clicking or locking of the knee secondary to loose cartilage in the knee but often have pain only on walking, particularly going up or down stairs. Pain along the joint line is sensitive for meniscal tears in 76% of patients, and findings of the McMurray test (as described in the case presentation) are specific for this condition in 97% of patients.

Ligamentous damage usually occurs as a result of forceful stress or direct blows to the knee while the extremity is bearing weight. A valgus stress (i.e., force applied to the lateral aspect of the knee) injures the medial collateral ligament; a varus stress (i.e., force applied to the medial aspect of the knee) injures the lateral collateral ligament. Hyperextension injures the posterior cruciate ligament, and excessive medial rotation with a planted foot stresses the anterior cruciate ligament. A popping or tearing sensation is also frequently reported in patients with ligamentous damage. As noted above, ligamentous tears tend to produce immediate swelling, whereas meniscal tears cause less swelling that is more delayed in onset.

Anserine bursitis is characterized by pain and tenderness over the anteromedial aspect of the lower leg below the joint line of the knee. The location of the patient's pain and her abnormal physical examination findings do not support the diagnosis of anserine bursitis. Patellofemoral pain syndrome is the most common cause of knee pain in active adults younger than 45 years of age. The exacerbation of the pain by going down steps and the development of knee stiffness and pain at rest when the knee is flexed for an extended period of time are clues to the diagnosis. Reproducing the pain by firmly moving the patella along the femur confirms the diagnosis. Patellofemoral pain syndrome is self-limited and responds to rest and nonsteroidal anti-inflammatory drugs.

KEY POINTS

- Patients with meniscal tears describe a twisting injury with the foot in a weight-bearing position in which a popping or tearing sensation is often felt, followed by severe pain.

- Pain along the joint line is sensitive for meniscal tears in 76% of patients, and findings of the McMurray test are specific for this condition in 97% of patients.

Bibliography

1. Jackson JL, O'Malley PG, Kroenke K. Evaluation of acute knee pain in primary care. Ann Intern Med. 2003;139:575-88. [PMID: 14530229]

Item 6   Answer: B

This patient's history and physical examination are classic examples of findings associated with the patellofemoral pain syndrome, the most common cause of knee pain in active adults younger than 45 years of age. The exacerbation of the pain by going down steps and the development of knee stiffness and pain at rest when the knee is flexed for an extended period are clues to the diagnosis. Reproducing the pain by firmly moving the patella along the femur confirms the diagnosis. Patellofemoral pain syndrome is self-limited and responds to rest and nonsteroidal anti-inflammatory drugs.

Prepatellar bursitis is nearly always unilateral and often asymptomatic. Typically, there is a history of knee trauma or crawling preceding the knee pain. On palpation, there is tenderness over the entire bursal sac and a collection of fluid directly over the patella; these findings are absent in this patient, excluding this diagnosis. Sciatica is characterized by back pain with shooting or lancinating pains radiating down the posterior leg to the knee. Referred sciatic pain is not associated with knee findings on physical examination; the patient's abnormal knee findings exclude this diagnosis. The patient is young for the diagnosis of osteoarthritis, and there is no history of worsening pain over the course of the day that is typical for osteoarthritis. Patients with knee osteoarthritis may have crepitus with joint movement and bone tenderness and enlargement. The absence of these signs and symptoms excludes the diagnosis of osteoarthritis in this patient.

KEY POINTS

- The patellofemoral pain syndrome is the most common cause of knee pain in adults younger than 45 years of age.
- The typical patient with patellofemoral pain syndrome is an active young woman with anterior knee pain worsened by going down steps.

Bibliography

1. Dixit S, Difiori J, Burton M, Mines B. Management of patellofemoral pain syndrome. Am Fam Phys 2007; 75:194-203 [PMID pending].

Item 7   Answer: D

Because this patient meets none of the criteria for a fracture according to the Ottawa Knee Rules, the most appropriate next step in management is reassurance and symptomatic treatment. Acute treatment for a knee sprain consists of rest, ice, compression, and elevation (RICE). After application of ice and when the area is thoroughly cooled, an elastic wrap should be applied to compress the injury, and anti-inflammatory medication may be used for pain relief. The patient should be advised to cease running for at least 2 weeks and to stop if pain recurs once running is resumed.

The Ottawa Knee Rules suggest obtaining a knee radiograph in patients who meet any of the following criteria: 1) age older than 55 years, 2) tenderness at the head of the fibula or patella, or 3) an inability to flex to 90 degrees or to bear weight both immediately after the injury and during evaluation. Because this patient does not meet these criteria, knee radiography is not necessary. Although these rules are highly sensitive, patients who receive symptomatic care should be instructed to return for re-evaluation if knee pain persists. Crutches and a knee brace are not necessary in the absence of laxity or significant pain with stressing of the knee ligaments. MRI has been found to be slightly more sensitive, but less specific, than physical examination for detecting meniscal and ligamentous injuries. Additionally, MRI frequently finds abnormalities that are of no clinical significance. Given the lack of evidence of a meniscal or ligamentous injury in this patient's history or physical examination, any MRI findings would likely not be associated with his current problem and might instead be associated with his history as a long-term runner. However, if the patient's symptoms do not respond to symptomatic treatment, MRI might be considered.

KEY POINT

- The Ottawa Knee Rules suggest obtaining a knee radiograph in patients with acute knee pain who are older than age 55 years, have tenderness at the head of the fibula or patella, or have an inability to flex to 90 degrees or to bear weight both immediately and during evaluation.

Bibliography

1. Jackson JL, O'Malley PG, Kroenke K. Evaluation of acute knee pain in primary care. Ann Intern Med. 2003;139:575-88. [PMID: 14530229]

Item 8   Answer: E

Rotator cuff tendinitis, an inflammation of the supraspinatus and/or infraspinatus tendon that can also involve the subacromial bursa, is a common overuse injury. This injury is characterized by subacromial tenderness and impingement—painful compression of the rotator cuff tendons and subacromial bursa between the humeral head and the acromion with arm elevation. Pain in patients with rotator cuff tendinitis often occurs with reaching overhead and when lying on the shoulder. The passive painful-arc maneuver assesses the degree of impingement. The examiner places one hand on the acromion and the other on the forearm and abducts the arm while preventing the patient from shrugging. Subacromial pain at 60 to 70 degrees of abduction suggests moderate impingement, while pain at 45 degrees or less suggests severe impingement. Pain with resisted mid-arc abduction is a specific finding for rotator cuff tendinitis. Appropriate treatments for acute tendinitis include nonsteroidal anti-inflammatory drugs, ice, and exercises; overhead reaching and lifting should be limited.

Adhesive capsulitis (frozen shoulder) is characterized by a decreased range of shoulder motion predominantly resulting from stiffness rather than from pain or weakness. Bicipital tendinitis is also an overuse injury in which the bicipital groove may be tender, and anterior shoulder pain is elicited with resisted forearm supination or elbow flexion. Glenohumeral arthritis is often related to trauma and the gradual onset of pain and stiffness over months to years. A torn rotator cuff usually results in arm weakness, particularly with abduction and/or external rotation. A positive drop-arm test (inability to smoothly lower the affected arm from full abduction) is a very specific but relatively insensitive method for diagnosing rotator cuff tear.

KEY POINT

- Rotator cuff tendinitis is characterized by subacromial tenderness and impingement; pain often occurs with reaching overhead and when lying on the shoulder.

Bibliography

1. Koester MC, George MS, Kuhn JE. Shoulder impingement syndrome. Am J Med. 2005;118:452-5. [PMID: 15866244]

Item 9   Answer: B

The radiograph of this patient's knee shows linear calcium deposits in the articular space consistent with chondrocalcinosis secondary to deposition of calcium pyrophosphate dihydrate crystals. Calcification of the cartilage, particularly the fibrocartilage of the knee meniscus, symphysis pubis, and glenoid and acetabular labra and the triangular cartilage of the wrist, is pathognomonic for calcium pyrophosphate deposition disease (CPPD), or pseudogout. This condition may coexist with osteoarthritis and cause worsening swelling and pain.

Patients with CPPD may be asymptomatic or have recurrent attacks of acute monoarticular or oligoarticular arthritis. This patient's exacerbations are consistent with the latter manifestation. Involvement in atypical locations, such as the wrist, elbow, metacarpophalangeal, or shoulder joints, in the absence of an inciting trauma also should raise clinical suspicion for CPPD.

The medial joint-space narrowing visible on radiography suggests osteoarthritis, which may coexist with CPPD. However, osteoarthritis progression usually is insidious, not episodic. This patient's discrete worsening and significant episodic swelling suggest an inflammatory condition most compatible with a crystal-induced arthropathy, such as CPPD with a pseudogout presentation. Osteoarthritis alone would not be expected to cause periodic flares with inflammatory effusions.

Anserine bursitis, which also may coexist with osteoarthritis, may be an unrecognized cause of pain in the medial knee area.

However, this patient's effusion and radiographic findings are not consistent with this condition. Anserine bursitis typically causes pain 2 to 3 cm distal to the medial knee joint margin overlying the anterior tibia.

Gout and pseudogout have similar presentations, although pseudogout is characterized by the presence of calcium pyrophosphate crystals on synovial fluid analysis and chondrocalcinosis on radiography. Joint aspiration would establish the differential diagnosis between these conditions, but the presence of chondrocalcinosis in the fibrocartilage of the knee raises strong clinical suspicion for pseudogout. Sepsis always should be suspected in patients with acute monoarticular arthritis, although it is unlikely in a patient with recurrent episodes that resolve without antibiotic treatment. Nevertheless, arthrocentesis during an acute event is indicated to establish a diagnosis of CPPD and exclude infection. Calcium pyrophosphate and sodium urate crystals may coexist, as may calcium pyrophosphate crystals with concomitant infection.

KEY POINT

- Calcification of the cartilage, particularly the fibrocartilage of the knee meniscus, symphysis pubis, glenoid and acetabular labra, and the triangular cartilage of the wrist, is pathognomonic for calcium pyrophosphate deposition disease.

Bibliography

1. Cassetta M, Gorevic PD. Crystal arthritis. Gout and pseudogout in the geriatric patient. Geriatrics. 2004;59:25-30. [PMID: 15461235]

Item 10   Answer: D

This patient most likely has tophaceous gout involving the second and third distal interphalangeal joints. Tophaceous gout involving the distal interphalangeal joints is particularly common in postmenopausal women taking diuretics. Nonsteroidal anti-inflammatory drug therapy most likely had been suppressing the number of attacks of gout, as well as her chronic joint stiffness due to osteoarthritis, but had not been affecting the urate deposition into the tophi.

Psoriatic arthritis and inflammatory osteoarthritis may involve the distal interphalangeal joints but do not cause tophi or ulceration as seen in this patient. Similarly, rheumatoid arthritis does not involve the distal interphalangeal joints, although it is associated with the development of subcutaneous nodules over bony prominences, at extensor surfaces, and at juxta-articular sites.

KEY POINT

- Postmenopausal women who use diuretics have an increased risk for tophaceous gout of the distal interphalangeal joints.

Bibliography

1. Monu JU, Pope TL Jr. Gout: a clinical and radiologic review. Radiol Clin North Am. 2004;42:169-84. [PMID: 15049530]

Item 11   Answer: C

This patient's allopurinol dose should be increased. In addition, repeat urate measurement is indicated several weeks afterwards to assure that the urate concentration is decreasing. This patient has tophaceous gout with infrequent but persistent attacks. His total body stores of urate are elevated, and the presence of tophi demonstrates that he has abnormal urate deposition.

Even if this patient did not have attacks of gout, treatment to dissolve his tophi would be reasonable. Although this patient's urate level is within the reference range, it is not biologically normal. Reference values describe the distribution of urate levels in the population, which are two standard deviations around the population mean value. However, in patients with uric acid levels >6.8 mg/dL, urate will continue to be deposited in tissues. Therefore, the target of hyperuricemic therapy is to obtain a uric acid level of approximately 6 mg/dL to dissolve detected tophi and other urate deposits in the tissues. If allopurinol is discontinued, uric acid levels will increase to the pretreatment levels and the tophi and gouty attacks will return.

Because decreasing a patient's uric acid level may induce a gouty attack, continuation of colchicine therapy is indicated while the allopurinol dose is increased. In some patients, however, colchicine may be discontinued once the uric acid level is decreased and stabilized and the patient has been free of gouty attacks for approximately 6 months. Measuring the 24-hour urine urate excretion is not needed before adjusting the allopurinol dose. The target uric acid level is approximately 6 mg/dL, regardless of the level of urate excretion. Adding a second drug, probenecid, to increase urine urate excretion is not indicated; simply increasing the allopurinol dose is the most effective method to reduce body urate stores.

KEY POINT

• Uric acid levels in patients with tophaceous gout should be reduced to 6 mg/dL to dissolve tophi and other urate deposits in the tissue.

Bibliography
1. Keith MP, Gilliland WR. Updates in the management of gout. Am J Med. 2007;120:221-4. [PMID: 17349440]

Item 12   Answer: D

This patient most likely has iron overload secondary to hereditary hemochromatosis and should be screened with a measurement of transferrin saturation. Although the disease is classically described as "bronze diabetes," patients today usually present with arthropathy, fatigue, impotence, and liver chemistry test abnormalities. The arthropathy generally develops in the second and third metacarpophalangeal joints, but may involve large joints as well. The impotence results from hypogonadotropic hypogonadism. Iron deposition in the liver may cause findings ranging from mild aminotransferase ele-

vations to cirrhosis. The most appropriate initial screening test for a patient with suspected hemochromatosis is a transferrin saturation measurement. A value ≥45% is an indication for further testing for hemochromatosis.

Although a thyroid-stimulating hormone determination could be done because of the fatigue and abnormal liver chemistry test results, an underlying thyroid condition is less likely to cause arthropathy, impotence, and diabetes. Wilson's disease should always be considered when evaluating a patient with liver chemistry test abnormalities. However, this patient's age and the absence of other findings associated with Wilson's disease (e.g., fatigue, anorexia, abdominal pain, tremors, poor coordination, spastic dystonia, and psychiatric conditions) make this diagnosis unlikely. Therefore, measurement of ceruloplasmin is not indicated. Noninvasive studies to rule out vascular disease may be useful when evaluating a patient with impotence. However, this patient's strong pedal pulses, absence of other risk factors for vascular disease, and presence of other systemic findings make a vascular disorder unlikely.

KEY POINT

• Patients with hereditary hemochromatosis usually present with abnormal liver chemistry test results, arthropathy, fatigue, and impotence.

Bibliography
1. Whitlock EP, Garlitz BA, Harris EL, Beil TL, Smith PR. Screening for hereditary hemochromatosis: a systematic review for the U.S. Preventive Services Task Force. Ann Intern Med. 2006;145:209-23. [PMID: 16880463]

Item 13   Answer: E

This patient most likely has osteoarthritis, and no additional studies are needed. She has knee pain that worsens with ambulation and morning joint stiffness that lasts <30 minutes (indicating lack of significant inflammation), which are consistent with osteoarthritis. The joints most commonly involved in osteoarthritis are the knee, hip, distal and proximal interphalangeal, and first carpometacarpal joints. This condition may involve a single joint or multiple joints. Joint crepitus, a reduction in joint range of motion, and pain in weight-bearing joints also may occur in this setting.

In advanced osteoarthritis, physical examination findings typically include bony enlargement of the joint, Heberden's (distal interphalangeal) and Bouchard's (proximal interphalangeal) nodes, restricted range of motion in joints, and pain on passive range of motion. Joint deformity, such as angulation of the distal and proximal interphalangeal joints and varus alignment of the knees, also frequently is visible. Because osteoarthritis is primarily a noninflammatory arthropathy, results of laboratory studies are typically normal in this setting. Diagnosis of this condition is based on the history and clinical examination. If needed, radiography may confirm the diagnosis but would not contribute greatly to understanding the source of this patient's pain.

Crystal or inflammatory arthritis may be associated with an elevated erythrocyte sedimentation rate, but these diagnoses are unlikely in a patient with chronic knee pain and no inflammatory signs on physical examination or history of previous inflammatory flares. Patients with osteoarthritis may have laboratory abnormalities such as an elevated erythrocyte sedimentation rate and anemia that are unrelated to osteoarthritis. These abnormalities are present in this population because of the prevalence of osteoarthritis, particularly among elderly patients. Therefore, abnormal laboratory findings would not exclude a diagnosis of osteoarthritis.

Systemic lupus erythematosus may cause joint swelling and symmetrical, nondeforming involvement of the small joints, but this patient has no other symptoms suggestive of this condition. Therefore, an antinuclear antibody assay is not warranted. Moreover, positive findings on this assay would not establish a diagnosis of systemic lupus erythematosus or exclude osteoarthritis.

Joint involvement that spares the metacarpophalangeal joints but affects the distal interphalangeal joints is not characteristic of rheumatoid arthritis. Morning stiffness in a patient with an inflammatory process such as rheumatoid arthritis also typically lasts >45 minutes. A rheumatoid factor assay is therefore not appropriate. In addition, rheumatoid factor positivity alone would not establish a diagnosis of rheumatoid arthritis.

Several studies show a strong association between positive findings on anti–cyclic citrullinated peptide antibody assay and rheumatoid arthritis. This assay most likely has the best predictive value when combined with rheumatoid factor assay. However, an anti–cyclic citrullinated peptide antibody assay is not needed to establish the most likely diagnosis in this patient, which is osteoarthritis.

KEY POINTS

- The most common joints involved in osteoarthritis are the knee, hip, distal and proximal interphalangeal and first carpometacarpal joints.

- Osteoarthritis is characterized by pain that worsens with activity and morning joint stiffness that lasts <30 minutes.

Bibliography
1. **Hunter DJ.** In the clinic. Osteoarthritis. Ann Intern Med. 2007;147:ITC8-1-ITC8-16. [PMID: 17679702]

Item 14   Answer: C

This patient's synovial fluid findings are minimally inflammatory and most consistent with osteoarthritis. Synovial fluid in this setting usually is clear, viscous, and noninflammatory, with a typical leukocyte count of <2000/µL. Synovial fluid analysis is not necessary to diagnose osteoarthritis, but this study supports the diagnosis. Synovial fluid analysis is particularly useful if the diagnosis is uncertain and is essential to exclude infection in patients with acute worsening of symptoms, unexplained inflammation and effusion, or fever.

Gout and calcium pyrophosphate deposition disease (pseudogout) are both inflammatory conditions characterized by a synovial fluid leukocyte count between 2000/µL and 50,000/µL, but the value may be higher. In addition, polarized light microscopy of synovial fluid in these patients typically reveals crystals. The synovial fluid leukocyte count for other inflammatory arthritis syndromes is also between 2000/µL and 50,000/µL. The synovial fluid leukocyte count in septic arthritis is highly variable but usually is moderately inflammatory (10,000/µL to 50,000/µL) or highly inflammatory (50,000/µL to 100,000/µL).

KEY POINTS

- Synovial fluid in osteoarthritis usually is clear, viscous, and non-inflammatory with a leukocyte count <2000/µL.

- Gout and calcium pyrophosphate deposition disease (pseudogout) are associated with inflammatory synovial fluid with a leukocyte count between 2000/µL and 50,000/µL.

- Synovial fluid in septic arthritis is generally highly inflammatory with a leukocyte count between 10,000/µL and 50,000/µL and is often higher.

Bibliography
1. **Swan A, Amer H, Dieppe P.** The value of synovial fluid assays in the diagnosis of joint disease: a literature survey. Ann Rheum Dis. 2002;61:493-8. [PMID: 12006320]

Item 15   Answer: A

Acetaminophen is an effective, inexpensive treatment for osteoarthritis. This agent also is safe, particularly compared with nonsteroidal anti-inflammatory drugs (NSAIDs). This patient has squaring of the first carpometacarpal joints and bony hypertrophy in several distal interphalangeal joints, which are characteristic findings in osteoarthritis.

Double-blind, placebo-controlled clinical trials have shown that acetaminophen effectively manages symptoms of osteoarthritis in many patients. However, the relative efficacy of acetaminophen and NSAIDs remains controversial among many experts. Some experts believe that acetaminophen should be the drug of choice for osteoarthritis, whereas others believe that recent data prove the superiority of NSAIDs in relieving symptoms.

A study testing a program in which physicians were educated to discontinue use of NSAIDs for osteoarthritis in elderly patients showed that these agents could be replaced with acetaminophen without worsening of pain. These results suggest that patients with osteoarthritis who have a high risk for NSAID-induced complications may use alternative therapy with acetaminophen without compromising pain control.

Methotrexate is appropriate for management of rheumatoid arthritis. However, rheumatoid arthritis is not associated with involvement of the distal interphalangeal joints, which is clearly present in this patient.

Corticosteroids, such as prednisolone, are potent anti-inflammatory agents. However, use of these agents would not benefit this patient, because osteoarthritis is not a systemic inflammatory disease. In addition, long-term use of corticosteroids is associated with significant adverse side effects. Etanercept is appropriate for the management of patients with rheumatoid arthritis but is not indicated for those with osteoarthritis.

KEY POINTS

• Characteristic findings in osteoarthritis include squaring of the first carpometacarpal joints and bony hypertrophy in the distal interphalangeal joints.

• Acetaminophen is an effective, safe, and inexpensive treatment for osteoarthritis.

Bibliography
1. **Hunter DJ.** In the clinic. Osteoarthritis. Ann Intern Med. 2007;147:ITC8-1-ITC8-16. [PMID: 17679702]

Item 16   Answer: C

Osteoarthritis is the most likely cause of this patient's knee pain. Her risk factors for osteoarthritis include age over 50 years and obesity. The quality of the pain in osteoarthritis is often described as a deep aching sensation. The pain usually occurs initially with exertion, but as the disease progresses the pain occurs at rest. Typically, patients have no systemic symptoms. Laboratory evaluation of synovial fluid shows a mildly elevated leukocyte count <2000/uL, consistent with inflammation but not infection.

Gouty arthritis may be clinically similar to osteoarthritis or may be severe enough to resemble a septic arthritis. The first metatarsophalangeal joint is most often affected in gout, but any joint may be involved. The onset of gout is usually acute, but it can cause chronic arthritis. Patients with chronic gouty arthritis typically have a history of previous acute attacks of monoarthritis. Like osteoarthritis, chronic gout may be associated with bony enlargement of joints, but tophi may be present on examination. Synovial fluid analysis in gout shows negatively birefringent needle-shaped monosodium urate crystals.

Rheumatoid arthritis is classically characterized as a symmetric polyarthritis primarily affecting the fingers, hands, wrists, and feet. Soft tissue swelling rather than bony enlargement of the joints is a characteristic difference between osteoarthritis and rheumatoid arthritis. Inflammatory signs (fatigue, prolonged morning stiffness) are present with rheumatoid arthritis and absent in osteoarthritis. The fact that this patient experiences pain in only one knee, has no evidence of synovial thickening, and does not have morning stiffness makes rheumatoid arthritis much less likely.

Although a meniscal tear can present with unilateral pain, there is no history of acute trauma and the pain in the knee was of gradual onset. Additionally, the patient does not report a "clicking" or "catching" sensation, which often occurs in meniscal tears.

Septic arthritis is associated with a synovial fluid leukocyte count >50,000/uL consisting primarily of neutrophils. The joint is usually erythematous, swollen, and warm. Symptoms are typically acute in onset, not gradually increasing over 1 month, as in this patient.

KEY POINT

• Osteoarthritis of the knee is associated with a synovial fluid leukocyte count <2000/uL and no crystals.

Bibliography
1. **Felson DT.** Clinical practice. Osteoarthritis of the knee. N Engl J Med. 2006;354:841-8. Erratum in: N Engl J Med. 20068;354:2520. [PMID: 16929000]

Item 17   Answer: A

This patient needs a trial of acetaminophen, weight loss, and exercise. Weight loss has been shown to reduce the risk for symptomatic osteoarthritis in women. The Arthritis, Diet, and Activity Promotion Trial, a randomized, single-blind clinical trial, showed that diet and exercise are associated with overall improvements in self-reported measures of function and pain and in performance measures of mobility in older, overweight, and obese adults with knee osteoarthritis. Patients with knee osteoarthritis who perform quadriceps muscle strength training exercises show modest improvements in decreasing pain and improving function. The degree of adherence to the exercise regimen correlates with the amount of improvement in pain and functional status experienced. Acetaminophen also has been shown to alleviate pain in knee osteoarthritis. Randomized controlled trials comparing 4 weeks of acetaminophen, 4000 mg/d, with ibuprofen, 1200 mg/d and 2400 mg/d, as well as 2 years of acetaminophen, 2600 mg/d, with naproxen, 750 mg/d, have shown equivalent efficacy in the management of this condition.

Because this patient has had recent upper gastrointestinal bleeding, use of diclofenac or indomethacin suppositories is not advisable. A randomized controlled trial comparing arthroscopic lavage and arthroscopic lavage plus débridement with a sham procedure for knee osteoarthritis showed no benefit associated with this intervention.

KEY POINTS

• Diet and exercise lead to improvement in function and alleviation of pain in older, overweight and obese adults with knee osteoarthritis.

• Acetaminophen is equally effective as nonsteroidal anti-inflammatory drugs in the treatment of osteoarthritis.

Bibliography
1. **Hunter DJ.** In the clinic. Osteoarthritis. Ann Intern Med. 2007;147:ITC8-1-ITC8-16. [PMID: 17679702]

Item 18   Answer: B

A recent double-blind, controlled clinical trial demonstrated the effectiveness of intra-articular corticosteroid injections in relieving symptoms of knee osteoarthritis. These agents are therefore indicated for acute exacerbations of knee pain due to osteoarthritis, particularly in patients with signs of local inflammation and joint effusion. However, synovial fluid analysis is vital in this setting because intra-articular corticosteroids are contraindicated if joint infection is suspected.

Oral corticosteroids, such as prednisone, are potent anti-inflammatory agents, but osteoarthritis is not a systemic inflammatory disease. Therefore, systemic administration of these agents is not indicated in this situation, particularly since long-term use of these drugs is associated with significant side effects. In a randomized trial, intervention with arthroscopic lavage and arthroscopic lavage plus surgical débridement was not shown to be more beneficial for patients with knee osteoarthritis compared with a sham procedure. In the United States, topical nonsteroidal anti-inflammatory drugs are available only through a compounding pharmacist. Moreover, the effectiveness of these agents has not been established.

KEY POINT
- Intra-articular corticosteroid injections effectively relieve symptoms of knee osteoarthritis.

Bibliography
1. **Raynauld JP, Buckland-Wright C, Ward R, Choquette D, Haraoui B, Martel-Pelletier J, et al.** Safety and efficacy of long-term intraarticular steroid injections in osteoarthritis of the knee: a randomized, double-blind, placebo-controlled trial. Arthritis Rheum. 2003;48:370-7. [PMID: 12571845]

Item 19   Answer: A

A careful evaluation for an occult malignancy is indicated for this patient, beginning with routine age- and sex-appropriate screening tests, including colonoscopy, mammography, pelvic examination, and Papanicolaou smear. Dermatomyositis and polymyositis in older patients have been shown to be associated with various forms of malignancy. The malignancy often is evident at the onset of the myositis, although it may occur up to several years later in some patients. A search for malignancy in young patients is not indicated.

Some experts recommend repeated testing for malignancy every 6 to 12 months for a few years. In older patients and in those with dermatomyositis, endoscopic and imaging studies are recommended to exclude pharyngeal, gastrointestinal, pulmonary, intra-abdominal, and pelvic malignancies. In Asian patients in particular, referral for otorhinolaryngology consultation is warranted to evaluate for nasopharyngeal cancer.

Liver biopsy is unlikely to identify an occult malignancy unless an imaging study reveals a liver mass. Cystoscopy and renal ultrasonography would be appropriate tests in the presence of urinary symptoms or unexplained hematuria but otherwise have low yield in patients with inflammatory myositis.

KEY POINT
- The risk for malignant disease is increased in patients with dermatomyositis and polymyositis and in those with inclusion-body myositis.

Bibliography
1. **Buchbinder R, Hill CL**. Malignancy in patients with inflammatory myopathy. Curr Rheumatol Rep. 2002;4:415-26. [PMID: 12217247]

Item 20   Answer: D

This patient's subacute onset of proximal muscle weakness and elevated muscle enzyme levels strongly suggests polymyositis. Patients usually present with fatigue and generalized weakness, and a directed inquiry is necessary to bring into focus the pattern of proximal muscle weakness caused by myositis. Proximal muscle weakness is the cardinal sign of myopathy, and patients without demonstrable proximal muscle weakness are unlikely to have polymyositis. Proximal muscle weakness and certain characteristic rashes (for example, Gottron's papules and periorbital heliotrope rash) are characteristic of dermatomyositis. Patients may also have signs of respiratory insufficiency because of respiratory muscle weakness, dyspnea because of cardiomyopathy, and pharyngeal and gastrointestinal dysmotility with regurgitation and aspiration. The serum creatine kinase concentration is typically elevated to 10 to 50 times above normal in patients with polymyositis. A combination of a high creatine kinase level and objective proximal muscle weakness establishes the presence of a muscle disorder and indicates the need for further testing with a muscle biopsy, electromyography, or both, to diagnose polymyositis and dermatomyositis.

Fibromyalgia is not associated with weakness unless it is due to disuse atrophy, in which case the weakness has a generalized distribution rather than being limited to the proximal muscles. Patients with fibromyalgia also have diffuse tender points on examination that are absent in polymyositis. The creatine kinase concentration is normal in fibromyalgia. Myasthenia gravis is a disorder of the neuromuscular junction that typically is associated with weakness that worsens with activity and improves with rest. Extraocular and eyelid muscles are often involved early in the course of the disease, which does not occur in polymyositis. The creatine kinase level is not elevated. Polymyalgia rheumatica typically occurs in persons older than 50 years and is characterized by hip and shoulder girdle pain and stiffness, especially in the morning. Weakness is not typical unless related to pain or muscle disuse. Patients almost always have a significantly elevated erythrocyte sedimentation rate but a normal creatine kinase level. Syringomyelia is characterized by the finding of upper cervical dissociated sensory loss; i.e., loss of pain and temperature sensation with preserved light touch, vibratory sense, and joint position sense. These findings are found in the arms, along with weakness, wasting, and upper motor neuron signs (e.g., spasticity and hyperreflexia). These findings are not present in this patient, making syringomyelia unlikely.

- Proximal muscle weakness is the cardinal sign of myopathy.

- A combination of a high creatine kinase level and proximal muscle weakness indicates the need for further testing with a muscle biopsy, electromyography, or both, to diagnose polymyositis and dermatomyositis.

Bibliography
1. **Dalakas MC, Hohlfeld R.** Polymyositis and dermatomyositis. Lancet. 2003;362:971-82. [PMID: 14511932]

Item 21   Answer: D

This patient most likely has rheumatoid arthritis. The evaluation of a patient's joint complaints is based on recognizing the distribution and timing of joint involvement and matching these findings to the characteristics of specific arthropathies. Rheumatoid arthritis causes symmetric polyarthritis (joint swelling) involving the proximal interphalangeal (PIP) joints, metacarpophalangeal (MCP) joints, wrists, elbows, shoulders, hips, knees, ankles, metatarsophalangeal (MTP) joints, and cervical spine. However, rheumatoid arthritis typically spares the carpometacarpal (CMC) and distal interphalangeal (DIP) joints and thoracic, lumbar, and sacral spine. The diagnosis of rheumatoid arthritis requires the presence of four of the following seven classification criteria: (1) morning stiffness in and around joints lasting at least 1 hour before maximal improvement; (2) soft tissue swelling of three or more joint areas observed by a physician (PIP, MCP, wrist, elbow, knee, ankle, MTP); (3) swelling of the PIP, MCP, or wrist joints; (4) symmetric joint swelling; (5) subcutaneous nodules over a bony prominence or extensor surface or in juxta-articular regions; (6) positive test for rheumatoid factor; and (7) radiographic periarticular osteopenia and/or marginal (where the joint capsule attaches to the bone) erosions in the hand or wrist joints. This patient has five of the seven criteria.

Gonococcal arthritis is the most common arthritis in sexually active women between the ages of 15 and 40 years. It typically manifests as a migratory arthritis or tenosynovitis, finally affecting a single joint, which this patient does not have. Gout is an episodic acute arthritis with significant joint swelling, redness, warmth, and pain. Gout attacks typically last 5 to 7 days before spontaneously abating. Any joint can be affected; however, the typical target joints are the great toe MTP joint, the ankle, and the knee. An individual attack can be monoarticular, oligoarticular, or polyarticular. Older women frequently present with gout as a polyarticular symmetric pseudorheumatoid arthritis. Endogenous estrogens appear to protect premenopausal women from gout attacks. Therefore, unless a woman has a proliferative disorder associated with high cell turnover that increases purine metabolism and uric acid production (such as psoriasis or malignancy) or a condition that interferes with urate excretion (such as effects of drugs, alcohol abuse, renal dysfunction, or enzyme deficiency), a premenopausal woman would not have gout.

Osteoarthritis most commonly affects women older than 40 years of age; it is associated with morning joint stiffness that commonly lasts less than 1 hour. The joints most commonly affected include the DIP, PIP, CMC, MTP, hip, knee, and spine joints. The joints that are typically spared include the MCP, wrist, and ankle joints. Physical findings typically include bony enlargement and malalignment.

- Rheumatoid arthritis is characterized by a symmetric polyarticular arthritis involving the proximal interphalangeal and metacarpophalangeal joints, wrists, elbows, shoulders, hips, knees, ankles, metatarsophalangeal joints, and cervical spine.

Bibliography
1. **Arnett FC, Edworthy SM, Bloch DA, McShane DJ, Fries JF, Cooper NS, Healey LA, Kaplan SR, Liang MH, Luthra HS, et al.** The American Rheumatism Association 1987 revised criteria for the classification of rheumatoid arthritis. Arthritis Rheum. 1988;31:315-24. [PMID: 3358796]

Item 22   Answer: B

This patient has symptoms, signs, and radiographic changes consistent with rheumatoid arthritis. The key radiographic changes include marginal erosions and juxta-articular osteopenia. This patient's hand radiograph shows soft-tissue swelling and ulnar styloid erosion consistent with erosive rheumatoid arthritis.

Viral arthritis is highly unlikely in a patient with rheumatoid arthritis–like, symmetrical joint inflammation that persists for >3 months. Moreover, patients with chronic viral arthritis, such as hepatitis C, do not develop erosive joint disease. Systemic lupus erythematosus may cause prominent and persistent rheumatoid arthritis–like, symmetrical joint inflammation in the hands and feet. However, this presentation usually is accompanied by extra-articular disease manifestations, such as fever, serositis, rash, renal disease, and cytopenia. In addition, patients with systemic lupus erythematosus do not develop erosive joint disease.

Psoriatic arthritis commonly manifests with psoriatic skin changes, nail pitting, often onycholysis, and asymmetrical polyarthritis that involves fewer than four lower-extremity large joints and causes distal interphalangeal joint inflammation in the hands. Radiography of the hands in this setting may show erosions, but the affected joints differ from those in rheumatoid arthritis. Erosions in psoriatic arthritis are associated with periostitis and bone whittling, not juxta-articular osteopenia.

- Characteristic radiographic changes associated with rheumatoid arthritis include juxta-articular osteoporosis and marginal erosions.

Bibliography
1. **Babyn P, Doria AS.** Radiologic investigation of rheumatic diseases. Pediatr Clin North Am. 2005;52:373-411. [PMID: 15820373]

Item 23   Answer: A

Ceftriaxone therapy should be started in this patient. Sexually active patients who develop migratory arthralgias and subsequent oligoarthritis and present with wrist tenosynovitis have strong clinical suspicion for disseminated gonococcal infection. Skin lesions may not be present, and cultures may be negative. Antibiotic response in this setting may not be rapid, and 72 hours may be required for a complete response to therapy. Screening for chlamydial infection, HIV, and other sexually transmitted diseases should be performed once gonorrhea is established. In patients with negative culture findings, a complete response to appropriate antibiotic therapy often is the gold standard for establishing a diagnosis of disseminated gonorrhea.

Terminal complement component deficiency is a rare disorder that is characterized by recurrent episodes of disseminated neisserial infection. Therefore, evaluation for this condition is not indicated on initial presentation of a patient with suspected gonorrhea. Vancomycin and doxycycline will not adequately treat disseminated gonorrhea and are not indicated; furthermore doxycycline is contraindicated during pregnancy.

KEY POINT

• Sexually active adults with acute monoarticular arthritis should be treated for disseminated gonorrhea.

Bibliography

1. **Rice PA**. Gonococcal arthritis (disseminated gonococcal infection). Infect Dis Clin North Am. 2005;19:853-61. [PMID: 16297736]

Item 24   Answer: B

This patient most likely has disseminated gonococcal infection, as manifested by dermatitis, tenosynovitis, and asymmetrical arthritis. Antimicrobial therapy should be directed specifically towards *Neisseria gonorrhoeae* pending culture results and in vitro susceptibility testing, and ceftriaxone is the most appropriate of the antibiotics listed. The Centers for Disease Control and Prevention (CDC) recently advised against the use of fluoroquinolones in men who have sex with men and emphasized that determination of the infected person's likely locale of infection (i.e., sex in a locale known to have high prevalence of fluoroquinolone-resistant gonorrhea or with a person from such a locale) is critical to help determine the appropriate choice of therapy. Because fluoroquinolone resistance has been observed in the Pacific Rim and Hawaii, ciprofloxacin should not be used as empiric therapy until in vitro susceptibility test results of the isolated organism are known. Penicillin G should never be used as empiric therapy because of the high incidence of penicillinase-producing *N. gonorrhoeae*. Resistance to trimethoprim–sulfamethoxazole also occurs. Cefazolin is inappropriate because it is not active against *N. gonorrhoeae*. This patient should also be screened for possible HIV infection and other sexually transmitted diseases in conjunction with appropriate counseling.

KEY POINTS

• Ceftriaxone provides effective empiric therapy for patients with possible disseminated gonococcal infection.

• Fluoroquinolone resistance in patients with gonorrhea has been observed in the Pacific Rim and Hawaii.

Bibliography

1. **Centers for Disease Control and Prevention, Workowski KA, Berman SM.** Sexually transmitted diseases treatment guidelines, 2006. MMWR Recomm Rep. 2006;55(RR-11):1-94. Erratum in: MMWR Recomm Rep. 2006;55:997. [PMID: 16888612]

Item 25   Answer: C

This patient most likely has septic arthritis caused by *Staphylococcus aureus*. Gram-positive bacteria (staphylococci and streptococci) are the most common causes of nongonococcal septic arthritis in adults. *S. aureus* accounts for 37% to 65% of all cases, but the percentage is much higher (approximately 75%) in patients with underlying rheumatoid arthritis. Some series have suggested that more than 90% of patients with rheumatoid arthritis and septic arthritis have had *S. aureus* infection. Infection by the other pathogens listed is highly unlikely.

KEY POINTS

• Gram-positive bacteria (staphylococci and streptococci) are the most common causes of nongonococcal septic arthritis in adults.

• In some series, more than 90% of patients with rheumatoid arthritis and septic arthritis have had *S. aureus* infection.

Bibliography

1. **Kherani RB, Shojania K.** Septic arthritis in patients with pre-existing inflammatory arthritis. CMAJ. 2007;176:1605-8. [PMID: 17515588]

Item 26   Answer: C

Acute joint pain and fever should raise suspicion for septic arthritis and should be evaluated with joint aspiration and synovial fluid analysis and culture. Septic arthritis is an urgent problem; the longer it goes unrecognized, the greater the potential for permanent damage to the joint and risk for developing a chronic infection. Instrumentation of the genitourinary tract and recurrent genitourinary tract infections are risk factors for development of septic arthritis and vertebral osteomyelitis. Other potential contributors are diabetes mellitus, contiguous decubitus ulcers, and certain hardware or prosthetic joints. Radiographic evidence is usually delayed 7 to 10 days in the acute setting but should not delay diagnosis. Joint aspiration with culture is essential and may be combined with blood cultures. Analysis of synovial fluid from joint aspiration helps to differentiate from among hemarthrosis, gout, or calcium pyrophosphate deposition disease (pseudogout) as alternative diagnoses. This patient's condition should be treated as a medical emergency because of the potential for bone destruction.

Gonococcal arthritis is a sexually acquired infection presenting with a complex of symptoms, including polyarthralgia (at times migratory), tenosynovitis, arthritis, and rash, usually on extensor surfaces of the skin. It generally affects those at risk for other sexually transmitted diseases. This patient does not have other symptoms and is not at high risk for this infection. For patients at high risk, mucosal culture demonstrating infection with *Neisseria gonorrhoeae* may confirm the diagnosis, because synovial fluid and blood culture results are usually negative. Although rheumatologic disorders such as systemic lupus erythematosus and rheumatoid arthritis may present with hip pain, the constellation of a recent genitourinary tract procedure and acute pain and fever is more supportive of septic arthritis. Fever may complicate the diagnosis of autoimmune processes by confusing them with infection, but in a patient with recent instrumentation of his genitourinary tract, infection must be ruled out first. Bone scan is sensitive for defining osteoblastic activity in the bone but is not specific and will not differentiate between septic arthritis and other destructive bone processes.

KEY POINT

- Acute joint pain and fever should raise suspicion for septic arthritis.

Bibliography

1. **Margaretten ME, Kohlwes J, Moore D, Bent S**. Does this adult patient have septic arthritis? JAMA. 2007;297:1478-88. [PMID: 17405973]

Item 27   Answer: A

This patient needs a diagnostic arthrocentesis of the sternoclavicular joint. She has the classic findings associated with septic arthritis, including fever, joint pain, joint swelling, and a source of bacteremia (recent injection drug use). Septic arthritis is monoarticular in 80% to 90% of patients but can be polyarticular in 10% to 20%. Therefore, patients with acute or subacute arthritis, particularly monoarticular arthritis, should be assumed to have septic arthritis, and urgent analysis of the synovial fluid is necessary to confirm a diagnosis and select treatment. Sternoclavicular septic arthritis accounts for only 1% of bone and joint infections. Concurrent osteomyelitis is common, occurring in over 50% of patients. Men and injection drug users are mainly affected, and the infection usually has a subacute presentation. Septic arthritis of the sternoclavicular joint may be difficult to diagnose. This condition is often associated with infection of contiguous structures and occasionally results in unusual presentations. For example, septic sternoclavicular joint arthritis has been reported to manifest as a breast abscess.

Migratory arthralgia or arthritis settling in one inflamed joint and the presence of tenosynovitis (wrist or ankle) and/or typical dermatitis (tender necrotic pustules on an erythematous base, especially on the distal extremities) in a sexually active and healthy young adult suggests gonococcal arthritis. The diagnosis of gonococcal septic arthritis is confirmed by the isolation of microorganisms from the synovial fluid, blood, skin lesions, or urethral/cervical, rectal, or throat specimens. The patient's presentation involving a single axial joint is very unusual for gonococcal arthritis, and cultures are not indicated at this point. Joint imaging is helpful to establish the baseline status of the joint, pre-existing arthritis, soft tissue calcification, chondrocalcinosis, foreign body, primary bone tumor, fracture, abscess, metastatic bone lesion, or evidence of loosening of a total joint replacement. Changes seen on imaging of the joint and bone damage due to infection are relatively late findings. In acute septic arthritis, soft tissue fullness and joint effusions are often the only initial findings. Bone scans are more sensitive for detecting inflammatory lesions in bones and joints but are not specific for infection. MRI of the affected joint is especially useful in detecting avascular necrosis, soft tissue masses, and collections of fluid not detectable by other imaging modalities, but no imaging procedure replaces synovial fluid analysis and culture as the gold standard for diagnosis and guide to antimicrobial therapy. Empiric antimicrobial therapy is not initiated; the diagnosis must be established by arthrocentesis and all cultures (blood, joint, and potential sites of extra-articular infection) should be obtained.

KEY POINTS

- Septic arthritis is monoarticular in 80% to 90% of patients but can affect more than one joint in 10% to 20%.

- Arthrocentesis and joint fluid analysis are needed in all patients with acute, particularly monoarticular, arthritis.

Bibliography

1. **Gupta MN, Sturrock RD, Field M.** A prospective 2-year study of 75 patients with adult-onset septic arthritis. Rheumatology (Oxford). 2001;40:24-30. [PMID: 11157138]

Item 28   Answer: A

Intravenous antibiotics and adequate joint drainage are indicated for this patient, who likely has a "closed-space" infection. Until a diagnosis of infection is excluded, treatment for septic arthritis should be administered in a patient with acute inflammatory monoarticular arthritis, particularly if there is a neutrophil predominance in the synovial fluid. Drainage with needle aspiration is possible in most peripheral joints and may need to be performed daily. If adequate drainage cannot be achieved, arthroscopic or open drainage is indicated. A delay in recognizing and initiating therapy for septic arthritis may cause future joint dysfunction.

If crystals are not seen on polarized light microscopy, crystal-induced arthritis is highly unlikely, even in the setting of a family history of gout. Therefore, nonsteroidal anti-inflammatory drug therapy is not indicated. Moreover, although these agents have not been shown to worsen the course of septic arthritis, they may decrease the inflammatory response and falsely imply that a patient is responding to antibiotics or that a patient's condition is self-limited. Oral antibiotics are not appropriate in a closed-space infection, such as nongonococcal septic arthritis, because these conditions may rapidly lead to joint destruction. Radiography of an acutely inflamed joint usually does not reveal the cause of the inflammatory response.

KEY POINT

- Treat acute inflammatory monoarthritis with antibiotics until an alternative diagnosis is definitively established or infection is excluded.

Bibliography

1. Margaretten ME, Kohlwes J, Moore D, Bent S. Does this adult patient have septic arthritis? JAMA. 2007;297:1478-88. [PMID: 17405973]

Item 29   Answer: A

This patient has aggressive new-onset diffuse cutaneous systemic sclerosis with extensive skin involvement. A diagnosis of systemic sclerosis is established in patients with thickening of the skin involving the fingers or sclerodactyly that extends beyond the proximal metacarpophalangeal joints. Diagnosis may also be established if patients present with two of the following features: sclerodactyly, digital pitting, and basilar fibrosis on chest radiograph. Systemic sclerosis is classified according to the degree of skin involvement. Patients with systemic sclerosis with limited skin involvement, CREST syndrome (calcinosis, Raynaud's phenomenon, esophageal dysmotility, sclerodactyly, and telangiectasias) present with skin thickening distal to the elbows and knees. Conversely, systemic sclerosis with diffuse cutaneous involvement is associated with skin thickening proximal to the elbows and knees. Both diffuse and limited systemic sclerosis may involve the face. This patient has skin thickening involving the arms, chest, and abdomen, in addition to the extremities, and therefore has diffuse systemic sclerosis.

Skin thickening is not a manifestation of systemic lupus erythematosus. Mixed connective tissue disease is a connective tissue disorder characterized by the presence of high-titer anti-ribonucleoprotein antibodies in combination with clinical features commonly seen in patients with systemic lupus erythematosus, systemic sclerosis, and polymyositis. Most patients have skin involvement, typically Raynaud's phenomenon. Swollen digits and total hand edema are also distinctive features. However, patients with mixed connective tissue disease do not have skin thickening involving the chest, abdomen, or arms.

KEY POINTS

- Systemic sclerosis is classified according to the degree of skin involvement.

- Limited systemic sclerosis presents with skin thickening distal to the elbows and knees; diffuse systemic sclerosis is associated with skin thickening proximal to the elbows and knees.

Bibliography

1. Wollheim FA. Classification of systemic sclerosis. Visions and reality. Rheumatology (Oxford). 2005;44:1212-6. [PMID: 15870151]

Item 30   Answer: E

This patient may have systemic lupus erythematosus (SLE). The approach to patients with joint complaints is based on recognizing the pattern of joints involved and extra-articular manifestations characteristic of the individual arthropathies. This patient has a symmetric polyarthritis involving her wrists, metacarpophalangeal joints, elbows, and knees. Additionally, she has a rash, a mucosal ulcer, and constitutional symptoms. Rheumatologic syndromes compatible with this clinical presentation include SLE, rheumatoid arthritis, and viral infection. Tests to differentiate these entities include a complete blood count; urinalysis; and assays for anti-cyclic citrullinated peptide antibodies (anti-CCP), rheumatoid factor, and antinuclear antibodies.

Behçet's disease is a multisystem inflammatory condition that is prevalent in persons of Asian and Eastern Mediterranean descent. This condition is characterized by recurrent aphthous oral ulcers and at least two of the following features: recurrent genital ulcers, inflammatory eye disease, cutaneous lesions, and positive findings on pathergy test (development of an erythematous papular or pustular lesion >5 mm 24 to 48 hours after skin prick by a needle). Although this patient has an oral ulcer, she has no other findings to support the diagnosis of Behçet's disease.

Manifestations of disseminated gonococcal infection in women may include tenosynovitis, oligoarthritis, and dermatitis. A finding of acute nontraumatic monoarticular arthritis, particularly in a sexually active young woman, should prompt consideration of disseminated gonococcal arthritis. However, this patient has a several-month history of symmetric polyarthritis, making disseminated gonococcal arthritis unlikely.

Fibromyalgia is thought to represent pain related to stress and depression, the misperception of pain, or abnormal pain signals. Fibromyalgia is not associated with objective findings such as mucosal ulcers, synovitis, or rash, making this diagnosis unlikely.

Reactive arthritis can be precipitated by infection with one of several different organisms, including *Chlamydia*, *Escherichia coli*, *Salmonella*, *Campylobacter*, and *Yersinia*. Common clinical manifestations include urethritis, conjunctivitis, keratoderma blennorrhagica (a rash similar to psoriasis) on the palms or soles, and arthritis. Heel pain with enthesitis is a common presentation. In reactive arthritis, unlike SLE, the arthritis is typically oligoarticular and asymmetric and is found more commonly in the lower extremities than in the upper extremities.

- The approach to patients with joint complaints is based on recognizing the pattern of joints involved and extra-articular manifestations characteristic of the individual arthropathies.

- Symmetric polyarthritis, rash, mucosal ulcer, and constitutional symptoms are compatible with systemic lupus erythematosus, rheumatoid arthritis, and viral infections.

Bibliography
1. **D'Cruz DP**. Systemic lupus erythematosus. BMJ. 2006;332:890-4. [PMID: 16613963]

Item 31   Answer: B

This patient most likely has systemic lupus erythematosus (SLE), as manifested by the characteristic malar rash, symmetric nondeforming synovitis, and pancytopenia and past history consistent with serositis (pleurisy). The diagnosis of SLE is guided by the presence of 11 SLE classification criteria, which can be remembered by the mnemonic SOAP BRAIN MD: *S*erositis (pleuritis, pericarditis); *O*ral or nasopharyngeal ulcerations (painless); *A*rthritis (nonerosive) involving more than two peripheral joints with synovitis; *P*hotosensitivity; *B*lood dyscrasias (Coombs'-positive hemolytic anemia with reticulocytosis or leukopenia <4000/µL on more than two occasions, or lymphopenia <1500/µL on two occasions, or thrombocytopenia < 100,000/µL); *R*enal disease (persistent proteinuria >500 mg/day or cellular casts in the absence of infection); *A*ntinuclear antibody (titer of >1:80); *I*mmunologic disorder (anti–double-stranded DNA antibody, anti-Smith antibody, antiphospholipid antibody, positive lupus anticoagulant, or false-positive rapid plasma reagin [RPR] or VDRL test); *N*eurologic disorder (seizures or psychosis); *M*alar rash; *D*iscoid rash (erythematous raised patches with scaling and follicular plugging).

Antinuclear antibody (ANA) is classically associated with SLE; 95% of all patients with SLE have a positive ANA at a titer ≥1:80. However, ANA is not specific for SLE and is detected in many patients with infection, malignancy, liver disease, other autoimmune diseases, and up to 10% to 15% of the normal population. Anti–double-stranded DNA antibody (also known as the anti–native DNA antibody) is found in less than 50% of patients with SLE but is considered highly specific; a positive test in a patient with a high pretest probability of SLE helps confirm the diagnosis.

The presence of an elevated erythrocyte sedimentation rate and C-reactive protein levels only reflects acute inflammation caused by viral and bacterial infection, malignancy, and all autoimmune diseases and does not help with this patient's diagnosis.

Patients with SLE can produce multiple autoantibodies, including rheumatoid factor; therefore, a positive rheumatoid factor does not distinguish between rheumatoid arthritis and SLE. The anti–cyclic citrullinated peptide antibody is specific for rheumatoid arthritis, and its presence is strong evidence for rheumatoid arthritis; however, its absence does not confirm the presence of SLE.

Elevated uric acid concentration and the presence of HL-B27 are not helpful because these laboratory abnormalities are not associated with SLE.

- Anti–double-stranded DNA antibody is highly specific for systemic lupus erythematosus; a positive test in a patient with a high pretest probability helps confirm the diagnosis.

Bibliography
1. **D'Cruz DP**. Systemic lupus erythematosus. BMJ. 2006;332:890-4. [PMID: 16613963]

Item 32   Answer: C

This patient most likely has giant cell arteritis, which is characterized by inflammation involving the extracranial branches of the carotid artery and typically affects the elderly population. Clinical manifestations of this condition include headaches, optic nerve ischemia, and accompanying polymyalgia rheumatica. Additional features that may occur in giant cell arteritis are scalp tenderness, carotidynia, and jaw claudication. Although most patients with giant cell arteritis have an elevated erythrocyte sedimentation rate, as does this patient, this rate is low or normal in 10% to 24% of patients.

This patient does not have muscle weakness or elevated levels of creatine kinase; therefore, she does not have polymyositis. Carotid artery dissection can be associated with ipsilateral head pain in one or more of the following areas: orbit, forehead, and side of the head. The pain of carotid artery dissection is acute and severe and can be associated with ischemic stroke, but it does not cause muscle stiffness or scalp tenderness and is an unlikely diagnosis in this patient.

- Clinical manifestations of giant cell arteritis include headaches, optic nerve ischemia, and accompanying polymyalgia rheumatica.

Bibliography
1. **Unwin B, Williams CM, Gilliland W.** Polymyalgia rheumatica and giant cell arteritis. Am Fam Physician. 2006;74:1547-54. [PMID: 17111894]

Item 33   Answer: E

Multiple mononeuropathies, as seen in this patient with involvement of the right radial and left peroneal nerves, most commonly occur in patients with diabetes mellitus and vasculitis. Vasculitic neuropathies (mononeuritis multiplex) typically present with the acute onset of asymmetrical weakness and sensory loss associated with severe pain. Multiple mononeuropathies have been reported in patients with systemic lupus erythematosus, polyarteritis nodosa, leprosy, sarcoidosis, amyloidosis, and a genetic disease known as hereditary neuropathy with predisposition to pressure palsies

(HNPP) but have not been described in association with Lyme disease.

Although Guillain–Barré syndrome and toxic neuropathies may present acutely, the distribution of weakness and sensory loss is usually symmetrical. Motor neuron disease can present with asymmetrical weakness but is not associated with pain or sensory symptoms and muscle fasciculations are typically present.

KEY POINT

- Peripheral nervous system vasculitis usually presents with asymmetrical weakness and sensory loss in specific nerve distributions.

Bibliography

1. **Younger DS**. Vasculitis of the nervous system. Curr Opin Neurol. 2004;17:317-36. [PMID: 15167068]

Item 34   Answer: B

This patient most likely has polymyalgia rheumatica. This diagnosis is supported by the history of pain and morning stiffness in the axial joints and proximal muscles and the absence of marked muscle weakness and joint swelling, pain, warmth, or restricted movement. Patients with polymyalgia rheumatica are typically >50 years of age, and approximately 90% of these patients have an erythrocyte sedimentation rate elevated above the age-adjusted normal range.

A diagnosis of rheumatoid arthritis is less likely because this patient has no findings consistent with an inflammatory arthritis. Findings suggestive of rheumatoid arthritis include symmetrical pain, swelling, tenderness, and stiffness involving the small joints of the hands and feet, as well as morning stiffness of these joints. Occasionally, rheumatoid arthritis of the elderly may initially appear similar to acute polymyalgia rheumatica. Polymyositis is unlikely because proximal muscle weakness predominates in inflammatory muscle disease. Conversely, pain and stiffness, which this patient has, predominate in polymyalgia rheumatica. This patient does not have an elevated creatine kinase level, which is a typical finding in polymyositis.

A history of fatigue and poor sleep habits in the absence of obvious synovitis or joint deformity, as well as multiple characteristic tender points, suggests a diagnosis of fibromyalgia. However, this patient has no other tender points associated with this condition, and fibromyalgia would not cause an elevated erythrocyte sedimentation rate or characteristic proximal localized morning stiffness and pain.

KEY POINT

- Polymyalgia rheumatica is characterized by a history of pain and morning stiffness in the axial joints and proximal muscles, no evidence of joint inflammation or muscle weakness, and an elevated erythrocyte sedimentation rate.

Bibliography

1. **Mandell BF**. Polymyalgia rheumatica: clinical presentation is key to diagnosis and treatment. Cleve Clin J Med. 2004;71:489-95. [PMID: 15242304]

Item 35   Answer: D

This patient most likely has polymyalgia rheumatica (PMR), and treatment with prednisone is indicated. This condition typically develops in patients >50 years of age, manifests as proximal pain, sometimes is accompanied by a sense of weakness of the upper and lower extremities, and usually is associated with an elevated erythrocyte sedimentation rate. Higher doses of prednisone or a corticosteroid equivalent are indicated if features of giant cell arteritis, such as headache, disturbance in vision, jaw claudication, or neck pain (carotidynia), are present. However, these symptoms are absent in this patient. Corticosteroid therapy often resolves symptoms of PMR and giant cell arteritis within 24 hours and 1 week, respectively. A population-based, long-term observational study of 232 patients diagnosed with PMR showed that, of 175 patients treated with corticosteroids, the mean duration of therapy was 2.4 years at an average dose of 9.6 mg/d.

Methotrexate is beneficial in patients with inflammatory arthritis, such as rheumatoid arthritis, but is not indicated in a patient without signs of synovitis on examination. Methotrexate also may be used as a steroid-sparing agent later in the course of certain inflammatory diseases but is not required in the treatment of PMR and may not be effective in giant cell arteritis. Etanercept is approved for the management of rheumatoid and psoriatic arthritis. However, this patient's lack of peripheral synovitis involving the small joints excludes these conditions. Hydroxychloroquine is an immunomodulator commonly used to treat arthritis and photosensitivity related to systemic lupus erythematosus and milder arthritis in patients with rheumatoid arthritis but is not beneficial for PMR or giant cell arteritis.

KEY POINT

- Corticosteroid therapy often resolves polymyalgia rheumatica symptoms within 24 hours.

Bibliography

1. **Spiera R, Spiera H**. Inflammatory diseases in older adults: polymyalgia rheumatica. Geriatrics. 2004;59:39-43. [PMID: 15615159]

NORMAL LABORATORY VALUES
MKSAP® for Students 4

U.S. traditional units are followed in parentheses by equivalent values expressed in S.I. units.

Blood, Plasma, and Serum Chemistries

Acetoacetate, plasma — Less than 1 mg/dL (0.1 mmol/L)
Alpha-fetoprotein, serum — 0-20 ng/mL (0-20 µg/L)
Aminotransferase, alanine (ALT, SGPT) — 0-35 U/L
Aminotransferase, aspartate (AST, SGOT) — 0-35 U/L
Ammonia, plasma — 40-80 µg/dL (23-47 µmol/L)
Amylase, serum — 0-130 U/L
Antistreptolysin O titer — Less than 150 units
Ascorbic acid (vitamin C), blood — 0.4-1.5 mg/dL (23-86 µmol/L); leukocyte — less than 20 mg/dL (< 3.5 µmol/L)
Bicarbonate, serum — 23-28 meq/L (23-28 mmol/L)
Bilirubin, serum
  Total — 0.3-1.2 mg/dL (5.1-20.5 µmol/L)
  Direct — 0-0.3 mg/dL (0-5.1 µmol/L)
Blood gases, arterial (room air)
  P_{O_2} - 80-100 mm Hg
  P_{CO_2} - 35-45 mm Hg
  pH - 7.38-7.44
Calcium, serum — 9-10.5 mg/dL (2.2-2.6 mmol/L)
Carbon dioxide content, serum — 23-28 meq/L (23-28 mmol/L)
Carcinoembryonic antigen — Less than 2 ng/mL (2 µg/L)
Carotene, serum — 75-300 µg/dL (1.4-5.6 µmol/L)
Ceruloplasmin, serum — 25-43 mg/dL (250-430 mg/L)
Chloride, serum — 98-106 meq/L (98-106 mmol/L)
Cholesterol, total, plasma — 150-199 mg/dL (3.88-5.15 mmol/L), desirable
Cholesterol, low-density lipoprotein (LDL), plasma — Less than or equal to 130 mg/dL (3.36 mmol/L), desirable
Cholesterol, high-density lipoprotein (HDL), plasma — Greater than or equal to 40 mg/dL (1.04 mmol/L), desirable
Complement, serum
  C3 - 55-120 mg/dL (550-1200 mg/L)
  Total - 37-55 U/mL (37-55 kU/L)
Copper, serum — 70-155 µg/dL (11-24.3 µmol/L)
Creatine kinase, serum — 30-170 U/L
Creatinine, serum — 0.7-1.3 mg/dL (61.9-115 µmol/L)
Delta-aminolevulinic acid, serum — 15-23 µg/dL (1.14-1.75 µmol/L)
Ethanol, blood — less than 50 mg/dL (11 nmol/L)
Fibrinogen, plasma — 150-350 mg/dL (1.5-3.5 g/L)
Folate, red cell — 160-855 ng/mL (362-1937 nmol/L)
Folate, serum — 2.5-20 ng/mL (5.7-45.3 nmol/L)
Glucose, plasma — Fasting, 70-105 mg/dL (3.9-5.8 mmol/L); 2 hours postprandial less than 140 mg/dL (7.8 mmol/L)
Homocysteine, plasma — Male: 4-16 µmol/L; female: 3-14 µmol/L
Immunoglobulins
  IgG - 640-1430 mg/dL (6.4-14.3 g/L)
    IgG_1 - 280-1020 mg/dL (2.8-10.2 g/L)
    IgG_2 - 60-790 mg/dL (0.6-7.9 g/L)
    IgG_3 - 14-240 mg/dL (0.14-2.4 g/L)
    IgG_4 - 11-330 mg/dL (0.11-3.3 g/L)
  IgA - 70-300 mg/dL (0.7-3.0 g/L)
  IgM - 20-140 mg/dL (0.2-1.4 g/L)
  IgD - Less than 8 mg/dL (80 mg/L)
  IgE - 0.01-0.04 mg/dL (0.1-0.4 mg/L)
Iron, serum — 60-160 µg/dL (11-29 µmol/L)
Iron binding capacity, serum — 250-460 µg/dL (45-82 µmol/L)
Lactate dehydrogenase, serum — 60-100 U/L
Lactic acid, venous blood — 6-16 mg/dL (0.67-1.8 mmol/L)
Lead, blood — Less than 40 µg/dL (1.9 µmol/L)
Lipase, serum — Less than 95 U/L
Magnesium, serum — 1.5-2.4 mg/dL (0.62-0.99 mmol/L)
Manganese, serum — 0.3-0.9 ng/mL (300-900 ng/L)
Methylmalonic acid, serum — 150-370 nmol/L
Osmolality, plasma — 275-295 mosm/kg H_2O
Phosphatase, acid, serum — 0.5-5.5 U/L
Phosphatase, alkaline, serum — 36-92 U/L
Phosphorus, inorganic, serum — 3-4.5 mg/dL (0.97-1.45 mmol/L)

Potassium, serum — 3.5-5 meq/L (3.5-5 mmol/L)
Protein, serum
  Total – 6.0-7.8 g/dL (60-78 g/L)
  Albumin - 3.5-5.5 g/dL (35-55 g/L)
  Globulins - 2.5-3.5 g/dL (25-35 g/L)
    $Alpha_1$ - 0.2-0.4 g/dL (2-4 g/L)
    $Alpha_2$ - 0.5-0.9 g/dL (5-9 g/L)
    Beta - 0.6-1.1 g/dL (6-11 g/L)
    Gamma - 0.7-1.7 g/dL (7-17 g/L)
Rheumatoid factor — less than 40 U/mL (less than 40 kU/L)
Sodium, serum — 136-145 meq/L (136-145 mmol/L)
Triglycerides — Less than 250 mg/dL (2.82 mmol/L), desirable
Urea nitrogen, serum — 8-20 mg/dL (2.9-7.1 mmol/L)
Uric acid, serum — 2.5-8 mg/dL (0.15-0.47 mmol/L)
Vitamin B_{12}, serum — 200-800 pg/mL (148-590 pmol/L)

Cerebrospinal Fluid

Cell count — 0-5 cells/µL ($0-5 \times 10^6$ cells/L)
Glucose — 40-80 mg/dL (2.5-4.4 mmol/L); less than 40% of simultaneous plasma concentration is abnormal
Protein — 15-60 mg/dL (150-600 mg/L)
Pressure (opening) — 70-200 cm H_2O

Endocrine

Adrenocorticotropin (ACTH) — 9-52 pg/mL (2-11 pmol/L)
Aldosterone, serum
  Supine - 2-5 ng/dL (55-138 pmol/L)
  Standing - 7-20 ng/dL (194-554 pmol/L)
Aldosterone, urine — 5-19 µg/24 h (13.9-52.6 nmol/24 h)
Catecholamines — Epinephrine (supine): less than 75 ng/L (410 pmol/L); norepinephrine (supine): 50-440 ng/L (296-2600 pmol/L)
Catecholamines, 24-hour, urine — Less than 100 µg/m² per 24 h (591 nmol/m² per 24 h)
Cortisol
  Serum - 8 am: 8-20 µg/dL (221-552 nmol/L); 5 pm: 3-13 µg/dL (83-359 nmol/L);
  1 h after cosyntropin; greater than 18 µg/dL (498 nmol/L); usually 8 µg/dL (221 nmol/L) or more above baseline overnight suppression test: less than 5 µg/dL (138 nmol/L)
  Urine free cortisol - less than 90 µg/24 h (248 nmol/24 h)
Dehydroepiandrosterone sulfate, plasma — Male: 1.3-5.5 mg/mL (3.5-14.9 µmol/L); female: 0.6-3.3 mg/mL (1.6-8.9 µmol/L)
11-deoxycortisol, plasma — Basal: less than 5 µg/dL (145 nmol/L); after metyrapone: greater than 7 µg/dL (203 nmol/L)
Estradiol, serum — Male: 10-30 pg/mL (37-110 pmol/L); female: day 1-10, 50-100 pmol/L; day 11-20, 50-200 pmol/L; day 21-30, 70-150 pmol/L
Estriol, urine — Greater than 12 mg/24 h (42 µmol/d)
Follicle-stimulating hormone, serum — Male (adult): 5-15 mU/mL (5-15 U/L); female: follicular or luteal phase, 5-20 mU/mL (5-20 U/L); midcycle peak, 30-50 mU/mL (30-50 U/L); postmenopausal, greater than 35 mU/mL (35 U/L)
Growth hormone, plasma — After oral glucose, less than 2 ng/mL (2 µg/L); response to provocative stimuli: greater than 7 ng/mL (7 µg/L)
17-hydroxycorticosteroids, urine (Porter-Silber) — Male: 3-10 mg/24 h (8.3-28 µmol/24 h); female: 2-8 mg/24 h (5.5-22.1 µmol/24 h)
Insulin, serum (fasting) — 5-20 mU/L (35-139 pmol/L)
17-ketosteroids, urine — Male: 8-22 mg/24 h (28-77 µmol/24 h); female: up to 15 µg/24 h (52 mmol/24 h)
Luteinizing hormone, serum — Male: 3-15 mU/mL (3-15 U/L); female: follicular or luteal phase, 5-22 mU/mL (5-22 U/L); midcycle peak, 30-250 mU/mL (30-250 U/L); postmenopausal, greater than 30 mU/mL (30 U/L)

Metanephrine, urine — Less than 1.2 mg/24 h (6.1 mmol/24 h)
Parathyroid hormone, serum — 10-65 pg/mL (10-65 ng/L)
Progesterone
    Luteal — 3-30 ng/mL (0.1-0.95 nmol/L)
    Follicular — less than 1 ng/mL (0.03-nmol/L)
Prolactin, serum — Male: less than 15 ng/mL (15 mg/L); female: less than 20 ng/mL (20 mg/L)
Renin activity (angiotensin-I radioimmunoassay), plasma
    Normal diet: supine, 0.3-1.9 ng/mL per h (0.3-1.9 µg/L per h); upright, 0.2-3.6 ng/mL per h (0.2-3.6 µg/L per h)
Sperm concentration — 20-150 million/mL (20-50 × 10^9/L)
Sweat test for sodium and chloride — Less than 60 meq/L (60 mmol/L)
Testosterone, serum — Adult male: 300-1200 ng/dL (10-42 nmol/L); female: 20-75 ng/dL (0.7-2.6 nmol/L)
Thyroid function tests (normal ranges vary)
    Thyroid iodine (^{131}I) uptake - 10% to 30% of administered dose at 24 h
    Thyroid-stimulating hormone (TSH) - 0.5-5.0 µU/mL (0.5-5.0 mU/mL)
    Thyroxine (T_4), serum
        Total - 5-12 µg/dL (64-155 nmol/L)
        Free - 0.9-2.4 ng/dL (12-31 pmol/L)
        Free T_4 index - 4-11
    Triiodothyronine, resin (T_3) - 25%-35%
    Triiodothyronine, serum (T_3) - 70-195 ng/dL (1.1-3.0 nmol/L)
Vanillylmandelic acid, urine — Less than 8 mg/24 h (40.4 µmol/24 h)
Vitamin D
    1,25-dihydroxy, serum - 25-65 pg/mL (60-156 pmol/L)
    25-hydroxy, serum - 15-80 ng/mL (37-200 nmol/L)

Gastrointestinal

D-xylose absorption (after ingestion of 25 g of D-xylose) — Urine excretion: 5-8 g at 5 h (33-53 mmol); serum D-xylose: greater than 20 mg/dL at 2 h (1.3 nmol/L)
Fecal urobilinogen — 40-280 mg/24 h (68-473 µmol/ 24 h)
Gastric secretion — Basal secretion: male: 4.0 ± 0.2 meq of HCl/h (4.0 ± 0.2 mmol/h); female: 2.1 ± 0.2 meq of HCl/h (2.1 ± 0.2 mmol/h); peak acid secretion: male: 37.4 ± 0.8 meq/h (37.4 ± 0.8 mmol/h); female: 24.9 ± 1.0 meq/h (24.9 ± 1.0 mmol/h)
Gastrin, serum — 0-180 pg/mL (0-180 ng/L)
Lactose tolerance test — Increase in plasma glucose: greater than 15 mg/dL (0.83 mmol/L)
Lipase, ascitic fluid — Less than 200 U/L
Secretin-cholecystokinin pancreatic function — Greater than 80 meq/L (80 mmol/L) of HCO_3 in at least 1 specimen collected over 1 h
Stool fat — Less than 5 g/d on a 100-g fat diet
Stool nitrogen — Less than 2 g/d
Stool weight — Less than 200 g/d

Hematology

Activated partial thromboplastin time — 25-35 s
Bleeding time — Less than 10 min
Coagulation factors, plasma
    Factor I - 150-350 mg/dL (1.5-3.5 g/L)
    Factor II - 60%-150% of normal
    Factor V - 60%-150% of normal
    Factor VII - 60%-150% of normal
    Factor VIII - 60%-150% of normal
    Factor IX - 60%-150% of normal
    Factor X - 60%-150% of normal
    Factor XI - 60%-150% of normal
    Factor XII - 60%-150% of normal
Erythrocyte count — 4.2-5.9 million cells/µL (4.2-5.9 x 10^{12} cells/L)
Erythrocyte survival rate (^{51}Cr) — T½ = 28 days
Erythropoietin — less than 30 mU/mL (30 U/L)
D-dimer — less than 0.5 µg/mL (500 mg/L)
Ferritin, serum — 15-200 ng/mL (15-200 mg/L)
Glucose-6-phosphate dehydrogenase, blood — 5-15 U/g Hgb (0.32-0.97 mU/mol Hgb)

Haptoglobin, serum — 50-150 mg/dL (500-1500 mg/L)
Hematocrit — Male: 41%-51%; female: 36%-47%
Hemoglobin, blood — Male: 14-17 g/dL (140-170 g/L); female: 12-16 g/dL (120-160 g/L)
Hemoglobin, plasma — 0.5-5 mg/dL (0.08-0.8 µmol/L)
Leukocyte alkaline phosphatase — 15-40 mg of phosphorus liberated/h per 10^{10} cells; score = 13-130/100 polymorphonuclear neutrophils and band forms
Leukocyte count — Nonblacks: 4000-10,000/µL (4.0-10 × 10^9/L); Blacks: 3500-10,000/µL (3.5-10 x 10^9/L)
Lymphocytes
    CD4$^+$ cell count — 640-1175/µL (0.64-1.18 × 10^9/L)
    CD8$^+$ cell count — 335-875/µL (0.34-0.88 × 10^9/L)
    CD4: CD8 ratio — 1.0-4.0
Mean corpuscular hemoglobin (MCH) — 28-32 pg
Mean corpuscular hemoglobin concentration (MCHC) — 32-36 g/dL (320-360 g/L)
Mean corpuscular volume (MCV) — 80-100 fL
Osmotic fragility of erythrocytes — Increased if hemolysis occurs in over 0.5% NaCl, decreased if hemolysis is incomplete in 0.3% NaCl
Platelet count — 150,000-350,000/µL (150-350 × 10^9/L)
Platelet life span (^{51}Cr) — 8-12 days
Protein C activity, plasma — 67%-131%
Protein C resistance — 2.2-2.6
Protein S activity, plasma — 82%-144%
Prothrombin time — 11-13 s
Reticulocyte count — 0.5%-1.5% of erythrocytes; absolute: 23,000-90,000 cells/µL (23-90 × 10^9/L)
Schilling test (oral administration of radioactive cobalamin-labeled vitamin B_{12}) — 8.5%-28% excreted in urine per 24-48 h
Sedimentation rate, erythrocyte (Westergren) — Male: 0-15 mm/h; female: 0-20 mm/h
Volume, blood
    Plasma - Male: 25-44 mL/kg (0.025-0.044 L/kg) body weight; female: 28-43 mL/kg (0.028-0.043 L/kg) body weight
    Erythrocyte - Male: 25-35 mL/kg (0.025-0.044 L/kg) body weight; female: 20-30 mL/kg (0.020-0.030 L/kg) body weight

Pulmonary

Forced expiratory volume in 1 second (FEV$_1$) — Greater than 80% predicted
Forced vital capacity (FVC) — Greater than 80% predicted
FEV$_1$/FVC — Greater than 75% (0.75)

Urine

Amino acids — 200-400 mg/24 h (14-29 nmol/24 h)
Amylase — 6.5-48.1 U/h
Calcium — 100-300 mg/d (2.5-7.5 mmol/d) on unrestricted diet
Chloride — 80-250 meq/d (80-250 mmol/d) (varies with intake)
Copper — 0-100 µg/24 h (0-1.6 µmol/d)
Coproporphyrin — 50-250 µg/24 h (76-382 nmol/d)
Creatine — Male: 4-40 mg/24 h (30-305 mmol/24 h); female: 0-100 mg/24 h (0-763 mmol/24 h)
Creatinine — 15-25 mg/kg per 24 h (133-221 mmol/kg per 24 h)
Creatinine clearance — 90-140 mL/min (0.09-0.14 l/min)
5-hydroxyindoleacetic acid (5-HIAA) — 2-9 mg/24 h (10.4-46.8 µmol/d)
Osmolality — 38-1400 mosm/kg H_2O
Phosphate, tubular resorption — 79%-94% (0.79-0.94) of filtered load
Potassium — 25-100 meq/24 h (25-100 mmol/24 h) (varies with intake)
Protein — Less than 100 mg/24 h
Sodium — 100-260 meq/24 h (100-260 mmol/24 h) (varies with intake)
Uric acid — 250-750 mg/24 h (1.48-4.43 mmol/24 h) (varies with diet)
Urobilinogen — 0.05-2.5 mg/24 h (0.08-4.22 µmol/24 h)

American College of Physicians
190 N. Independence Mall West, Philadelphia, PA 19106-1572

Color Plates

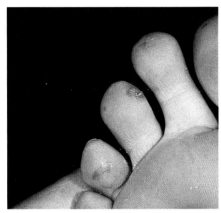

Figure 1
Cardiovascular Medicine 1

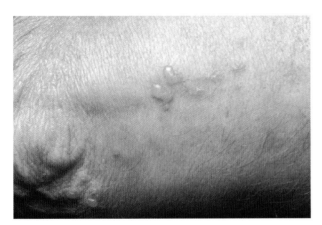

Figure 2
Gastroenterology and Hepatology 18

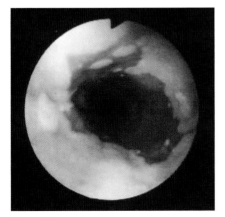

Figure 3
Gastroenterology and Hepatology 30

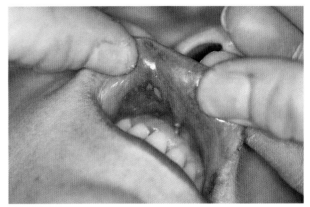

Figure 4
General Internal Medicine 46

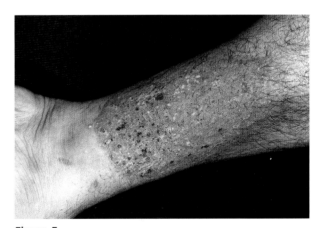

Figure 5
General Internal Medicine 47

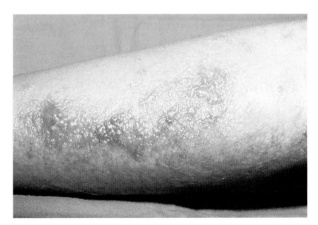

Figure 6
General Internal Medicine 49

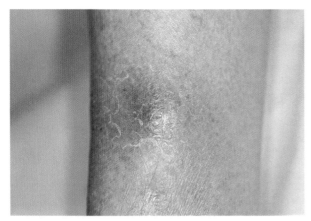

Figure 7
General Internal Medicine 50

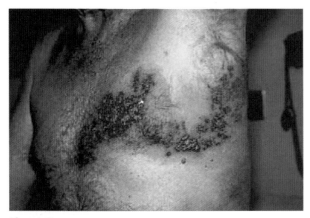

Figure 8
General Internal Medicine 51

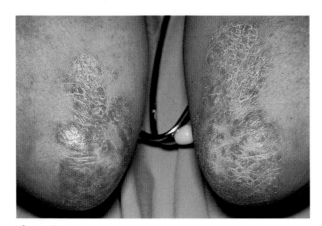

Figure 9
General Internal Medicine 53

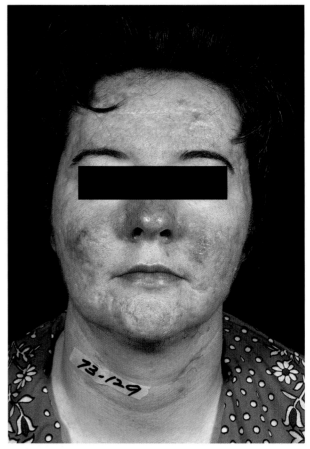

Figure 10
General Internal Medicine 54

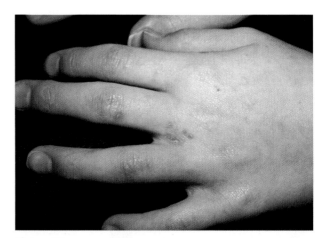

Figure 11
General Internal Medicine 55

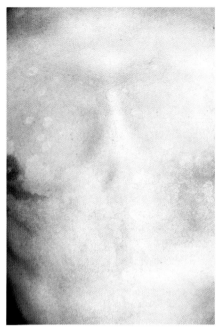

Figure 12
General Internal Medicine 56

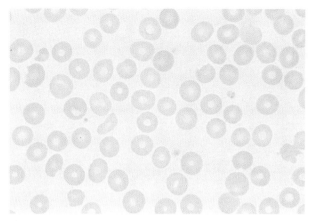

Figure 15
Hematology 06

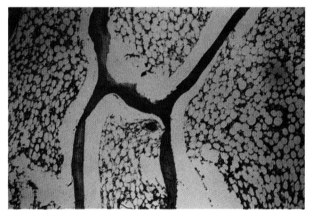

Figure 13
Hematology 03

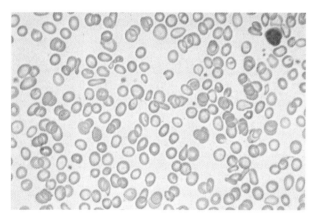

Figure 16
Hematology 07

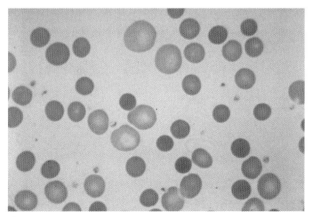

Figure 14
Hematology 04

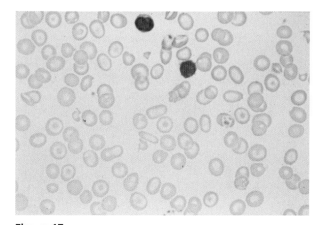

Figure 17
Hematology 08

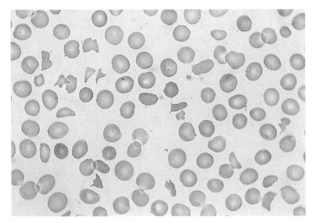

Figure 18
Hematology 22

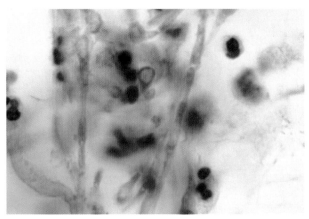

Figure 21
Infectious Disease Medicine 03

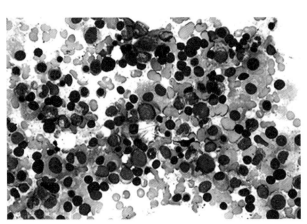

Figure 19
Hematology 28

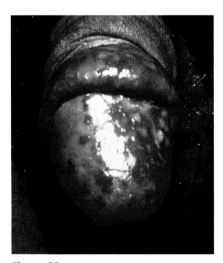

Figure 22
Infectious Disease Medicine 14

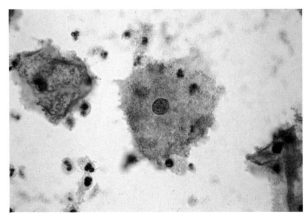

Figure 20
Infectious Disease Medicine 02

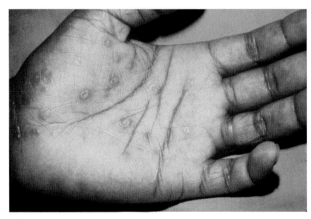

Figure 23
Infectious Disease Medicine 16

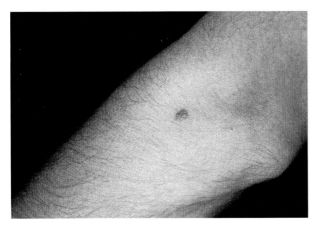

Figure 24
Infectious Disease Medicine 20

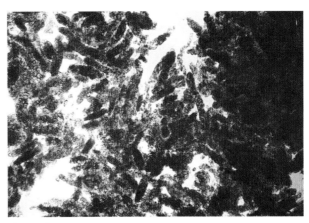

Figure 27
Nephrology 08

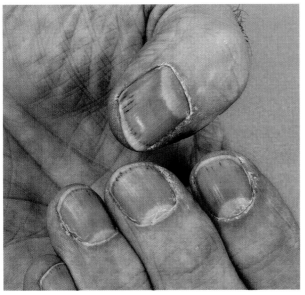

Figure 25
Infectious Disease Medicine 44

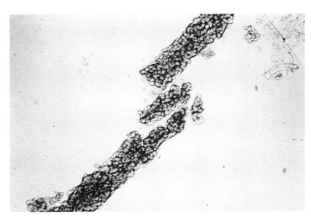

Figure 28
Nephrology 09

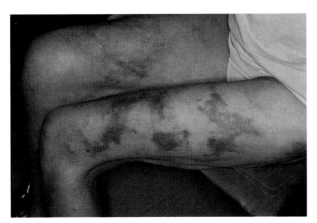

Figure 26
Nephrology 03

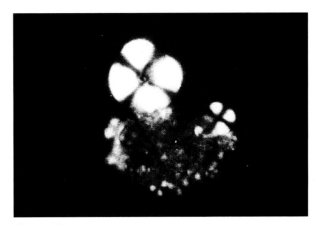

Figure 29
Nephrology 15

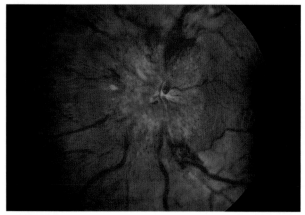

Figure 30
Neurology 09

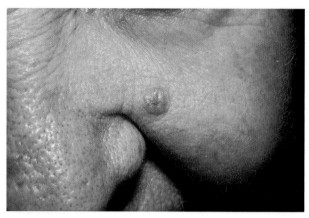

Figure 32
Oncology 23

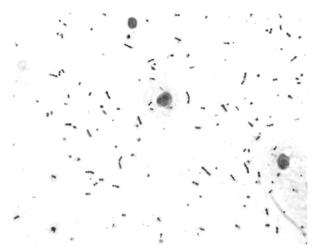

Figure 31
Neurology 17

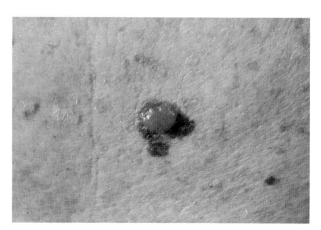

Figure 33
Oncology 24

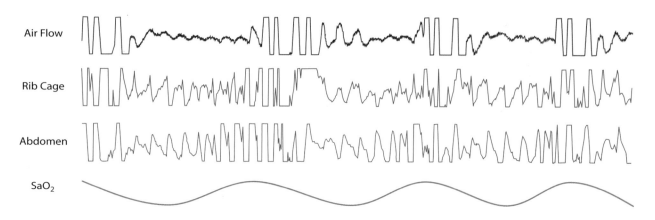

Figure 34
Pulmonary Medicine 25

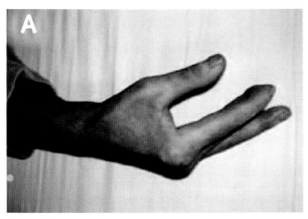

Figure 35
Pulmonary Medicine 27

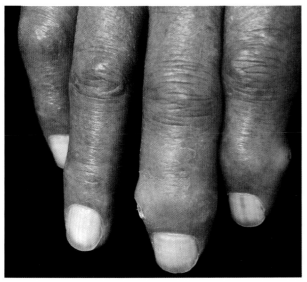

Figure 36
Rheumatology 10

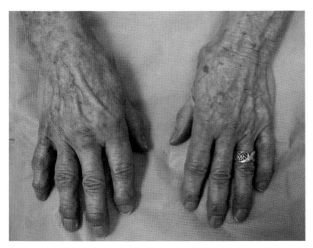

Figure 37
Rheumatology 15